Clinical Haematology

Clinical Haematology

Edited by

Christopher A. Ludlam

BSc (Hons) PhD FRCP (Edin) FRCPath
Consultant Haematologist and Director, Haemophilia Centre,
Royal Infirmary of Edinburgh; Part-time Senior Lecturer,
Department of Medicine, University of Edinburgh, Edinburgh, UK

CHURCHILL LIVINGSTONE
EDINBURGH LONDON MELBOURNE AND NEW YORK 1990

CHURCHILL LIVINGSTONE
Medical Division of Longman Group UK Limited

Distributed in the United States of America by Churchill
Livingstone Inc., 1560 Broadway, New York, N.Y. 10036,
and by associated companies, branches and representatives
throughout the world.

First published 1990

ISBN 0-443-03834-1

British Library Cataloguing in Publication Data
Clinical haematology.
   1. Man. Blood. Therapy
   I. Ludlam, Christopher A.
   616.1′506

Library of Congress Cataloging in Publication Data
Clinical haematology / edited by Christopher A. Ludlam.
     p. cm.
   1. Blood--Diseases. 2. Hematology. I. Ludlam,
   Christopher A. [DNLM: 1. Hematologic
Diseases--diagnosis. 2. Hematologic
Diseases--therapy. WH 100 C6395]
RC633.C57 1990
616.1′5--dc20

Produced by Longman Singapore Publishers (Pte) Ltd.
Printed in Singapore.

Preface

Haematology is one of the most rapidly advancing fields in medicine today and because it covers such diverse diseases it has become increasingly difficult for any individual to keep abreast of all developments. For the practising clinician, and for those in training, however, it is essential to have a working knowledge of most aspects of the specialty. It is to such individuals that this book is aimed. The emphasis, therefore, is placed on clinical assessment and management rather than laboratory methods.

To this end the first nine chapters are given over to the evaluation of patients presenting with common haematological problems e.g. anaemia, paraproteinaemia and excessive bleeding. Thereafter follow three sections reviewing disorders systematically. Although the emphasis is on the patient and his management, to do this effectively it has become increasingly important to have a working knowledge of molecular biology as applied to haematology and a chapter on this topic is included.

Many treatments are common to different haematological diseases. Bone marrow transplantation, for example, is carried out for an increasing number of disorders and rather than have repetitive descriptions of the procedure under different diseases a whole chapter is devoted to all aspects of the procedure. Other topics considered in this way are cytotoxic drugs and the varied causes, both congenital and acquired, of reduced immunity to infection.

Many patients with malignant haematological conditions are often made profoundly pancytopenic with chemotherapy either to treat disease or in preparations for bone marrow transplantation. The support of such individuals requires considerable expertise. The final section of the book contains chapters addressing the management of the many difficulties that arise. Successful therapy requires psychological support of the patient and this is discussed in a separate chapter.

Although this is not a text book of paediatric haematology, there are a number of problems that occur in the neonate and small child which are of importance to all with an interest in the specialty. Several chapters therefore deal exclusively with aspects of the subject which occur uniquely in the young.

I hope the reader will find that the bibliographies at the end of each chapter provide a useful lead into the literature.

I should like to thank all who have contributed to the book's production. The staff of Churchill Livingstone must be thanked for their tact, kindness and gentle perseverance in putting this book together. The help of Mrs Pat Stewart with the manuscript was invaluable. My family, Molly, Naomi and Michael deserve a special note of appreciation for their support and forbearance whilst I have been preoccupied with the preparation of this book.

Edinburgh, 1990   C.A.L.

Contributors

Alastair J. Bellingham FRCP FRCPath
Professor of Haematology, Department of
Haematology, King's College School of Medicine,
London, UK

Robert J. G. Cuthbert MB BCh BAO MRCP
Senior Registrar, Department of Haematology, City
Hospital, Nottingham, UK

Charles D. Forbes MD DSc FRCP
Professor of Medicine and Honorary Consultant
Physician, Ninewells Hospital, Dundee, UK

Karen S. Froebel BSc PhD
Senior Scientist, H.I.V. Immunology Laboratory,
Department of Medicine, University of Edinburgh,
Edinburgh, UK

George Galea MRCP
Consultant in Transfusion Medicine, Aberdeen and
North East Scotland Blood Transfusion Service,
Aberdeen Royal Infirmary, Aberdeen, UK

Donald S. Gillett BSc MRCP MRCPath
Consultant Haematologist, Pembury Hospital,
Tunbridge Wells, UK

R. David Hutton MB ChB MRCPath
Senior Lecturer in Haematology, University of Wales
College of Medicine; Honorary Consultant
Haematologist, South Glamorgan Health Authority,
Cardiff Royal Infirmary, UK

Mary Judge MB ChB MRCP
Formerly Lecturer in Haematology, Department of
Haematology, University of Wales, Cardiff, UK

Elizabeth A. Letsky MB BS FRCPath
Consultant Haematologist, Queen Charlotte's Hospital
for Women, London, UK

David C. Linch BA MB BChir FRCP
Professor of Clinical Haematology, University College
and Middlesex School of Medicine, London, UK

Geoffrey G. Lloyd MD FRCP FRCPsych
Consultant Psychiatrist, Royal Free Hospital,
London, UK

Gordon D. O. Lowe MD FRCP
Senior Lecturer, Department of Medicine, Royal
Infirmary, Glasgow, UK

Christopher A. Ludlam BSc(Hons) PhD FRCP(Ed) FRCPath
Consultant Haematologist and Director, Haemophilia
Centre, Royal Infirmary of Edinburgh; Part-time
Senior Lecturer, Department of Medicine, University
of Edinburgh, Edinburgh, UK

Michael J. Mackie MD MRCPath FRCP
Consultant Haematologist, Western General Hospital,
Edinburgh, UK

Alistair C. Parker BSc (Hons) FRCP(Ed) FRCPath
Senior Lecturer in Medicine, Royal Infirmary of
Edinburgh, Edinburgh, UK

Stephen A. Schey MB BS MRCP MRCPath FRACP
Senior Lecturer; Honorary Consultant Haematologist,
Guys Hospital, London, UK

R. Alexander Sharp MRCP MRCPath
Senior Registrar, Department of Haematology,
Ninewells Hospital, Dundee, UK

Thomas Sheehan MB ChB MRCP MRCPath
Consultant Haematologist, Victoria Infirmary,
Glasgow, UK

Michael Steel MB ChB PhD DSc MRCP MRCPath
Assistant Director, MRC Human Genetics Unit,
Western General Hospital, Edinburgh, UK

Stan J. Urbaniak BSc MB ChB PhD FRCPE MRCPath
Regional Director, Aberdeen and North East Scotland
Regional Transfusion Centre, Aberdeen Royal
Infirmary; Clinical Senior Lecturer, University of
Aberdeen, Aberdeen, UK

Heather H. K. Watson BSc PhD
Senior Biochemist, Aberdeen Royal Infirmary,
Aberdeen, UK

J. A. Whittaker MD FRCP FRCPath
Reader in Haematology, University of Wales College of
Medicine; Honorary Consultant, University Hospital of
Wales, Cardiff, UK

Contents

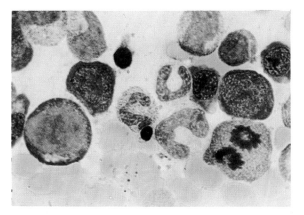

Plate 1 Marrow with megaloblasts and giant metamyelocytes.

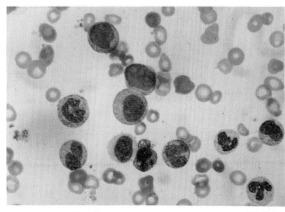

Plate 2 The blood film from a 26-year-old man with AML showing a mixed population of myeloblasts and hypogranular neutrophils.

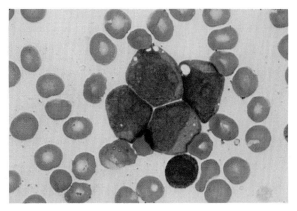

Plate 3 The bone marrow from a patient with M1 AML.

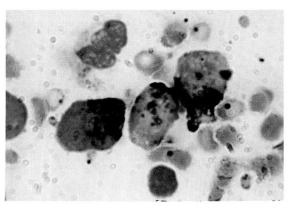

Plate 4 Sudan Black B positivity in M1 bone marrow blasts.

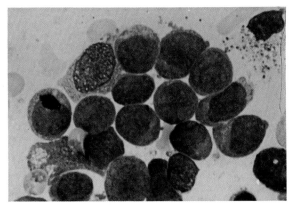

Plate 5 The bone marrow from a patient with M2 AML.

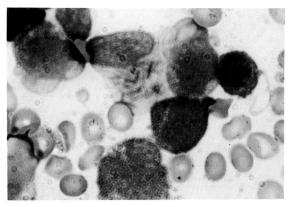

Plate 6 Multiple Auer rods (faggots) in M3 AML.

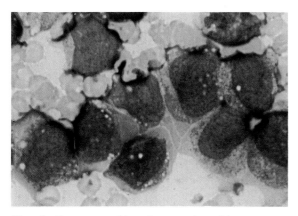

Plate 7 Bone marrow blasts from a patient with acute myelomonocytic leukaemia (M4).

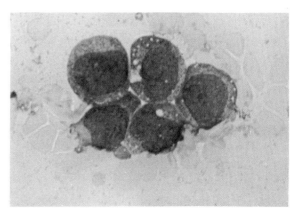

Plate 8 Bone marrow blasts from a patient with acute monoblastic leukaemia (M5).

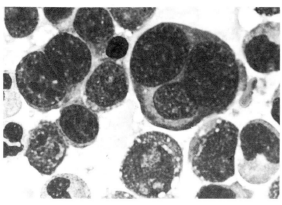

Plate 9 Erythroblasts from a patient with acute erythroleukaemia (M6). Note the trinucleate cell showing bizarre dyserythropoietic change.

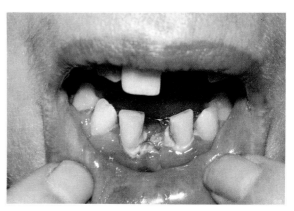

Plate 10 Gingival hypertrophy in a woman with M4 AML.

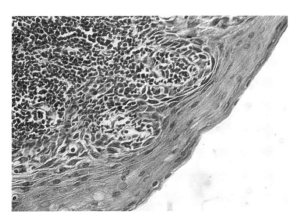

Plate 11 Section of the testis of a 14-year-old boy with testicular relapse of ALL.

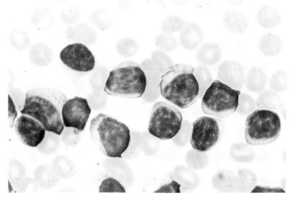

Plate 12 Blood film in chronic lymphatic leukaemia.

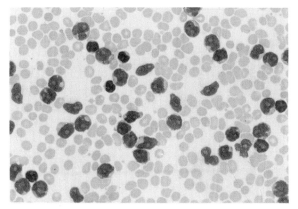

Plate 13   Peripheral blood in prolymphocytic leukaemia.

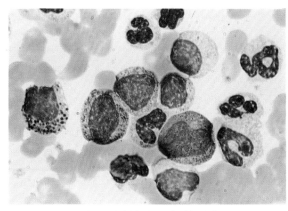

Plate 14   Chronic myeloid leukaemia blood film.

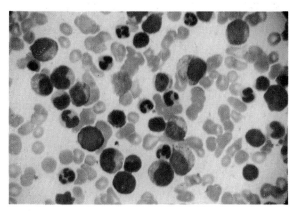

Plate 15   Chronic myelomonocytic leukaemia blood film.

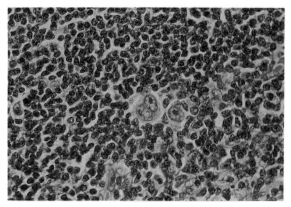

Plate 16   Lymphocyte-predominant Hodgkin's disease. Lymph-node histology showing two large Reed Sternberg cells surrounded by lymphocytes.

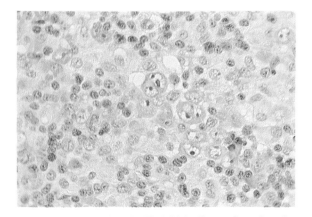

Plate 17   Mixed cellularity Hodgkin's disease. Lymph-node histology showing several Reed Sternberg cells surrounded by a mixture of reactive cells including lymphocytes and plasma cells.

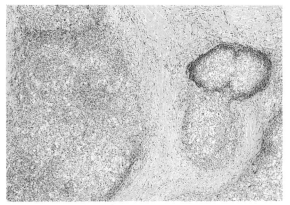

Plate 18   Nodular sclerosing Hodgkin's disease. Lymph-node histology showing broad bands of collagen and nodules containing a mixture of cells including prominent lacunar cells.

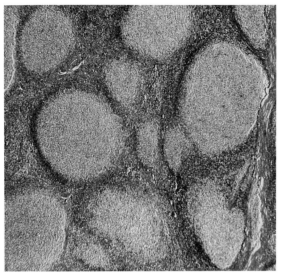

Plate 19 Follicular lymphoma. Low-power view of involved node showing numerous large well-defined nodules.

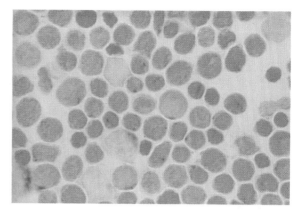

Plate 20 Peripheral blood film from a patient with T-cell ALL showing characteristic focal red staining with acid phosphatase.

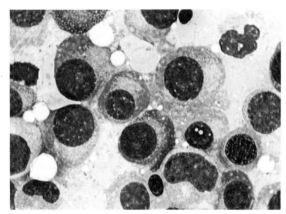

Plate 21 Plasma-cell infiltration in bone marrow.

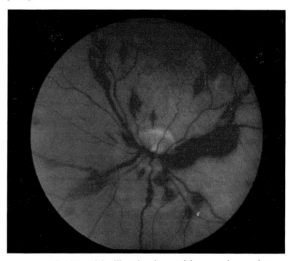

Plate 22 Retina with dilated veins and haemorrhages due to hyperviscosity secondary to a paraprotein.

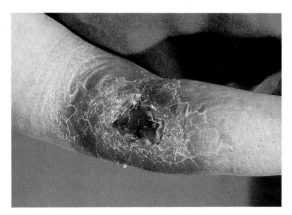

Plate 23 Ulcer due to extravasation of adriamycin.

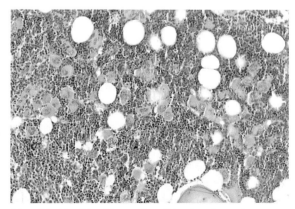

Plate 24 Trephine biopsy of proliferative phase of myelofibrosis with megakaryocytic proliferation.

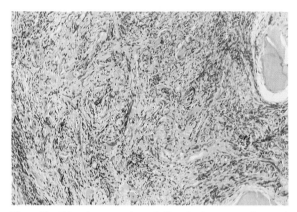

Plate 25 Fibrotic stage of myelofibrosis (haemotoxylin and eosin).

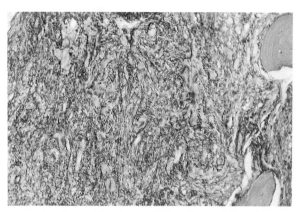

Plate 26 Dense fibrosis revealed by silver staining of section in Plate 24.

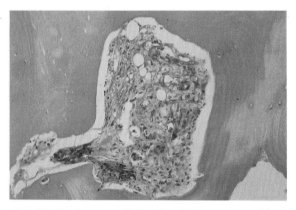

Plate 27 Carcinomatous infiltration of bone marrow with fibrotic reaction.

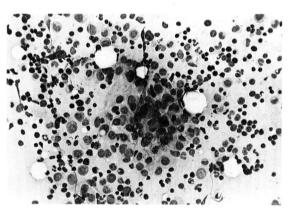

Plate 28 Marrow aspirate reveals clump of carcinoma cells.

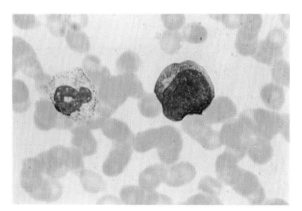

Plate 29 Activated 'atypical' lymphocyte as seen in infectious mononucleosis.

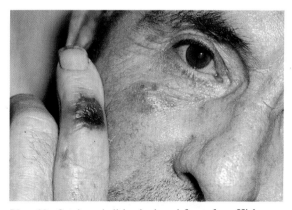

Plate 30 Septic emboli in cheek and finger from Hichman line infected with staphylococcus aureus.

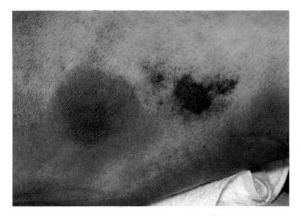

Plate 31 Pseudomonal septic lesion arising from haematogenous spread.

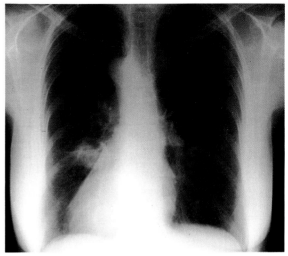

Plate 32 Radiograph of solitary lesion which at post mortem (Plate 33) revealed aspergillus (Plate 34) and an embolic lesion in the cerebral cortex (Plate 35).

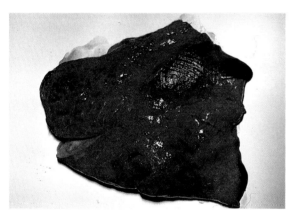

Plate 33 Pulmonary aspergillus (see Plates 32, 34 and 35).

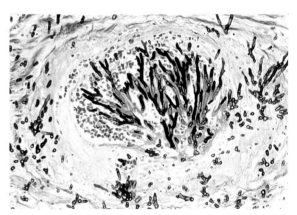

Plate 34 Pulmonary aspergillus (see Plates 32, 33 and 35).

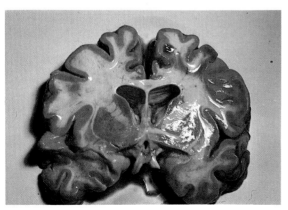

Plate 35 Embolic focus of aspergillus in cerebral cortex from pulmonary lesion in Plate 32.

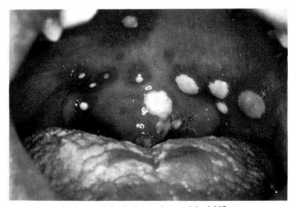

Plate 36 Oral candidiasis in patient with AML.

Clinical assessment and investigation

1. Assessment of patient with anaemia

R. D. Hutton

Anaemia is defined as a condition in which the blood is deficient in haemoglobin and therefore, by assumption, also deficient in oxygen-carrying capacity. The diagnosis of anaemia relies primarily on the estimation of the haemoglobin concentration of a venous blood sample. In most situations this provides an adequate guide to its oxygen delivering capacity. Based on population studies, reference ranges have been defined in relation to age, sex and altitude such that if a person's haemoglobin concentration is below a certain value they are said to be anaemic. For practical purposes a normal adult haemoglobin lies between 13–18 g/dl for men and 11.5–16.5 g/dl for women. Relative anaemia occurs when tissue oxygenation is inadequate, despite the haemoglobin concentration being within the 'normal' range. The circumstances in which this may occur are shown in Table 1.1.

It is not entirely clear how the body determines the optimum haemoglobin concentration under different circumstances but it is known that a major part of the mechanism relates to intrarenal oxygen delivery and the

Table 1.1 Situations in which the haemoglobin concentration may wrongly estimate the oxygen delivering capacity of the blood.

Changes in blood volumes	Acute blood loss
	Compartmental fluid shifts
	Burns
	Pregnancy
	Splenomegaly
	Paraproteinaemia
Hypoxia	Living at high altitude
	Respiratory dysfunction
	Cardiac disease
	High affinity haemoglobins
	Non-functional haemoglobins
	Alkalosis
Abnormal blood rheology	Decreased red cell flexibility
	Increased nucleated cell count
	Paraproteinaemia

effect of this on production of the hormone erythropoietin.

Some individuals have variant haemoglobins with either high or low oxygen affinity. In such cases the individual may have a haemoglobin concentration which is outside of the range found in people with normal haemoglobin.

Oxygen delivery falls exponentially as the distance between the nutritive capillary and the respiring cells increases. Oxygen delivery is, therefore, dependent upon the number of perfused nutritive capillaries. Besides autonomic control, the number of perfused capillaries is dependent on the blood volume and the number of such capillaries blocked by slowly deforming white cells. The rate of flow through the capillaries is also important and this may be markedly reduced in some pathological states.

The patient who has recently bled may have a normal haemoglobin concentration but will have a decreased red cell mass and therefore a decreased oxygen delivery. Conversely, in pregnancy and also in some cases of splenomegaly and paraproteinaemia, the peripheral haemoglobin concentration may be decreased but the total red cell mass and/or blood volume is increased. The increase in the number of capillaries perfused at any one time will have an important beneficial effect on tissue oxygen delivery and hence on symptoms of anaemia.

It is apparent from the above that the degree of anaemia can only be absolutely determined if blood volumes are measured. This obviously will be performed only rarely. The introduction of new non-radioactive techniques for such measurements may, however, lead to an increasing place for this in the investigation and understanding of apparent anaemia in many conditions.

Hypoxia may result from many different causes. Whatever the cause, patients with hypoxia require an increased red cell mass to maintain normal oxygen supply. This will often, but not always, be reflected by an increased haemoglobin concentration. They may well become symptomatically anaemic even though their haemoglobin concentration remains within the reference range for normal people living at, or near, sea level.

It would appear that when there is an abnormality leading to increased blood viscosity, the body is able to sense that a normal haemoglobin concentration would lead to sub-optimum oxygen delivery. This is well illustrated by the anaemia of thalassaemia trait, where measurements of erythroid iron turnover show that most cases have decreased erythropoiesis, despite their anaemia. Another example is chronic granulocytic leukaemia, where the haemoglobin concentration shows an inverse relationship to the white cell count. This is not just due to marrow replacement, as is shown by the increase in the haemoglobin concentration that follows reducing the blood viscosity by repeated leukopheresis. A high nucleated cell count will not only result in an increase in bulk viscosity but, depending upon the type of cells, may also lead to decreased oxygenation by the plugging of nutritive capillaries with slowly deforming cells. This is most commonly seen again in chronic granulocytic leukaemia.

When to investigate

As there are many inter-relating factors affecting the haemoglobin concentration for any individual, it is best to use reference values only as a guide. The fact that the haemoglobin concentration falls within accepted values does not exclude developing or relative anaemia.

It may be obvious that a low normal haemoglobin concentration is abnormal for an individual, because a higher than average haemoglobin would have been expected due to chronic hypoxia, or because of their smoking or drinking habits.

Developing anaemia may be apparent from historical data showing that the haemoglobin concentration has decreased significantly from a previous value. It would be foolish to delay investigating the cause until the result was below the 'normal' range.

A third reason why attention may be drawn to the presence of relative or developing anaemia is the finding of abnormal red cell indices. Even if the haemoglobin concentration is apparently 'normal', it is important to note macrocytosis, which may be due to B_{12} or folate deficiency. Microcytosis and a normal haemoglobin concentration may indicate either an iron-deficient polycythaemic state or a haemoglobinopathy (most commonly thalassaemia trait).

In some epidemiological studies the absence or presence of anaemia has been looked for by observing the response to haematinic supplements. It could be argued that the only certain way of ensuring that an individual is not anaemic would be by – as far as is possible – excluding contributory factors, which would include giving haematinic supplements.

Symptomatology

The signs and symptoms of anaemia are related to three major components. The first is tissue hypoxia. This may present as light-headedness and fainting secondary to the brain not receiving adequate oxygen, and as easy fatigue and sometimes pain (claudication and angina) by other tissues. The second is related to the respiratory system. An increased respiratory rate and a sense of air hunger develop in an effort to compensate for the hypoxia. The third component arises secondary to adaptive changes in the cardiovascular system. Initially, the patient may be aware of increased cardiac activity, experienced through tachycardia, palpitations, thumping in the chest and noises in the head due to increased flow rates. Increased flow may also lead to, or accentuate, flow murmurs and bruits. The increased forces within the vascular tree can lead to the rupture of small blood vessels and this may be seen as retinal haemorrhages even when the platelet count is unaffected. Later, the heart is unable to maintain optimum function and signs of failure will ensue. This may present as peripheral oedema, or in more severe cases by generalised oedema, including pulmonary oedema and paroxysmal nocturnal dyspnoea, gut oedema leading to anorexia and malabsorption, hepatic congestion leading to liver dysfunction (raised enzymes, jaundice, decreased vitamin K dependent factors etc.), hepatic enlargement and tenderness. The load on the right side of the heart is also reflected in a raised jugular venous pressure.

The onset of signs and symptoms is variable and depends on:

1. The speed of onset

A sudden onset of anaemia from blood loss will lead to severe symptomatology. Death can occur when only 30% of the circulating haemoglobin mass is acutely lost. This is due to decreased perfusion. Larger losses can be tolerated provided the circulating volume is maintained. There are many compensatory mechanisms that take place when anaemia develops slowly. These include:

a. An increased flow rate. This is partly due to the decreased viscosity of the anaemic blood and also to increased cardiac work.
b. An increased respiratory rate to maintain optimum oxygenation of the faster moving blood.

c. Biochemical adaptations, the most well known of which is the 'shift to the right' of the oxygen dissociation curve largely caused by increased amounts of 2, 3-diphosphoglycerate within the red cells.

Through these adaptations some patients are able to tolerate extremely low haemoglobin concentrations with only minimal symptoms.

2. Other complicating pathology

If the patient already has ischaemic heart disease, peripheral vascular disease, respiratory disease, etc., symptoms related to decompensation will obviously appear earlier.

3. The underlying cause or causes for the anaemia

The patient may present from other complications related to the underlying pathology before he has developed symptomatic anaemia. Examples of this would be neuropathy or dementia in B_{12} deficiency, purpura in marrow failure, hyperviscosity in paraproteinaemia or high white count in leukaemia, etc.

History

A well taken history may give vital clues as to the cause of anaemia. It is often valuable to obtain a history from somebody close to the patient, as well as from the actual patient, particularly if there is any doubt as to whether they are capable, or willing, to give full details of diet, drug ingestion, alcohol intake, etc.

Rate of onset of symptoms

It is important to attempt to assess how quickly the patient's symptoms of anaemia have developed. It is often helpful to enquire as to whether the patient has had previous blood counts or been a blood donor.

Gastrointestinal disturbance

A careful and thorough history of any gastrointestinal symptoms is invaluable. Enquiry should be made about any dysphagia, dyspepsia, pain, alteration of bowel habit, steatorrhoea or melaena. Bleeding haemorrhoids may occasionally give rise to iron deficiency.

Diet

Protein as well as iron, B_{12} and folate are needed for normal erythropoiesis. Food faddists, vegans, the poor and the mentally disturbed may not eat a reasonably balanced diet. During the rapid growth spurt of adolescence, children may outgrow iron reserves and become anaemic.

Menstrual and reproductive history

Menorrhagia is the commonest cause of iron deficiency in women between the ages of 15 and 45 years. Sequential pregnancies, in rapid succession, may exhaust the mother's iron reserves, particularly in the case of twins.

Drugs and toxins

A detailed history of all drugs must be obtained. Specific enquiry should be made about non-prescribed medicines which may contain aspirin. Exposure to potential toxins can also occur at work or from a hobby.

Family history

Specific enquiry should be made to determine whether there is a family history of anaemia. This is particularly important for haemolytic anaemias, thalassaemias and haemoglobinopathies. It may also be useful for patients with possible pernicious anaemia who may have relatives with either this disorder or another autoimmune condition.

Past history

Enquiry should be made as to whether the patient has been anaemic in the past and what investigations and treatment were given. Has the patient had an operation to the gastrointestinal tract?

Examination

As almost any medical condition may present with anaemia, all patients should be very carefully, thoroughly and systematically examined. Some of the most important abnormalities to search for are described.

Superficial examination

The degree of pallor does not accurately reflect the severity of the anaemia; it is traditional to examine the conjunctiva and palmar creases. A patient who is obviously pale usually has a significant degree of anaemia. The mouth, lips and finger tips should be searched for evidence of hereditary haemorrhagic telangiectasia. Inspection of the mouth may also reveal angular stomatitis, ulcers and the glossitis of pernicious anaemia. Jaundice may be due to a haemolytic anaemia, lymphoma, liver disease, leukaemia or myeloproliferative disorder.

Examination of the hands may reveal koilonychia of iron deficiency; leukonychia and clubbing are associated with liver disease and other disorders that cause anaemia.

Evidence of local or systemic infection or the presence of purpura or ecchymosis would implicate a leukocyte defect or thrombocytopenia.

Cardiovascular system

Tachycardia due to a reduced haemoglobin reflects a clinically significant degree of anaemia. With more severe anaemia the pulse volume increases to become bounding as stroke volume rises to increase the cardiac output. Systolic cardiac flow murmurs may be heard.

Lymphoreticular system

Splenomegaly may be associated with a haemolytic anaemia as well as leukaemia, lymphoma or liver disease. Almost any of the many causes of lymphadenopathy may result in anaemia.

Abdominal examination

A careful evaluation of the abdomen will often be rewarding. Anaemia may be found with nearly every condition resulting in hepatosplenomegaly. A particular search should be made for any evidence of malignancy in the form of an abdominal mass or ascites.

No abdominal examination can be considered complete without a rectal examination, with sigmoidoscopy to search for pelvic or colo-rectal disease. Care should be taken to ascertain whether internal haemorrhoids are present. Vaginal examination is appropriate for menorrhagia, intermenstrual or post-menopausal bleeding.

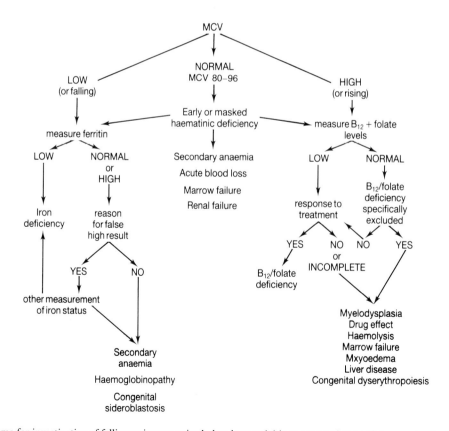

Fig. 1.1 Schema for investigation of falling or inappropriately low haemoglobin concentration or of abnormal red cell indices.

Leg ulcers

These may be found in congenital intrinsic red cell disorders, e.g. sickle cell disease.

Table 1.2 Peripheral blood red cell abnormalities

Microcytes
Iron deficiency
Thalassaemias
Sideroblastic anaemias

Macrocytes
B_{12} and folate deficiency
Chemotherapy
Liver disease
Hypothyroidism
Myeloma
Aplastic anaemia

Target cells
Liver disease
Thalassaemia
Post-splenectomy
Iron deficiency
Sickle cell
Haemoglobin C disease

Spherocytes
Autoimmune haemolytic anaemia
Hereditary spherocytosis
Microangiopathic haemolytic anaemias
Disseminated intravascular coagulation
Post-splenectomy

Fragmented erythrocytes
Microangiopathic haemolytic anaemias
Disseminated intravascular coagulation

Rod cells
Iron deficiency
Hereditary elliptocytosis

Tear drop cells
Myelofibrosis
Marrow infiltration

Nucleated red blood cells
Marrow infiltration
Severe haemolysis
Myelofibrosis

Burr cells
Renal failure

Howell-Jolly bodies
Post-splenectomy/hyposplenism
Dyshaemopoietic states, e.g. megaloblastic anaemia

Basophilic stippling
Dyshaemopoietic states, e.g. megaloblastic anaemia

Rouleau
High plasma fibrinogen
Paraprotein

Agglutination
Cold agglutinins

Arthritis

If present may indicate the presence of SLE, rheumatoid arthritis or other collagenosis.

Investigations

Full blood count

The result of a complete blood count performed as part of a general screen for disease often provides the first indication that a patient is anaemic. If the history or examination suggests the possibility of anaemia, then a blood count should be the first investigation. The haemoglobin should be interpreted taking into account all the information known about the patient. Do they have a lower haemoglobin concentration than you would expect, or has their haemoglobin concentration fallen? Anaemias can be classified (Fig. 1.1) initially on the basis of the mean corpuscular volume (MCV). A blood film may reveal red cell abnormalities characteristic of particular disorders (Table 1.2 and Fig. 1.2).

A reticulocyte count will reflect the bone marrow's response to anaemia. These cells are identified by staining residual ribosome-associated RNA with brilliant cresyl blue. A low reticulocyte count is found in bone marrow hypoplasia whereas a reticulocytosis is seen in situations where the marrow is able to respond (Table 1.3).

Table 1.3 Common causes of reticulocytosis and Heinz bodies

Reticulocytosis
Haematinic therapy
Bleeding
Haemolysis
Marrow infiltration
Sudden severe hypoxia

Heinz Bodies
Enzymopathies, e.g. G6PD deficiency
Oxidants, e.g. sulphonamides
Unstable haemoglobins, e.g. Hb Leiden
Post-splenectomy

A Heinz body stain with methyl violet demonstrates the presence of denatured haemoglobin. This is observed either if the red cell contains an unstable haemoglobin that is readily denatured and precipitates, or if there is a lowering of the reducing capacity of the cells because of an enzymopathy, e.g. glucose 6 phosphate dehydrogenase deficiency. Ingestion of oxidising drugs may also result in the appearance of Heinz bodies.

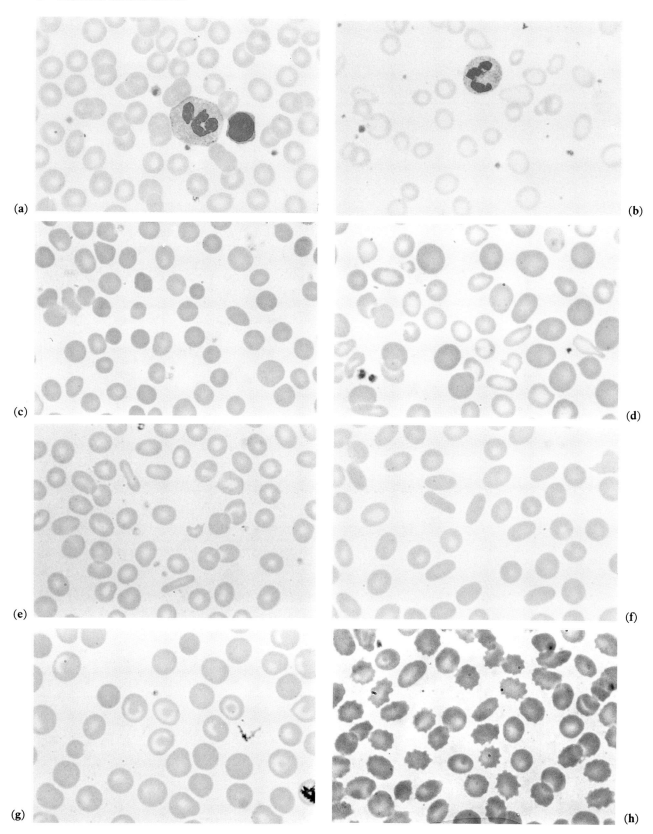

(a)

(b)

(c)

(d)

(e)

(f)

(g)

(h)

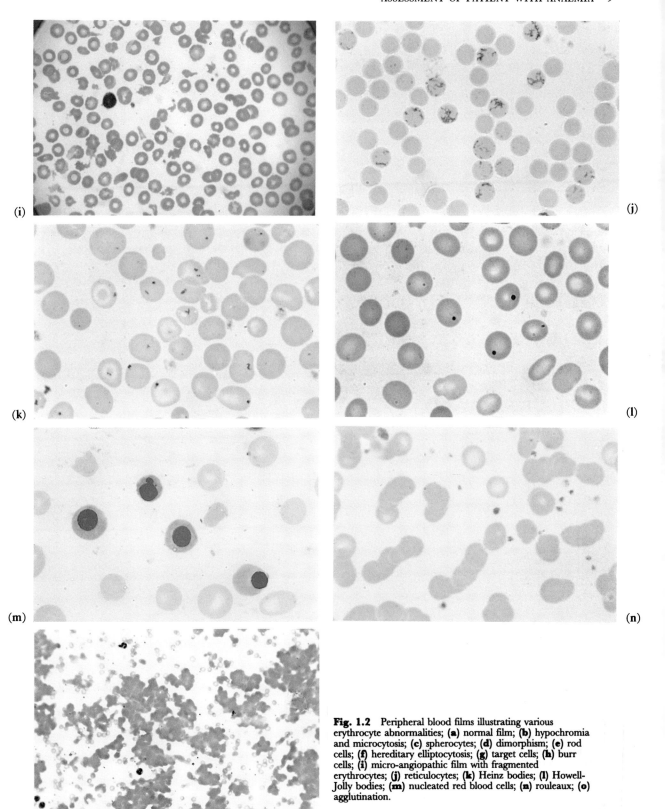

(i)

(j)

(k)

(l)

(m)

(n)

(o)

Fig. 1.2 Peripheral blood films illustrating various erythrocyte abnormalities; (a) normal film; (b) hypochromia and microcytosis; (c) spherocytes; (d) dimorphism; (e) rod cells; (f) hereditary elliptocytosis; (g) target cells; (h) burr cells; (i) micro-angiopathic film with fragmented erythrocytes; (j) reticulocytes; (k) Heinz bodies; (l) Howell-Jolly bodies; (m) nucleated red blood cells; (n) rouleaux; (o) agglutination.

Bone marrow

An aspirate should be undertaken if it is suspected that there may be a primary marrow disorder causing the anaemia, e.g. megaloblastosis, myelodysplasia, sideroblastic change or leukaemia. A trephine biopsy will be more informative if an infiltrative condition is suspected, e.g. lymphoma or carcinoma.

Haematinic assays

Evaluation of the iron status, by measurement of serum ferritin, as well as serum B_{12} and folate, should be considered for all patients whatever the principal cause of the anaemia. This is necessary because many anaemias, particularly those associated with general medical diseases, are of multifactorial origin and iron or folate deficiency may be exacerbating factors. Furthermore, in patients with combined iron and folate deficiency, the lack of iron may mask the megaloblastic change due to the deficiency of folate.

Further investigation

The results of the history, examination and investigations as set out above should provide sufficient clues to direct appropriate further investigation. It should be remembered that the majority of patients with anaemia have this secondary to another disorder or to haematinic deficiency rather than a primary disease of the marrow. Additionally many anaemias are due to several different contributory causes; for example in liver disease there may be haemolysis, bleeding, folate deficiency and splenic pooling of red cells.

2. Assessment of patient with polycythaemia

C. A. Ludlam

A patient may have a raised haemoglobin either because the circulation contains an increased number of red cells (true polycythaemia) or because the plasma volume is reduced (relative or apparent polycythaemia). A high haemoglobin may be an incidental finding during a routine blood count check or during the investigation of apparently unrelated disorders. Acutely ill patients admitted to hospital may have relatively high haemoglobins due to dehydration and therefore a repeat estimation is essential, after appropriate fluids, before embarking on further investigations to elucidate the cause. The causes of polycythaemia are given in Table 2.1.

True polycythaemia is diagnosed when the high haemoglobin is due to an increase in the total circulating red cell mass; this usually results from increased

Table 2.1 Causes of polycythaemia

True polycythaemia
    Primary proliferative polycythaemia (polycythaemia rubra vera)

Secondary polycythaemia
    Tissue hypoxia
        Pulmonary disease
        Cardiac disease
        Congenital methaemoglobinaemia
        Abnormal haemoglobins
        Smoking
        Erythrocyte metabolic defects
        Altitude

Inappropriate erythropoietin secretion
    Renal
        Cysts
        Carcinoma
        Hydronephrosis
    Hepatoma
    Cerebellar haemangioblastoma
    Uterine fibroids
    Phaeochromocytoma
    Bronchogenic carcinoma
Hypertransfusion

Table 2.2 Red cell mass and plasma volume changes in polycythaemia*

	Red cell mass	Plasma volume
True polycythaemia	Increased	Normal
Relative polycythaemia	Normal	Decreased

* For absolute values see Table 26.2

erythrocyte production by the bone marrow (Table 2.2). This excessive production may arise from a primary marrow disorder in which there is increased and autonomous production of erythrocytes, i.e. primary proliferative polycythaemia (PPP or polycythaemia rubra vera), which may be accompanied by an increase in leukocytes and platelets. This condition is one of the myeloproliferative disorders and as such it has features in common with essential thrombocythaemia, chronic myeloid leukaemia and myelofibrosis. On the other hand, increased erythropoiesis may be secondary to raised levels of erythroprotein. Such secondary polycythaemias are most commonly associated with chronic hypoxia and renal abnormalities.

Relative polycythaemia can be diagnosed when the total circulating mass of red cells is normal but the plasma volume is reduced. This may be observed in patients with dehydration, those on diuretics or those who consume large amounts of alcohol.

To distinguish between true and relative polycythaemia it is necessary to measure the total circulating red cell mass and plasma volume. This is usually accomplished by labelling a sample of the patient's erythrocytes with ^{51}Cr; following re-injection the total red cell mass can be calculated by a simple dye dilution technique. Plasma volume is measured by injecting a known amount of ^{125}I-albumin and measuring its dilution. Both the red cell mass and plasma volume are divided by the lean body mass (calculated from the patient's height and weight) to standardise the results. Normal values are given in Table 26.2.

History

Plethoric appearance

Has the patient, or relative, noticed an increasing ruddy complexion?

Thrombosis

Does the patient have an acute arterial, e.g. stroke, or venous thrombosis? Has one occurred in the past? Usually large arteries are the most vulnerable to thrombosis but occlusion of digital vessels particularly in the toes may cause local gangrene. This is especially seen when the platelet count is raised as in PPP.

Hyperviscosity

A feeling of fullness in the head and persistent headaches, along with blurring of vision may indicate stagnating blood flow. Patients sometimes notice increasing intellectual impairment.

Bleeding

Gastrointestinal haemorrhage may be a presenting feature of PPP partly due to hyperviscosity but it may be exacerbated by associated platelet functional abnormalities found in this condition. Haematuria may indicate a renal lesion causing secondary polycythaemia.

Pruritus

An episodic itch, particularly after a hot bath, may be a presenting feature of PPP or it may develop during the course of the illness. It often affects the limbs and back. Although excessive histamine release from basophils has been blamed, the use of antihistamines does not often alleviate this distressing symptom. Treatment of the underlying disorder usually ameliorates the pruritus.

Gout

The high marrow turnover of cells in PPP causes a rise in the plasma urate level and acute gout may be precipitated. Occasionally chronic gouty tophi may be observed.

Respiratory symptoms

Enquiry should be made about dyspnoea and other symptoms of respiratory disease. Chronic bronchitis and emphysema are common causes of secondary polycythaemia.

Altitude

Has the patient recently lived in a high mountainous region where hypoxia could have stimulated erythropoiesis?

Hypertransfusion

Occasionally patients are given an excessive number of units of red cells to correct an anaemia. In the newborn a twin-twin transfusion may be observed.

Cigarettes and alcohol

Smoking may not only result in loss of pulmonary function and hypoxia but the circulation may contain up to 10% carboxyhaemoglobin which is unable to carry oxygen. This will tend, therefore, to raise the haemoglobin further. 'Stress', or relative polycythaemia (Gaisbock's syndrome), is associated with a high alcohol and cigarette consumption particularly in stressed individuals who often have mild hypertension and clinical evidence of atherosclerosis, e.g. intermittent claudication.

Examination

Plethoric appearance

A ruddy complexion is often observed; its absence does not exclude a diagnosis of polycythaemia.

Thrombosis

This may be the presenting complaint and should be assessed as outlined in Chapter 9. Gangrene of the toes, with palpable peripheral pulses, is observed with small vessels occlusion as in essential thrombocythaemia, diabetes or vasculitis.

Respiratory system

Are there any features of hypoxia, e.g. cyanosis, or chronic pulmonary insufficiency?

Abdominal examination

The finding of splenomegaly is strongly indicative of PPP. Care must also be taken to palpate for the kidneys in case one of the many renal causes is responsible for the polycythaemia.

Optic fundi

Polycythaemia may cause distension of retinal veins. Superficial flame shaped haemorrhages may be seen, as may papilloedema in severe cases.

Investigations

A scheme for investigating patients with a high haemoglobin is given in Figure 2.1.

Full blood count

A persistently raised haemoglobin (over 18 g/dl in a male and 16.5 g/dl in a female) is an indication for further assessment. The MCV is usually normal although the finding of a normal haemoglobin with a reduced MCV is indicative of an iron-deficient polycythaemia (or thalassaemia trait). A raised granulocyte count is characteristic of PPP, although occasionally this may be observed secondary to the underlying disorder causing the polycythaemia, e.g. chronic bronchitis during exacerbation. A thrombocytosis favours a diagnosis of PPP but again can occur secondary to other pathology.

Red cell mass and plasma volume

These should be measured when the patient is in a haemodynamically stable condition by using autologous ^{51}Cr labelled erythrocytes and homologous ^{125}I-albumin. Interpretation of the results is given in Table 2.2.

Bone marrow

This should be considered if the red cell mass is raised. The appearances are those of panhyperplasia reflecting the peripheral blood: stainable iron may be absent. A trephine biopsy has the advantage of demonstrating the

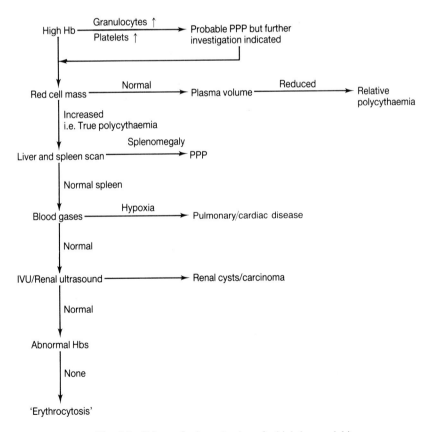

Fig. 2.1 Scheme for investigation of a high haemoglobin

overall cellularity of the marrow which may be markedly increased in PPP, as well as indicating the presence of increased fibrosis, a feature of myeloproliferative disorders.

Leukocyte alkaline phosphatase

This enzyme, characterised by histochemical staining, is normal or increased in PPP. It is sometimes useful to help distinguish this disorder from chronic myeloid leukaemia in which it is usually very low.

Plasma urate

An increased uric acid level favours a diagnosis of PPP rather than a secondary cause for the polycythaemia. Individuals with 'stress' polycythaemia not infrequently have a raised urate.

Liver and spleen isotope scan

An objective assessment of splenomegaly is useful as, if present, it is strongly indicative of PPP. Early PPP may be associated with an enlarged, but impalpable, spleen. The associated liver scan image may indicate whether the splenomegaly may be secondary to chronic liver disease, e.g. cirrhosis, or whether the polycythaemia could be due to a previously unsuspected hepatoma.

Blood gases

Unless the patient clearly has PPP it is necessary to assess objectively whether arterial hypoxia could be the cause of the polycythaemia.

Assessment of renal pathology

If it is not possible to make an unequivocal diagnosis of PPP and the patient is not hypoxic, an IVU or renal ultrasound is indicated. Either investigation will demonstrate all renal causes of secondary polycythaemia.

Abnormal haemoglobins

Occasional cases of polycythaemia may be due to abnormal high affinity haemoglobins, e.g. Hb Chesapeake, or a haemoglobin which results in excessive methaemoglobin, e.g. HbM. Rarely, an erythrocyte enzyme defect may result in polycythaemia.

If the previous investigations fail to reveal the cause of the polycythaemia, then investigation for abnormal haemoglobins or enzymopathies may be justified.

A grossly elevated serum vitamin B_{12} concentration supports a diagnosis of PPP. A serum erythropoietin estimation may assist the diagnosis, as in PPP it will be low, while it is characteristically raised in secondary polycythaemia.

In some patients with true polycythaemia all the above investigations to elucidate the cause yield normal results. The patient is then said to have an isolated erythrocytosis; some individuals may be entirely normal merely having a haemoglobin outside the normal ranges 95% confidence limits. In others, however, the erythrocytosis is the first manifestation of PPP and if the patient is followed up for a prolonged period other features of this disorder will become apparent.

3. Assessment of patient with white cell disorder

J. A. Whittaker

In almost all blood diseases, a careful history and thorough general examination of the patient is an essential basis for correct diagnosis and is particularly crucial where disorders of white blood cells are possible. These disorders are more often secondary than primary (Tables 3.1, 3.2 and 3.3), for example the result of inflammatory disease, infection and carcinoma, whereas primary disorders such as leukaemia and lymphoma, although frequently seen in haematological practice, are in fact relatively uncommon.

History

There is no substitute for a good history. The patient must be allowed to relate this without undue interruption, but with guidance towards areas of potential importance and specific questioning afterwards for the following:

Weight loss

Generally important in debilitating diseases, but especially important in secondary carcinoma and in lymphomas where, if greater than 10%, it is included in staging schemes as a 'B' symptom. Patients with acute leukaemia do not usually lose weight initially, but do so nearly always after chemotherapy.

Fever

This is common in infections and in lymphomas where, if persistent, it should be regarded as a 'B' symptom in the absence of an alternative cause. Fever in leukaemia is nearly always due to infection (see Ch. 4).

Pain

Bone pain occurs especially in myeloma, where it is often due to pathological fractures at the site of deposits in the axial skeleton. Sudden expansion of malignant cells can cause excruciating bone pain with exquisite tenderness, characteristically in patients with acute leukaemia and usually as a terminal event.

The shoulder-tip pain of splenic infarction is seen in patients with large spleens, especially those with chronic myeloid leukaemia. It is a sharp, severe pain, often made worse by deep inspiration and sometimes associated with a rub audible over the spleen.

Joint pain may be due to secondary gout in large joints, especially the ankle and knee, related to increased uric acid production. It occurs following cytoreduction of a high WBC in patients not protected with allopurinol, but also occasionally in untreated high WBC turnover such as that which may occur in CML.

Abdominal pain, especially in the loins, may be due to urinary tract infection, which occurs frequently in neutropenic patients.

Skin rashes

Skin itching and skin rashes are especially seen in patients with Hodgkin's disease and non-Hodgkin's lymphoma.

Family history

Inherited WBC disorders are rare and family history taking relates more to the identification of potential donors of HLA matched platelets and bone marrow.

Drugs and chemicals

Drugs frequently cause reductions in WBC and their use is seldom volunteered. Specific questions must be asked for analgesics, anti-inflammatory agents, stimulants, sedatives and tranquillisers which may have been taken for years (Table 3.1). Contact with organic chemicals occurs in certain occupations and in hobbies (e.g. gardening, model aircraft), household pest control and the use of cosmetics and hair dyes.

Table 3.1   The common causes of drug-induced neutropenia

Analgesics:	Aminopyrine*
Antibiotics:	Semi-synthetic penicillins
	Cephalosporins
	Chloramphenicol
	Sulphonamides
	Co-trimoxazole
Anti-convulsants:	Diphenylhydantoin
	Phenytoin
	Ethosuximide
Anti-inflammatory agents:	Aspirin
	Phenylbutazone
	Oxyphenbutazone
	Indomethacin
	Ibufen
	Gold salts
Anti-thyroid drugs:	Carbimazole
Phenothiazines:	All phenothiazines, but particularly
	Chlorpromazine
	Promazine
	Prochlorperazine
Sedatives:	Chlordiazepoxide
	Diazepam
	Imipramine
Others:	Benzene*
	Phenindione

* Sale in chemists shops banned in most Western countries, but available widely elsewhere.

Examination

Particular attention should be paid to the mouth, respiratory system, abdomen (including the liver and spleen), lymph nodes and skin.

Mouth

Ulceration and candida infections are common in all neutropenic patients, especially leukaemic patients receiving treatment. Gum hypertrophy occurs in some patients with acute myeloid leukaemia, particularly of the monocytic (M5) or myelomonocytic (M4) subtypes.

Bruising and bleeding

Petechiae, ecchymoses, epistaxis, and bleeding in the fundi, mucous membranes and elsewhere occur commonly in patients with low platelet counts, especially those with acute leukaemia. This topic is more fully discussed in Chapter 7.

Skin

Cutaneous deposits are seen particularly in M4 and M5 AML and in non-Hodgkin's lymphoma. They are usually rose-red to purple in colour and often multiple, less than $\frac{1}{2}$ cm diameter, but may be larger and occur singly or in small groups in non-Hodgkin's lymphoma. Secondary carcinoma deposits are usually subcutaneous and easily palpable.

The skin may be the site of a multitude of non-specific allergic or infective rashes of which those associated with gram negative sepsis are the most important. *Pseudomonas pyocyanea* septicaemia is a life-threatening infection in neutropenic patients, often associated with skin foci of varying size, usually but not always tender with a well-defined, inflamed centre.

Respiratory system

Pneumonia may occur initially and is the presenting feature in 15% of myeloma patients.

Lymph nodes

The lymph node-bearing areas should be examined carefully, especially for enlarged or tender nodes in the neck (including occipital areas), axillae and groins. Remember that Waldeyer's ring is often involved, and look particularly at the throat and tonsils. Nodes in the neck and axillae are more often pathological, but small nodes in the groins occur in some young adults and are easily detected in those who are underweight.

If there are palpable nodes, which cannot be attributed to infection, consideration should be given to radiological examination of the abdomen and mediastinum with computerised tomography.

Spleen

This is usually about twice its normal size (i.e. >300 g) before it is palpable and, therefore, a palpable spleen is always of significance. Masses in the stomach, colon, kidney and pancreas may occasionally mimic a spleen and radiological confirmation is sometimes helpful.

Liver

An enlarged liver is of less certain value than an enlarged spleen and in normal subjects the liver edge may be palpable. Liver deposits in non-Hodgkin's lymphoma and Hodgkin's disease are not usually associated with enlargement and are unlikely to be detected except on open biopsy as part of a staging laparotomy.

Skeletal system

Tenderness in the axial skeleton occurs at the site of myeloma deposits and secondary to bone marrow expansion as an end-stage feature in the acute leukaemias. Myeloma is also often characterised by kyphosis and loss of height secondary to vertebral body collapse, and very occasionally by arthritis and carpal tunnel syndrome as a result of amyloid deposition.

Investigations

The history and examination may indicate a leukocyte defect, but in patients where there is no clinical help a leukocyte defect will usually be identified or suggested by a full blood count (including a differential WBC) and examination of a blood film. Any alteration in the *number* of leukocytes in the differential WBC or the detection of abnormal cells indicates the need for a bone marrow aspirate.

Neutropenia

The most frequent defect is neutropenia (Tables 3.1 and 3.2), when patients usually give a history of infections, especially if the neutrophil count is less than $0.5 \times 10^9/l$.

Laboratory diagnosis is usually straightforward and depends on the demonstration of a persistently low neutrophil count in blood and marrow aspirates. Blood neutrophil counts should be done two or three times a week for one to two months to exclude cyclical neutropenia. Occasionally, acute leukaemia presents as a chronic neutropenia; cytogenetic analysis of blood or bone marrow will often establish the diagnosis of leukaemia and cell culture studies may help. However, cell marker studies are not practical in the absence of overt leukaemic change.

Identification of drugs causing neutropenia (Table 3.1) is difficult, largely because patients are treated with multiple agents. The most common mechanism is a dose-related interference with cell proliferation seen most frequently with phenothiazines, phenylbutazone and sulphonamides, but also with semi-synthetic penicillins and anti-thyroid drugs. Patients with allergies or previous drug reactions are prone to drug-induced hypersensitivity reactions which are more frequent in older women and possibly of genetic origin (e.g. slow

Table 3.2 Causes of neutropenia not associated with drugs

Hereditary stem cell disorders	Acquired stem cell disorders
Cyclical neutropenia	Preleukaemia Histiocytic medullary reticulosis Marrow failure (tumour, leukaemic, fibrosis) Aplastic anaemia
T- and B-cell disorders Dysgammaglobulinaemia	*T- and B-cell disorders* T-cell lymphoma
	Antibody related Autoimmune neutropenia SLE

Other
Familial agranulocytosis
Chronic neutropenia of childhood
Chediak-Higashi syndrome
	Other
	Feltys syndrome
	Splenic neutropenia
	Viral infection
	Bacterial infection
	    Typhoid fever
	    Brucellosis
	    Whooping cough
	Protozoan infections
	Megaloblastic anaemia

acetylators of sulphonamides, levamisole and the HLA-B27 genotype).

Drug-induced neutropenia is often severe with counts less than $0.5 \times 10^9/l$, when it may be associated with the sudden onset of fever, rigors or overt signs of infection (see Chapter 16) and mortality rates of 20% have been reported. However, if the diagnosis is recognised promptly and the drug withdrawn, most patients will recover uneventfully.

The commonest cause of hereditary neutropenia (Table 3.2) is cyclical neutropenia, probably due to intermittent multipotential stem cell failure, inherited as an autosomal dominant and developing in infancy or childhood. Periods of severe neutropenia occur approximately every 21 days, but although initially counts are very low, the disorder is not usually fatal and tends to become milder with time.

Causes of acquired neutropenia not associated with drugs are listed in Table 3.2 and many of these are described elsewhere in this book.

Leukocytosis

Leukocytosis in adult Caucasians due to neutrophilia occurs when blood neutrophil counts exceed $7.5 \times 10^9/l$.

Table 3.3 Causes of leukocytosis

Physiological:	Exercise
	Heavy smokers
	Pregnancy (third trimester)
	Changes in body temperature
	Anoxia
	Blood loss
	Post-splenectomy
Drugs:	Glucocorticoids
	Hydroxyethyl starch
	Anaesthetic agents
	Etiocholanalone
	Lithium salts
Infections:	Bacterial (including tuberculosis)
	Viral (acute phase of measles, chicken pox, poliomyelitis, infectious mononucleosis)
	Systemic mycotic and protozoan
Chronic inflammation:	Rheumatoid arthritis
	Collagen diseases
	Chronic skin disorders
Tissue damage:	Azotemia
	Diabetic acidosis
	Glomerulonephritis
	Hepatic necrosis
	Thyroid crisis
Malignancy:	Cancer, especially of lung, stomach or kidney
Primary haematological:	Myelofibrosis
	Chronic myeloid leukaemia
	Primary proliferative polycythaemia
Inherited or genetic defects:	Downs syndrome
	Hereditary neutrophilia
	Familial myeloproliferative disease
	Familial urticaria

In the newborn, counts of up to $12 \times 10^9/l$ are normal.

The main causes of neutrophilia are shown in Table 3.3. The term 'leukaemoid reaction' is used when the blood picture of leukaemia is simulated, usually as a response to tumour, bone marrow infiltrates, severe infections or inflammation. Often, in addition to band and segmented neutrophils, immature cells are present in blood and bone marrow. Leukaemoid reactions are most often due to tumours, especially bronchial carcinoma, but occur also in gastric and renal tumours. Disseminated tuberculosis is said to cause leukaemoid reactions, but this is now so rare a cause as to be discountable, while diagnosis of those leukaemoid reactions secondary to other infections or severe inflammation is usually obvious. However, cancer is not only the most frequent cause, but because it is often associated with leuko-erythroblastic anaemia or thrombocytopenia, presents the most difficult differential diagnosis. Cytochemical stains help when blast cells are prominent and cytogenetic studies often show diagnostic anomalies in leukaemia patients. The leukocyte alkaline phosphatase level is helpful when chronic myeloid leukaemia is suspected, it being low or absent in this disorder, but nearly always raised in leukaemoid reactions.

4. Assessment of infection in the immunocompromised patient

M. J. Mackie

Infection is a very important cause of morbidity and mortality in the immunocompromised and its diagnosis and treatment is crucial for the successful management of the patient. Virtually every organ in the body can be affected, so infection can give rise to a wide range of symptomatology. Often a difficulty is to determine whether signs and symptoms are due to infection, the disease or complications of therapy. A variety of organisms may be involved which tend to reflect the defect in the host's defence mechanisms. Opportunistic infection is common and the prevalence of particular infections is influenced by the type of therapy given to

the patient. Cytotoxic drugs cause neutropenia which predisposes to bacterial infection; use of steroids enhances susceptibility to fungi. Central venous lines are associated with colonisation, particularly with *Staphylococcus albus*. Haemophiliacs who have been users of factor VIII concentrate, especially if of non-UK origin, may be infected with HIV and susceptible to a number of opportunistic infections.

The wide range of organisms which can affect compromised hosts is shown in Tables 4.1 and 4.2. The former shows how the type of infection can often be predicted on the basis of the immune deficit. This can

Table 4.1 Examples of potential pathogens occurring in particular defects in the host's defences in patients with primary haematological disease

Deficit	Disease	Likely organisms		
Neutropenia	Acute leukaemia	Bacteria	Gram +	*Staphylococcus aureus* *Staphylococcus albus* *Streptococci*
			Gram −	*E. coli* *H. influenza* *Klebsiella* *Pseudomonas*
		Fungi		*Candida* *Aspergillus Mucor*
Immunoglobulin	Multiple myeloma Chronic lymphatic leukaemia Congenital agammaglobulinaemia	Bacteria	Gram + and − (as above)	
Cellular immunity	Hodgkin's Disease Non-Hodgkin's lymphoma	Viruses (*Herpes zoster*) Protozoa (*Pneumocystitis carinii* *Toxoplasma gondii*) *Cryptococcus neoformans*		
		Viruses	*Herpes simplex* and *zoster*; cytomegalovirus,	
		Bacteria	mycobacteria, salmonella, legionella, *Streptococcus pneumonia*, *Haemophilus influenzae*, *Staphylococcus aureus*	
	Haemophilia (anti-HIV positive)	Parasites	*Pneumocystis carinii* *Toxoplasma gondii* *Cryptosporidium*	
		Fungus	*Candida*	

Table 4.2 Likely organisms causing organ infections in various haematological disorders

Organ/system involved	Disease	Likely organism
	Acute non-lymphoblastic leukaemia	Bacteria, fungi
Chest	Acute lymphoblastic leukaemia	Bacteria *Pneumocystis carinii*
	Bone marrow transplant	
	Early	Bacteria, fungi
	Later	*Pneumocystis carinii*, Cytomegalovirus
CNS	Hodgkin's	*Listeria monocytogenes Cryptococcus neoformans Toxoplasma gondii*
	AIDS	*Cryptococcus neoformans Toxoplasma gondii* Cytomegalovirus
Mouth	Acute leukaemia	*Candida Herpes simplex* Anaerobic bacteria
Peri-anal area	Acute leukaemia	Gram negative bacteria and anaerobes
Skin	Acute leukaemia	*Staphylococcus Pseudomonas Candida*
	Lymphoproliferative disorders	*Herpes zoster*

alter temporarily, as for example following bone marrow transplantation when during the initial stages bacterial infections secondary to neutropenia are common, whereas later protozoa and virus infections occur when the neutropenia has resolved but cellular immunity is impaired. Treatment (cytotoxic drugs, radiotherapy) and management procedures (insertion of central lines, splenectomy) can impose further defence deficits on the patient and render him susceptible to a particular range of organisms. Table 4.2 illustrates the organisms which should be considered when signs and/or symptoms suggest infection at a particular site. The nature of the underlying disease determines the prevalence of the type of organism involved. It is very important to liaise with the microbiology department over the collection of the specimen, its rapid transit to the laboratory and what organisms should be specifically sought.

History

Causes of immunodeficiency

Two situations require consideration; first the evaluation of infection in a patient known to have a disorder predisposing to infection, and secondly the patient who presents with recurrent or persistent infection in whom an underlying haematological disorder is not obvious. A patient in the first category may present with an infection but it is usually apparent after the history, examination and some basic investigations that the predominant diagnosis is haematological.

Previous infections. All previous infections should be carefully documented and so far as possible the organism and site noted. Is the patient prone to bacterial, viral or fungal infections? Have these been localised and recurrent at one site or have they been systemic? Even if the patient presents with fever alone, careful questioning and examination will often reveal the potential origin of the fever. Enquiry should be made concerning classical sites – chest, abdominal and urinary tract symptoms. Both the mouth, skin and perianal areas are important foci for infection. The central nervous system should also be evaluated. It must be remembered that in severely neutropenic patients the signs and symptoms of infection often appear minor. Such patients are not able to mount the normal degree of inflammatory response; thus a slightly painful infected throat or minimal reddening around an intravenous cannulae site are often significant.

Specific enquiry should be made about tuberculosis and fungal infections, particularly if the individual has lived in an area where these may be endemic.

Symptoms of marrow failure. Anaemia and thrombocytopenia will give rise to tiredness, dizziness, palpitations and dyspnoea and bleeding respectively.

Lymphoreticular system. Has the patient noted lymphadenopathy? It is important to enquire as to whether the patient has had a splenectomy and if so the reason for the operation.

Drugs. A scrupulous drug history is essential as the ingestion of many drugs may result in leukopenia which will predispose to infection. Red cell and platelet production may also be compromised.

HIV infection. Could the patient be infected with the immunodeficiency virus? Intravenous drug abuse, multiple sexual partners, particularly homosexual, and haemophilia are associated with an increased chance of being infected.

Family history. Some congenital immunodeficiency syndromes are familial and a careful history as to whether other family members have recurrent infections can be useful.

Examination

Superficial examination

On examination of the patient the infection involved may be obvious (e.g. *Herpes zoster* or *simplex*) but more frequently the purpose of the physical examination is to try to determine the site of origin of the infection. The skin may be the primary site of infection as in the cases of *Herpes simplex* or *zoster*, or an inflamed intravenous line site. However, the skin should be routinely and regularly examined as the appearance of lesions may be related to disseminated bacterial or fungal infection; their biopsy with culture and microscopy often provides the definitive diagnosis.

In neutropenic patients, the local signs of infection may not be dramatic. Thus any degree of erythema and discomfort in the mouth, around intravenous cannulae, or perianally is likely to be significant.

Fever

It is important to remember that in severely neutropenic patients fever is usually the first and often the only sign of infection despite a thorough examination. Its evaluation should include the potential role of drugs in its production, and its relationship to the administration of blood products. Patients receiving bleomycin or amphotericin often have fever or rigors which occur and usually resolve within the five hours following their administration; fever may be due to drug allergy. Repeated transfusions may sensitise the patient to white cells and fever may occur whilst a patient is receiving blood or platelets. However, care must always be exercised when ascribing fever to a non-infectious cause; certainly the absence of the conventional clinical parameters of shock should not be used as an excuse to withhold investigation and treatment.

Investigations

An outline sequence for investigating patients is illustrated in Fig. 4.1. The complete blood count indicates the presence and severity of neutropenia as well as the presence of anaemia or thrombocytopenia. This should be repeated as an increase in the neutrophil count is an important factor in determining the patient's response to treatment.

Microbiology

The following routine cultures should be taken:

1. Blood cultures (aerobic, anaerobic bottles)
2. Swab throat, IV sites, perianal areas
3. Mid-stream specimen of urine
4. Sputum if available
5. Viral cultures for cytomegalovirus.

It may be difficult to be sure that an organism detected by the laboratory is the real cause of the infection rather than a commensal. An interesting example is the detection of *Aspergillus* in the sputum which has a poor correlation with invasive lung infection in

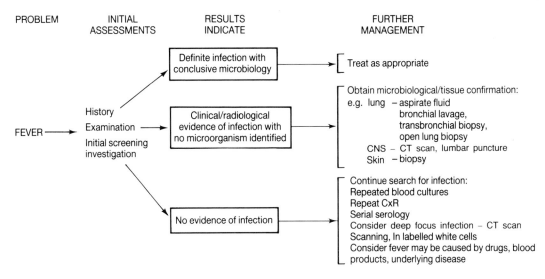

Fig. 4.1 An approach to the investigation of fever in immunocompromised patients.

non-compromised subjects. However it is a much stronger pointer to tissue infection in neutropenic patients. Generally, organisms isolated from the blood are clinically very relevant. Recently, with the increase in the use of indwelling central lines, skin commensals, in particular *Staphylococcus epidermidis*, have become a frequent cause of line infection and septicaemia in neutropenic patients. In the non-compromised the detection of *Candida* species in the blood may be the result of candidaemia due to a colonised intravenous cannula which should be removed. Systemic antifungal therapy may not be required; but in a febrile neutropenic patient, particularly one who is unresponsive to antibiotics, antifungal treatment should be started in the presence of *Candida* in the blood. In the compromised there is a much higher correlation with candidaemia and invasive infection.

Generally the incidence of positive blood cultures is low (approximately 20%) in neutropenic patients with fever but it is important to repeat these cultures at least every 48 hours if the patient remains febrile without a microbiological diagnosis.

Chest X-ray

This may be informative if the patient has a local or generalised pneumonia. In individuals with severe neutropenia, however, very little inflammation or consolidation may be present because of the lack of leukocytes to mount an adequate response.

Serology

There are a number of drawbacks as regards the serological diagnosis of infection in the immunocompromised. The patient may not produce a good antibody response and there is always a delay in confirming the diagnosis as serial samples are required to demonstrate a rising titre suggesting recent infection. Passive transfer of antibody may be a problem in some situations (e.g. anti-cytomegalovirus). Thus most available tests suffer from low sensitivity and specificity, e.g. fungal precipitins. A frequent problem is the inability to ascribe a definite infectious origin to a fever. The demonstration of a significant elevated C-reactive protein has been shown to correlate with the presence of bacterial infection.

Tissue diagnosis

The best diagnostic approach is to try to identify the organism in the tissues. *Herpes simplex* and *zoster* viruses can be speedily identified in material from lesions by

electron microscopy and grow relatively quickly in culture. However, cytomegalovirus grows slowly in culture, although recently rapid diagnosis has been achieved by the detection of the first products of the genetic replication process, i.e. well before the production of intact virions. Material obtained from bronchoscopy (cells from lavage fluid are quite satisfactory) can be stained with appropriate antisera. The organism may be identified directly in histological section (owl's eye inclusion cell with *Cytomegalovirus* pneumonitis; demonstration of *Pneumocystis carinii* with silver staining). Material obtained by biopsy should not only be examined histologically but also sent for culture. Occasionally it is necessary to resort to open lung biopsy in a patient with pulmonary infiltrates which remain undiagnosed following a negative bronchoscopy. It is important to remember that patients with haematological problems often have associated thrombocytopenia and/or coagulation abnormalities which require correction before biopsy is undertaken. It is also most important to liaise directly with the relevant laboratory department concerning prompt delivery of the specimen and the detailed investigations which should be performed in view of the clinical situation.

Body fluids

The accessibility of tissue fluids provides a further route, when appropriate, for diagnosis. Pleural and ascites fluid should be tapped and the fluid sent not only for culture but also for cytological examination. Cerebro-spinal fluid should be examined for sugar, protein and cell content of sample sent for cultures. If the disease status of the patient (see Table 4.2) predisposes him to an organism which requires special staining or culture techniques, then it is particularly important to discuss the case with the laboratory.

Other investigations may be required to identify deep foci of infection. CT scanning of the head and/or body may be useful. Indium labelled white cells can also be used to reveal infected sites. Gallium scanning will also detect areas of inflammation but will be positive in areas of lymphoma involvement. The excretion of gallium into the colon limits the test's usefulness in the abdomen.

Investigation of a patient presenting with recurrent and/or resistent infection caused by possible underlying immunodeficiency state

Infection may be the presenting feature of a haematological disorder which may be readily diagnosed from a full blood count. A more difficult diagnostic problem is the occurrence of recurrent infections in patients, often children, who do not have an obvious underlying haematological disorder. The history, in particular the sites of infection and any familial involvement, is important. The pattern of the micro-organisms involved may suggest a particular type of deficit. The following is an appropriate list of investigations:

1. Full blood count and examination of blood film (giant cytoplasmic granules in white cells in Chediak-Higashi Syndrome; thrombocytopenia with small platelets in Wiskott Aldrich Syndrome)

2. Immunoglobulin levels
3. Complement levels
4. Sweat test for cystic fibrosis
5. Neutrophil function tests for mobility
   migration
   ingestion
   oxygen metabolism – (chronic granulomatous disease)
6. Assay of T- and B- cells in peripheral blood
7. Assessment of delayed hypersensitivity by skin tests.

5. Assessment of patient with paraproteinaemia

S. A. Schey   D. C. Linch

The term 'Paraprotein' was first used by Apitz in 1940 to describe an immunoglobulin that has been secreted by a single clone of B-cells in abnormal amounts. Paraproteinaemia is therefore defined as any condition giving rise to the presence of a paraprotein circulating in the blood. The term 'gammopathy' has been used interchangeably with 'paraproteinaemia' because the vast majority of paraproteins will travel in the γ – region on serum protein electrophoresis. Although technically incorrect, paraproteinaemia is used to describe light-chain disease, where light-chains are excreted in the urine and in the presence of normal renal function there is an absence of circulating paraprotein (Bence-Jones proteinuria).

The presence of a paraproteinaemia implies the existence of a monoclonal proliferation of B lymphocytes which may be either malignant or reactive (Table 5.1). In most cases of benign monoclonal gammopathy (page 183) no underlying cause is apparent and the disease appears to be a primary B cell disorder. The emergence of a clone of B cells will result in the production of a spectrum of cells at different stages of differentiation. Depending on the disease entity there will be a relative accumulation of cells at different stages of development such that only a small number of immunoglobulin-secreting cells may be present. In CLL, for instance, a paraprotein is found only in a small proportion of cases; its presence does not indicate bulk disease but suggests a further degree of differentiation of some of the cells of the malignant clone.

It should be noted that more than one apparently monoclonal band can be present in a serum sample. Rarely, this represents a biclonal or even tri-clonal disease; alternately, a monoclonal proliferation may produce two immunoglobulins of different heavy-chain isotypes and the same light-chain isotype.

The incidence of paraproteinaemia is undoubtedly underestimated and will vary depending upon how intensively it is looked for. Paraproteinaemia should not be considered to be a diagnosis in itself but a product of underlying disorders such as primary lympho-proliferative disorders, non-lymphoid neoplasms and a variety of inflammatory and infective diseases (Table 5.1). Its discovery, therefore, should prompt a search for one of the known predisposing conditions.

The presence of a paraprotein in any of these conditions, as well as in idiopathic paraproteinaemia, is often

Table 5.1 Aetiology of paraproteinaemia

A *Lymphoproliferative disorders*
   – Plasma cell myeloma
   – Waldenstrom's macroglobulinaemia
   – Chronic lymphocytic leukaemia
   – Lymphoma
   – Heavy-chain disease
   – Primary amyloidosis

B *Benign monoclonal gammopathies*
   a) Reactive
   – Non-lymphoid neoplasms, e.g. Ca colon
   – Infection, e.g. CMV, Myc. tuberculosis
   – Autoimmune disease, e.g. SLE, myasthenia
   – Liver disease, e.g. hepatitis, cirrhosis
   – Lichen myxoedematosus
   – Misc. including Gaucher's
   b) Idiopathic

Table 5.2 Pathophysiological effects of paraproteins

1. Autoimmune activity
   – CHAD (anti-I activity)
   – Haemochromatosis (transferrin binding activity)
   – Xanthomata (Lipoprotein binding activity)
   – Peripheral neuropathy (anti-myelin activity)

2. Cold precipitation

3. High intrinsic viscosity

4. Haemostatic abnormalities
   – Platelet dysfunction
   – Coagulation abnormalities
   – Vascular

5. Formation of amyloid fibrils

6. Hyperviscosity

brought to light by the clinical manifestations caused by the abnormal clinico-pathological properties of the protein. (Table 5.2).

PROPERTIES OF THE PARAPROTEIN

Antibody activity

The majority of paraproteins are secreted as complete immunoglobulins and therefore exhibit activity against specific antigen binding sites in exactly the same way as normal immunoglobulins. A large literature describes paraprotein activity against a vast number of microbiological, chemical and auto-antigens, although in any individual case it is usually not possible to determine the antibody specificity. Autoimmune phenomena such as immune haemolysis are common in those conditions associated with paraproteins but this is usually due to the immune dysregulation created by the underlying disorder rather than by the paraprotein per se.

Cold precipitation

Between 5 and 10% of myeloma proteins and 10 and 20% of macroglobulinaemia proteins are cryoprecipitable but only half of these will cause symptoms. In myeloma the paraprotein is usually an IgG protein but cryoprecipitable IgA and Bence-Jones protein have been described. In Waldenstrom's macroglobulinaemia and other lymphoproliferative disorders, however, the cryoglobulin is more usually an IgM.

A number of biochemical features have been described to account for the cryoprecipitability of these paraproteins, including an over-abundance of hydrophobic residues, an abnormal tyrosine-tryptophan ratio in the molecule and a paucity of sialic acid residues. To date, however, no consistent feature has been described.

The clinical features are varied and include Raynaud's phenomenon, skin changes, glomerulonephritis, haemorrhages (into skin, retina, epistaxis, haemoptysis and melaena), thromboses (of pulmonary, renal and mesenteric arteries), peripheral neuropathy and articular manifestations. In addition, constitutional symptoms such as fever or chill may be provoked by exposure to the cold.

Haemostatic abnormalities

Haemostatic abnormalities have been reported to occur in 15% of IgG myeloma, 40% of IgA myeloma and 60% of IgM macroglobulinaemias. Thrombotic complications occur less frequently and have been variously reported in 3–24% of patients. The pathogenesis of haemostatic complications is complex, involving many different aspects and a combination of factors is probably responsible for the final clinical picture.

Coagulation factors

Numerous reports have demonstrated in-vitro inhibitors to coagulation factors V, VII, VIII, XI and XII but the most commonly described inhibitor has been one that acts by interfering with fibrin monomer polymerisation. There is not a strong correlation, however, between these in-vitro abnormalities and clinical bleeding, and often other co-existing abnormalities are present, such as uraemia or thrombocytopaenia, making interpretation difficult.

Platelet defects

Although thrombocytopaenia is often described in association with paraproteinaemia, it rarely is severe enough to cause bleeding and a more common cause is an associated qualitative defect of platelet function. The qualitative defects have been ascribed to the fact that in these conditions increased membrane-bound IgG can be demonstrated which is thought to interfere with platelet function.

Vascular abnormalities

Vascular damage due to toxic or autoimmune damage by the abnormal protein may not uncommonly give rise to purpura. A condition known as primary hypergammaglobulinaemic purpura, most commonly occurring in women, is associated with a polyclonal paraproteinaemia and purpura. It is a benign condition affecting mainly the extremities and is characterised by premonitory itching, stinging and erythema with associated deposition of pigment which over the years may result in the legs becoming swollen and brown from haemosiderin deposition. A number of studies have shown that with prolonged follow-up a significant proportion of patients will develop Sjogren's syndrome or a variety of other disorders.

Cryoglobulinaemia and cryofibrinogenaemia produce similar clinical pictures in which purpura is a prominent feature. Lesions are commonest in exposed areas such as nose, ears, face and extremities. They are thought to be due to precipitation of the proteins on exposure to cold with resulting vascular damage.

Hyperviscosity syndrome

Viscosity is defined as the ability of a fluid to resist flow. The viscosity of whole blood is dependent on both the cellular compartment and the serum compartment, and in-vivo viscosity varies at high and low shear rates, a factor dependent on the internal diameter of the blood vessels through which the blood flows.

The viscosity of serum is primarily a function of the concentration and physico-chemical properties of the serum proteins. The large size and intricate shape of the IgM immunoglobulins imparts a high intrinsic viscosity to this class of immunoglobulin. IgG has a much lower intrinsic viscosity, with the exception of IgG_3, which has a tendency to form unstable complexes, hence the intrinsic viscosity of this sub-class.

IgA immunoglobulins have an intermediate viscosity because of their tendency to form polymers. The hyperviscosity syndrome occurs most frequently, therefore, in patients with IgM-paraproteins, whilst the second commonest cause is IgA paraproteins. On the other hand, the syndrome is not seen in IgG paraproteinaemia unless there is a very high concentration of protein or the paraprotein is of the IgG_3 sub-class.

Viscosity can be measured by determining the time taken for a fluid to pass through a measured length of capillary tube at standard temperatures and pressures. This method measures viscosity at high shear rates but does not reflect the influence of protein-cell interactions which occur at low shear rates. It is, however, perfectly satisfactory for measuring plasma viscosity and is the technique of choice in most laboratories.

History

Lassitude, fever, weight loss and dehydration

Patients with paraproteins may have non-specific systemic symptoms because of their underlying disorder. Greater than 10% weight loss or otherwise unexplained fever constitute 'B' symptoms which usually indicate more generalised disease. Dehydration is often apparent at presentation. This may be due to decreased fluid intake because of generalised malaise and nausea but renal failure and hypercalcaemia are important contributing factors.

Symptoms of anaemia

Part of the lassitude may be due to an accompanying low haemoglobin. Anaemia may be due to marrow infiltration, renal failure, bleeding or haemodilution due to increased plasma volume resulting from the increased oncotic effect of the paraprotein.

Infection

Respiratory and urinary infections are commonly observed and relate to the degree of immunoparesis.

Symptoms of hyperviscosity

Increased plasma viscosity resulting in a sluggish circulation often manifests itself in fluctuating neurological abnormalities such as headache, vertigo and somnolence. Occasionally fits or coma may occur, particularly if there is accompanying hypercalcaemia. Occlusion of vasa nervora may produce progressive peripheral neuropathy (Bing-Neal Syndrome). Blurring of vision may be reported due to sluggish retinal blood flow.

Skeletal pain

In myeloma severe bony pain is a common presenting feature. It usually results from destruction of bones in the axial skeleton. Vertebral collapse induces severe localised pain sometimes with associated nerve root compression and referred pain in the distribution of an intercostal nerve. Lytic lesions invading the cortex of ribs may be associated with pleuritic pain whilst such lesions in the skull are usually asymptomatic.

Bleeding manifestations

Haemorrhagic manifestations, usually of mucosal type, occasionally occur and are more common with IgM and IgA paraproteins. These may complex with various coagulation factors but there is a poor correlation between factor assay levels in vitro and clinical manifestations. Platelet function is also compromised by coating with the paraprotein. Bleeding may also be exacerbated by accompanying renal failure and thrombocytopenia. This low platelet count, along with microvascular changes due to toxic or autoimmune damage may induce purpura. If this appears on exposed areas, e.g. nose, ears or extremities of limbs, cryoglobulinaemia or cryofibrinogenaemia may be present.

Local effect of plasmacytoma

Local pressure or destruction of surrounding tissues may cause a wide variety of clinical manifestations depending upon the site involved. A common site is within the spinal column with cord compression and resultant paraplegia.

Thrombosis and Raynaud's phenomenon

Both arterial and venous thrombosis may occur with paraproteinaemias, although their frequency is rare.

Examination

General appearance

Although many patients look and may feel well, some will present with an acute systemic debilitating illness for the reasons enumerated above. It is particularly important to assess the patient for dehydration and weight loss.

Haemorrhagic manifestations

The skin and mouth should be carefully inspected for purpura or echymoses.

Hyperviscosity

Has the patient clinical evidence of sluggish cerebral circulation as manifest by slowness of thought or stupor? Fundal examination may reveal distended tortuous veins along with superficial haemorrhages and exudates (Plate 22).

Bony lesions

Any site of skeletal pain or swelling should be carefully inspected.

Focal neurological signs

Is there evidence of peripheral neuropathy, either from nerve compression or occlusion of the vasa nervosa? Signs of spinal cord compression should be sought in a patient with leg, bladder or bowel symptoms.

Lymphadenopathy and hepatosplenomegaly

These should be carefully looked for because they may indicate the presence of an underlying immunoproliferative disorder.

Investigations

Full blood count

This may reveal anaemia, which may be macrocytic, neutropenia or thrombocytopenia. Rouleau are prominent in the presence of whole immunoglobulin or heavy-chain but may not be observed with a light-chain secreting tumour (Fig. 1.2). Agglutination of erythrocytes indicates presence of a cold agglutinin. Approximately 10% of patients with myeloma have a leukoerythroblastic anaemia at presentation. The presence of circulating plasma cells indicates plasma cell leukaemia and is a poor prognostic finding. The blood film may reveal evidence of underlying pathology, e.g. chronic lymphocytic leukaemia.

Immunoglobulins and Bence-Jones proteinaemia

Each immunoglobulin type should be quantitated as well as the concentration of the paraprotein assessed. In the presence of a cryoglobulin the blood sample will need to be transported to the laboratory in a 37°C water bath for centrifugation at this temperature. Urinary light-chains should be characterised and quantitated.

Urea, electrolytes and calcium

At presentation the urea may be raised by many different mechanisms, e.g. dehydration, hypercalcaemia, deposition of light-chains in renal tubules and renal amyloid.

Bone marrow aspirate

The finding of greater than 20% of plasma cells is strongly indicative of myeloma. The number of plasma cells, although usually less than 5%, rises with age and the presence of any chronic inflammatory condition. If there is doubt as to whether the plasma cells are reactive or malignant, immunophenotyping with labelled anti-k or anti-λ antibodies will distinguish between a reactive polyclonal and a malignant monoclonal population.

Skeletal survey

Plain X-rays of the axial skeleton, skull along with femora, humeri and a chest X-ray should be examined. Generalised osteoporosis is commonly seen but vertebral crush fractures are characteristic. Lytic lesions may be observed in any bones but are most commonly seen in the skull, ribs, pelvis and proximal long bones.

Biopsy

Consideration should be given to biopsying any ap-

proachable tumour to achieve a tissue diagnosis of either a plasmacytoma or other pathology. In the case of suspected amyloid, a rectal or renal biopsy may be necessary.

6. Investigation of patient with lymphadenopathy or splenomegaly

T. Sheehan   A. C. Parker

Lymphadenopathy occurs in an extremely diverse group of disorders (Table 6.1) and numerous investigations, some more invasive than others, are available which may enable the clinician to identify the underlying cause (Table 6.2). While it is not possible to lay down blanket guidelines for the investigation of such a heterogeneous group of patients, certain basic principles can be outlined.

An important principle is that the investigational approach in an individual case depends entirely on the clinical circumstances. Investigations selected must be

Table 6.1   Causes of lymphadenopathy

Infective	
Bacterial	Tonsillitis (cervical lymphadenopathy)
	Syphilis (inguinal lymphadenopathy in
	primary; generalised in secondary)
	Tuberculosis (human or bovine)
	Brucellosis
	Atypical mycobacterial infections
	Cat-scratch fever
Chlamydia	Lymphogranuloma venereum
Viral	Epstein Barr virus
	Cytomegalovirus
	Infectious hepatitis
	Rubella
	Measles
	HIV
Fungal	Histoplasmosis
Protozoan	Toxoplasmosis
Immunological	SLE
	Rheumatoid arthritis
	Sarcoidosis
	Thyrotoxicosis
Malignant	Hodgkin's disease
	Non-Hodgkin's lymphoma
	Chronic lymphocytic leukaemia
	Acute lymphoblastic leukaemia
	Metastic carcinoma
	Acute myeloid or monocytic leukaemia
	Chronic myeloid leukaemia

Table 6.2   Investigations available for lymphadenopathy

Blood film
Monospot
Viral serology (EBV, CMV, HIV)
Toxoplasma titre
ANF
Rheumatoid factor
VDRL
Kveim test
Marrow aspirate
Trephine biopsy
Chest X-Ray (well penetrated film or tomogram)
CT scan
Lymphangiogram
Liver/spleen scan
Gallium scan
Lymph node aspirate
Lymph node biopsy

dictated by the results of a carefully taken clinical history and thorough physical examination. The indiscriminate use of a battery of tests is wasteful, unrewarding and potentially hazardous.

Following clinical assessment a series of investigations should be planned in a way which is most likely to give a specific diagnosis with the minimum of risk to the patient.

History

General

The age and social circumstances of the patient, including occupation, will provide important diagnostic pointers.

Infectious mononucleosis associated with Epstein Barr virus infection is uncommon in the elderly for example, while HIV infection would have to be considered in a young drug abuser or haemophiliac.

Character of nodal enlargement

The character and rate of progression of lymph node

enlargement is important. Rapid lymph node enlargement is usually seen in infective states or occasionally with highly aggressive neoplastic disorders such as Burkitt's lymphoma. Malignant lymphadenopathy is usually painless and progressive, although some fluctuation of nodal size is occasionally seen in Hodgkin's disease or non-Hodgkin's lymphomas. Painful adenopathy suggests an infective or inflammatory cause. Alcohol-induced pain is rare and entirely non-specific.

Associated symptoms

The presence of 'B' symptoms (unexplained weight loss of greater than 10% during the preceding six months, unexplained fever of greater than 38°C on more than one occasion or unexplained night sweats) is of major prognostic importance in Hodgkin's disease and non-Hodgkin's lymphoma and must be sought by direct questioning in all cases. Pruritus may also occur in these disorders but is not of prognostic significance.

Symptoms suggestive of thyrotoxicosis or a multisystem collagen disorder may be highly relevant.

Physical examination

Site and character of lymph nodes

A search for enlarged nodes in the epitrochlear, preauricular and popliteal regions should not be forgotten, and formal assessment of the lymphoid tissue of Waldeyer's ring may be necessary.

Not only the location and extent of lymphadenopathy but also its character should be documented. Lymphadenopathy associated with infection may be tender and there may be local erythema and warmth of the overlying skin. In most reactive or lymphomatous states the nodes are discrete, rubbery and non-tender. Hard or fixed nodes are suggestive of metastic carcinoma.

While localised or regional lymphadenopathy may occur in Hodgkin's disease or non-Hodgkin's lymphoma, in such instances a careful search for a primary infective or neoplastic lesion in the region drained by the enlarged nodes is indicated. Unexplained cervical lymphadenopathy should prompt a thorough search for nasopharyngeal carcinoma for example, while the presence of hard nodes in the left supraclavicular fossa should immediately raise suspicions of gastric carcinoma.

Physical findings in other systems

Physical findings in other systems may provide useful diagnostic clues, e.g. erythema nodosum in sarcoidosis, a butterfly rash in systemic lupus erythematosus, finger clubbing in bronchogenic carcinoma or subcutaneous nodules and joint deformities in rheumatoid disease.

Investigations

Full blood count

Examination of a peripheral blood film is a simple procedure and may provide helpful information. Mature lymphocytosis with numerous 'smear' cells is characteristically seen in B cell CLL. Lymphoblasts can be found in the peripheral blood in the majority of cases of acute lymphoblastic leukaemia while atypical lymphocytes may point to a diagnosis of infectious mononucleosis due to Epstein Barr virus infection, or less commonly, cytomegalovirus or toxoplasmosis. In a minority of cases of non-Hodgkin's lymphoma abnormal cells are present in the peripheral blood.

Lymphopenia, when present, is an important prognostic factor in Hodgkin's disease. In bacterial infections or metastic disease neutrophilia is a common finding and is occasionally of marked degree, mimicking chronic myeloid leukaemia ('leukaemoid reaction').

Eosinophilia is occasionally seen in Hodgkin's disease or acute lymphoblastic leukaemia and leukoerythroblastic blood films are seen in some patients with advanced metastatic carcinoma.

Bone marrow

In cases of suspected carcinoma, lymphoma or granulomatosis disease, trephine biopsy should be performed in addition to bone marrow aspiration. Where indicated, samples of marrow should be sent to the appropriate laboratory for microbiological or immunohistological analysis.

Other blood tests

As can be seen from Table 6.2 a range of serological tests are available. They should be used selectively and the limitations of some of these tests should be borne in mind when evaluating the results. False negative results may be obtained if samples are taken too early during the course of an infective illness, and serological tests in general are often unreliable in immunosuppressed patients who may fail to mount normal antibody responses. The presence of IgG class antibodies does not necessarily indicate current infection, and a rising titre of such antibodies or the appearance of IgM antibodies directed against the pathogen in question are of greater diagnostic value. In cases of unexplained lymphocytosis, sophisticated investigations are now available to identify the subsets of lymphocytes involved and to demonstrate clonality.

Radiology

A well-penetrated chest X-Ray should be performed to exclude lung pathology, or mediastinal, hilar or paratracheal lymphadenopathy. Tomograms may increase the sensitivity of the investigation and the distribution of lymphadenopathy may suggest a specific diagnosis (e.g. bilateral hilar and paratracheal lymphadenopathy in sarcoidosis). Intra-abdominal lymphadenopathy can be assessed either by lymphangiography or CT scanning. The theoretical advantage of lymphangiography is that normal-sized but pathological nodes may be delineated, but the procedure is cumbersome, painful and not without hazard, particularly in patients with respiratory pathology. In many centres CT scanning has replaced lymphangiography as the investigation of choice.

Liver/spleen isotope scans or gallium scans may prove useful in selected instances. Ultrasound scanning can be very useful particularly to assess spleen size.

Lymph node biopsy

In many cases this procedure is required for definitive diagnosis. Lymph nodes can usually be removed under local anaesthetic and in all instances the largest nodes which can be safely removed should be sent intact and without fixative to the pathology department where the appropriate investigations can be performed.

Lymph node aspiration is a technically simpler procedure and may be of great value where infection or metastatic carcinoma is suspected but is not recommended for diagnosis in non-Hodgkin's lymphoma or Hodgkin's disease, since in these conditions an assessment of nodal architecture forms an integral part of the histological diagnosis.

SPLENOMEGALY

The list of causes of splenomegaly is long and formidable (Table 6.3). If there is coincidental lymphadenopathy, then the investigational approach should be that previously described for the investigation of lymphadenopathy. Isolated splenomegaly, however, poses a different set of diagnostic problems. It is usually possible to be confident on clinical grounds that a left hypochondrial mass which is dull to percussion, moves downwards and medially on inspiration and has a well-

Table 6.3 Causes of splenomegaly

Haematological	
Chronic haemolysis	Congenital spherocytosis
	Hereditary elliptocytosis
	Sickle cell disease
	Thalassaemia
	G6PD deficiency
	Pyruvate kinase deficiency
	Acquired warm antibody type
	Haemolytic anaemia
	Pernicious anaemia
Myeloproliferative disorders	Primary proliferative polycythaemia
	Chronic myeloid leukaemia
	Essential thrombocythaemia
	Myelofibrosis
Lymphoreticular malignancies	Acute lymphoblastic leukaemia
	Chronic lymphocytic leukaemia
	Prolymphocytic leukaemia
	Non-Hodgkin's lymphoma
	Hodgkin's disease
	Hairy cell leukaemia
Infective	
Bacterial	Septicaemia
	Infective endocarditis
	Salmonellosis
	Tuberculosis
	Brucellosis
	Syphilis
Viral	Infectious mononucleosis (EBV)
	Cytomegalovirus
	Viral hepatitis
Fungal	Histoplasmosis
Protozoan	Toxoplasmosis
	Malaria
	Leishmaniasis
	Trypanosomiasis
Congestive	Congestive cardiac failure (uncommon)
	Hepatic cirrhosis
	Budd-Chiari syndrome
	Veno-occlusive disease
	Portal vein thrombosis
Storage diseases	Gaucher's disease
	Niemann-Pick
	Histocytosis X
Non-haematological malignancies	Carcinoma
	Sarcoma
	Melanoma
Miscellaneous	Amyloid
	Cysts

defined palpable notch is an enlarged spleen. If there are diagnostic doubts, these can be settled by appropriate radiological investigations. A plain X-ray of abdomen is relatively cheap and non-invasive and may resolve the issue. If not, a liver/spleen scan, ultrasound or, where appropriate, an intravenous pyelogram can be performed. The history and physical findings will often suggest the diagnosis or at least appropriate avenues of investigation.

Massive splenomegaly

Truly massive splenic enlargement, extending below the umbilicus or even below the pelvic brim should immediately suggest myelofibrosis, chronic myeloid leukaemia, or a 'tropical' infection such as malaria or Leishmaniasis (kala-azar). In these circumstances a blood film may provide a diagnosis (e.g. malaria) or suggest a myeloproliferative disorder, the further elucidation of which may be aided by relatively simple investigations such as neutrophil alkaline phosphatase score (low in CML) or bone marrow aspirate (dry tap in myelofibrosis, Leishman-Donovan bodies in kala-azar).

Moderate or mild splenomegaly

Moderate or marked splenomegaly in a ruddy faced patient who complains of pruritus should prompt investigations for primary proliferative polycythaemia – full blood count (raised haematocrit and often leukocytosis or thrombocytosis), red cell mass and plasma volume studies.

In a patient with a history of alcohol abuse, splenomegaly is likely to be congestive in origin, resulting from the portal hypertension which occurs in hepatic cirrhosis.

A careful search for other clinical stigmata of chronic liver disease, such as palmar erythema, flapping tremor and spider naevi, would be warranted. Thereafter, biochemical tests of liver function and a barium swallow to demonstrate oesophageal varices may be performed.

The hypertensive patient with pallor, jaundice and modest splenomegaly could well have autoimmune haemolytic anaemia, e.g. induced by methyldopa therapy. Scrutiny of a peripheral blood film for spherocytes and polychromasia, and a direct Coomb's test would be appropriate in such a case.

The minor degree of soft, and sometimes tender, splenomegaly which can be seen in the septicaemic patient is usually overshadowed by other signs of overwhelming infection, although in elderly people the pyrexial response may be impaired or absent and mild splenomegaly may be a useful pointer to the infective nature of an otherwise obscure illness.

Similarly, infective endocarditis may be extremely difficult to diagnose, particularly in elderly patients who have no prior history of valvular disease and whose valves may have become colonised after a relatively minor procedure. In such patients, splenomegaly may be one of the subtle clinical signs which should alert the astute physician to the possible diagnosis.

Clearly in these 'infective' circumstances the splenomegaly requires no investigation in its own right but is often an extremely useful physical sign pointing the way to appropriate investigation of the underlying disorder.

Hyposplenism

Splenic absence or hypofunction can often be inferred from the presence of numerous Howell-Jolly bodies in the peripheral blood film; target cells, leukocytosis and thrombocytosis may also be present.

If the spleen has not been surgically removed congenital splenic absence, sickle cell disease or coeliac disease should be considered. Hyposplenism in sickle cell disease results from recurrent infarction.

7. Assessment of bleeding patient

C. A. Ludlam

The initial arrest of haemorrhage is brought about during primary haemostasis by adhesion of platelets to damaged endothelium and subendothelial structures (Fig. 30.1) with subsequent formation of a platelet plug (see Chapter 30). During secondary haemostasis the coagulation system is activated resulting in the depo-

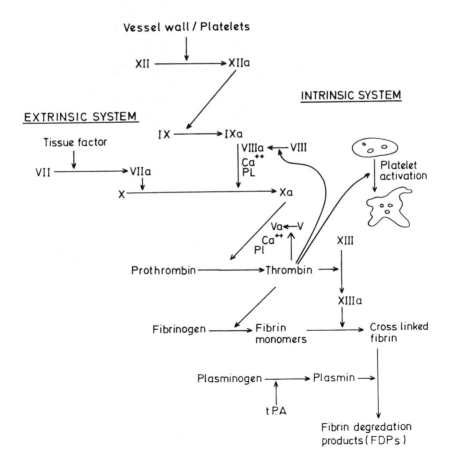

Fig. 7.1 Coagulation cascade

Table 7.1 Summary of common causes of platelet, coagulation and vessel wall disorders which predispose to excessive bleeding

Thrombopathies	
Congenital	Bernard Soulier syndrome
	Thrombasthenia
	Storage pool disorders
Acquired	Drugs
	Paraproteinaemias
	Uraemia
Thrombocytopenia	
Congenital	Wiscott Aldrich
Acquired	Idiopathic thrombocytopenic purpura
	Infections – viral
	– bacterial
	Drugs
	Thrombotic thrombocytopenic purpura
	Disseminated intravascular coagulation
	Aplastic anaemia
	Marrow infiltration
	Megaloblastic anaemia
	Splenomegaly
Thrombocytosis	Myeloproliferative disorders
	Reactive to infection
	malignancy
	bleeding
	collagenosis
	post-splenectomy
Coagulation disorders	
Congenital	Haemophilia A and B
Acquired	Anticoagulants
	Liver disease
	Disseminated intravascular coagulation
	Paraproteinaemia
Vessel wall abnormalities	Marfan syndrome
	Hereditary haemorrhagic telangiectasia
	Vasculitis

sition of fibrin which consolidates the platelet plug (Fig. 7.1). Causes of congenital and acquired bleeding disorders are summarised in Table 7.1.

In assessing a patient with a potential, or an actual, bleeding state it may be quite easy to distinguish between a congenital and an acquired disorder, particularly if bleeding has been recurrent and severe. For an individual presenting with only occasional or recent symptoms suggestive of a mild bleeding state, it may be difficult to know whether he has a congenital or acquired disorder. The diagnostic difficulty is compounded because a patient with mild symptoms usually has only mild abnormalities on repeat testing and these can sometimes be difficult to distinguish from results

obtained in normal individuals. Therefore a thorough, carefully assessed, history is needed to allow a clinical decision to be made as to whether the patient is likely to have a bleeding disorder.

History

Site of bleed

Haemarthroses and muscle haematoma indicate a defect in the coagulation cascade, whereas purpura, prolonged bleeding from superfical cuts, epistaxis, gastrointestinal haemorrhage and menorrhagia indicate a failure of platelets or von Willebrand factor to secure primary haemostasis. Recurrent bleeding at a single site suggests the presence of a structural lesion.

Duration of bleeding

Are the bleeding symptoms of recent origin? The aim is to assess whether the patient has a congenital or acquired haemorrhagic diathesis. In a severe bleeding disorder it is usually quite clear whether it is of recent origin or of longstanding duration. Difficulty may arise with mild disorders in which there may be excessive bleeding only after the occasional tooth extraction.

Precipitating causes

Does the bleeding occur spontaneously or is it only observed following trauma or surgery? Clearly, bleeding that appears to arise without provocation indicates a more severely affected individual than one in whom haemorrhage only follows trauma.

Surgery

Is there excessive post-operative bleeding? It is useful to ask about tonsillectomy, dental extraction and circumcision, as all these are potent tests of haemostasis. Does bleeding start immediately or is it delayed after surgery? A defect in primary haemostasis does not allow the formation of an adequate platelet plug and bleeding is therefore observed immediately after surgery or trauma. In a coagulation disorder platelet plug formation is normal but fibrin reinforcement is defective and after several hours the friable plug disintegrates leading to haemorrhage.

Family history

The absence of a family history does not exclude the presence of a hereditary bleeding disorder. With a good history in a large family it may be possible to identify the mode of inheritance.

Other systemic illness

Has the patient any underlying systemic medical disorder that could predispose to excessive bleeding? It is particularly important to consider whether a patient has hepatic or renal failure, a paraproteinaemia or a collagenosis. An acutely ill patient may have multiple factors predisposing to haemorrhage, e.g. septicaemia and uraemia.

Drugs

Almost any medicine can potentially produce a bleeding disorder, either by depressing the bone marrow with resultant thrombocytopenia, or by interacting with warfarin. Check that the patient is not on a heparin infusion or taking warfarin. Non-steroidal anti-inflammatory drugs inhibit platelet function and the effect of aspirin may last up to 10 days following the ingestion of a single tablet.

Examination

Superifical examination

Carefully inspect the skin for purpura and bruises and the mucous membranes of the mouth for evidence of bleeding. Apparently spontaneous bruising around the head or neck should arouse a suspicion that it may in fact be post-traumatic and in the case of a child represent a non-accidental injury. Telangiectasis around the lips and on the tongue indicate a diagnosis of hereditary haemorrhagic telangiectasia. Scars over the elbows and knees are characteristic of factor XIII deficiency due to the poor healing of wounds. A diagnosis of Ehlers Danlos should be considered in any individual with excessive skin folds and pliable joints. All joints should be carefully examined, particularly the knees, ankles and elbows, in a patient who has had joint swelling that could have been an haemarthrosis.

General examination

A full medical examination is essential to search for evidence of disorders which might predispose to bleeding. Particular attention should be paid to whether there are any cutaneous stigmata of liver disease. Lymphadenopathy and hepatosplenomegaly should be sought as evidence of malignancy or lymphoma. In an acutely ill patient, neurological signs, if recent, are suggestive of disseminated intravascular coagulation, thrombotic thrombocytopenic purpura or an intracranial bleed. Septicaemia, particularly due to gram negative organisms, often results in a degree of consumptive coagulopathy.

Local lesion

Any bleeding point should, if possible, be carefully inspected to exclude a structural lesion. Such an assessment may require investigation by endoscopy to visualise the site of haemorrhage.

Investigations

The history and examination should give an indication as to the nature and severity of the possible bleeding diathesis.

Screening tests

All patients should have a full blood count including platelets and film, prothrombin time, APTT,

Table 7.2 Screening investigtions to detect a haemorrhagic state

	Components assessed	Conditions in which test is abnormal
Primary haemostasis		
Platelet count	Platelets	See Table 7.1
Bleeding time	Platelet function von Willebrand factor	See Table 7.1 von Willebrand's disease
Secondary haemostasis		
Prothrombin time	II V VII X	Warfarin Liver disease Congenital factor deficiencies DIC SLE inhibitor
Activated partial thromboplastin time (APTT)	V VIII IX X XI XII	Heparin DIC Congenital factor deficiencies Anti-factor VIII and inhibitors
Fibrinogen concentration	Fibrinogen	DIC Congenital hypofibrinogenaemia Severe liver disease
Fibrin degradation products (FDPs)	Lysis of fibrin	DIC

fibrinogen, FDPs and template bleeding time (provided the platelet count is over about $50 \times 10^9/l$. The interpretation of these investigations is given in Table 7.2.

Specialised investigations

Depending on the history and the results of the screening tests individual coagulation factors should be assayed or platelet function assessed. If screening tests are normal but the history is strongly suggestive of a bleeding disorder, further investigation is indicated. The screening tests for the coagulation system are only sensitive to factor levels below approximately 25% of normal and therefore if a deficiency of one of these is suspected they should be assayed individually starting with factors VIII and IX. The screening tests do not assess factor XIII deficiency and this should be specifically assayed if there is a good clinical history suggestive of a bleeding diathesis.

Clinically significant platelet disorders may have normal bleeding times. Therefore, if from the history platelet function is considered defective, further tests of their function in vitro should be undertaken.

8. Assessment of patient with platelet disorder

C. A. Ludlam

THROMBOCYTOPENIA

A reduced platelet count may arise by one of three mechanisms: under-production of platelets by the marrow, excessive consumption within the circulation, or sequestration within an enlarged spleen. Platelets are responsible for the initial arrest of haemorrhage by forming an occlusive plug in the leaking vessel. Thrombocytopenia therefore leads to a failure of this primary haemostatic process with purpura and other manifestations of mucocutaneous haemorrhage. Purpura due to thrombocytopenia must be distinguished from vasculitis; the latter may have a characteristic distribution, being slightly papular, and is usually accompanied by a normal platelet count. Thrombocytopenia may be observed as an isolated event in an otherwise apparently healthy person, or as a manifestation of a systemic disorder in which the patient is clearly unwell (Table 7.1). Initially it is important to ascertain whether there are other haemostatic abnormalities and assessment of the coagulation system is advisable.

History

Site of bleeding

Does the patient have a history of mucocutaneous haemorrhage? Purpura and spontaneous bruising usually indicate a platelet count of less than $30 \times 10^9/l$ although in paraproteinaemias and occasionally in thrombopathies the count may be much higher. Recurrent bilateral epistaxis, gastrointestinal haemorrhage, including mucous membrane bleeding visible in the mouth, and persistent menorrhagia commonly result from thrombocytopenia. Cut fingers may bleed for prolonged periods. Visual disturbance following fundal haemorrhage indicates a critical haemorrhagic state and may be premonitory of a more catastrophic intracranial bleed.

Muscle and particularly joint haematoma are charac-teristic of coagulation abnormalities and are virtually never the result of thrombocytopenia.

Precipitating factors

Have the bleeds arisen spontaneously or only after trauma? Clearly the latter indicates a less severe degree of impaired haemostasis than apparently spontaneous bruising.

Duration of symptoms

It is important to ascertain the duration of the haemorrhagic state so as to distinguish a congenital from an acquired disorder. In some patients with congenital thrombocytopenia the bleeding manifestations may be relatively mild with symptoms appearing only in adult life.

Surgery

Has the patient had previous surgery? Tonsillectomy, dental extraction and circumcision are all excellent stress tests for the haemostatic system and if an individual has had these performed without excessive bleeding it is unlikely that significant thrombocytopenia was present at that time.

Drugs

A history of all drug ingestion is mandatory because of the large number of drugs that may depress megakaryocytic maturation in the bone marrow. Aspirin and non-steroidal drugs inhibit platelet function and may exacerbate the haemorrhagic diathesis resulting from thrombocytopenia.

Family history

Congenital thrombocytopenias can be both dominantly

and recessively inherited. Although other family members may be asymptomatic, it is often worthwhile to arrange for platelet counts to be carried out on parents, siblings and children of the patient.

Examination

Superficial examination

Careful inspection should be made of skin, mouth and occular fundi for purpura and bruising. If the bruises are of varying ages it suggests that the patient has not developed the thrombocytopenia very recently.

Spleen

Palpable splenomegaly should be assiduously sought. Approximately a third of the platelets are pooled in a normal-sized spleen and the proportion increases with increasing spleen size. Up to 90% of the platelets may be sequestered in a large spleen resulting in thrombocytopenia.

General examination

Full general medical examination is essential particularly to seek evidence of a collagenosis, liver disease or malignancy. The possibility of an infective cause should always be considered.

Investigations

Full blood count

A haemoglobin, white and platelet count and examination of a blood film will allow visual confirmation of the reduced platelet count as well as assessment of their morphology. By inspecting the erythrocytes and leukocytes it is possible to ascertain whether a more extensive haematological disorder may be present (Table 8.1).

Coagulation screen

An APTT, prothrombin time, fibrinogen and FDPs should be measured to identify whether thrombocytopenia is part of a general coagulopathy.

Bone marrow

An aspirate or trephine biopsy will indicate whether megakaryocytes are present in normal or increased members when peripheral destruction is the cause of the

Table 8.1 Interpretation of blood film in patient with thrombocytopenia

	Abnormalities	Interpretation
Erythrocytes	Normal	Immune or congenital thrombocytopenia
	Fragmented cells	Disseminated intravascular coagulation Thrombotic thrombocytopenic purpura Renal failure
	Macrocytic	B_{12} or folate deficiency Myeloma
	Target cells	Liver disease
Leukocytes	Normal	Immune or congenital thrombocytopenia
	Blasts or myelocytes	Leukaemia
	Leuko-erythroblastic	Marrow infiltration Myelofibrosis
	Döhle bodies	May-Hegglin anomaly
	Inclusions	Chediak-Higashi syndrome
Platelets	Giant platelets	May-Hegglin anomaly Bernard Soulier syndrome Recovering bone marrow
	Agranular platelets	Grey platelet syndrome
	Small platelets	Wiscott-Aldrich syndrome Iron deficiency

thrombocytopenia or whether they are reduced reflecting decreased production by the marrow. The presence of an infiltrate of non-haematological cells will be more apparent in the trephine biopsy.

Bleeding time

If mucocutaneous bleeding is observed at a platelet count of greater than $50 \times 10^9/l$, a bleeding time may be useful. Spontaneous bruising is rare at this level of platelets and if present suggests a degree of thrombopathy, as in a paraproteinaemia, which may be demonstrated by observing a disproportionately long bleeding time compared to platelet count.

Assessment of platelet survival

Radio-isotope platelet lifespan studies may sometimes be useful to determine whether thrombocytopenia is due to either shortened platelet survival within the circulation or excessive splenic sequestration. A normal platelet survival, in the absence of splenomegaly, indicates that the thrombocytopenia is secondary to decreased platelet production by megakaryocytes in the bone marrow.

THROMBOCYTOSIS

The platelet count may increase in response to inflammation, malignancy, bleeding or splenectomy. Such a reactive thrombocytosis must be distinguished from a malignant proliferation of megakaryocytes as in essential thrombocythaemia. This disorder is part of the myeloproliferative spectrum which also includes chronic myeloid leukaemia, primary proliferative polycythaemia and myelofibrosis in which there is clonal proliferation of other cell lines. The platelets in these conditions often have abnormal function which predisposes to bleeding or thrombosis. In the majority of patients with a reactive thrombocytosis the cause is usually obvious (Table 8.2) but in a minority it may be difficult to distinguish from essential thrombocythaemia.

History

Systemic disorder

Does the patient have one of the many causes of a reactive thrombocytosis (Table 7.1)? If the patient is systemically ill it is likely that the thrombocytosis is secondary to an underlying medical disorder. If the patient is apparently well, and the high platelet count was an incidental finding in a full blood count, a full and detailed history will be required. It is often useful to enquire about fever, night sweats, weight loss and melaena as indicators of systemic disease or bleeding.

Splenectomy

Although the platelet count rises promptly after removal of the spleen, it usually subsides to normal within several months. In a few patients the platelets remain mildly elevated.

Bleeding

If there has been haemorrhage, the elevated platelet count is usually due to the bleeding but occasionally patients with essential thrombocythaemia may bleed because the platelet function is defective.

Thrombosis

Arterial or venous thrombo-embolism indicates that the high platelet count is more likely to be due to essential thrombocythaemia; occlusions are not normally seen with a reactive thrombocytosis.

Specific enquiry should be made about digital ischaemia, particularly of the toes, or transient visual disturbance, e.g. amaurosis fugax. These, when associated with a high platelet count, strongly suggest a diagnosis of essential thrombocythaemia.

Drugs

Occasionally some drugs increase the platelet count, e.g. vincristine. After myelosuppressive chemotherapy causing thrombocytopenia a rebound thrombocytosis may occur in the bone marrow recovery phase.

Examination

Physical examination

A full general examination is essential in an attempt to detect one of underlying secondary causes of the raised platelet count (Table 8.2).

Table 8.2 Summary of causes of thrombocytosis

Malignant thrombocytosis
Essential thrombocythaemia
Primary proliferative polycythaemia
Myelofibrosis
Chronic myeloid leukaemia
Reactive thrombocytosis
Chronic inflammatory disorders
Malignancy
Tissue damage
Haemolytic anaemias
Post-splenectomy
Rebound post-thrombocytopenia
Post-haemorrhage
Drug-induced, e.g. vincristine

Hepatosplenomegaly

The presence of an enlarged spleen or liver is strongly indicative of a myeloproliferative disorder. Some patients, however, with essential thrombocythaemia have splenic atrophy at presentation as a result of repeated small asymptomatic infarcts.

Vascular occlusions

Digital ischaemia, often symmetrical, with palpable peripheral pulses, may be found in essential thrombocythaemia. It is also important to exclude causes of vasculitis and diabetes mellitus. The patient should be assessed clinically for the presence of a venous thrombosis.

Investigations

Full blood count

A complete blood count and film are often very informative (Table 8.3). Serial platelet counts are useful to assess whether the numbers are rising or falling.

Table 8.3 Interpretation of blood film in patient with thrombocytosis

	Abnormality	Interpretation
Erythrocytes s	Microcytosis	Iron deficiency If Hb normal consider iron-deficiency PPP
	Leuko-erythroblastosis (With tear drop cells)	Marrow infiltration Myelofibrosis
	Acanthocytes Target cells Howell-Jolly bodies	Splenectomy Hyposplenism
Leukocytes	Blasts or myelocytes	Chronic myeloid leukaemia Chronic myelomonocytic leukaemia
	Neutrophilia	Infection Malignancy
Platelets	Large bizarre forms	Myeloproliferative disorder especially essential thrombocythaemia
	Normal morphology	Any cause of thrombocytosis

Bone marrow

A trephine biopsy allows assessment of megakaryocyte numbers and morphology which is often abnormal in essential thrombocythaemia. A malignant infiltrate, as a cause of the thrombocytosis, will be more apparent in a trephine biopsy than an aspirate.

Bleeding time

An estimate of the template bleeding time may be useful as in essential thrombocythaemia it may be prolonged because of defective platelet function. A normal bleeding time does not exclude this diagnosis.

Platelet function

Platelet aggregation studies are often helpful. Reduced responses, particularly to adrenaline, support a diagnosis of essential thrombocythaemia.

Chromosomes

Studies of chromosomes are sometimes helpful, as the finding of an abnormal karyotype is indicative of a myeloproliferative disorder.

Other investigations

Any investigation deemed appropriate by the history and examination to diagnose a condition predisposing to a reactive thrombocytosis.

A full history, examination and investigation in most instances will allow a reactive thrombocytosis to be distinguished from the malignant disorder of essential thrombocythaemia. On rare occasions a tentative provisional diagnosis of essential thrombocythaemia may have to be made and the patient observed over a period of time to see whether another underlying medical disorder becomes apparent.

9. Assessment of patient with acute or recurrent thrombosis

G. D. O. Lowe

Arterial and venous thromboembolism are both common disorders in the western world and are a major cause of morbidity and mortality. When assessing a patient presenting with an apparent thrombosis it is important to establish whether thrombus is present or not, and if so to define its site and extent. It is also necessary to determine whether there are any underlying conditions predisposing to thrombosis. In addition it is important to ascertain whether the patient has any contraindication to anticoagulant, antiplatelet or thrombolytic drugs.

In this chapter separate consideration is given firstly to assessing whether a patient has a prothrombotic condition, i.e. one that makes it more likely he will develop a clinical thrombus, and secondly to evaluating an acute venous or peripheral arterial thrombosis.

PROTHROMBOTIC STATE

Clinical, biochemical and haematological factors predisposing to thromboembolism are listed in Table 9.1. Some are easy to determine from the history and examination of the patient; others require specialised laboratory investigation. Apart from vessel wall abnormalities, e.g. atherosclerosis, increases in any of the cellular blood components or in plasma viscosity may result in thrombosis. There are also a number of well characterised congenital disorders of plasma proteins that predispose to thrombus formation. In this chapter, guidance will be offered as to which patients merit extensive laboratory tests and in which a full blood count alone is adequate. It is important to distinguish between arterial and venous occlusive events because, in general, haematological abnormality is more likely to result in venous thrombosis, whereas vessel wall changes, e.g. atherosclerosis, are more likely to lead to arterial events.

History

Type of thrombus

In the past has the patient had arterial or venous throm-

Table 9.1 Predisposing factors to thromboembolism

Mainly arterial	Arterial and venous	Mainly venous
Smoking	SLE	
Rheumatic heart disease	Behcet's disease	Malignancy
Prosthetic heart valves	Homocystinaemia	Pregnancy
Hypertension		Obesity
Hypercholesterol-aemia	Oestrogens	Trauma
Diabetes		Surgery
Atrial fibrillation		Paroxysmal nocturnal haemoglobinuria (PNH)
Chronic renal failure	Primary proliferative polycythaemia	Immobility/paralysis
Lupus anticoagulant		Heart failure
Essential thrombocythaemia		Nephrotic syndrome
	Myelofibrosis	Varicose veins
	Decreased fibrinolytic activity	
		Deficiencies of: Antithrombin III Proteins C and S Plasminogen Dysfibrinogen-aemias

bosis? An arterial lesion usually presents suddenly with catastrophic consequences, e.g. stroke or myocardial infarction. Occlusion of a major limb artery causes the constellation of pallor, pain, pulselessness, paraesthesia and paralysis. From the history and examination alone it should have been possible to make a reasonably accurate assessment of the site of the lesion. Venous thrombosis on the other hand results in the more gradual onset of symptoms, usually over several days, with pain, swelling, warmth and distended veins being common features. Unlike arterial thrombosis, it is usually not possible to make a definitive diagnosis on history alone and further investigation should have been undertaken to demonstrate the presence, as well as the extent, of the occlusion. It is useful to know whether the patient was receiving oral anticoagulation at the time the thrombosis became apparent. Particularly for patients with venous disease, a thrombus that develops despite anticoagulation, assuming adequate dosage, probably reflects the presence of a more severe prothrombotic state than one that arises in the absence of anticoagulation.

Symptoms suggestive of pulmonary embolism should be sought, e.g. dyspnoea, pleuritic or central chest pain (depending upon size of embolus) and haemoptysis.

Systemic disorders

As will be seen from Table 9.1 a range of medical conditions predisposes to thrombosis. A full general history is therefore important particularly to exclude the presence of hyperviscosity or a vasculitis. Furthermore, enquiry should be made to ascertain whether the patient might have a condition which would be a contraindication to anticoagulation, e.g. liver or renal disease.

Family history

There is a hereditary predisposition to atherosclerosis and consequent arterial thromboembolism. A familial incidence of venous thrombosis, particularly in a young individual, is more suggestive of an underlying congenital plasma abnormality predisposing to the thrombosis, e.g. antithrombin III deficiency.

Drugs

Oral contraceptives and other preparations of oestrogens predispose to both arterial and venous thrombosis. As well as enquiring about oral anticoagulation, it is necessary to ask whether other drugs which might interfere with the degree of anticoagulation are also being taken. If, for example, the patient has been stabilised on warfarin whilst taking another drug that potentiates its action and this latter medicine is withdrawn, without subsequently checking the prothrombin time and in- creasing the warfarin dose, the patient will become inadequately anticoagulated.

Examination

The principal aim of examining a patient who may have a hypercoagulable state is to ascertain whether there is any evidence of a local or systemic disorder which may have predisposed to a thrombosis. For patients who have presented with a venous thrombosis it is necessary to be satisfied that there is no lesion causing pressure on an adjacent vein, e.g. a pelvic mass resulting in compression of an external iliac vein. Any clinical evidence for disorders listed in Table 9.1 should be sought. Particular care should be taken to look for signs of malignancy, collagenosis and myeloproliferative disorders.

Investigations

The extent of investigation of an individual patient will vary enormously depending upon the history and examination. All patients should have a full blood count and ESR (or plasma viscosity) which will identify those with a possible myeloproliferative disorder. If underlying malignancy is suspected this should be assiduously looked for by appropriate investigation.

Further investigation will depend upon the strength of the history. Individuals within the following categories require further investigation.

1. Venous thrombosis without apparent precipitating cause under 40 years of age
2. Recurrent thrombosis without apparent cause
3. Strong family history of thrombosis

The investigations to be considered are shown in Table 9.2. These are listed in descending order of importance. The chance of making a definitive diagnosis depends upon the strength of the history and the age of onset of thrombosis. In approximately 5–10% of individuals an abnormality will be apparent. It is likely that further plasma, and possibly endothelial cell, abnormalities, will be identified in future. There is increasing evidence that disorders of the fibrinolytic system may be important in predisposing to both arterial and venous thrombosis.

ACUTE THROMBOEMBOLISM

The assessment of arterial and venous thromboembolism presents distinct clinical challenges. This section considers the evaluation of an individual presenting with a possible venous or pulmonary thromboembolism or

Table 9.2 Investigations to detect prothrombotic state

Haemoglobin	High in polycythaemia Low may indicate malignancy
Platelets	High in myeloproliferative disorders
ESR (or plasma viscosity)	High in paraproteinaemias and vasculitis
Activated partial thromboplastin time (APTT)	Factor XII deficiency Lupus anticoagulant
Thrombin time and reptilase time	Dysfibrinogenaemia
Dilute prothrombin time	Lupus anticoagulant
Functional and immunological assays of Antithrombin III Protein C Protein S Plasminogen	Congenital or acquired deficiencies
Euglobulin lysis time or fibrin plate lysis before and after venous occlusion	Assessment of fibrinolytic potential
Plasminogen activator inhibition	High levels are usual cause of low fibrinolytic potential

Table 9.3 Contra-indications to anticoagulant and thrombolytic therapy

Known bleeding disorder	Haemophilia von Willebrand's disease Thrombocytopenia
Medical conditions	Liver disease Renal failure Gastrointestinal ulcers Severe hypertension Malignancy especially intracranial Proliferative retinopathy Endocarditis Active infection, e.g. TB Cerebrovascular accident
Surgery	Any operation within 10 days esp. to CNS or eye Arterial puncture Lumbar puncture Organ biopsy Paracentesis
Drugs	Warfarin if previously caused haemorrhage Drugs potentiating warfarin Heparin, especially with history of thrombocytopenia or arterial thrombosis (use ancrod instead) Aspirin

peripheral arterial occlusion. The assessment of patients presenting with a stroke or myocardial infarction will not be considered in the following discussion.

Part of the assessment of a patient presenting with a possible thrombosis requires the evaluation as to the suitability of the individual for treatment with anti-coagulants or fibrinolytic therapy. Contra-indications to anticoagulation are given in Table 9.3.

VENOUS THROMBOSIS

History

The symptoms of pain, swelling, discoloration and in-crease in local temperature are the usual presenting features of a venous thrombosis. When these symptoms are present in the distal limb only, these non specific symptoms are a very poor guide as to the presence of a thrombus. Only one third of such patients have a thrombus at venography. Muscle strain, superficial thrombophlebitis, cellulitis, haemorrhage or ruptured Baker's cyst at the knee may all mimic a venous throm-bosis. When the symptoms are noted to extend proximal to the knee or elbow they are a better guide to the presence of an underlying venous thrombosis; however,

venography is still desirable to establish the need for thrombolytic therapy or long-term anticoagulants.

Examination

As in the history, if the signs of increased temperature, swelling, muscle tenderness and distended veins are limited to the distal limb, clinical diagnosis is inaccurate. When such symptoms are present in the proximal limb, clinical diagnosis is often more reliable. In an extensive proximal thrombosis the distal limb may become cool and cyanosed from arterial spasm and sluggish venous return. This may be manifested as 'white leg', or phleg-masia alba dolens, or the more severe 'blue leg', or phlegmasia caerulea dolens.

Investigations

The clinician must be satisfied that a venous thrombosis is present prior to instituting appropriate therapy. If the whole lower limb is swollen with all the features of ex-tensive venous thrombosis, then it may be reasonable to proceed to anticoagulation prior to further investigation. In the majority of instances, however, further investi-gation will be necessary either to determine whether a thrombosis is in fact present or to delineate its extent. It may also be appropriate to determine whether the patient has had a pulmonary embolus (see below).

A variety of techniques are available and each has its value in particular clinical settings.

Venography

This is the recommended and reference technique against which others are assessed. With experienced operators, and the use of image intensifiers and television monitors, it is possible to dynamically view the flow of radio-opaque contrast in the veins. However, this is time-consuming and static films are usually adequate. Distal and proximal thrombi can be accurately viewed (Fig. 9.1), but thrombus in the external iliacs and inferior vena cava may only be seen in a third of cases when the dye is infused peripherally. If there is the possibility of thrombosis in these sites, contrast may have to be injected centrally, e.g. retrograde venography.

Fibrinogen uptake test

This technique is useful for serially assessing over a few days a patient at high risk of developing a thrombus. It is used most extensively for post-operative detection of early DVT formation. It is not as useful for evaluating a patient presenting with symptoms or signs of a thrombus. The test is carried out by injection of ^{125}I-fibrinogen and measuring radioactivity, with a sodium iodide crystal and photomultiplier, daily in the legs. The ^{125}I-fibrinogen is incorporated into developing thrombus; if this is found to increase locally by approximately 20% and is sustained for at least 24 hours, the test is said to be positive. It is necessary to use the radioactive counter with the legs slightly elevated to reduce venous pooling which might give a false positive result. The fibrinogen uptake test is reliable at diagnosing peripheral thrombi; it is less useful for detecting isolated proximal thrombus, e.g. in common femoral or external iliac veins.

Impedance plethysmography (IPG)

In this technique a cuff is placed around the proximal thigh and inflated. Following release of the cuff the maximum outflow of blood from the leg is measured by the rate of reduction of calf blood volume. In the presence of occlusive venous thrombi, particularly in proximal vessels, the outflow of blood is reduced. The technique is useful in detecting an individual with an occlusive proximal thrombus, but it is insensitive to

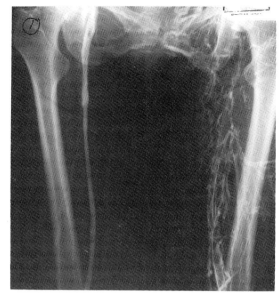

(a)

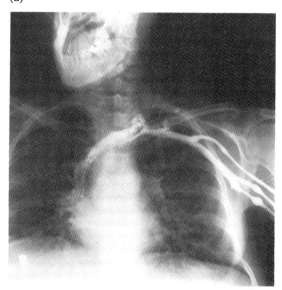

(b)

Fig. 9.1 Bilateral ascending venogram (**A**) demonstrating extensive clots (filling defects) resulting in obstruction and collateral flow on left compared to normal venous drainage clot in innominate vein and superior vena cava. (Reproduced by permission of Dr D. Readhead)

small distal thrombi or those which only partially occlude a major vein. External pressure, e.g. pelvic mass, may give a false positive result and if good collaterals are present a false negative result may be obtained. It can be used together with ^{125}I-fibrinogen scanning for diagnosis of suspected thrombus in patients in whom venography is contra-indicated or unsuccessful; or in screening high-risk patients.

Ultrasound

A beam of ultrasound is directed at the femoral vein. The rate of venous outflow of the lower limb is detected by measuring the change in frequency of the reflected signal brought about by the Doppler effect. Squeezing the calf should augment the received signal if the vein is patent. This technique has similar uses, limitations and difficulties of interpretation to impedance phlebography. A negative test can be interpreted as demonstrating that the proximal veins are patent; a positive result should be confirmed by venography. Recently, two-dimensional Doppler imaging has been used to visualise proximal thrombi, but this technique is still under investigation.

Thermography

This simple non-invasive technique, uses an infra-red camera to detect variation in temperature in the limbs. In the presence of thrombus the increased temperature or the delayed cooling on exposure to air is increased. It is not sensitive to pelvic or inferior vena caval thromboses. False positive results will be seen in the presence of cellulitis, superficial thrombophlebitis and extensive varicose veins. The method is expensive and available only in a few centres.

PULMONARY EMBOLISM

The clinical presentation of pulmonary embolism is very varied and careful consideration must be given to the history and clinical findings. The course of investigations will depend upon interpretation of the acute presentation in the light of relevant past history. The diagnosis may be much harder to make with a high degree of certainty in an individual with prior cardiopulmonary disease.

History and examination

Dyspnoea

The patient usually appears unduly breathless or tachypnoeaic. Air hunger may be a prominent feature of major embolism. The degree of apprehension is often greater than the apparent physical disability and is a symptom worth taking the time to elicit. Occasionally patients may present with syncope.

Cough

This is usually dry, repetitive and nonproductive. Sometimes a pulmonary infarct becomes infected or an individual with a primary pneumonic lesion develops a pulmonary embolism and in both these instances the sputum may be purulent.

Chest pain

In an individual without previous chest disease the occurrence of pleuritic pain in the absence of a respiratory infection is strongly suggestive of a pulmonary infarct. It is a feature of small to moderate emboli and is not usually seen with large vessel occlusion. When this occurs with a massive embolus, central chest discomfort can occur, partly due to reduced coronary artery perfusion consequent on hypotension.

Haemoptysis

This is a relatively uncommon symptom but when it is present is strongly suggestive of an underlying pulmonary infarct, especially if accompanied by pleuritic pain.

Cyanosis

A major embolus will result in gross hypoxia and cyanosis. When present it indicates major embolism in the absence of other causes.

Chest signs

Lung fields will often be clear and it is rare to find a pleural rub. Bronchospasm is sometimes heard.

Cardiovascular signs

A tachycardia of over 100 beats/min is a common finding; a loud P_2 indicates pulmonary hypertension, and S_3 and S_4 are features of right ventricular strain. A raised jugular venous pressure is strong evidence favouring a diagnosis in the absence of any other obvious cause.

Investigations

The most appropriate investigations depend on the presentation. If the symptoms and signs are suggestive of a small infarct, then it may be appropriate to expeditiously arrange the necessary tests prior to anticoagulation. If, however, the patient presents with classical features of a major pulmonary embolus, then in the absence of contra-indications immediate heparin therapy may be appropriate.

Chest X-ray

This will often be normal but features of consolidation, effusion or infiltration may be present. Elevation of a hemidiaphragm may be seen.

ECG

Non-specific changes are quite common with atrial and ventricular ectopics and paroxysmal atrial tachycardia. Non-specific ST and T wave changes and right bundle branch block are common features. The S1 Q3 T3 triad is said to be observed in only 10% of cases.

Arterial blood gases

The degree of hypoxia is proportional to the size of the embolus. The pCO_2 is usually reduced.

Lung scan

A perfusion scan is usually the single most informative investigation, particularly in an individual with a normal chest X-ray. In at least 30% of patients the scan will be difficult to interpret but the presence of multiple defects, particularly if these appear segmental, is strongly suggestive of emboli. A normal scan virtually excludes embolism. In cases of doubt an accompanying ventilation scan may be helpful. When compared to the perfusion scan it will demonstrate areas of normal ventilation by reduced perfusion. Difficulties may be encountered in the presence of pre-existing cardiopulmonary disease; in such patients bilateral leg venography or pulmonary angiography should be considered.

Pulmonary angiography

This is the definitive investigation but is usually indicated only in patients thought to have had a major life-threatening embolus who may be candidates for pulmonary embolectomy, or in patients in whom a ventilation/perfusion scan has given equivocal results (Fig. 9.2). Injection of the radio-opaque dye into the main pulmonary artery will demonstrate intravascular filling defects or pulmonary artery cut off. It is also possible to measure pulmonary artery pressure and if this is greater than 40 mHg the dose of contrast may have to be reduced or selective views only obtained.

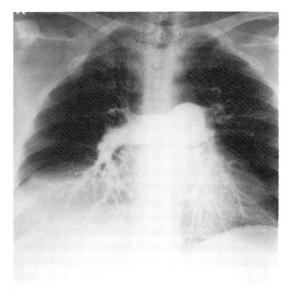

(a)

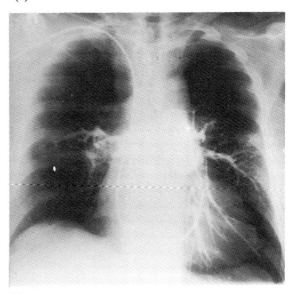

(b)

Fig. 9.2 Pulmonary angiograms illustrating emboli in left upper lobe vessels (**A**) and more major thrombo-embolism with large clot in the right pulmonary artery and small ones on the left side (**B**). (Reproduced by permission of Dr D. Readhead)

ARTERIAL THROMBOSIS

Occlusion of an artery can usually be diagnosed accurately from the history and examination. The following discussion is confined to thromboembolism in peripheral arteries; cerebrovascular accidents and myocardial infarction are not considered further.

History

Presentation

Symptoms of limb pain, pallor, coldness, paraesthesia and paralysis are the cardinal symptoms of an arterial occlusion. The extent of the symptoms is often a reliable guide as to the site of the occlusion.

Predisposing factors

Classical conditions associated with arterial thrombosis are listed in Table 9.1. If there is the possibility of a primary embolic event its origin should be considered. The majority arise in the heart, either from mural thrombi developing in akinetic regions (e.g. left atrium with atrial fibrillation, ventricular aneurysm) or occasionally from 'paradoxical' venous emboli traversing a patent foramen ovale.

Examination

Careful examination of peripheral pulses along with the extent of the pallor, coolness and cyanosis will give an indication as to the site of occlusion. If thrombosis has occurred at a previous stenosis, then collateral vessels may provide an adequate arterial supply, thus minimising the symptoms and signs. As evidence of underlying chronic arterial disease there may be a history of claudication, atrophic changes (e.g. loss of hair), or early gangrene in the toes or feet.

Investigation

This should be undertaken in conjunction with a vascular surgeon and radiologist. Arterial angiography will demonstrate precisely the site of thrombosis and also allow assessment of collateral vessels. If the angiography is undertaken shortly after the symptoms appear, and the thrombus is therefore relatively fresh, it may be possible to lyse it by infusion of a small local dose of streptokinase (repeated angiograms through the catheter will show lysis). If this is unsuccessful, then catheter embolectomy, arteriotomy or later reconstructive surgery may be appropriate.

Red cell disorders

10. Macrocytic anaemias

R. D. Hutton

Erythrocytes are described as macrocytic when their mean corpuscular volume (MCV) is raised; this may, or may not, be associated with anaemia. The causes of macrocytosis are listed in Table 10.1. The MCV, as derived from an automated blood counter, may truly reflect a macrocytosis but it may conceal a subpopulation of macrocytic cells (Fig. 10.1).

As the developing erythroblast matures, each cell division results in daughter cells smaller than the mother cell. Classically Stohlman has hypothesised that macrocytosis and microcytosis are related to an imbalance between nuclear and cytoplasmic maturation. He suggested that the cessation of nuclear division results from

the intracellular haemoglobin concentration reaching a critical level. If either nuclear maturation is delayed (due to a defect in DNA synthesis) or the cytoplasmic maturation is accelerated (increased erythropoietin drive), then the cells will reach their critical haemoglobin concentration earlier and hence undergo fewer divisions resulting in macrocytic cells (Fig. 10.2).

The term 'megaloblastic' refers to specific morphological changes seen in the erythroblasts in severe B_{12}/folate deficiency (Plate I) and in some other conditions (Table 10.1). As well as being abnormally large,

Table 10.1 Conditions that may result in macrocytosis

B_{12}/folate deficiency
Cytotoxic drugs
Myelodysplasia
Myeloid leukaemia
Congenital dyserythropoietic syndromes
Orotic aciduria
Lesch-Nyhan syndrome
Other vitamin deficiencies
Other enzyme deficiencies

Liver disease
Alcohol
Reticulocytosis
Hypoplastic anaemia
Marrow replacement syndromes
Hypothyroidism

Table 10.2 Clinical situations associated with B_{12}/folate deficiency, $^*B_{12}$ deficiency only

Megaloblastic anaemia
Bowel disturbance
General debility
Weight loss
Fever
Infertility*
Neuropathy*
Dementia*

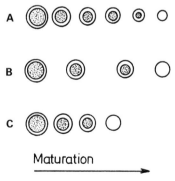

Maturation

Fig. 10.2 Schematic representation of erythroblast maturation. (**A**) Normal reduction in cell size with each division produces normocytes. (**B**) Megaloblastosis. Nuclear division is delayed but cytoplasmic maturation is normal producing macrocytes. (**C**) Increased erythropoietin drive. Nuclear division is normal but cytoplasmic maturation is enhanced leading to skipped divisions and macrocytes.

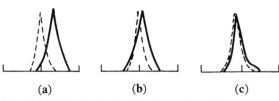

(a)   (b)   (c)

Fig. 10.1 Red cell size distribution graphs; with macrocytosis (**a**); normal MCV but concealing a macrocytosis due to high red cell distribution width (**b**); and normal MCV concealing a subpopulation of macrocytic cells (**c**); (normal size distribution).

the nucleus of the megaloblast has an open, finely stippled chromatin pattern. There is also a dissociation between the nuclear and cytoplasmic maturation such that cells that are well haemoglobinised may retain early nuclear features. With the introduction of modern blood cell counters increasing numbers of patients are found with macrocytosis at a stage of their condition when the classical features of megaloblastosis are not yet fully developed. The term megaloblastoid is sometimes used where there are features, but not classical ones, of megaloblastosis and on occasions to describe megaloblastic changes that are refractory to B_{12}/folate therapy.

PATHOPHYSIOLOGY OF B_{12} AND FOLATE METABOLISM

The biochemical lesion that produces the haematological abnormalities seen in both B_{12} and folate deficiency is a lack of 5,10-methylenetetrahydrofolate. This is required for the conversion of deoxyuridylate to deoxythymidylate, a rate limiting step in DNA synthesis. Deficiencies of 5,10-methylenetetrahydrofolate may arise from different causes, some of which are illustrated in Fig. 10.3.

The exact mechanism by which B_{12} deficiency leads to a lack of 5,10-methylenetetrahydrofolate is still not entirely clear. It is certainly not entirely due to a failure to demethylate methyl-tetrahydrofolate but it may be due to a deficiency of methionine which causes a deficiency of active formate. The latter is required for efficient polyglutamate formation and it is the polyglutamate form of folate which is required for many of the biochemical reactions involving folate.

Drugs causing megaloblastic change by interfering with the conversion of dihydrofolate to tetrahydrofolate include methotrexate, trimethoprim, triamterene and pyrimethamine.

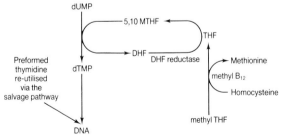

Fig. 10.3 B_{12}/folate pathways involved in thymidine synthesis.

  dUMP = deoxyuridine monophosphate
  dTMP = deoxythimidine monophosphate
  DHF = dihydrofolate
  THF = tetrahydrofolate
  5,10-MTHF = 5,10-methylenetetrahydrofolate

B_{12} is also required for the isomerisation of methylmalonyl CoA to succinyl CoA which explains the appearance of methylmalonic aciduria in B_{12} deficiency. The biochemical abnormality that results in the neurological damage seen in the absence of normal levels of active B_{12} largely remains unexplained.

Folate participates in various forms in a large number of biochemical reactions, many of which require the transfer of single carbon units from one compound to another as in the methylation of deoxyuridylate to deoxythymidylate. Other important pathways in which folates participate are purine synthesis, amino acid interconversion and formate activation.

OTHER BIOCHEMICAL ABNORMALITIES RESULTING IN MEGALOBLASTIC CHANGE

Many drugs are chosen to interfere specifically with DNA synthesis (antimetabolites) along pathways not involving folate. Examples of these are cytarabine, fluorouracil, mercaptopurine, thioguanine and azathioprine. These induce dyserythropoietic changes in developing red cell precursors which resemble megaloblastic change.

Other drugs interfere non-specifically, or by poorly defined mechanisms, with DNA replication but again may result in similar appearances to those seen in B_{12}/folate deficiency. These include alkylating agents (cylophosphamide, melphalan, mustine, etc.) and hydroxyurea.

There are rare congenital deficiencies that result in abnormalities of DNA synthesis independent of folate pathways. For example orotic aciduria (deficiency of orotidylic pyrophosphorylase and orotidylic decarboxylase) results in a deficiency of uridine, leading to megaloblastic anaemia and mental retardation, and the Lesch-Nyhan syndrome (hypoxanthine-phosphoribosyl transfere deficiency) leads to gout, self-mutilation and megaloblastic anaemia.

Presentation of macrocytosis

Since the advent of automated blood cell counters most cases of macrocytosis are picked up by chance. The fact that the individual may not be anaemic or have relevant symptoms is irrelevant to further investigation and diagnosis. It is obviously preferable to diagnose a condition such as B_{12} deficiency while it is symptomless rather than wait for the patient to re-present with severe life-threatening anaemia or irreversible neurological damage. The irrelevancy to the final diagnosis of the haemoglobin concentration is clearly shown in Fig. 10.4.

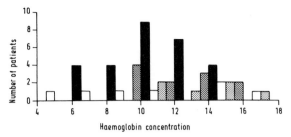

Fig. 10.4 Distribution of the haemoglobin concentration in 100 patients with macrocytosis. Folate deficiency ■ , B_{12} deficiency □, ethanol related ▨ , other causes ◩ .

Often, regardless of the underlying pathological process leading to macrocytosis, a patient will present purely with symptoms related to anaemia. In such a case the presenting features will be as described in Chapter 1. B_{12} and folate deficiency, however, affects all dividing cells and additionally B_{12} deficiency may result in neurological complications.

Investigation of the patient with macrocytosis

It is vital that B_{12}/folate deficiency is excluded in all cases of macrocytosis. A scheme for investigation is shown in Fig. 10.5. The exact division between 'urgent' and 'non-urgent' cases and the investigations performed will, to some extent, depend upon local circumstances. Urgent cases will include those which require some action to be taken before the results of the B_{12}/folate

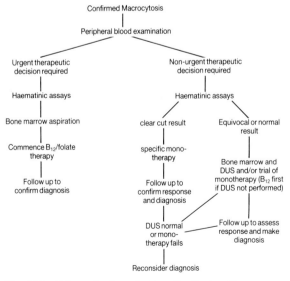

Fig. 10.5 Scheme for investigation of patients with macrocytosis. DUS = deoxyuridine suppression test

assays are available, for instance patients with severe symptomatology related to their anaemia or patients who require urgent surgery. Conversely, non-urgent cases are those who are not at any great risk from waiting for the results of their assays.

A bone marrow aspirate will allow a quick diagnosis of megaloblastic change to be made. It may also reveal any other underlying marrow pathology which may cause a macrocytosis, e.g. myelodysplasia.

Diagnosis of B_{12} and folate deficiency

Blood film appearances

Classically in B_{12}/folate deficiency the FBC will show a raised MCV and MCH, anaemia and possibly a leukopenia and thrombocytopenia. In addition a blood film will reveal macrocytic erythrocytes and hypersegmented neutrophils. None of these features is unique to B_{12}/folate deficiency and may be found in any condition which causes abnormalities in DNA synthesis. These features are also dependent on the degree of anaemia, such that in a non-anaemic patient the only blood film abnormalities may be a uniform macrocytosis with hypersegmented neutrophils (right shift). Where there is co-existing iron deficiency or another condition that produces microcytosis, apart from occasional larger cells the only features suggesting the possibility of a DNA synthetic defect may well be hypersegmented neutrophils (which can themselves be seen in severe iron deficiency) with possibly a leukopenia and/or thrombocytopenia. In acute folate deficiency, developing in an acutely ill patient, the only changes may be rapidly progressive cytopenias.

Bone marrow appearances

As with the peripheral blood, the abnormalities in the red cell series become more marked with increasing anaemia and the classical appearances of megaloblastosis may be masked by conditions that normally tend to produce microcytosis. In severe cases there is a marked erythroblastic hyperplasia with a preponderance of early forms. Megaloblasts (Plate 1) show a finely speckled chromatin pattern and frequently there are other abnormalities of DNA replication such as multiple Howell-Jolly bodies and failed divisions. Mitoses are frequent and often abnormal. Cytoplasmic maturation is relatively unaffected, so that cells may be well haemoglobinised but retain early nuclear features. Pathological sideroblasts are common, including occasional ring forms. Macrophage iron is usually increased in proportion to the degree of anaemia.

Nuclear abnormalities are present in all the developing cells and are possibly best seen in the metamyelocytes, where giant forms may precede other more overt marrow changes. Megakaryocyte nuclei are frequently hypersegmented with widely separated lobes.

B_{12}/folate assays

The first assays for measuring serum B_{12} were based on the growth requirement for this vitamin by certain microbiological organisms. These have been replaced by tests that utilise intrinsic factor as the binding protein and these assays give results similar to the original biological assays.

Occasionally a serum B_{12} assay will give a misleading result. Whichever methodology is used there is still a fundamental problem with B_{12} assays (Table 10.3 and Fig. 10.6). An assay for B_{12} not only measures the physiologically active B_{12} which is bound to transcobalamin II (TCII) and represents usually less than 10% of the measured serum B_{12}, but it also measures B_{12} bound to TCI and TCIII. These latter proteins are largely derived from myeloid cells and have no obvious physiological role. The difficulties that this causes are uncommon but very important. They are highlighted by the fact that in TCII deficiency there is a life-threatening physiological lack of B_{12} but the serum levels are usually normal due to B_{12} bound to TCI and III, whereas in congenital deficiency of these, the serum B_{12} is extremely low but there is no evidence of megaloblas-

Fig. 10.6 Possible results of B_{12}/folate assays in normal subjects, patients with B_{12} deficiency, and patients with folate deficiency.

N	=	usually normal
n	=	sometimes normal
↑	=	usually increased
↟	=	sometimes increased
↓	=	usually decreased
↡	=	sometimes decreased

For explanation see text and Table 10.3

tic change. Another area of importance is where the myeloid mass is increased, particularly in myeloproliferative disorders, but also in chronic infection or inflammation, where an increased basal level of B_{12} bound to TCI and TCIII may mask a deficiency of the physiologically important TCII B_{12}. What is really required is a simple assay that only measures TCII B_{12}.

Even accepting these uncommon situations, a low serum B_{12} does not necessarily mean physiological deficiency of the vitamin. In many clinical situations folate deficiency is the commonest cause of a low B_{12} concentration. The exact mechanism for this is uncertain but the levels return to normal within days of commencing folate therapy. Levels may also be low in vegans, in the latter stages of normal pregnancies, in severe iron deficiency, post-partial gastrectomy and in other situations. Because of this it is essential that further tests are performed before labelling a patient as B_{12}-deficient requiring life-long supplements.

Assays of folate have progressed in a similar way to those for B_{12}. The original assays were microbiological but have now been almost entirely replaced by radio-isotope assays. The serum level reflects recent folate status and may be low before physiological folate deficiency has developed; conversely, it will rise quickly if the factors that led to folate deficiency are reversed. For example, a patient admitted to hospital with dietary folate deficiency may have resumed a folate-rich diet before assays are taken and hence the levels may be normal. The red cell levels, however, reflect long-term folate status and so will be normal in acute folate deficiency but will remain abnormal even some time

Table 10.3 Reasons for misleading assay results

False* low serum B_{12}	Folate deficiency Pregnancy Vegan Atrophic gastritis Deficiency of TCI/TCIII
False high serum B_{12}	Myeloproliferative disease Chronic inflammatory/infective disorder (increased myeloid mass) TCII deficiency
False low serum folate	Recent intake of ethanol Recent lack of intake B_{12} deficiency
False high serum folate	Recent intake of folates Rare enzyme deficiencies
False low red cell folate	B_{12} deficiency
False high red cell folate	Blood transfusion Reticulocytosis

*NB 'False' is used in the sense of being clinically misleading.

after therapy has been instituted or the precipitating events reversed.

As the circulating haemoglobin concentration decreases, so the amount of storage iron increases. This results in high levels of serum iron and high transferrin saturations. The serum ferritin level increases in proportion to the fall in haemoglobin. Due to ineffective erythropoiesis there is an increase in circulating bilirubin levels (giving the classic lemon yellow tinge) and also in the serum levels of some intracellular enzymes, in particular lactate dehydrogenase. The haemoglobin released as a consequence of defective erythropoiesis reduces the serum levels of haptoglobins and will result in other tests for intravascular haemolysis being positive.

B_{12} DEFICIENCY

It is difficult to know precisely how commonly B_{12} deficiency occurs. Some cases thought to be B_{12} deficiency are almost certainly misdiagnosed cases of folate deficiency as, particularly in elderly or very ill patients, an absolute diagnosis is not made. There also appears to be marked geographical variation, although for the United Kingdom it is thought that the average incidence is about 0.1% of the population.

Sources of B_{12}

B_{12} is derived originally from microbiological sources as it cannot be synthesised by higher plants or animals. It becomes concentrated in animals and it is from this source that most people derive what they require (levels are particularly high in liver and kidney). An average mixed diet contains 5–30 μg per day and the physiological requirement is 1–3 μg daily. Body stores are relatively large, about 2–5 mg. Contaminating microorganisms provide small amounts of B_{12} from plant and water sources. This source is most important for vegans and if only 'clean' fruit and vegetables and 'purified' water are taken, then B_{12} deficiency is likely to occur.

It may be expected from the level of stores and the daily requirements of vitamin B_{12} that it would be very many years before deficiency occurred even if there was a total failure of supply or absorption. There is, however, an enterohepatic circulation of around 5 μg a day which will be lost to the body if there is a failure in absorption. Hence B_{12} deficiency will occur much quicker if there is a failure of absorption (e.g. following total gastrectomy) than if there is a change in intake. Even so, it still usually takes several years before B_{12} deficiency does occur.

Absorption of B_{12}

Dietary B_{12} is absorbed by an active mechanism in the terminal ileum only after it has combined with intrinsic factor (IF), a specific binding protein produced by the parietal cells of the stomach. In the absence of IF severe malabsorption of B_{12} will occur that can only be overcome if milligram amounts are taken by mouth, so ensuring that enough is absorbed by passive diffusion. For optimum absorption of B_{12}, normal gastric and pancreatic function are required in order to make dietary B_{12} maximally available to IF. Normal pancreatic function is also required to provide an alkaline environment for maximal absorption in the ileum.

A list of causes of B_{12} malabsorption is shown in Table 10.4 and discussed below. In all cases if clinical deficiency is present this is initially managed with B_{12} injections and where possible by treating the underlying condition. Where the latter cannot be done life-long parenteral therapy will be required.

Lack of intrinsic factor

Adult and childhood pernicious anaemia are discussed more fully below. IF may be deficient following gastric resection, the deficiency being proportional to the mass of parietal cells resected. Total gastrectomy will of course result in total IF deficiency, whereas the incidence of clinically significant malabsorption following partial gastrectomy depends on the site and size of the resection and increases with the length of time since the resection. Atrophic gastritis (sometimes secondary to severe iron deficiency) also reduces IF production but is seldom severe enough to result in clinical deficiency.

Table 10.4   Causes of B_{12} malabsorption

Gastric causes	Congenital abnormality of IF
	Pernicious anaemia
	Gastrectomy
	Atrophic gastritis
Intestinal causes	Bacterial overgrowth
	Ileal resection
	Ileal disease
	Tropical sprue
	Coeliac disease
	Imerslund–Gräsbeck disease
	Fish tapeworm
	Severe pancreatitis
	Zollinger–Ellison syndrome
	B_{12}/folate deficiency
	Certain drugs including ethanol

Ileal disease

Disease or resection affecting several feet of the terminal ileum will result in B_{12} malabsorption. Diseases that can affect the absorption of B_{12} in the ileum include Crohn's disease, tropical sprue, severe coeliac disease and radiation damage. Both B_{12} deficiency and folate deficiency also cause ileal malabsorption of B_{12} which can take several weeks to return to normal following therapy. Imerslund-Gräsbeck syndrome is a recessive autosomally inherited disorder due to a specific ileal defect in B_{12} absorption and/or transport. It is usually associated with a benign non-progressive proteinuria and presents usually within the first few years of life, although some cases have presented as late as the second decade.

Bacterial overgrowth

The small bowel is usually relatively free from bacteria but in some conditions (such as small bowel diverticulosis, stricture, blind loop, fistula with the large bowel, etc.) large numbers may be present. The bacteria utilise available B_{12} resulting in a deficit of the vitamin for absorption. Symptoms of the underlying condition often predominate and the nature of the condition can be shown by an improvement in B_{12} absorption following a course of a broad spectrum antibiotic.

Infestation with the fish tapeworm

The parasite (*Diphyllobothrium latum*) competes for available B_{12} and occasionally can lead to clinical deficiency. It is common where fish is eaten raw or under-cooked.

Acid pH in the ileum

As the ileal pH falls further below 6, the ileal uptake of IF-B_{12} complex is reduced. Malabsorption secondary to this cause can be demonstrated in severe pancreatic disease or resection, due to the failure of bicarbonate production, or secondary to excessive acid production in the Zollinger-Ellison syndrome. Slow-release potassium chloride may cause sufficient acidification of the ileal contents to incur malabsorption. It may also occur in chronic biochemical acidotic states. Rarely is it severe enough to cause clinical deficiency.

Drugs

Many drugs, including ethanol, neomycin, colchicine and metformin, have been shown to interfere with B_{12} absorption but again clinical deficiency states secondary to them are uncommon.

Adult pernicious anaemia

Anaemia is not required to make the diagnosis of pernicious anaemia (PA), a fact which can cause confusion. It is the commonest cause of physiological B_{12} deficiency.

This is an autoimmune disorder that results in the immune destruction of parietal cells mainly through the cellular arm of the immune system. It is the parietal cells that produce acid and intrinsic factor and so their destruction results in diminution in the production of both. There is also immune destruction of secreted intrinsic factor by antibodies appearing in the gastric juice.

Various other autoimmune disorders are frequently associated and include thyroid disease, premature greying of the hair, vitiligo, hypoparathyroidism and Addison's disease. These may be observed in the patient with PA or in close relatives. It occurs more commonly in those who have selective IgA deficiency or complete hypogammaglobulinaemia. It is also more common in people with blood group A and those with blue eyes.

Clinical presentation

This is very variable, particularly because since the introduction of modern automated blood cell counters it is an increasingly chance diagnosis made during the investigation of a high MCV. It is commoner in the elderly with a peak incidence in the sixth decade of life. Presentation may occur through any of the problems listed in Table 10.2 but is commonest with anaemia, sometimes of marked severity. It is important to realise, however, that such complications as neurological problems or infertility may be completely dissociated from anaemia, although macrocytosis is usually present.

Investigation

A scheme for investigation is shown in Fig. 10.7. Many people do not consider it essential to make a diagnosis of PA in all cases of apparent B_{12} deficiency – particularly in the elderly. However, it is possible to present a strong case for making a precise diagnosis, firstly on economic grounds, as it has been shown that many patients receive life-long supplements of B_{12} unnecessarily at considerable expense, and secondly on the grounds that there may be another diagnosis which has been missed and which requires separate investigation and treatment.

A low serum assay result does not in itself mean the subject has B_{12} deficiency and similarly a normal or even a high result does not exclude it (see section on B_{12}/folate assays). However, where the result of assays, or therapeutic trial suggests such a deficiency, further in-

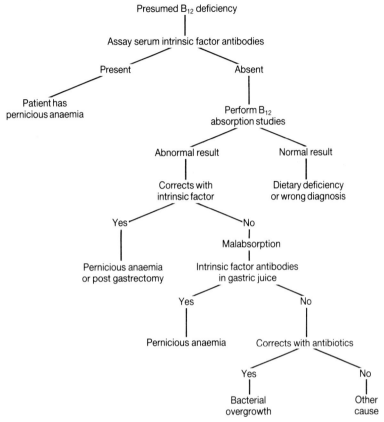

Fig. 10.7 Scheme for the diagnosis of pernicious anaemia.

vestigations are required to confirm or refute the diagnosis.

A logical approach to the diagnosis is firstly to look for the presence of intrinsic factor antibodies in the serum. These are present in about half the patients and together with evidence of B_{12} deficiency virtually guarantee the diagnosis, making further investigation unnecessary. If the result is negative, it is usual to proceed to a measure of B_{12} absorption by a modified form of Schilling test. This should, however, be delayed until the deficiency has been adequately treated, as both B_{12} and folate deficiency cause malabsorption of B_{12} due to their effects on the dividing enterocytes. The original version relied upon the collection of urine which is extremely unreliable and has now been modified to include serum measurements, liver counting or whole body retention.

In the Schilling test or its modifications, radioactively labelled B_{12} is administered by mouth and the amount absorbed measured. The test may be repeated with labelled B_{12} bound to IF. In pernicious anaemia there is malabsorption of the unbound B_{12} and normal absorption of the B_{12}-IF complex. Similar results will of

course be given if there is a deficiency of IF for other reasons, so results can only be suggestive and not diagnostic. If malabsorption is not improved by the addition of IF, this does not exclude the diagnosis as in some cases high levels of precipitating antibodies are present which destroy both IF and the IF-B_{12} complex. Improvement in absorption following a course of broad-spectrum antibiotics is suggestive of bacterial overgrowth in the small bowel.

Other diagnostic tests

Tests of gastric function used to be almost routine in the investigation of patients with possible PA but despite their usefulness are now seldom performed. Gastric juice is collected after a maximal stimulus for acid production has been given. The aspirate should be tested for maximal acidity and for the presence of IF and IF antibody. This antibody is present in about 80% of patients and its presence can be considered as diagnostic. Normal amounts of IF or hydrochloric acid will discount a diagnosis of adult PA. In association with the achlorhydria there is usually a raised level of serum gastrin.

Tests for serum parietal cell antibodies are occasionally performed but can only provide supporting evidence. Some 90% of people with PA have these in their blood but they are also present in many people, particularly the elderly, with no other evidence of the condition.

It is claimed that tests of cellular immunity against IF have a very high rate of positivity but they are not generally available.

Steroid therapy and other therapies used in the management of autoimmune diseases may produce a remission by modifying the underlying autoimmune mechanisms.

Therapeutic trial of B$_{12}$. In some cases the diagnosis may still remain in doubt, in which case administering daily doses of 2 μg of B$_{12}$ either intramuscularly or intravenously will, if leading to a full haematological response, support the diagnosis of B$_{12}$ deficiency. It does not, however, make a diagnosis of PA and can also be misleading if there are other changes brought about by the patient being under scrutiny, i.e. their diet may improve or their alcohol intake decrease!

Childhood pernicious anaemia

There are really two separate diseases. The first is merely an early onset form of adult pernicious anaemia and is often accompanied by other autoimmune conditions. The considerations for diagnosis are as above. The second is due to abnormalities of the genes controlling the production of IF which are normally inherited as autosomal recessive disorders. They may result in a qualitive and/or a quantitative defect in IF production. Very severe cases will present within the first year of life but some variants have not presented until much later. Gastric acid production is normal and there are no associated autoimmune phenomena. Studies of gastric juice may show absent or reduced IF. Sometimes it is normally reactive immunologically but can be shown to be defective functionally. B$_{12}$ absorption studies show defective absorption corrected by ingestion of normal intrinsic factor.

Other abnormalities resulting in functional B$_{12}$ deficiency

Transcobalamin II deficiency has been discussed under B$_{12}$/folate assays. This is a rare autosomal recessive disorder presenting in infancy, usually with severe megaloblastosis and failure to thrive. Serum B$_{12}$ levels are usually normal and should not prevent a therapeutic trial of high dose intramuscular or intravenous B$_{12}$. A

diagnosis can be made by fractionation of the different transcobalamins by physical methods. What is not generally recognised is that carriers for this condition, because they only have half the normal amounts of TCII, may become physiologically B$_{12}$ deficient while their total serum levels remain within the normal reference range.

There are several rare inherited disorders of B$_{12}$ utilisation. Defective synthesis of adenosyl B$_{12}$ results in B$_{12}$ responsive methylmalonic aciduria without megaloblastosis, whereas defective synthesis of methyl B$_{12}$ results in homocystinuria and megaloblastosis. Conditions also exist where the production of both adenosyl and methyl B$_{12}$ are defective, resulting in both homocystinuria and methylmalonic aciduria with megaloblastosis. The results of B$_{12}$ therapy have been variable.

Nitrous oxide irreversibly damages B$_{12}$. Chronic exposure will lead to neuropathy and megaloblastosis. Even short term exposure during surgery can be shown to have an effect on otherwise normal bone marrow by producing abnormalities in the deoxyuridine suppression test. It can be envisaged that in patients with already compromised B$_{12}$/folate status exposure to nitrous oxide may be the final straw leading to a breakdown in the marrow's ability to cope with the extra stress of surgery. For this reason macrocytosis should be investigated and treated prior to surgery.

Management of B$_{12}$ deficiency

Wherever there is a clinical suspicion of B$_{12}$ deficiency it is essential to give a trial of B$_{12}$ regardless of the other laboratory findings. Failure of response can only be determined after careful follow-up over a period of several months, particularly if the patient is non-anaemic.

Standard therapy for all cases of B$_{12}$ deficiency is by regular intramuscular injections of B$_{12}$, usually in the form of hydroxocobalamin in a 1 mg dose administered at 2- to 3-monthly intervals. Therapy may need to be repeated much more often in the inherited metabolic disorders of B$_{12}$ but there is no evidence to support the use of more frequent therapy when deficiency results from malabsorption or inadequate intake. In patients with inadequate dietary intake supplements may be given by mouth. Obviously if there is a treatable underlying condition this should be managed separately.

FOLATE DEFICIENCY

Folates appear in a wide variety of dietary forms, some of which are more readily available for absorption than others. A normal western diet provides some 600–800 μg a day, the richest sources being liver, yeast, some green vegetables, nuts and chocolate. It is present in most foods but is easily destroyed by cooking, particularly in large amounts of water and in an alkaline environment. Daily requirements vary considerably and are largely related to cell turnover. A healthy adult will need about 100 μg but this can increase severalfold if cellular turnover is increased by pregnancy, growth, infection, ineffective haemopoiesis or exfoliative conditions. Body stores are usually between 5 and 10 mg and hence are sufficient for only a few months.

Causes of folate deficiency (See Table 10.5)

Dietary deficiency

This is the commonest form seen in the UK and often results from consumption of 'convenience foods'. It is particularly common amongst the elderly, the socially deprived, alcohol abusers, the chronically sick, infants (particularly those given goats milk which is very low in folate and those born prematurely) and the psychiatrically disturbed. Careful dietary assessment and advice will often be required in suspected cases. Patients admitted to hospital may respond simply through their change in diet.

Table 10.5 Causes of folate deficiency

Dietary insufficiency
Malabsorption
Excess utilisation
Increased loss
Antifolate drugs
Ethanol abuse

Malabsorption of folate

Malabsorption is seen commonly in tropical sprue, coeliac disease and dermatitis herpetiformis. It is less common in Crohn's disease and in those who have had gastric or jejunal resections. It also occurs in lymphoproliferative conditions involving the upper small bowel and where the bowel wall is affected by oedema in severe congestive heart failure. There is a rare specific malabsorption of folate described. It is also described in association with the use of certain drugs including ethanol, anticonvulsants and oral contraceptives but often the evidence for the association is poor.

Increased demand

Physiological requirements are increased during periods of growth (especially common in premature infants), pregnancy and lactation. Requirements are increased in many pathological conditions in which there is increased cellular turnover, e.g. haemolytic anaemias, myeloproliferative conditions, dyshaemopoietic syndromes, malignant diseases, skin diseases associated with increased exfoliation, chronic inflammatory and infective disorders, and in rare metabolic conditions such as homocystinuria.

Increased losses

These occur in liver disease, congestive heart failure and renal dialysis.

Use of drugs with antifolate properties

Drugs such as methotrexate, trimethoprim and pyrimethamine are specifically designed to have antifolate activity. In the case of many drugs, however, these are unintended side effects and may occur through increased utilisation or direct interference in metabolic pathways. Such drugs include triamterene, many anticonvulsant drugs and ethanol. The use of cytotoxic drugs is coincidently often associated with folate deficiency through many mechanisms of which the associated anorexia is probably the most important.

Multiple aetiologic factors

Many cases of folate deficiency probably have multiple aetiologic factors. A careful consideration of the full history, examination and laboratory findings is required to assess their relative importance.

Clinical features

The clinical features of folate deficiency are those associated with any underlying pathology together with the effects on the haemopoietic system as previously described for B_{12} deficiency. Folate deficiency has not been definitely linked to neurological changes, although disturbances of mood are often improved following therapy. The progress of the haematological abnormalities is, however, often very much more rapid than that seen in B_{12} deficiency because so frequently the underlying condition increases the actual demand for the vitamin. In addition the underlying condition may itself be suppressing normal erythropoiesis so that the classical peripheral blood changes may be minimal or absent. Acute deficiency states may in fact present with a severely sick pancytopenic patient with no classical blood film features. Marrow changes may also not be so marked as they are in B_{12} deficiency, again due to the rapidity of onset.

Investigation

This generally follows the scheme illustrated in Fig. 10.5.

Management

Wherever possible the underlying problem should be reversed. Specific therapy is usually with folic acid by mouth, 5 mg daily being an adequate dose. Where oral therapy is not possible folate should be given intramuscularly or intravenously and if inhibition at the level of dihydrofolate reductase is suspected (e.g. following methotrexate), therapy should initially be with folinic acid. It is essential that in the very ill patient or where there are rapidly developing cytopenias therapy is not delayed. In patients with malignant disease therapy should not be withheld for fear of 'feeding the cancer'. Not only will the patient benefit symptomatically from treatment but in some cases specific treatment of the malignancy is only possible after blood counts have improved after giving folate. It is important in treatment regimes that depend upon the level of the blood count that treatment is not unnecessarily delayed because of the coincidental effects of folate deficiency.

In some cases regular prophylactic folate therapy is appropriate. It is usually given to women with multiple pregnancies and to patients with chronic disorders increasing basal requirements, such as anaemias with an ineffective or haemolytic component and myelofibrosis.

It is usual practice to give both B_{12} and folate to patients in whom B_{12} deficiency has not yet been excluded, both to avoid a delay in essential therapy and to prevent further deterioration in patients with neurological problems secondary to B_{12} deficiency states.

Rare metabolic abnormalities of folate metabolism

There are many, often isolated, case reports of patients with megaloblastic anaemia responsive to folic acid alone or folic acid in combination with B_{12}. There are frequently other associated abnormalities, particularly mental retardation. In most cases the metabolic abnormality has not been defined but in one case a deficiency of 5-methyltetrahydrofolate-transferase has been described.

BIBLIOGRAPHY

Chanarin I 1979 The megaloblastic anaemias, 2nd edn. Blackwell Scientific Publications, Oxford
Chanarin I, Deacon R, Lumb M, Muir M, Perry J 1985 Cobalamin-folate interrelations: a critical review. Blood 66: 479–489
Hoffbrand A V, Wickremasinghe R G 1982 Megaloblastic anaemia. Recent Advances in Haematology 3: 22–44

11. Haemolytic anaemias

D. S. Gillett   A. J. Bellingham

The term 'haemolysis' refers to an increased rate of red cell destruction with shortening of the red cell lifespan. The latter occurs not only in the classical haemolytic anaemias (Table 11.1) but also in conditions where there is also ineffective erythropoiesis, such as the megaloblastic anaemias and thalassemias, but it represents only a minor aspect of the clinical picture and these conditions are considered separately (see Chs. 10 and 12). The normal mean red cell life is 110–120 days after which destruction is effected by bone marrow and splenic macrophages. Any reduction in the mean cell life will lead to erythropoietin-induced erythroid hyperplasia with an increase in red cell production of up to ten times normal. Increased erythropoiesis will often compensate for the reduced red cell life and the haemoglobin remains normal. Anaemia occurs particularly if the onset of haemolysis is abrupt with no time for marrow compensation. It may also occur in severe chronic haemolysis when the mean cell life is very short and, rarely, when there is an associated decrease in haemoglobin oxygen affinity.

The mean cell life is affected by alterations in the red cell membrane and the molecular configuration of the haemoglobin. Abnormalities of either can decrease the deformability of the cell, which slows its passage between splenic macrophages increasing the risk of phagocytosis.

CLINICAL FEATURES OF HAEMOLYSIS

History

General features that may indicate the presence of haemolysis

Jaundice. This is generally mild and is often not noticed by the patient.

Symptoms of anaemia. The severity to some extent depends on the rate of onset of anaemia. The duration of the symptoms may give a clue as to whether the dis-

Table 11.1   Classification of haemolytic anaemias

Genetic disorders	

Membrane	Hereditary
	  Spherocytosis
	  Elliptocytosis
	  Pyropoikilocytosis
	  Stomatocytosis

Haemoglobin	Haemoglobinopathies, e.g. HbS Unstable haemoglobins Thalassaemias

Enzymes	Hexose monophosphate shunt
	  e.g. G6PD deficiency
	Embden – Meyerhof pathway
	  e.g. PK deficiency

Milieu	Abeta–lipoproteinaemia
Acquired disorders	
Immune	Isoimmune, e.g. haemolytic disease of the newborn Autoimmune, warm or cold antibody Drugs
Mechanical	March haemoglobinuria Burns Micro-angiopathic haemolytic anaemia Valve prostheses
Infections	Malaria *Cl. welchii* Bartonella
Toxins	Arsenic Copper
Dyserythropoietic	Megaloblastosis Paroxysmal nocturnal haemoglobinuria
Milieu	Liver disease Hypophosphataemia

order is of recent onset or is of long-standing duration, possibly congenital.

Urine. This is of normal colour (acholuric) but may darken on standing due to oxidation of urobilinogen. Heinz body haemolytic anaemia may give rise to dark urine. Haemoglobinuria may be observed with intravascular haemolysis.

Symptoms of cholelithiasis. Chronic haemolysis, as in hereditary spherocytosis, leads to the accumulation of pigment gallstones which may cause symptoms.

Splenic pain. This may occur if the spleen rapidly enlarges in size as a result of acute onset haemolysis or if the organ develops an infarct.

Recent infections. Particularly important are mycoplasma, cytomegalovirus, infectious mononucleosis and malaria.

Specific features which may suggest a cause of haemolysis

Family history. See Table 11.1

Age of onset of symptoms. Is there a history of neonatal or episodic jaundice such as may be observed in G6PD deficiency or hereditary spherocytosis?

Initiating factors. Do any particular drugs, infections or dietary constituents precipitate a haemolytic episode? Exposure to cold may precipitate haemolysis in paroxysmal cold haemoglobinuria or cold haemagglutinin disease. Jogging or marching may result in symptoms in march haemoglobinuria.

Geographical and racial origin. Enzymopathies, e.g. G6PD deficiency, thalassaemias and haemoglobinopathies originate, in many instances, in particular geographical locations.

Related disorders. Does the patient have an underlying systemic disorder, e.g. SLE, lymphoma or thymoma, that may be associated with a haemolytic anaemia.

Examination

General features indicating haemolysis

Jaundice and anaemia. Unless haemolysis is severe, neither pallor nor icterus may be observed but with markedly shortened erythrocyte lifespan the patient will usually be pale and jaundiced.

Splenomegaly. The spleen enlarges to a moderate degree in response to haemolysis. The presence of a very large spleen indicates the presence of a predisposing disorder, e.g. lymphoma.

Signs of systemic disease. A full general medical examination is essential to determine whether there is any evidence of a disease or lesion that might predispose to haemolysis, e.g. prosthetic heart valve infection, collagenosis or lymphoma.

Cholelithiasis. This will be asymptomatic unless cholecystitis or obstruction supervenes.

Leg ulcers. These are observed on the legs in patients with intrinsic red cell disorders, e.g. sickle cell disease.

Skeletal hypertrophy. Enlargement of the maxillary bones and frontal bossing may be observed in some severe congenital haemolytic anaemias and thalassaemias.

Laboratory investigations

The investigation of a haemolytic anaemia requires assessment of the severity of the haemolytic process and identification of the cause.

Recognition of haemolysis

a. Detection of increased erythrocyte breakdown
   i.   Unconjugated bilirubinaemia – up to about 50 μmol/L
   ii. Urobilinogen excretion in urine increased – dip stick test
   iii. Haptoglobins decreased – not a very good test as they are acute phase reactants
   iv. Lactate dehydrogenase increased – occasionally helpful but many other causes
   v. ^{51}Cr red cell survival – quantitate rate and site of destruction.

b. Detection of increased erythrocyte production
   i.   Reticulocytosis – stain with new methylene blue
   ii. Blood film may reveal polychromasia and nucleated red blood cells
   iii. Erythroid hyperplasia in bone marrow aspirate
   iv. Radiological changes in congenital haemolytic anaemias – hair on end appearance in skull X-ray.

c. Features specific to intravascular haemolysis
   i.   Haemoglobinaemia when haptoglobins and haemopexins exhausted
   ii. Methaemoglobinaemia – detected by Schumm's test
   iii. Haemoglobinuria
   iv. Haemosiderinuria – iron shed by tubular cells.

Recognition of cause of haemolysis

a. Peripheral blood film – see Table 11.2
b. Miscellaneous investigations – see Fig. 11.1

The following groups of tests should be undertaken to confirm a suspected disorder.
   i.   Immune haemolysis – direct and indirect antiglobulin test (Coomb's test) with antibody specificity

ii. Haemoglobinopathy
   a. sickle cell disorder – haemoglobin solubility test and electrophoresis
   b. Unstable haemoglobin – Heinz body preparation along with isopropanol and heat stability tests
   c. Abnormal oxygen dissociation – P_{50}
iii. Enzyme defect – measure enzyme activity and kinetics along with glycolytic pathway intermediates
iv. Membrane defects – measure osmotic fragility, sucrose lysis and Ham's test.

Table 11.2 Red cell morphology in haemolytic anaemias

	Possible diagnosis
Sickle cells	Sickling disorders
Elliptocytes	Hereditary elliptocytosis
Parasites	Malaria
	Bartonella
Spherocytes	Hereditary spherocytosis
	Autoimmune haemolytic anaemia
	Post-splenectomy
	ABO haemolytic disease of newborn
	Burns
Target cells	Hb SC
	Liver disease
Bitten out cells	G6PD deficiency
Prickle cells	PK deficiency
Acanthocytes	Abeta-lipoproteinaemia
Cold agglutinins	Chronic cold agglutinin disease
RBC fragments	Micro-angiopathic haemolytic anaemia

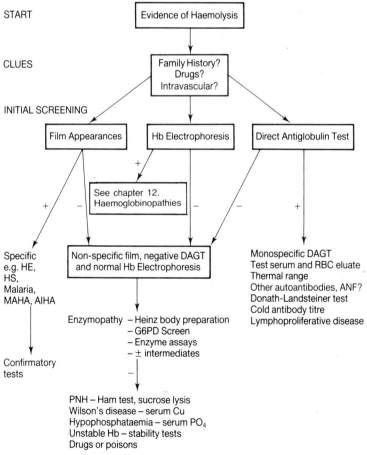

Fig. 11.1 Investigation of haemolysis (DAGT, Direct antiglobulin test; AIHA, Autoimmune haemolytic anaemia; MAHA, Microangiopathic haemolytic anaemia)

CONGENITAL HAEMOLYTIC ANAEMIAS

MEMBRANE DISORDERS

Hereditary spherocytosis

Hereditary spherocytosis (HS) is the commonest congenital haemolytic anaemia in northern Europeans. Inheritance is by autosomal dominant transmission but in about 25% of cases there are no affected family members and these have presumably arisen through new mutation or by variable penetrance. The exact nature of the red cell defect in HS is uncertain and may vary from one kindred to another. There is usually a subnormal level of spectrin in the membrane cytoskeleton and a high rate of cation flux with increased ATP utilisation.

There is considerable variability in the clinical expression of the disease and also in the demonstrable laboratory findings. One quarter of those with the disease have little or no evidence of haemolysis or splenomegaly. A haemolytic episode may, however, be initiated by infections or by pregnancy. Two thirds are chronically anaemic with variable jaundice and splenomegaly and the condition may be detected postnatally because of prolonged neonatal jaundice. Ultrasound examination will usually reveal modest splenomegaly and often the premature development of biliary calculi resulting from increased bilirubin excretion. Rarely patients are encountered with severe transfusion-dependent anaemia.

Diagnosis

The spherocytes have lost surface area relative to volume and characteristically show decreased ability to withstand osmotic stress. Not all the cells are spheres, so the osmotic fragility curve may just show a 'tail' where osmotic lysis is increased (Fig. 11.2). The test may be made more sensitive by the pre-incubation of red cells at 37°C for 24 hours. The antiglobulin test is negative and reticulocytes generally 5–25%. The MCHC is often slightly raised. The autohaemolysis test gives a type I result. It is essential to perform family studies.

Treatment

Splenectomy should be performed in most cases. This practically returns the red cell survival to normal by preventing trapping of spherocytes by splenic macrophages. Splenectomy generally abolishes aplastic or haemolytic episodes, reduces the risk of pigment gallstones and will often ameliorate chronic leg ulceration. It should if possible be postponed until adolescence because of the increased risk of overwhelming post-splenectomy infec-

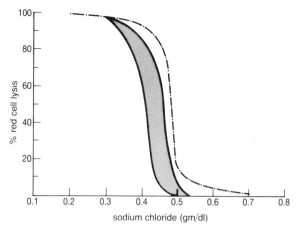

Fig. 11.2 Osmotic fragility test. Graph of red cell lysis versus Na Cl concentration. Hatched area = normal range. Dotted line diagnostic of hereditary spherocytosis. Note 'tail'.

tion in children. Folate supplements may be required as in any chronic haemolytic state.

Hereditary elliptocytosis

Hereditary elliptocytosis (HE) is a heterogeneous group of disorders in terms of clinical expression, red cell morphology and molecular pathology. Both common, benign HE and haemolytic HE are transmitted by a dominant gene with variable expression within families and in some cases there is linkage with the genes determining Rh blood group. Common or benign HE is little more than a morphological curiosity with variable red cell shape (from ovalocytes to rods) and osmotic fragility. In haemolytic HE a few red cell fragments and spherocytes are often seen and in infants these appearances may be marked with pyknocytosis. The management of HE is the same as for HS but splenectomy is rarely necessary.

Hereditary stomatocytosis

Erythrocytes with slit-like central pallor occur in a variety of haematological disorders and their significance is uncertain. In hereditary stomatocytosis, a dominantly transmitted disorder, 10–40% of cells show such slits and there may be mild haemolysis. The red cell cation content can be shown to be abnormal.

Hereditary pyropoikilocytosis

In this rare disorder erythrocytes fragment in vitro at a lower temperature than normal. The blood film shows marked pyknocytosis and fragmentation of red cells.

DEFECTS OF RED CELL METABOLISM

Such a defect should be suspected in any case of non-spherocytic haemolytic anaemia where there is no obvious acquired cause. Most general haematology laboratories do not have the facilities for the biochemical assays of all the enzymes, reaction products and intermediates but in practice the commonest enzymopathy is glucose-6-phosphate dehydrogenase (G6PD) deficiency. Simple screening tests are available for this and for pyruvate kinase deficiency.

Normal red cell metabolism

This is relatively simple in that glucose is the only substrate and is used to provide energy in the form of ATP via the Embden-Meyerhof (glycolytic) pathway (EMP) (Fig. 11.3). The Krebs cycle is active only in reticulocytes. There are many enzymes in the mature erythrocyte but only 25 are required for the EMP and pentose phosphate pathways (PPP) and their associated reactions. There is great variation in the specific activity of the enzymes but hexokinase shows the least and therefore this step is rate limiting. The reactions involving hexokinase, phosphofructokinase and pyruvate kinase are essentially irreversible and, together with the concentrations of the adenine nucleotides, they regulate the EMP.

The red cell needs ATP to maintain water and cation balance, achieved through a membrane bound Na^+ and K^+ dependent ATPase. There is also a similar Ca^+, Mg^+ ATPase which removes calcium ions against a concentration gradient utilising ATP. Cation and water homeostasis are essential to maintain red cell size, shape and flexibility and between 10 and 20% of the energy produced by glycolysis is required for the sodium pump. The EMP, via its Rapoport-Luebering shuttle, also maintains a high concentration of 2,3-diphosphoglycerate (2,3-DPG) which interacts with haemoglobin and regulates oxygen affinity. Hypoxia stimulates 2,3-DPG production with a resultant shift to the right of the oxygen dissociation curve, so enhancing tissue oxygen release.

NADH and NADPH are produced by the EMP and PPP respectively and play important roles in maintaining the status quo within the erythrocyte by preventing Hb oxidation. NADH is the cofactor for NADH methaemoglobin reductase which reconverts methaemoglobin to haemoglobin. Without it methaemoglobin would accumulate at a rate of 3% per day. NADPH is required to maintain glutathione (GSH), a tripeptide of glycine, cysteine and glutamate in its reduced form. GSH acts as a reducing agent to

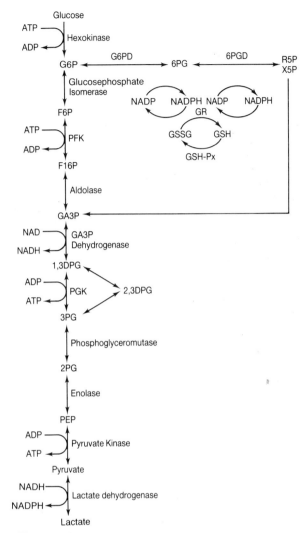

Fig. 11.3   Red cell metabolism. Abbreviations: G6P Glucose 6-phosphate. F6P Fructose 6-phosphate. F1,6P Fructose 1, 6-diphosphate. GA3P Glyceraldehyde 3-phosphate. 2, 3-diphosphoglycerate. 3PG 3-phosphoglycerate. 2PG 2-phosphoglycerate. PEP phosphoenolypyruvate. 1, 3DPG 1, 3-diphosphoglycerate. GPI glucosephosphate isomerase. PFK phosphofructokinase. 6PG 6-phosphogluconate. X5P Xylulose 5-phosphate. R5P Ribulose 5-phosphate. PGK Phosphoglycerokinase. G6PD Glucose 6-phosphate dehydrogenase. 6PG 6 Phosphogluconate dehydrogenase. GSSG Oxidised glutathione. GSH Reduced glutathione. GR Glutathione reductase. GSH-Px Glutathione peroxidase.

protect protein (especially Hb) SH groups from oxidation to disulphide bridges. Methaemoglobin formation can liberate free oxygen radicals which produce hydrogen peroxide; GSH, and therefore NADPH, are necessary for the breakdown of hydrogen peroxide.

Pentose phosphate pathway enzymopathies

These deficiencies are much commoner than deficiencies of enzymes involved in the EMP but their clinical effects are usually mild in comparison. Deficiencies of G6PD, 6PGD, GSH, GSH peroxidase and GSH reductase will all lead to the production of Heinz bodies. These are irregular red cell inclusions attached to the membrane which stain with methyl violet. They represent insoluble aggregates of partially denatured haemoglobin. In contrast to EMP enzyme defects the ATP concentration is normal and haemolysis is often initiated or increased by oxidant drug ingestion. The PPP is responsible for generating reducing power in the form of reduced glutathione and NADPH which counteract oxidant stresses exerted on the red cell by drugs and infections. Such stresses may result in haemolysis in individuals with PPP enzymopathies where this protective mechanism is less efficient.

G6PD deficiency

The gene for this enzyme is carried on the X chromosome so that full phenotypic expression is exhibited by hemizygous males and homozygous females. Over 180 variants of the enzyme have been described, some with greater and some with lesser activity than the commonest type which is G6PD B. The A variant occurs in 18% of Africans and has been useful in the identification of clonal disorders in heterozygous females. The A− variant is also of African origin and although young cells show normal activity of the enzyme it is unstable and cells become deficient on ageing. This African type of G6PD deficiency is considerably milder than the Mediterranean type in which cells of all ages are affected and the variant enzyme also has an abnormal Km value. Erythrocytes deficient in the enzyme are relatively resistant to *P. falciparum* parasitisation but the mechanism of protection remains obscure.

Most individuals with G6PD deficiency are symptomless but there is great variability in susceptibility to stimuli which will produce haemolysis. Favism, which refers to episodic haemolysis initiated by eating the *Vicia faba* bean or inhaling its pollen, has been recognised around the Mediterranean for centuries as a familial jaundice particularly affecting young boys. It is not a feature of the African form of the disease but haemolysis can be precipitated by infections or drugs in most of the variants where G6PD activity is deficient (Table 11.3). Drugs induce a dose-dependent haemolysis by stimulating hydrogen peroxide and superoxide radical formation, thereby depleting GSH which cannot be replenished without NADPH. In normal individuals

Table 11.3 Common drugs causing haemolysis in G6PD-deficient subjects

Antimalarials
Chloroquine
Primaquine
Quinine

Antipyretics
Paracetamol
Aspirin
Phenacetin

Sulphonamides
Sulphadiazine
Sulphadimidine
Sulphanilamide
Sulphapyridine

Nitrofurans
Nitrofurantoin

Sulphones
Dapsone

Other drugs
Ascorbic acid
L-Dopa
Quinidine
GTN
Vitamin K

PPP activity can be increased up to forty-fold to cope with such oxidant stress. Cases frequently present with prolonged neonatal jaundice in which the precipitating factor is not known. Deficiency can rarely produce a chronic haemolytic anaemia.

Many of the drugs in Table 11.3 can be prescribed safely in all but the most severely deficient subjects and failure to give the drug may be more hazardous than the often minor degree of haemolysis caused. The blood picture should be observed during such therapy in case severe haemolysis is precipitated.

Diagnosis. The common, oxidant stress-induced haemolysis is intravascular. If G6PD-deficient RBC are incubated with phenylhydrazine for 2 hours, Heinz bodies are produced. This non-specific test may give false positive results. In performing any red cell enzyme assay two points should be remembered. Firstly, the enzyme activity depends on red cell age with the highest activity in reticulocytes. Secondly, in neonates enzyme levels are generally increased. Thus quantitative assays should preferably be performed when the reticulocytosis has abated. Comparison of the activity of one enzyme with another may assist interpretation of so-called normal results. The fluorescent spot screening test is based upon production of NADPH which fluoresces under UV light. It is excellent for low level hemizygotes but heterozygotes may not be detected and A−hemizygotes may also give a normal result if the reticulocyte count is raised.

Treatment. Generally no treatment is needed other than advice concerning drug avoidance. Transfusions may be necessary for severe haemolysis and supportive care for acute renal failure in rare instances. Exchange transfusions may be needed for neonatal jaundice. Fava beans and oxidant drugs must be avoided in susceptible individuals.

GSH deficiency

A low level of reduced glutathione results from deficiency of one of the two enzymes responsible for its synthesis; gamma-L glutamylcysteine synthetase and GSH synthetase. Deficiency of the latter may produce a chronic non-spherocytic haemolytic anaemia, in some cases associated with metabolic acidosis and oxyprolinuria.

Enzymopathies of the Embden-Meyerhof pathway

These rare and generally autosomal recessive disorders produce a congenital non-spherocytic haemolytic anaemia of variable severity exacerbated by infections but unaffected by drug administration. The morphological features are non-specific but small numbers of prickle cells may be seen. Pyruvate kinase (PK) deficiency is the least rare of the glycolytic pathway enzymopathies.

Pyruvate kinase deficiency

Normal PK catalyses the conversion of phosphoenolpyruvate to pyruvate with the simultaneous production of ATP. PK-deficient red cells are deficient in ATP, which is normally only produced by the EMP, and their lifespan is shortened. Reticulocytes, however, have an alternative source of ATP via the Krebs cycle and are often markedly increased in PK deficient subjects. Many kinetic variants of PK have been described showing different Km values for PEP, abnormal pH optima curves, increased thermal lability or other features. Many cases of PK deficiency are due to double heterozygosity for abnormal variants. Not surprisingly the disorder shows considerable variation in its clinical expression and severity. Jaundice, splenomegaly and haemolysis may be the presenting features in early infancy but many cases are not detected until adult life. The haemoglobin concentration ranges from 5 gm/dl up to near normal values with a variable reticulocytosis which increases after splenectomy. Owing to the position of PK in the EMP there is a build up of 2,3-DPG

with a resultant reduction in oxygen affinity so the anaemia is relatively well tolerated.

The diagnosis rests on the demonstration of reduced PK activity but full kinetic studies may be required. Increased levels of intermediate metabolites, especially 2,3-DPG provide supportive evidence for PK deficiency.

Treatment consists of blood transfusion when necessary and splenectomy should be considered for patients who need regular transfusions. The haemoglobin does not return to normal following splenectomy. Folate supplements are advisable.

Hexokinase deficiency

Hexokinase has the lowest specific activity of all the glycolytic enzymes and is the prime determinant of glycolytic rate. It yields G6P from glucose in an irreversible step and when deficient there is reduced glucose consumption and 2,3-DPG production. The resultant increase in oxygen affinity causes a greater erythropoietin drive and a higher haemoglobin than in other causes of haemolysis. It is likely that at a given haemoglobin such patients are more symptomatic.

NADH-linked methaemoglobin reductase deficiency

This enzyme, also known as diaphorase, is responsible for the reduction of Met Hb which accumulates in deficient individuals to produce cyanosis. There is no associated haemolysis and indeed compensatory erythrocytosis may occur. The condition may be differentiated from Hb M disease which also presents with cyanosis but in which ascorbate or methylene blue fail to reduce the level of Hb M. In diaphorase deficiency methylene blue will stimulate the PPP and increase the level of NADPH-linked Met Hb reductase activity which corrects the methaemoglobinaemia although this enzyme normally has no known function. Vitamin C acts as a direct reducing agent for Met Hb.

ACQUIRED HAEMOLYTIC ANAEMIAS

IMMUNE MEDIATED HAEMOLYSIS

This is effected by the attachment of antibody to the red cell surface. The rate and site of haemolysis and therefore the clinical manifestations depend on the type of antibody attached and on its propensity to fix complement. The antibodies are usually IgG (often subclass 1 or 3) or IgM but occasionally IgA can be detected. The optimal temperature for binding of antibody to red cell is important. In most cases IgG antibodies are 'warm' in that they attach best 37°C, whereas IgM antibodies are cold-reacting and dissociate at body temperature. Cells coated with IgG1 or IgG3 can be removed directly and preferentially by splenic macrophages which bear Fc receptors. Both IgG and IgM can fix complement but usually only part of the sequence is fixed and thus intravascular haemolysis is avoided. Nevertheless cells coated with activated C3 can be removed rapidly by macrophages throughout the entire RE system but this component has a short half-life and gives rise to C3d to which macrophage receptors are insensitive. Part of the membrane of the red cells may be stripped off during immune adherence. This gives rise to the spherocytes that are a feature of warm AIHA. Cold-reacting IgM antibodies are more likely to trigger the entire complement cascade giving rise to intravascular haemolysis.

The antiglobulin tests

The direct AGT, or direct Coomb's test as it is often called, makes use of antibodies to human immunoglobulins which have been raised in animals. These polyspecific reagents are still in general use and are designed to react with cells bearing IgG and complement. IgM always binds complement so it is unnecessary for the reagent to contain anti-IgM. In the direct test, washed red cells are mixed directly with the antiglobulin reagent and the presence of attached antibodies is detected by an agglutination reaction which can be graded. The test is positive in nearly all cases of AIHA. Rarely the concentration of Ig molecules on the red cells is too low to be detected by this method. Monospecific reagents demonstrate IgG alone or together with C3 in idiopathic AIHA and in cases secondary to lymphoproliferative disease. In the immune haemolysis associated with SLE, IgG is detected together with C3 in most cases, whereas only C3 is present in cold antibody states. Occasionally IgA can be detected but generally together with IgG.

The indirect antiglobulin test (IDAT) is used to detect free antibody (allo-antibody or auto-antibody) in the serum using cells with known antigenic characteristics. It is of most use in compatibility testing but is often positive in severe AIHA. An eluate of antibody from the patient's cells can be used in an IDAT with red cells of known type to determine whether there is any antigenic specificity.

Idiopathic AIHA

As with other autoimmune diseases there is a higher incidence in females and it occurs most commonly after middle age. The mode of presentation varies from the insidious onset of anaemia over several months to the

Table 11.4   Conditions associated with immune haemolysis

Non-Hodgkin's lymphoma
Chronic lymphocytic leukaemia
Systemic lupus erythematosus
Rheumatoid arthritis
Thyrotoxicosis
Myasthenia gravis
Pernicious anaemia
Ulcerative colitis
Autoimmune hepatitis
Hypogammaglobulinaemia
Wiscott–Aldrich syndrome
Thymoma
Post-viral AIHA (particularly in children)
Post-malaria
Ovarian teratoma
Dermoid cyst

almost explosive development of severe anaemia with jaundice. The history and examination are vital, bearing in mind the diseases which are associated with warm AIHA. Only about 50% of cases of warm AIHA are idiopathic and the majority of these exhibit modest splenomegaly. Marked splenomegaly raises the suspicion of a lymphoproliferative disorder with associated immune haemolysis. Many idiopathic cases are found to have an underlying cause in the course of time (Table 11.4).

Additional investigations

The blood film characteristically shows numerous spherocytes, polychromasia and possibly circulating nucleated red cells with an associated neutrophilia and sometimes thrombocytosis (Fig. 11.4). Free antibody may be detected in the serum with the same

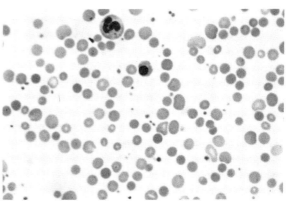

Fig. 11.4   Autoimmune haemolytic anaemia film with spherocytes, polychromasia and nucleated red blood cells.

specificity as that eluted from the red cells. This specificity is only relative but in 70% of cases is directed towards antigens in the Rh system. Red cells coated with IgG are destroyed extravascularly by the liver and the spleen and occasionally ^{51}Cr labelled red cell studies will be helpful in predicting the response to splenectomy.

Management and prognosis

Most adults respond to prednisolone 40–100 mg daily. There may be difficulties in obtaining compatible blood for transfusion but this should not cause undue delay. Nevertheless it should be remembered that auto-antibodies may mask the presence of acquired allo-antibodies in transfused patients. After a short course of high dose prednisolone the dose may be tailed to the minimum required to prevent haemolysis. Patients who do not respond or who require a high dose of steroid after 6 months of treatment should be considered for splenectomy. Cytotoxic drugs, e.g. azathioprine, are also effective, either alone or as a means of reducing the dose of prednisolone. The risks of immunosuppression need to be weighed against the side effects of steroids. Splenectomy should, if possible, be preceded by vaccination with polyvalent pneumococcal antigen and followed by prophylactic penicillin V, 250 mg BD., for life.

DRUG-INDUCED HAEMOLYTIC ANAEMIAS

These may be divided into two broad categories: firstly those cases in which the patient's serum will only react with normal red cells the in the presence of the offending drug, and secondly those in which the drug triggers off an autoimmune process in which, once initiated, it plays no part in the reaction between red cell and antibody (Table 11.5).

Table 11.5 Drugs provoking immune haemolysis

Quinidine
Quinine
Nomifensine
Phenacetin
Paracetamol
Penicillin
Sulphonamides
Sulphonylureas
Salazopyrine
Cephalosporins
Rifampicin

Acute intravascular haemolysis

This type of reaction is exemplified by chlorpropamide or quinidine induced haemolysis in which the drug provokes antibody formation and the resulting immune complex is loosely adsorbed onto the red cell where it can fix complement which is detectable by the DAGT. The haemolysis is often abrupt in onset and occurs on second or subsequent exposure to the drug. It is not possible to demonstrate immune complexes or the drug on the red cell surface, so the proposed mechanism has been described as the innocent bystander mechanism.

Slow onset of haemolytic anaemia

The prime example of this type of reaction is that induced by penicillin when given in high dosage, e.g. 20 MU per day. The drug is firmly bound to the red cell and IgG antibody directed to the drug then attaches leading to extravascular destruction of coated erythrocytes. The drug may act as a hapten and only provoke antibody formation after attachment to the red cell. Cephalosporins can cause immune haemolysis in the same manner but in some cases complement is fixed and intravascular haemolysis ensues. The DAGT is positive and if test red cells are pre-incubated with the drug the indirect test is also positive.

Autoimmune haemolysis induced by drugs

This was first reported in association with methyldopa, an agent which has now been largely superseded, but mefenamic acid, flufenamic acid and L-dopa may cause haemolysis by a similar mechanism. After at least four months of treatment 15–20% of patients on methyldopa develop a positive DAGT due to IgG coating but less than 1% of patients show evidence of haemolysis. As with idiopathic AIHA most sera and red cell eluates exhibit antibodies with partial Rh specificity and it is not uncommon to find other auto-antibodies such as ANF, parietal cell antibodies, leuko-agglutinins and platelet antibodies. The mechanism of haemolysis is not well understood but there appears to be decreased T suppressor lymphocyte activity.

Management

Stopping the offending drug will rapidly halt haemolysis in those cases where the drug is directly implicated, although transfusions may be indicated at the time of presentation. Methyldopa-induced haemolysis may take longer to resolve and require a short course of prednisolone. The positive DAGT persists for over two years. It is usually not necessary to discontinue methyldopa administration in patients with a positive DAGT but without evidence of haemolysis.

COLD HAEMAGGLUTININ DISORDERS

This group of disorders is characterised by agglutination of red cells at temperatures below 37°C in association with specific clinical and laboratory manifestations. The illness may be acute in onset and short in duration when it is secondary to certain infections, or insidious in onset and chronic as idiopathic cold haemagglutinin syndrome.

Mechanisms and causes

Following infection with *Mycoplasma pneumoniae* about 50% of patients show a rise in the titre of anti-I, a cold antibody normally present in low titre. This is an IgM antibody, first discovered in the serum of a patient with cold haemagglutinin disease (CHAD) which reacts optimally with adult red cells in the cold. Neonatal erythrocytes express I antigen and are therefore not agglutinated. Following infectious mononucleosis a similar cold-reacting antibody, anti-i, is frequently produced which in rare cases can affect adult I red cells and cause a similar clinical picture. The cold antibodies produced secondary to these infections are polyclonal, they contain both lambda and kappa light-chains and serum protein electrophoresis shows a diffuse increase in IgM. In contrast the anti-I found in CHAD and cold haemagglutination secondary to lymphomas is a monoclonal paraprotein generally with kappa light-chain specificity. The low thermal amplitude of the antibody results in red cell agglutination in the cooler peripheral circulation of the hands, feet, nose and ears with complement fixation. IgM elutes from the cells on rewarming but if sufficient complement is bound intravascular haemolysis occurs.

Clinical features

The haemolysis associated with *Mycoplasma pneumoniae* infection generally occurs 2 to 3 weeks after the acute illness with the rapid onset of anaemia. The patient may notice red urine due to haemoglobinuria, particularly if the environment is cold. The patient with CHAD is generally elderly and may present with symptoms of anaemia or haemoglobinuria or of painful blue discoloration of the extremities, particularly during cold weather. The latter phenomenon is called acrocyanosis and may be distinguished from Raynaud's phenomenon by the sites affected (nose and ears in addition to hands), the absence of a blanching phase or of an erythematous phase on rewarming. The onset of these symptoms may precede or follow the diagnosis of lymphoma in those patients with secondary cold haemagglutination.

Investigations

It is imperative that blood samples be kept at 37°C to avoid agglutination and haemolysis. The DAGT shows complement coating only. The anti-I titre at 4°C is over 1 in 1000. The blood film shows agglutination unless made at 37°C and the MCV may be spuriously raised. Protein electrophoresis may show a paraprotein band which can be defined by immunofixation.

Management

The syndrome associated with infections is shelf-limiting and generally requires no treatment other than warmth and bed rest. CHAD, whether idiopathic or secondary, does not respond to steroids or to splenectomy. Most patients learn to avoid outdoor activities in winter and use warm clothing. Heated gloves and socks may be helpful. If these measures fail, chlorambucil in intermittent courses can be effective. Also, since the IgM antibody is entirely intravascular, the titre can be reduced and the symptoms ameliorated by regular plasmapheresis.

Paroxysmal cold haemoglobinuria

This rare disorder, which is also characterised by haemoglobinuria following cold exposure, was associated in the past with congenital syphilis. It also occurs in children in association with various viral infections and is caused by the Donath-Landsteiner antibody, a unique IgG antibody with a low thermal range and the ability to fix complement. The diagnosis rests on the demonstration of in vitro haemolysis when red cells and serum are first chilled and then rewarmed. The condition is generally self-limiting but transfusion may be required and although the antibody shows anti-P specifity it is safe to give warmed P1 positive blood. Chronic PCH may present, like CHAD, with episodes of haemoglobinuria associated with cold weather but generally no treatment is required.

Haemolysis caused directly by infections

Bacterial septicaemias can cause modest haemolysis even in the absence of proven DIC. The aetiology is obscure and the treatment is that of the underlying infection.

Malaria

The commonest acquired haemolytic anaemia is that caused by the protozoon *Plasmodium falciparum*. Lesser degrees of haemolysis are caused by the other members of the genus *Plasmodium*. Haemolysis occurs in most severe *P. falciparum* infections particularly when there are cerebral or respiratory symptoms, and in rare cases blackwater fever due to massive haemoglobinuria can occur. The degree of haemolysis is usually proportional to the parasitaemia but the anaemia is also caused by increased RES activity, DIC (most patients with falciparum malaria are thrombocytopenic) and dyserythropoiesis.

Diagnosis is by film inspection and treatment depends on the type of malaria, its geographical origin and the degree of parasitaemia. Chloroquine should be followed by primaquine for patients with non-falciparum malaria to eradicate protozoa in the exoerythrocytic phase and G6PD-deficient individuals should be monitored while taking the latter drug. Falciparum malaria from a resistance area should be treated with quinine. Exchange transfusion may be life-saving in cases of cerebral malaria or when there is a high degree of parasitaemia.

Clostridium welchii

This organism produces toxins with lecithinase-like activity causing rapid intravascular haemolysis with DIC, microspherocytosis and hyperkalaemia. It is an uncommon but often fatal cause of septicaemia requiring immediate parenteral penicillin and supportive care.

Bartonella bacilliformis

Infection with this organism, which occurs only in South America, causes Oroya fever or Carrion's disease. It is characterised by fever, aching limbs, generalised lymphadenopathy and rapid extravascular haemolysis. Inspection of the blood film reveals small red cell inclusions. The disease is often fatal if untreated but penicillin is curative.

Mechanical causes of haemolysis

Erythrocytes are uniquely flexible cells which deform many times during their lifespan to pass through small capillaries. However, when excessive shear stresses are applied, fragmentation occurs with resulting intravascular cell lysis or the formation of persistent red cell fragments.

Cardiac causes of mechanical haemolysis

In this situation the shear stresses are caused by turbulent blood flow in a high pressure system. This arises around prosthetic heart valves, particularly if the valve malfunctions. It is more common with aortic than mitral replacements and is occasionally seen in aortic stenosis and/or regurgitation. Teflon patch repair of atrial or ventricular septal defects can also give rise to fragmentation haemolysis.

Micro-angiopathic haemolytic anaemia (MAHA)

This is caused by small vessel abnormalities which impede blood flow. Such abnormalities are often associated with fibrin deposition, microthrombi and DIC. In the haemolytic uraemic syndrome there is endothelial damage with fibrin deposition in small vessels. The MAHA in thrombotic thrombocytopenic purpura is related to hyaline occlusion and aneurysmal dilation of small vessels. Other causes of MAHA include renal cortical necrosis, pre-eclampsia, vasculitis (PAN, Wegener's granulomatosis, SLE), carcinomatosis and giant cavernous haemangioma (Kasabach-Merritt syndrome).

Others

Direct mechanical damage to red cells in the small vessels of the feet can occur in some individuals during prolonged marching, giving rise to so-called march haemoglobinuria. Bouts of karate and other body contact sports are sometimes followed by transient haemoglobinuria due to intravascular mechanical haemolysis. Severe burns can produce a bizarre thermal injury to red cells which leads to fragmentation and very small microspherocytes.

A careful history and examination will often reveal the cause of mechanical haemolysis as indicated by the presence of red cell fragments in the peripheral blood. A Perl's stain of the urinary sediment shows the presence of iron; a useful test for any chronic low grade intravascular haemolysis when there is little evidence on blood film inspection. The coagulation screen may be abnormal with associated thrombocytopenia in many cases of MAHA due to chronic DIC.

Altered milieu leading to haemolysis

The lipids of the red cell membrane are in dynamic equilibrium with those of the surrounding plasma. The lipid content of the plasma therefore affects that of the red cell and may lead to changes in the shape and osmotic fragility of the cell.

Liver disease

Hepatocellular disease or biliary obstruction usually lead to the presence of target cells but not to haemolysis. In severe hepatocellular disease and alcoholic cirrhosis, however, spur cells and acanthocytes may be seen with evidence of reduced red cell survival. In Zieve's syndrome there is haemolytic anaemia with spherocytes, hyperlipidaemia and acute abdominal pain in association with alcoholic cirrhosis. Wilson's disease may present with a haemolytic anaemia of obscure aetiology.

Abeta-lipoproteinaemia

This is a rare, recessively inherited deficiency of beta lipoprotein which leads to an imbalanced distribution of membrane phospholipids. It is included in this section for completeness as it is the only inherited alteration in milieu which leads to haemolysis. Most of the circulating cells are acanthocytes with reduced life span.

Vitamin E deficiency

Alpha tocopherol is known to protect against non-enzymatic attack of molecular oxygen on polyunsaturated fatty acids in the red cell membrane. Deficiency has been implicated as the cause of a haemolytic anaemia with acanthocytosis seen in infants.

Hypophosphataemia

Starvation, parental nutrition or misuse of antacids can lead to depression of the serum phosphate with consequent depletion of intracellular phosphate which is necessary for ATP production. This leads to an acquired spherocytic haemolysis which is readily reversed by phosphate administration.

Chemical causes of haemolysis

Drug and chemical causes of haemolysis have already been discussed in the sections on enzymopathies and immune mediated haemolysis. Chemicals can also exert an oxidant effect on normal red cells to produce haemolysis (Table 11.6). Damage to membrane lipids, the production of disulphide bonds, methaemoglobin and Heinz bodies lead to loss of deformability and reduced survival. These oxidative stresses are countered by the reducing power generated mainly by the pentose phosphate shunt. Aspirin may facilitate the oxidant action of

Table 11.6 Chemicals and drugs causing haemolysis

Sulphonamides
Dapsone
Salazopyrine
Phenothiazine
Para-amino-salicylic acid
Water-soluble vitamin K analogues
Sodium or potassium chlorate
Naphthalene
Nitrites
Nitrobenzene derivatives
Arsine
Lead

other drugs by inhibition of PK and G6PD, although it will not cause haemolysis by itself. In many cases it is the drug metabolites which are oxidant. Metabolic variation is important. For example, dapsone is a drug which is acetylated and individuals who are slow acetylators are more prone to its oxidant effects. Renal or hepatic dysfunction may also aggravate such toxicity. Similarly, hepatic immaturity and lower enzyme levels in neonates increase susceptibility to these agents. Haemolysis has been caused in infants by water-soluble vitamin K analogues and by drinking water contaminated with fertiliser nitrites.

The clinical effects of oxidants are variable. Cyanosis from methaemoglobinaemia can occur with or without haemolysis and the latter may be chronic, as in patients on dapsone or salazopyrine, or acute as seen in those with severe G6PD deficiency. Very strong oxidising agents will also produce acute renal failure and DIC secondary to intravascular haemolysis.

Paroxysmal nocturnal haemoglobinuria

PNH is a rare stem cell disorder characterised by episodic intravascular haemolysis, venous thromboses, bouts of abdominal and back pain and bone marrow hypoplasia. The abnormal clone, usually co-existing with normal haemopoietic cells, results in abnormal cells of all three cell lines in the peripheral blood which are deficient in a membrane regulatory protein of complement known as decay-accelerating factor (DAF). DAF regulates C3 activation at the membrane and deficiency results in unusual sensitivity to lysis by autologous complement. The patient's red cells may be graded as type I to type III according to their complement sensitivity or DAF content. Their proportions will vary with time, with complement-sensitive type III cells often disappearing after an episode of haemolysis. The PNH defect is associated with other disorders of the bone marrow such as hypoplasia and myeloproliferative disorders.

Clinical features

Haemolysis. The peak incidence is in early adult life and the commonest presentation is with haemoglobinuria, classically on waking, which may be chronic or episodic. Exacerbating factors include infections, menstruation, pregnancy, vaccinations, blood transfusions and drugs, e.g. heparin, aspirin, iron and chlorpromazine. Iron initiates lysis by promoting erythropoiesis.

Thrombosis. Venous thrombosis may be the presenting feature in PNH. The abdominal pains are thought to be due to thrombosis of venules of the mesenteric veins but may presage the onset of the Budd-Chiari syndrome. Ilio-femoral thromboses also occur and may result in pulmonary emboli.

Bone marrow hypoplasia. The temporal relationship of PNH with aplasia is unpredictable. Hypoplasia may precede the onset of PNH but usually it develops insidiously as a sequel, often many years later. Rarely PNH may terminate in acute myeloid leukaemia.

The physical signs of PNH are variable. There may be features of iron deficiency due to chronic haemosiderinuria. Splenomegaly is unusual and there are no characteristic features on the blood film. The reticulocytosis may not be marked and there may be neutropenia and thrombocytopenia. Tests for IV haemolysis are positive and the neutrophil alkaline phosphatase score may be low (but rises if aplasia supervenes). The diagnosis is made by demonstrating a positive acidified serum lysis test (Ham's test). An initial negative result should not deter one from repeating the test if the diagnosis is still suspected.

Treatment

Iron deficiency is common but giving iron in the presence of anaemia has been reported to initiate haemolysis. This can be suppressed by judicious transfusion and the use of prednisolone. Transfusion must be with washed red cells or cryopreserved red cells as small amounts of transfused complement can induce haemolysis. Some patients have an improvement in their haemoglobin and clinical status when treated with androgenic steroids, particularly if there is bone marrow hypoplasia. Prednisolone in a dose of 1 mg/kg/day may be effective in aborting acute haemolytic episodes. It is important to maintain adequate hydration during these crises to avoid acute renal failure. Given the high risk of venous thrombosis, oral anticoagulation is recommended. If heparin is indicated it should be remembered that in some patients it triggers acute haemolysis. The overall median survival in PNH is about 10 years.

BIBLIOGRAPHY

Dacie J, Sir 1985 The haemolytic anaemias, vol. 1. Churchill Livingston, Edinburgh
Mollison P L 1986 Blood transfusion in clinical medicine. Blackwell, Oxford
The red blood cell membrane. 1 Feb 1985 Clinics in Haematology 14

12. Haemoglobinopathies

A. J. Bellingham   D. S. Gillett

The normal haemoglobin A molecule is a tetramer of two alpha and two beta globin chains each carrying a haem group which is responsible for the carriage of oxygen. Both globin chains are similar, consisting of a series of helices of amino acids, the beta chain having 146 and the alpha 141. The three-dimensional structure of the individual globin chains is similar. A small proportion of haemoglobin consists of Hb A_2 which is composed of two alpha and two delta chains. For the last few months of gestation the predominant haemoglobin species is haemoglobin F which has two gamma chains in place of the beta chains in haemoglobin A. At birth the production of gamma chains is switched to beta chains so that haemoglobin F is gradually replaced by haemoglobin A in the first few months of life. Earlier in fetal development other globin chains are produced so giving rise to other haemoglobin species which can be detected antenatally (see Ch. 28).

Haemoglobin function

Each haemoglobin molecule carries four molecules of oxygen each bound to one of the haem groups when fully saturated. The haemoglobin tetrameric structure is essential for normal oxygen transport as the co-operative movement of the four globin chains gives rise to the sigmoid-shaped oxygen dissociation curve. The molecule has two conformations associated with the oxy- and deoxygenated states respectively. During oxygenation the two beta chains move together to give a species more avid for oxygen. Hence as the initial oxygen is taken up by the haemoglobin it increases its affinity for oxygen to bind to the remaining haem groups on the molecule and so the allosteric oxygen binding curve results. The ability of 2,3-diphosphoglycerate (2,3-DPG) to reduce oxygen affinity is dependent on it stabilising the deoxygenated conformation by binding between the two beta chains. A fall in pH or a rise in temperature will also favour the deoxygenated conformation and so lower the oxygen affinity. Any structural change in the globin chain may interfere with the normal molecular movement and so modify the capacity for oxygen delivery. The capability of the blood to deliver oxygen to the tissues may be modified by one of these factors (usually 2,3-DPG) by altering the position of the oxygen dissociation curve or by a change in the haemoglobin content of the blood. Hence in anaemia the effect on tissue oxygen delivery caused by the low haemoglobin is partially compensated for by a rise in 2,3-DPG.

Molecular basis of the haemoglobinopathies

In recent years there has been an enormous increase in knowledge of the DNA coding responsible for globin chain production. Beta chains are coded by a gene on chromosome 11 in a cluster of all the non-alpha genes, which interestingly are in the same sequence on the chromosome in which they appear in phenotypic development. The alpha genes and their fetal precursors are similarly ordered on chromosome 16 but the former are duplicated resulting in four alpha genes in the normal individual.

Inherited defects of haemoglobin synthesis may be divided into two main groups:

a) The abnormal haemoglobins

Here there is usually a single amino acid substitution in one of the globin chains resulting from a single base change in the gene.

b) The thalassaemias

An imbalance of synthesis of the globin chains causes the clinical manifestations and there are several mechanisms by which this can occur. Gene deletion, loss of a section of the gene and errors of transcription are the most frequent.

THE ABNORMAL HAEMOGLOBINS

The abnormal haemoglobins result almost exclusively from a mutation in which there is a single base change. However, the resulting clinical consequences are extremely varied. Commonly there is no physiological or pathological effect; these silent haemoglobins are only identified coincidentally. The substituted amino acid may lead to instability of either the single globin chain or the tetrameric molecule. In either case the clinical manifestation is of haemolysis of varying severity. Usually independently but rarely in association with the globin instability there may be a tendency for the iron atom to oxidise so giving rise to methaemoglobinaemia. This occurs particularly if the substitution involves the haem pocket of the globin chain. Another possibility is that the tetrameric conformation of the haemoglobin is stabilised resulting in modification of oxygen affinity. Most commonly the oxy conformation is favoured, resulting in an increased affinity which, as a result of the impaired tissue oxygen delivery, manifests clinically as polycythaemia.

One of the most common abnormal haemoglobins, HbS, does not fit this classification. Although haemolysis is a major feature of the disease it results from the polymerisation of the haemoglobin molecule rather than its instability. This leads to red cell rigidity and consequently a tendency to block the microvasculature. Other abnormal haemoglobins will be encountered only rarely and in this discussion the broad clinical groups will be presented first, after which separate sections will deal with those few abnormal haemoglobins that occur occasionally.

Haemolysis

Those abnormal haemoglobins which cause instability of the haemoglobin present because of the haemolytic process. The age of presentation is dependent on the globin chain involved. Beta chain abnormalities, which are the most common, do not present until a few months of age, as until then there is insufficient abnormal chain produced. In contrast, alpha chain abnormalities are present at birth and therefore enter the differential diagnosis of haemolytic disease of the newborn. In this respect it is interesting to note that alpha chain abnormalities causing haemolysis tend to be milder and are less common. It is likely that a fetus with severe haemolysis due to alpha chain abnormality does not survive, as the alpha chain, unlike the beta chain, is essential for haemoglobin F production prior to birth (see above).

As the haemolysis is clinically manifest in the heterozygous state, most patients will have a positive family history, although in milder cases affected family members may only be detected by the enquiring physician. Owing to the instability of the haemoglobin and consequent predisposition to oxidation occasional patients present with an acute haemolytic crisis resulting from oxidant drugs similar to that seen in G6PD deficiency. Alternatively an intercurrent infection may aggravate the condition and the patient presents because of more profound anaemia. This is more common in childhood.

On examination, other than the signs of jaundice and anaemia, which are of variable severity, the spleen is commonly enlarged up to 4 cm below the costal margin. With the increase in folate required in these patients it is usual to give supplements and to advise on the effect of infections. Splenectomy has rarely been reported to be of benefit except in the most severely affected and because of the infective risk this procedure is best avoided if possible.

Diagnosis

The blood film usually shows the non-specific changes of haemolysis. The reticulocytes are raised to a variable degree but close inspection of this preparation may show Heinz bodies, although these are better shown on staining with brilliant cresyl blue. One or both the precipitation tests with heat or isopropyl alcohol are usually positive. For this reason it is usually worth performing both tests in a suspected case. Haemoglobin electrophoresis will normally show the variant haemoglobin but if it is particularly unstable then it may precipitate during the preparation of the haemolysate and hence be missed. For this reason, if an unstable haemoglobin is suspected, it is essential that all studies are performed on fresh blood. The substitution causing the instability may also cause a change in the oxygen affinity which is often a useful measurement in difficult cases.

Polycythaemia

As a cause of familial polycythaemia the abnormal haemoglobins have provoked an interest out of proportion to their incidence. Identification is particularly important as unnecessary treatment with potentially dangerous agents must be avoided. The condition is remarkably asymptomatic, consequently it is often discovered coincidentally on a routine blood count. Suspicion of the diagnosis should be raised if there is a lack of the usual features of polycythaemia rubra vera, the other causes of secondary polycythaemia are absent and particularly if there is a family history. As with the unstable haemoglobins the polycythaemia is manifest in the heterozygous state so dominant inheritance is the rule. From the relatively few cases reported the condition does not appear to result in shortened survival or to have the common complications of the more frequent myeloproliferative state. Many patients are asymptomatic with a long-standing haematocrit of the order of 60%. As a result it is difficult to advise firmly on the management strategy but some physicians appear to be unhappy to leave the haematocrit above 55% for long periods, particularly if the patient is over the age of 50 when the incidence of vascular degenerative disease will increase. It has often been stated that women with high affinity haemoglobins are more likely to have spontaneous abortions, as the maternal oxygen dissociation curve may be to the left of the fetal dissociation curve, opposite to the normal situation. This is not so, as is shown by the meagre clinical data available and in terms of oxygen delivery considerations. The polycythaemia compensates for the impaired oxygen delivery resulting from the increased oxygen affinity. However a person with a high affinity haemoglobin who has been venesected to reduce his haematocrit is 'anaemic' in terms of oxygen delivery capability. This is supported by the raised erythropoietin excretion reported in those patients whose haematocrit has been reduced to a normal value.

Diagnosis

Establishing the diagnosis rests on the demonstration of a raised whole blood oxygen affinity which is not due to reduced red cell 2,3-diphosphoglycerate. Although the abnormal haemoglobin may be detected on haemoglobin electrophoresis, the lack of an abnormal band does not exclude the diagnosis. There is usually no evidence of haemolysis.

Methaemoglobins

The abnormal haemoglobins causing methaemoglobinaemia are another rare but important group to recognise promptly in order to avoid unnecessary invasive investigations. The condition usually presents in childhood with the recognition of the persistent cyanotic hue. In the case of the alpha chain variants this will be present at birth and the baby runs a particular risk of being investigated for a cardiac defect. The beta chain variants only present after a few months of life. At the bedside the patient is not distressed and oxygen administration does nothing to improve the cyanosis. As the condition is manifest in the heterozygous state it is inherited as an autosomal dominant condition. This is

particularly important as the other inherited cause of methaemoglobinaemia, due to deficiency of the methaemoglobin reductase enzyme, is inherited as a recessive characteristic. The other, probably more common, cause of methaemoglobinaemia in childhood is due to drug or chemical ingestion and this must always be excluded first as a cause.

Having identified methaemoglobin as the cause of persistent cyanosis the main action is to inform the patient or relatives so as to avoid unnecessary medical intervention. No specific action is indicated and life expectancy is not affected.

Diagnosis

The identification of methaemoglobin is usually easily carried out spectrophotometrically but it may also be apparent on routine haemoglobin electrophoresis. Though the separation of the methaemoglobin as due to an abnormal haemoglobin from the oxidised normal haemoglobin occurring as a result of drugs or deficiency of the reductase enzyme is more subtle. A detailed spectral analysis of the haemoglobin usually resolves this problem.

Sickle cell disease

This is the most common disease caused by an abnormal haemoglobin. First described in 1910, it is now known to be due to a substitution of valine for glutamic acid at the sixth residue of the beta chain. This substitution causes the haemoglobin to polymerise when deoxygenated, forming strands of haemoglobin molecules which distort the red cell and make it rigid, so reducing its ability to negotiate the microvasculature.

The term 'sickle cell disease' (SCD) applies not only to the homozygous sickle cell anaemia (HbSS) but to mixed syndromes in which sickling occurs clinically due to HbS being in combination with another Hb, the most frequent being HbC; HbD; HbE; HbO and beta thalassaemia. The term 'sickle cell trait' applies to the clinically silent heterozygous state HbAS.

Classically the disease was described in those indigenous to West and Central Africa, where in some areas the gene frequency may reach one in three. There is a lower but nevertheless significant incidence in Greece, Turkey, Southern Italy and Arabia, whilst in some parts of India the incidence is higher than previously thought. Sickle cell disease is uncommon in the Asian population in the UK due to the uneven distribution of the gene in the Indian subcontinent. In the Afro-Caribbean population of the UK the incidence of the gene is about one in ten.

The hallmark of the disease is one of chronic haemolysis punctuated by crises of varying severity and type occurring in an unpredictable fashion but often precipitated by intercurrent infections. The types of crises are as follows:

Infarctive crisis. This occurs most frequently in the musculoskeletal system and fortunately does not usually result in long-term sequelae, although avascular necrosis of the hip and occasional permanent damage to other joints is well recognised. Infarction of any organ may occur but the spleen is often affected and by the time a patient has reached the late teens the spleen is usually reduced to a small fibrous remnant with no significant function. Under the age of 5 years a common presenting feature is bilateral dactylitis, which is rarely, if ever, seen in the older patient. Cerebral infarcts, thankfully rare, also have a predilection for childhood and have a tendency to recur. This latter phenomenon is unexplained but regular transfusion often gives protection from further episodes.

The reduced immunity in sickle cell disease is probably largely due to the early loss of splenic function and results in an increased propensity to infections, particularly bacterial. Osteomyelitis, frequently due to salmonella, is a well known complication of the disease. Pneumococcal infections are a particular hazard in childhood. There is clear evidence that prophylactic oral penicillin is of benefit in childhood but its value in the older patient is not proven. There is less evidence of the value of pneumococcal vaccine in children. This may in part be due to the strain of pneumococcus in the vaccine being inappropriate. The frequently quoted protection from malaria is only applicable to the first two years of life in sickle cell trait and then only from overwhelming falciparum infection. Consequently sickle patients should always receive malarial prophylaxis, as infection may precipitate a crisis. Recurrent upper respiratory tract infections and pneumonia from a variety of organisms are also common.

Aplastic crisis. As well as infarction patients with sickle cell disease are prone to other forms of crisis. Aplastic crisis occurs when the marrow is temporarily suppressed, commonly as a result of intercurrent infection. It has been shown in recent years that the most frequent infection causing aplastic crises is human parvovirus. Although the marrow suppression is usually only for a few days and selective for the red cell series, owing to the markedly shortened red cell life span the fall in haemoglobin concentration is often dramatic and may be life-threatening. Aplastic crisis may occur at any age but the incidence decreases with age owing to acquired immunity from infection. It is not uncommon for the infection to spread through a family, so leading to siblings with sickle cell disease being affected together.

Sequestration crisis. In young patients a sequestration crisis may also result in a sudden life-threatening drop in the haemoglobin concentration. The sequestration may be in the spleen or less commonly in the liver. In either case there is rapid, painful swelling of the affected organ over a few hours accompanied by dramatic worsening of the anaemia, requiring rapid intervention by transfusion. There is a significant risk of recurrence and in view of the life-threatening nature of splenic sequestration splenectomy should always be considered in this condition. Although rare, sequestration may occur in adults.

Acute chest syndrome. A particularly life-threatening complication is the acute chest syndrome, which may present with chest pain alone or mimicking pneumonia. The condition may rapidly progress to fulminating lung failure if prompt exchange transfusion is not instituted. Such action has to be taken before any result is available from the microbiologist. Likewise at this early stage the chest radiograph is often normal. With pneumonia being common in these patients identifying this syndrome calls for close observation of patients with chest symptom; any suggestion of progression should raise the possibility of acute chest syndrome in the physician's mind.

Other manifestations. Other complications, although less acute, nonetheless cause a significant morbidity in SCD. Leg ulcers are particularly common. They arise spontaneously and need diligent care, possibly including transfusion, if they are to heal quickly. The few that become intractable can cause contractures if the underlying tendons become involved and it is preferable to attempt skin grafting if this outcome appears likely. Retinal microinfarcts are also more common with increasing age and may occasionally be sufficiently severe to cause loss of sight. This complication is more common in patients with higher haematocrits, appearing to be a direct consequence of the rise in viscosity. Hyposthenuria is also more severe with increasing age and results from gradual papillary necrosis. This may be a distressing symptom and early identification and reassurance is of value as it rarely progresses to significant renal failure.

Management

The early intervention in crises not only shortens and relieves the patient's discomfort but also probably reduces the incidence of complications in the long term. The main factors needing early attention are:

Pain. The severity of the pain of an infarctive crisis is often underestimated by both medical and nursing staff. Earliest possible administration of analgesia not only brings relief but gives the patient confidence. As the patient has usually taken mild analgesics before seeking help, opiates are frequently required. Pethidine because of its short action is particularly useful but frequent repeated doses are needed in most cases, often as high as 150 mgm 2-hourly for a period until the pain subsides, when the drug should be gradually withdrawn.

Dehydration. Owing to their illness these patients are often dehydrated due to poor fluid intake, hyposthenuria and increased insensible loss if there is an associated fever. At least three litres of fluid every 24 hours should be maintained until the crisis abates and this usually has to be administered intravenously in a crisis severe enough to require hospital admission. Patients should be advised to increase fluids as a protective measure should they begin to develop a crisis or an intercurrent infection.

Hypoxia. As well as advising patients not to expose themselves to hypoxic stress, e.g. high altitude, hypoxia should be borne in mind as an aggravating factor in any patient in crisis, particularly if pneumonia or other lung complication is suspected. Adequate oxygenation is essential. Patients are often advised not to fly but most are able to fly in standard pressurised commercial aircraft with no problems, although there are undoubted cases of crises being precipitated by flying. Patients with SCD should be told to take plenty of fluids prior to and during flight to avoid the dehydration that normally occurs.

Infection. Due to the increased susceptibility to infections and the effect of fever in inducing sickling it is imperative to treat infection in SCD promptly and vigorously. First, as a prophylactic measure all children should have daily oral penicillin to protect against pneumococcal infection. The value of pneumococcal vaccine in this respect has recently been questioned and if the child can be relied on to take the antibiotic it is probably not so important. The age at which the penicillin may be stopped is much debated, although most patients, even if not advised to stop, do so in their teens. Any SCD patient who is feverish needs adequate investigation and prompt treatment of any infection. If there is already an established crisis, such treatment may have to be 'blind' until the microbiology is known. As crisis in SCD also causes fever, the problem of differential diagnosis is always present, but if in doubt antibiotics should be given.

Transfusion. As well as treating anaemia in crises, transfusion also helps in aborting severe crises. This is particularly important in life-threatening situations such as acute lung syndrome, where early intervention is often life-saving. The use of regular transfusion is much more debatable but because of the long-term complications, particularly iron overload, it should be avoided unless crises are so frequent as to cause a severe social disruption or impair academic progress.

Diagnosis

The clinical story outlined above coupled with confirmation of the haemolytic anaemia and a blood film showing the characteristic sickle cells usually indicates SCD, but identification of the type is important as some of the mixed syndromes are not stereotyped in presentation. In particular the haemoglobin concentration may be normal in HbSC disease but rarely is in HbSS disease. All patients with SCD have a raised reticulocyte count in the steady state. The initial test used is frequently the solubility test, which is simple and reliable if performed properly and interpreted by an experienced worker. Recent studies have shown this test to be unreliable if performed only occasionally by untrained staff, which may happen in emergencies. The results of all, including negative, solubility tests should be confirmed by haemoglobin electrophoresis as soon as possible. In spite of these reservations the solubility test is a valuable investigation for rapid specific identification of sickle haemoglobin but it does not differentiate between SCD and sickle trait, for which haemoglobin electrophoresis is required.

Haemoglobin electrophoresis is performed at acid pH usually on cellulose acetate. An abnormal band in the position of sickle haemoglobin must be confirmed with a positive solubility test as HbD has the same mobility. If the solubility test is negative, the abnormal haemoglobins should be confirmed as HbD on agar gel electrophoresis which separates it from haemoglobin S. It also separates HbC and E which have the same mobility on cellulose acetate. In HbSS the HbS is the predominant band with a band of HbF, the fraction of which is usually raised to between 5 and 15%, and occasionally as high as 20%. The fraction of HbA_2 is normal. If SCD is due to double heterozygous condition, then the two haemoglobins are present in equal proportions. The most common such condition is HbSC disease. More difficult to identify is HbSD disease, as the two haemoglobins have the same mobility on the standard electrophoresis and a positive solubility test. Identification requires agar gel electrophoresis which at diagnosis should be performed on all patients to exclude the presence of HbD.

SCD due to Hb-beta thalassaemia needs careful identification. In HbS-beta zero thalassaemia HbA is not produced, whilst in -beta plus thalassaemia the fraction of Hb in A is between 15 and 30%. It is necessary to measure the fraction of HbA and measure the red cell indices to ensure separation from HbAS. The interaction of either blood transfusion or iron deficiency must be considered in interpreting all these tests. Family studies are invaluable in clarifying difficult cases.

Sickle cell trait

The carrier state, sickle cell trait (HbAS), is practically asymptomatic and poses no threat to life expectancy. However, because its incidence is so high in some populations (see above), the chance of a couple being at risk of having a child with sickle cell disease is high. Rarely, sickle cell trait may cause spontaneous haematuria owing to the hyperosmolar stress on the red cells in the renal tubules being sufficient to cause papillary necrosis similar to that occurring in diabetes. Renal failure is not a usual sequel but HbAS clearly needs to be considered in the early investigation of haematuria.

The presence of approximately 45% sickle haemoglobin in the red cell may allow sickling to occur if the hypoxia is severe enough, as may happen in anaesthetic accidents or on exposure to very high altitude. For these reasons it is important that symptomless carriers are identified before operations under general anaesthetics or flying in unpressurised aircraft, although there is no reason why a sickle carrier should not fly in a standard pressurised commercial aircraft.

As there is frequently a need for urgent surgery and for the counselling of couples on the risk of having a child with SCD, it is beneficial to identify sickle carriers in the population. This latter aspect has taken on particular importance in the last few years with the development of techniques of antenatal diagnosis (see below). As a result there has been, in areas of high incidence of the gene in the UK, the development of a number of counselling centres where specially trained health visitors provide advice on both genetic and clinical aspects of SCD and also arrange for screening to be carried out. These centres have also provided an important educational service by talking to such groups as clubs, churches and schools. Such centres provide a valuable service, not only in identifying the carriers but in reassuring many people who have heard 'old wives tales' and are a valuable link between the hospital and the community.

Identification

Sickle cell trait does not cause anaemia or an abnormal blood film so, unlike thalassaemia trait, it is not detected on routine blood counts. Haemoglobin electrophoresis shows the presence of HbS in approximately equal proportions, although HbA is usually predominant and may be up to 60% of the total haemoglobin. The HbS may be distinguished from HbD using the solubility test and with agar gel electrophoresis.

The differentiation of sickle cell trait from sickle beta plus thalassaemia, in which the fraction of HbA may be as high as 25–30% of the haemoglobin, is afforded by the abnormal blood film and low red cell indices in the latter condition. Family studies when available are invaluable in this respect and iron deficiency complicating sickle cell trait should be borne in mind in the differential diagnosis.

ANTENATAL DIAGNOSIS OF HAEMOGLOBINOPATHIES

Antenatal diagnosis was first introduced in 1975 using the technique of cord blood sampling and chromatographic separation of the isotopically labelled haemoglobin chains, so enabling identification of both imbalanced chain synthesis and abnormal chains. The technique has proved to be very reliable for identifying SCD and thalassaemia if used between the eighteenth and twentieth week of pregnancy when production of beta chains is sufficient. The lateness in pregnancy has meant that the technique has not proved universally acceptable. The introduction of chorion villous sampling coupled with restriction analysis of the DNA has allowed diagnosis earlier. It may be applied between the eighth and twelfth week of pregnancy.

Restriction enzymes cut the DNA at specific sites determined by the base sequence, usually dependent on a sequence of four or six base residues. The resulting fragments are then separated and identified by electrophoresis similar to haemoglobin variants. This technique has proved relatively simple in the case of HbS, as several restriction enzymes recognise the new sequence provided by the abnormal substitution and not the sequence in the normal Hb. It is therefore possible to identify directly fetuses with sickle trait and SCD without the need for family studies.

In the case of beta thalassaemia the problem is more complicated, as there is a multitude of different DNA abnormalities that lead to thalassaemia. The most commonly used technique is restriction fragment length polymorphism analysis. This involves the study of the DNA of at least both parents and an affected sibling with restriction enzyme analysis in the hope of finding a specific restriction site linked with the abnormal phenotype. Using this method it is not always possible to give definitive advice to the parents as to whether the fetus is affected; it can only be presented as a probability. The statistics are usually improved by studying more family members, particularly other siblings or grandparents.

Chorion villous sampling with DNA analysis is more acceptable as it is performed so much earlier in pregnancy and data so far suggest that it is as safe and reliable as cord blood sampling. It does, however, require that the mother is seen at the earliest possible time in pregnancy so that the risk of her having an affected child is fully evaluated before undertaking a procedure which might, even if the risks are small, induce a miscarriage. The data so far do not indicate that the incidence of miscarriage is significantly increased by the procedure above the normal high rate at this stage of gestation. In the case of thalassaemia it is preferable to see the couple before the pregnancy so that any necessary family studies can be undertaken in good time and to enable counselling of the couple as to the risk of having an affected child. The 'walk in' counselling centres that have been opened in those areas with a high population at risk have proved invaluable in this respect. They have also played a major part in educating the various other health professionals of these changes in the management of the haemoglobinopathies in the child-bearing age group.

Owing to the widely differing perceptions, both by the patients and their professional advisors, as to which diseases justify termination of pregnancy, coupled with the unpredictably broad spectrum of the clinical severity of SCD, there is no firm advice as to which variants justify termination. This places a heavy burden on the doctor and other health professionals to be both well informed and impartial. This contrasts with thalassaemia major in which the clinical severity is usually predictable and on the whole more life-threatening.

OTHER HAEMOGLOBINOPATHIES

There are many abnormal haemoglobins reported but only those likely to be commonly encountered or with important clinical implications are dealt with here.

Haemoglobin C

This abnormal haemoglobin occurs in West Africa and is most common in Mali but is also not infrequently seen in northern Nigeria and Ghana. It often occurs in the Afro-Caribbean community in the UK. In the trait form it is asymptomatic but in the homozygous state gives rise to a mild haemolysis. Mild splenomegaly is common and the haemoglobin concentration is usually above 10 G/dl, although intercurrent infections and pregnancy may reduce this to values occasionally necessitating intervention.

The most important aspect of haemoglobin C is the interaction with HbS in the double heterozygous condition. Haemoglobin SC disease is one form of SCD with all the clinical implications outlined above. Hence in a population in which both haemoglobins are prevalent there is a need to recognise the genetic implications, particularly for antenatal counselling.

Laboratory diagnosis

The characteristic finding on the blood film of homozygous HbC disease is the presence of target cells, often as many as 60%. Crystals of HbC may also be seen on the blood film. Occasional target cells are also seen in the trait condition. In HbSC disease both target and sickle cells are found. On electrophoresis at alkaline pH on cellulose acetate HbC moves slower than haemoglobin S to the same position as HbA2 and HbE. Separation of HbS and C occurs on agar gel at acid pH.

Haemoglobin D

This haemoglobin, which is prevalent in parts of India, particularly the Punjab, is asymptomatic in both the trait and homozygous states. Its importance is that the doubly heterozygous condition with haemoglobin S gives rise to a particularly severe form of SCD. Since on electrophoresis at alkaline pH it has the same mobility as HbS, identification may be missed unless agar gel electrophoresis is done routinely on all SCD disease patients. Haemoglobin D is negative on the solubility tests for haemoglobin S.

Haemoglobin E

This variant is common in south east Asia. The trait form gives rise to mild microcytosis and hypochromia without anaemia. The homozygous state causes mild anaemia and splenomegaly with both hypochromia and target cells on the blood film. On electrophoresis HbE has the same mobility as HbC at alkaline pH but again separates on agar gel.

THALASSAEMIAS

The fundamental defect in the thalassaemias is a reduction in synthesis of one of the globin chains, resulting in an imbalance of chain synthesis. Reduction of alpha and beta chain synthesis causes alpha and beta thalassaemia respectively. Whilst there is a multitude of causes at the gene level of either form, the clinical expression of hypochromia and microcytosis is almost universal. Depending on the degree of chain imbalance so the clinical picture varies from a transfusion-dependent anaemia to a clinically silent feature which is usually detected coincidentally. Thalassaemia may involve the other globin chains which consequently have depressed synthesis but the two globin chains of paramount clinical importance are alpha and beta chains. In this necessarily brief review only those forms of thalassaemia commonly encountered in clinical practice will be considered.

Genetic basis

The alpha genes are duplicated on chromosome 16 and deletion of one or more of the four genes is the most common cause of alpha thalassaemia. In contrast the beta gene on chromosome 11 is not duplicated. There is a multitude of mechanisms, including point and nonsense mutations and partial deletions, causing beta thalassaemia which result in impaired or absent translation of the gene.

Owing to the varied number of possible alpha genes involved and the range of mechanisms involving the beta genes there is a wide spectrum of clinical expressions for the thalassaemias. Whilst worldwide there are many mechanisms causing thalassaemia, any one population group tends to have only one or at most a few abnormalities within it. This has proved valuable in applying molecular biological techniques to the diagnosis, particularly antenatal, of these disorders.

Clinical pathology

The hallmark of thalassaemia is the microcytosis and hypochromia of the red cells in the absence of iron deficiency. This reflects the poor haemoglobinisation due to the imbalance of globin chain synthesis.

In the mildest forms the haemoglobin concentration is maintained, whilst in the more severe forms it is so low that regular transfusion support is required. In the most severe forms the erythropoiesis is ineffective so the marrow, in its attempt to overcome the defect, expands to give the characteristic X-ray findings, particularly the 'hair on end' appearance in the skull. There is usually extramedullary haemopoiesis leading to massive hepatic and splenic enlargement. The marrow, if examined, shows hypercellularity, predominantly of the erythroid line. The greater the imbalance of globin chain synthesis the greater these pathological abnormalities. With increasing severity there is also a progressive shortening of red cell survival.

Since the first reports of thalassaemia it has been convential to describe the three forms as minor, intermedia and major based on the clinical severity, largely reflect-

ing the haemoglobin concentration. Now that the genetic basis is well defined as far as beta thalassaemia is concerned, the term 'intermedia' is probably best phased out as the condition has a multiplicity of causes at the genetic level (e.g. double heterozygotes). The terms 'minor' and 'major' are then reserved for the heterozygous and homozygous forms respectively.

Alpha thalassaemia

Alpha thalassaemia is particularly common in south east Asia and the Far East, less so but frequent in Africa and the Mediterranean, and rare in northern Europe. Chromosome 11 may have one or both alpha genes deleted (alpha 1 thalassaemia and alpha 0 thalassaemia respectively). Therefore two alpha genes are lost in both alpha 0 trait and homozygous alpha 1 trait. Loss of either one or two alpha genes gives rise to thalassaemia trait, the two forms being indistinguishable clinically although loss of two genes results in a lower average haemoglobin concentration. Double heterozygosity for alpha 1 and 0 thalassaemia results in loss of three alpha genes, causing haemoglobin H disease. Loss of all four alpha genes due to homozygous alpha 0 thalassemia causes hydrops fetalis. In south east Asia both alpha 0 and 1 thalassaemia are frequent, hence there occurs the total spectrum of clinical expression due to loss of between one and four genes. In Africa and the Mediterranean areas alpha 1 thalassaemia occurs almost exclusively, so the most severe clinical states of hydrops fetalis and haemoglobin H disease, which require the deletion of four and three genes respectively, are virtually unknown.

Alpha thalassaemia trait

The term alpha thalassaemia trait is applied to the loss of either one or two alpha genes. Commonly there is only a microcytic hypochromic blood film which is usually discovered coincidentally, often by the modern electronic cell counters. The patient may be mildly anaemic, but is still symptomless. If mild anaemia is present a misdiagnosis of iron deficiency may occur. The importance of identification lies both in avoiding unnecessary iron medication and in indicating a need for genetic counselling. This is particularly relevant in south east Asia where alpha 0 and alpha 1 thalassaemia are frequent and the possibility of haemoglobin H disease and hydrops fetalis is ever present.

Haemoglobin H disease

The loss of three alpha genes due to heterozygous alpha

0/alpha 1 thalassaemia gives a distinct clinical picture of chronic anaemia and splenomegaly with the thalassaemic blood picture. Being an alpha chain disorder the disease is present in the neonatal period when it may contribute to any jaundice present and cause anaemia which may require transfusion. As the child grows splenomegaly soon becomes evident. In both the child and the adult the haemoglobin lies between 8.00 and 11.00 gm/dl in the steady state and transfusion support is usually needed only in the case of intercurrent infections and during pregnancy. The spleen may become sufficiently large to require removal due either to its physical size or hypersplenism, which may also increase the transfusion support needed.

Hydrops fetalis

Owing to the need for some alpha chain synthesis for fetal haemoglobin (HbF) formation in the gestational period, the loss of all four alpha genes is incompatible with fetal survival. Death usually occurs at about the twenty-fourth week of pregnancy. As the condition is due to homozygous alpha 0 thalassaemia, it does not occur in Africa, whilst it is relatively common in the Far East where it is a recognised cause of recurrent late spontaneous abortions.

Beta thalassaemia

In contrast to alpha thalassaemia, beta thalassaemia occurs predominantly around the Mediterranean area, being very common in Greece and Turkey where the gene frequency reaches one in seven in some areas. Beta thalassaemia major, with its high morbidity and consequent heavy demand on health care resources, presents a severe economic problem to many countries. The advent of antenatal diagnosis in the past 15 years with an accompanying increase in awareness by the population at risk has resulted in an almost zero incidence of beta thalassaemia major in the newborn in many countries. This trend has been helped in the past 5 years by the increasing use of DNA analysis of chorion villous samples enabling the diagnosis to be established as early as the tenth week of pregnancy when termination of an affected fetus is more acceptable.

Beta thalassaemia trait

Clinically this condition is indistinguishable from alpha thalassaemia trait but there are important differences in the genetic counselling aspect. The risk of a couple who both have the trait having a child with thalassaemia major is one in four. Beta chain production normally increases to adult levels in the first few months of life, so the condition is not present at birth. The earliest diagnosis is usually possible around the age of 3 months but now, with the almost universal use of electronic counters, it is more frequently discovered coincidentally unless specific investigation is requested.

Beta thalassaemia major

This condition, also known as Cooley's anaemia, is the most severe form of thalassaemia seen in clinical practice. After being normal in the first month or two of life the child rapidly becomes transfusion-dependent with an enlarging spleen. Owing to the many genetic causes there is a wide spectrum in the clinical severity depending on whether there is no beta chain produced (beta 0) or reduced production (beta +). Without blood transfusion there is often difficulty in maintaining the haemoglobin even as high as 2–3 G/dl and the ineffective erythropoiesis results in marrow hypertrophy in its attempt to overcome the anaemia. The resulting bone changes give rise to the classical facies with the prominent frontal, parietal and maxillary bones with the associated typical radiological appearances. With the universal use of blood transfusion support these once characteristic signs of the condition are now rarely seen in the UK.

The current practice of maintaining the haemoglobin above 10 G/dl by regular transfusion has resulted in near normal growth and development. The spleen, however, continues to enlarge and frequently needs removal in childhood due to hypersplenism or occasionally because of its physical size. The regular transfusion regime leads to accumulation of iron and a chelation programme has to be commenced with the transfusions. Whilst it is clear that chelation results in a lower rate of iron accumulation and consequent improved survival, secondary failure of other organs, particularly endocrine, is still frequent. Thorough endocrine assessment is important throughout the patient's development, particularly around puberty when replacement hormonal therapy can improve the quality of life. The currently available chelating agents have to be given parenterally and the usual practice is for self-administration of desferrioxamine subcutaneously with an infusion pump overnight. This procedure in itself is off-putting and compliance, particularly during adolescence, is a problem. There are also frequent problems of discomfort at the site of injection and the need for an effective oral chelating agent is great. Current research trends are encouraging in this respect. Vitamin C should also be given to aid chelation and folic acid supplements are usual. After splenectomy prophylactic penicillin should be given for protection from pneumococcal infections. The role of pneumococcal vaccination is debated but may confer some benefit.

Laboratory diagnosis of thalassaemia syndromes

A summary of the findings in the commonly encountered forms of thalassaemia using the investigations discussed below are shown in Table 12.1. Coupled with clinical and family studies these tests resolve the diagnosis in the majority of cases.

Blood film

The initial finding of a microcytic hypochromic blood film in the absence of iron deficiency usually raises the possibility of the diagnosis. Whilst mild chain imbalance may cause only a minimal decrease in the MCV and MCH, it is usually detected by the modern electronic cell counters. The blood film also shows anisocytosis, poikilocytosis and target cells. The severity of the anaemia and red cell changes progresses with the degree of imbalance of chain synthesis, hence the trait forms show less severe abnormalities than thalassaemia major in which there is also a raised reticulocyte percentage and normoblasts are seen on the blood film.

Haemoglobin electrophoresis

The mainstay of diagnosis is haemoglobin electrophoresis at alkaline pH, commonly on cellulose acetate.

The hallmark of beta thalassaemia is a raised fraction of haemoglobin A_2 due to a relative decrease of beta chain production compared to delta chains. The increase in Hb A_2 may not occur in the mildest forms and it may also be normal if there is an associated iron deficiency, hence the need to be sure of the iron status before discarding the diagnosis on the basis of the haemoglobin

electrophoresis. In the trait HbF is usually not increased but on occasions may rise up to 5%. In untransfused homozygous beta 0 thalassaemia only HbF is found and small quantities of HbA and HbF in homozygous beta+ thalassaemia.

In alpha thalassaemia the non-alpha chains, both beta and gamma, combine to form an unstable tetramer HbH or Barts respectively; these species both migrate faster than haemoglobin A at alkaline pH. In the newborn period the fraction of haemoglobin Barts is raised progressively with increasing loss of alpha chain production, being up to 5% in alpha 1 thalassaemia to as high as 50% in HbH disease. The tetramer is unstable and if small quantities are present it may be missed on electrophoresis if the sample is old or the preparation of the haemolysate entails lengthy purification. After the neonatal period HbH is not found in alpha 0 and alpha 1 thalassaemia but clearly HbH persists if three genes are non-functional (HbH disease). Hence normal haemoglobin electrophoresis is found in alpha thalassaemia trait.

Other tests

'H bodies' are denatured haemoglobin and may be seen in HbH disease and alpha thalassaemia trait in blood films stained supravitally with new methylene blue.

In particularly difficult cases globin chain synthesis may be measured radio-isotopically. These techniques are also used for antenatal diagnosis but cannot be applied before the second trimester. As the genetic defect is increasingly better defined in the thalassaemias, first trimester is replacing second trimester diagnosis.

Whilst not defining the type of thalassaemia, isotope studies may be used to quantify red cell survival, hypersplenism and ineffective erythropoiesis, giving an assessment of the severity of the illness which may be useful in management, particularly in the decision as to whether to undertake splenectomy.

Table 12.1 The characteristic laboratory findings in the thalassaemias

Type	Hb conc	Hb electrophoresis
alpha trait 0,1,1+1	11–14	Neonate Hb Barts <10% Adult normal
alpha 1+0	8–10	Neonate Hb Barts 25% Adult HbH up to 25%
beta trait	11–14	Neonate normal Adult HbA$_2$ >3.5%
Beta major	<6	Neonate HbF only

Hereditary persistence of F

This condition is characterised by the persistence of HbF production into adult life. It is symptomless and occurs predominantly in Afro-Caribbeans. It is usually detected coincidentally on Hb electrophoresis. In combination with HbS it ameliorates the sickling process. It is important in the context of counselling to distinguish this condition from homozygous HbS with high HbF. This may be achieved by family studies and using the Kleihaur stain for HbF. In hereditary persistence of HbF the HbF is evenly distributed throughout all erythrocytes.

BIBLIOGRAPHY

Alter B P, 1988 Prenatal diagnosis: general introduction, methodology, and review. Hemoglobin 12: 763–772

Bank A, Markowitz D, Lerner N 1989 Gene transfer. A potential approach to gene therapy for sickle cell disease. Ann NY Acad Sci 565: 37–43

Brozovic M & Davies S 1987. Management of sickle cell disease. Postgrad Med J, 63: 605–609

Davies S C, Brozovic M, 1989 The presentation, management and prophylaxis of sickle cell disease. Blood Rev 3: 29–44

Embury S H, 1988 The different types of alpha-thalassemia-2: genetic aspects. Hemoglobin 12: 445–453

Fleming A F, 1989 The presentation, management and prevention of crisis in sickle cell disease in Africa. Blood Rev 3: 1–6

Higgs D R, Vickers M A, Wilkie A D, Pretorius I M, Jarman A P, Weatherall D J 1989 A review of the molecular genetics of the human alpha-globin gene cluster. Blood 73(5): 1081–1104

Hoffbrand A V, Wonke B 1989 Results of long term subcutaneous desferrioxamine therapy. Baillieres Clin Haematol 2: 345–362

Kazazian H H Jr, Boehm C D 1988 Molecular basis and prenatal diagnosis of beta-thalassemia. Blood 72: 1107–1116

Radin A I, Benz E J Jr 1988 Antenatal diagnosis of the hemoglobinopathies. Hematol Pathol 2(4): 199–220

Rodgers G P, Noguchi C T, Schechter A N 1989 Hemodynamic studies in sickle cell disease. Ann NY Acad Sci 565: 338–346

Schwartz E, Cohen A, Surrey S 1988 Overview of the beta thalassemias: genetic and clinical aspects. Hemoglobin 12: 551–564

Steinberg M H, 1988 Thalassemia: molecular pathology and management. Am J Med Sci 296: 308–321

Wainscoat J S, Thein S L, Weatherall D J 1987 Thalassaemia intermedia. Blood Rev 1(4): 273–279

Whitten C F and Bertles J F (Ed) 1989 Sickle Cell Disease. Ann NY Acad Sci 565: 1–346

Vichinsky E, Lubin B H 1987 Suggested guidelines for the treatment of children with sickle cell anemia. Hematol Oncol Clin North Am 1(3): 483–501

13. Iron deficiency and overload

R. D. Hutton

IRON DEFICIENCY

Iron is an essential constituent of haemoglobin and hence red blood cells require, compared to other cell types, large amounts. Symptoms of iron deficiency are mainly due to a deficit of haemoglobin and are therefore similar to those experienced in other types of anaemia. The degree of anaemia will depend upon the iron deficit, and the severity of symptoms, in the period over which it develops, together with other interacting factors including respiratory and cardiac function.

Iron deficiency is probably the commonest cause of anaemia throughout the world because the amount of iron in many diets is inadequate to keep pace with daily requirements. Every cell in the body contains iron and loss of any cell from the body (skin, gut, etc.) results in iron loss. This represents the so-called obligatory iron loss. There is also a continuous occult, and sometimes overt, loss of red cells from body surfaces. This iron must be replaced if a deficiency is not to occur. Additionally, there are extra requirements to meet the specific needs of growth, pregnancy and blood donation (Table 13.1). Pathological processes also add to this demand through blood loss, developing polycythaemia, increased exfoliation of cells from body surfaces, haemosiderinuria and pulmonary siderosis.

Pathophysiology

Iron is present in the diet in many forms which are absorbed at different rates. In a normal mixed diet haem iron is the most important source and because of this some vegetarians may need to supplement their dietary intake with non-organic iron. It is generally considered that a normal adult needs to take in about 15 to 20 mg of iron a day to remain in balance. The average western diet is usually only just adequate in this respect and indeed many manufactured foods have inorganic iron added in recognition of this.

Iron is normally absorbed into the body by active

Table 13.1 Average daily requirements of iron

Obligatory losses	0.5–1.0 mg
Normal menstrual loss	0.5–1.0 mg
Pregnancy (singleton)	2.0–3.0 mg
Lactation	0.5 mg
Growth	0.5 mg
Twice yearly blood donation	0.8–1.5 mg

To calculate the likely requirements for an individual, add together the relevant values.

transport across the wall of the duodenum and upper part of the jejunum. The mechanism is complex and incompletely understood but can be readily saturated by excess iron. Where very large amounts of inorganic iron are ingested (as in iron poisoning) the active transport mechanism is overtaken by passive diffusion across the gut wall. Disease of the upper small gut can lead to malabsorption of iron and this can be seen in coeliac disease and tropical sprue.

The amount of iron absorbed is normally closely controlled by the needs of the body. About 10% of the dietary iron is usually taken up by the body but this can be increased several-fold in iron deficiency, or reduced substantially if the body has surplus iron available. It is usual for the body to have some storage iron for times of increased need but this may vary from a few milligrams to a few grams.

Iron is best absorbed in the ferrous (reduced) form and absorption is improved by the presence of reducing substances such as ascorbic acid. Absorption is also increased by certain iron chelators and by alcohol. Hydrochloric acid in the stomach helps to maintain iron in the ferrous form and achlorhydria, whether due to gastrectomy, pernicious anaemia or therapy with antacids or H_2 receptor antagonists, will impair iron absorption. Other factors may decrease the amount of iron absorbed and these include the presence of phytates, tannic acid and tetracycline which form insoluble complexes with iron.

Table 13.2 The distribution of body iron in a healthy 70 kg male

Haemoglobin	2500 mg
Ferritin & haemosiderin	1000 mg
Myoglobin	140 mg
Iron-containing enzymes	10 mg
Serum iron	4 mg

Most of the iron in the body is in the form of haem. This is present in large amounts in red cells, muscle and liver where it is essential for the adequate supply of oxygen to respiring tissues. Iron (often in the haem form) is also present as an integral part of many enzyme systems and partakes in numerous biochemical pathways, particularly in electron transport systems and DNA synthesis. The protein transferrin actively binds and transports iron in the body and can be estimated by measuring the serum total iron binding capacity. The amount present is increased in iron deficiency and decreased in iron overload, liver disease, infection, malignancy and protein deficiency states. Excess iron is stored mainly in macrophages, inside which the protein ferritin can undergo degeneration to form haemosiderin. Serum ferritin normally contains very little iron but in health reflects the amount of storage iron. The distribution of iron in the body of a normal adult is shown in Table 13.2.

Clinical features

A good history is very important when assessing the cause of iron deficiency. Particular attention should be paid to the following points.

Previous history

Has the patient always been anaemic or has it been recurrent; or is this the first episode? Previous therapy and response, and results of specific investigations, if known, are useful. History of abdominal surgery along with type and extent of the pathology may provide invaluable information. Could the patient have a bleeding disorder?

Family history

Are there any familial complaints that may lead to iron deficiency, such as hereditary telangiectasia, polyposis coli, bleeding disorders, etc?

Diet.

Does the diet contain enough iron to meet physiological needs? Sometimes it is obvious that the diet is iron-deficient but in other cases expert assessment is required.

Blood loss

Is the patient aware of any increased blood loss? Specific enquiry must be made in women with regard to menstrual loss and pregnancies. It is difficult for many women to assess if their menstrual loss is or is not pathological. The best simple guide is the number of days that the patient bleeds; if this exceeds 7 days in 28 it is likely to be pathological. Sometimes specific measurements to reflect the quantity of blood loss need to be made.

The presence or absence of blood loss per rectum, or of black motions indicating higher gastrointestinal tract bleeding must be specifically asked about, but remembering that inorganic iron preparations will cause the patient's stools to become black. Many patients will not be aware that they are losing blood, whereas others have a greater curiosity about their bodily functions! This can result in patients saying that they do not lose blood per rectum or do not have black stools when they have never looked. None the less, it is possible to lose substantial amounts of blood into the gut without an obvious change in the appearances of the faeces. Blood loss from the urinary tract is more likely to be noticed but again some women may not look. Blood loss from the nose, respiratory system, or vomited blood will usually be noted by the patient, but again specific enquiry must be made. It may be appropriate to enquire specifically about residence in areas where parasitic diseases such as hookworm, whipworm or schistosomiasis are endemic.

Is the patient a recent or past blood donor? Approximately 150 to 250 mg of iron is lost for every unit of blood donated. Table 13.1 reveals why iron deficiency may easily occur in donors, particularly menstruating women, unless iron supplements are taken.

Disturbances of gastrointestinal function

Gut symptoms must be carefully enquired for, as bleeding is a frequent cause of iron deficiency. The amount of loss required to cause anaemia over a prolonged period is very small and may well not be observable by the patient. Heartburn, indigestion, regular taking of antacids, will point to an upper gastrointestinal cause for a deficiency, whereas a change in bowel habit, diarrhoea, intermittent constipation and diarrhoea, or passing slime per rectum, will indicate a loss in the lower bowel. The possibility of malabsorption should be considered where there is frequency of bowel action and/or steatorrhoea.

Drug history

Non-steroidal anti-inflammatory drugs invariably lead to increased occult bleeding from the stomach and occasionally to massive haemorrhage. Specific enquiry must be made about use of these drugs, particularly over-the-counter preparations, as many patients do not consider them drugs and even take them to aid sleep! Anticoagulants and antiplatelet agents are also likely to increase occult bleeding and menstrual loss.

Examination

Particular attention should be paid to markers of chronic deficiency such as koilonychia, angular stomatitis, atrophic glossitis and dysphagia. The gastrointestinal tract should always be examined carefully, starting at the mouth, looking for evidence of telangiectasia followed by a careful examination of the abdomen, and finishing at the anus where evidence of bleeding haemorrhoids or higher bowel disease may be revealed. Where gut blood-loss is suspected a rectal examination and proctoscopy and/or sigmoidoscopy must be performed. If possible any faeces should be observed for signs of overt abnormality and tested for occult blood. When there is evidence of pathological vaginal blood loss a full gynaecological examination should be performed.

Investigation

Iron deficiency is not a diagnosis but a symptom. It is essential that the underlying problem is diagnosed. All patients suspected of being iron deficient should have a full blood count performed. Further management and investigation is suggested in Fig 13.1.

Low risk patients are those in whom the most likely cause of deficiency is a simple imbalance between intake and requirements, or those in whom there is an obvious cause of pathological blood loss which can be easily

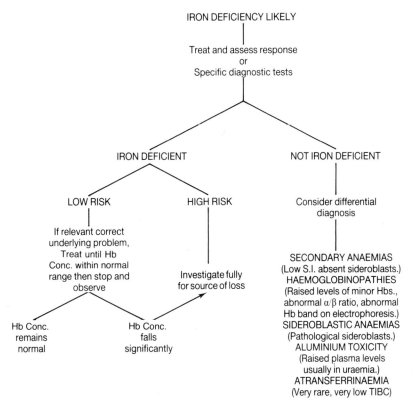

Fig. 13.1 Scheme for the further investigation of patients with apparent iron deficiency.

Table 13.3 Patient groups at low and high risk of having serious underlying pathology as the cause of their iron deficiency

Low risk patients
1. Males under 20 years of age
2. Pre-menopausal females and those within 2 years of the menopause
3. Patients in whom an easily remediable cause is identified

High risk patients
1. Those not fulfilling the above criteria
2. Those fulfilling the above criteria who have symptoms or signs suggesting serious disease

remedied (Table 13.3). High risk patients are more likely to have a serious underlying pathology and require full investigation to elucidate any disease process present.

Full blood count

This may be highly suggestive of iron deficiency but alone can never be diagnostic. As iron deficiency develops, the haemoglobin concentration falls with little change in the red cell indices, but with continued negative iron balance the indices become microcytic and hypochromic. In adults, if the MCH is below 27.5 pg, iron deficiency should be excluded. There is obviously no point in waiting until the MCV or the MCH fall to below the lower reference values, and any consistent fall should be investigated, as should cases of normochromic anaemia.

It is difficult to distinguish the appearances of iron deficiency from those that can occur in anaemia secondary to chronic inflammation, infection or malignancy. In such cases iron deficiency must be excluded. Complicating haematinic deficiencies are particularly likely where the haemoglobin concentration is lower than 9 g/dl. Occasionally very severe microcytic hypochromic anaemia is seen purely secondary to an inflammatory disease process.

The thalassaemia syndromes provide another cause of diagnostic difficulty with a microcytic hypochromic blood film, as may haemoglobinopathies. The frequency of such diagnostic confusion varies with geographical location and should be particularly considered in some parts of the world where thalassaemias are common. It may, however, arise in any population and should always be considered in the differential diagnosis. Thalassaemic syndromes are often suggested by the red count being relatively high compared to the haemoglobin concentration. Various 'discriminant functions' have been derived to try to assist in differentiating iron deficiency from thalassaemia trait but they

usually fail in cases of iron-deficient polycythaemia. In many cases of iron deficiency there is also a thrombocytosis. This is not very useful diagnostically as it often occurs in secondary anaemias.

The blood film appearances in iron deficiency are very variable, ranging from mild anisocytosis to gross anisopoikilocytosis with marked hypochromia and microcytosis. As noted previously there is often an accompanying thrombocytosis. The white blood cells are usually normal, but in severe deficiency sometimes there is a basophil leukocytosis and the neutrophils may show hyperlobulation of their nuclei. The presence of such features can only be suggestive, and not diagnostic, of iron deficiency.

Therapeutic trial of iron

In many cases this is the only investigation that is required to make a positive diagnosis of iron deficiency. Modern blood cell counters provide red cell histograms, and a response to therapy is usually obvious in a week or two by the appearance of a dual population. A rise in the haemoglobin concentration and in the red cell indices should also be readily apparent. A repeat FBC after two weeks oral iron therapy is far cheaper than requesting unnecessary haematinic assays. Reasons for failure to respond to iron are highlighted in Table 13.4 and will require further investigation.

Measurement of serum ferritin

In many centres this has now become a standard diagnostic test because the only known cause of a low value is iron deficiency. Normally the level of serum ferritin reflects the body iron stores to the extent that each 100 μg/l indicates approximately 800 mg of storage iron. A value of less than 15 μg/l is diagnostic of iron deficiency.

There are, however, circumstances in which the serum ferritin concentration is normal or even high despite iron deficiency. These include:

Liver dysfunction. The liver contains large amounts of ferritin even in iron deficiency. When the hepatocyte membrane is damaged, ferritin is released into the circulation, often in very large amounts. This liver ferritin

Table 13.4 Possible reasons for failure to respond to oral iron therapy

1. Therapy not being taken as prescribed
2. Continued blood loss
3. Other complicating conditions, e.g. uraemia
4. Severe malabsorption
5. Wrong diagnosis

is different from normal serum ferritin but routine testing assays both.

Increased haem turnover. This results in ferritin measurements that can substantially overestimate the body iron stores. Haem turnover will be increased wherever there is increased red cell breakdown. Apart from haemolysis, trauma (including surgical) will often leave substantial amounts of blood in tissues that will be metabolised. For this reason it is not uncommon to see a blood picture characteristic of iron deficiency in trauma patients who have normal ferritin levels.

Inflammatory lesions. It has been suggested that in the presence of malignancy, inflammation and infection the serum ferritin may be falsely high. For this reason some clinicians will treat such patients with oral iron if their serum ferritin is less than 40 μg/l.

Measurement of serum iron (SI) and total iron-binding capacity (TIBC).

In iron deficiency the SI level is low (less than 10 μmol/l) and the TIBC is usually raised (above 70 μmol/l). It is generally thought that erythropoiesis will become iron-deficient when the transferrin saturation (SI $\div$ TIBC $\times$ 100%) falls below 15%. Unfortunately the SI shows marked variation during the day, even in healthy subjects. A further diagnostic problem is that levels fall, often markedly, in the presence of infection or inflammation and so low readings do not always represent iron deficiency. The TIBC is also affected by nutrition and may be low in malnourished persons despite their being iron deficient. It is because of these problems that the serum ferritin is now so frequently the first line investigation when it is necessary to establish a diagnosis of iron deficiency.

The SI and TIBC remain very useful where there is reason to suspect that the ferritin result may be falsely high for the reasons discussed above. When iron deficiency is suspected from the FBC and the serum ferritin and iron is normal or raised, then a haemoglobinopathy should be excluded, or, rarely, a diagnosis of sideroblastic anaemia considered.

Bone marrow examination

The appearances of a Romanovsky stained marrow smear in iron deficiency are not unique. Similar appearances may be seen in secondary anaemias and in sideroblastic anaemias. For this reason Perls (Prussian blue) staining for iron in bone marrow aspirate is essential to the diagnosis.

In a normal bone marrow aspirate, stainable iron is usually evident within the macrophages and it can also be seen under high power within some of the developing erythroblasts (siderocytes). The absence of stainable iron indicates that the iron stores are low but it cannot be used to make a definitive diagnosis of iron deficiency. Conversely, the presence of stainable iron will exclude iron deficiency (exceptionally, following parenteral iron therapy, stainable iron may be observed in macrophages even when erythropoiesis is iron-deficient. The explanation for this is that the molecular complexes can not be broken down fast enough to supply the needs of the developing red cells).

The main use of a marrow aspiration is in clarifying a differential diagnosis. The presence of stainable iron normally excludes iron deficiency. Where there is plentiful macrophage iron, but virtually absent sideroblasts, this suggests secondary anaemia. When microcytosis is accompanied by plentiful sideroblasts, a haemoglobinopathy is suggested, or if the sideroblasts are ringed sideroblastic anaemia is probable.

Investigation of the cause of iron deficiency

As already highlighted iron deficiency is a symptom and the underlying cause should always be identified. In many cases the reason for the deficiency is obvious and easily treated. It should, however, always be considered that there may be more than one explanation for the deficiency and the patient reviewed appropriately. Many patients fall into a high risk group and do not have an easily identified cause for their problem. In such patients a methodical plan of investigation should be followed.

If blood loss studies are readily available, these can be extremely valuable in either distinguishing between inadequate intake and blood loss, or, in menstruating women, assessing the menstrual blood loss and ensuring that there is no pathological intermenstrual bleeding that requires investigation. An example of ^{59}Fe blood loss studies is shown in Fig 13.2.

All patients with unexplained iron deficiency must have a careful history and examination performed which should include a rectal examination and sigmoidoscopy. Faecal occult bloods can be useful in confirming that there is gastrointestinal tract bleeding but negative results should not delay further investigation as blood loss may be intermittent. Symptoms may suggest at which end of the gut investigations should begin but where they do not, a barium enema should be performed first, followed by a barium meal. It is important not to accept a benign lesion, such as diverticular disease or a hiatus hernia, as the source of blood loss without also excluding a more sinister lesion elsewhere in the gut. In some patients barium studies will not reveal a lesion and endoscopy will be required.

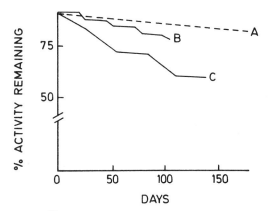

Fig. 13.2 ^{59}Fe blood loss studies showing: (**A**) Limit of normal loss, (**B**) Increased menstrual loss with normal intermenstrual loss, and (**C**) Intermittent blood loss in a patient with peptic ulceration.

Despite the above investigations the source of iron loss will remain unresolved in some patients. If gut loss is not obvious it is important to exclude haemosiderinuria by performing a Perl's stain on the patient's urinary sediment. If the diagnostic difficulty remains, then further specialised investigations such as a ^{99}Tc scan to look for a Meckel's diverticulum, a radiolabelled red cell scan or selective mesenteric angiography must be considered. Rarely a diagnosis may only be made at laparotomy.

If malabsorption is suggested by the patient's symptoms or by the finding of other deficiencies, particularly folate, small bowel biopsy will be required.

In some patients the diagnosis may still remain elusive and it should be remembered that a variation of the Munchausen syndrome is self-inflicted iron deficiency through blood letting. This may be extremely difficult to diagnose as patients can go to elaborate extremes to avoid detection.

Management

The treatment of iron deficiency is usually simple, whereas the management of the underlying cause may be much more difficult.

Oral therapy

There is normally no therapeutic advantage to using parenteral iron and as complications are more common compared to oral iron therapy, the latter is to be preferred. The Hb concentration should rise by between 0.1 to 0.2 g/dl a day regardless of the route of ad-

ministration. Reasons for therapeutic failure are given in Table 13.4. It should be noted that in cases of malabsorption it is usually possible to give adequate therapy by mouth.

Ferrous sulphate provides the most useful therapy. The standard adult dose is 200 mg twice daily. This provides 120 mg of elemental iron which is about the maximum that is tolerated without giving rise to symptoms. Giving higher doses is often counterproductive as patients may stop therapy because of gastrointestinal disturbances. To further reduce the incidence of side effects the iron should be administered with food. An alternative therapy is ferrous gluconate. A 300 mg tablet supplies 35 mg of elemental iron and so should be given three times a day for maximal effect. For children appropriate dose reductions should be made and liquid preparations may be easier to administer.

Where the aim is to prevent recurrent iron deficiency, smaller doses of iron may be sufficient and the minimum dose necessary should be ascertained. There is no therapeutic advantage in giving either slow release or combination preparations of iron but there is a cost disadvantage. Where there is a failure of response to a slow release preparation, there is often a satisfactory response to plain ferrous sulphate or gluconate. The explanation is that the slow release iron is probably being made available beyond the site of maximal absorption in the gut.

Oral iron therapy should not be administered with tetracycline, trientine, penicillamine, magnesium trisilicate or zinc salts, as this will result in decreased absorption of one or both substances. In all cases the patient and/or carer should be warned that the iron will result in the motions becoming black. Adequate warning must also be given of the toxic hazard from overdosage and advice given to keep iron therapy away from small children.

Parenteral iron therapy

This should only be prescribed when oral therapy has failed and a definite diagnosis of iron deficiency has been made. The latter is particularly important as it is easy to cause iron overload by giving inappropriate therapy. One or more of the following circumstances will normally be present:

1. Genuine gastrointestinal intolerance to oral iron therapy. This is usually associated with gut pathology
2. The rate of iron (blood) loss exceeds the rate at which iron can be absorbed from the gut

3. Severe malabsorption
4. Non-compliance.

Parenteral iron is usually given in the form of iron dextran but is also available as iron sorbitol. Only the dextran preparation is suitable for intravenous use and both preparations should be avoided in patients with liver disease and renal disease, particularly renal tract infections. Rarely the dextran preparation is associated with severe anaphylactic reactions and should be used with extreme caution in patients with a history of allergic disorders. The manufacturer's instructions should be carefully complied with. The intramuscular route is preferred but the intravenous route may be required in patients with coagulation disorders, small muscle mass or where frequent therapy would be required to keep pace with continued blood loss.

Blood transfusion

This should be reserved for the management of acute, potentially life-threatening haemorrhage, for patients who have severe symptomatology that will not respond to other therapy (e.g. diuretics for heart failure) and to prepare severely anaemic patients for emergency or acute surgery. It can seldom, if ever, be justified to transfuse a patient with iron deficiency simply for the convenience of the attending clinician (e.g. for routine cold surgery).

Duration of therapy

Where a patient is in a low risk group (see Table 13.3) treatment should be continued only until the haemoglobin concentration is back within the normal range. This should not take more than 4–6 weeks. If the Hb concentration is not within the normal range within this time, then a reason for the failure of response should be sought (see Table 13.4). Following this initial course of therapy iron supplements should be stopped and the patient observed over some months to ensure that there is no drop in the Hb concentration. If there is, then the patient should be investigated as a high risk patient.

Where a cause of iron loss has been established and rectified, treatment should continue for three months beyond the time when the Hb concentration becomes normal. This is to replenish the iron stores. In some patients iron deficiency is recurrent due to either deficient intake or a continuing source of loss that can not be easily rectified. In these patients long term supplements are justified and the minimum amount necessary to maintain iron balance should be prescribed. This is

so that other new additional causes of iron deficiency (e.g. gastrointestinal neoplasm) will not be masked.

IRON OVERLOAD

Storage iron is normally beneficial as it provides for circumstances when iron requirements exceed available dietary intake. This occurs most commonly following blood loss. Usually storage iron accounts for only a small proportion of total body iron, varying from a few to several hundred milligrams. Rarely does it exceed one gram.

There is no physiological mechanism for excretion of excess iron and control of stores relies entirely on mucosal absorption. Excessive storage iron may arise from inappropriate absorption, from red cell transfusions or the unnecessary parenteral administration of iron.

The terminology used to classify iron overload is confusing as the same name is used by different authors to describe various conditions. Hereditary haemochromatosis is a genetically determined disorder of iron handling; it is also called primary haemochromatosis. Secondary haemochromatosis, or haemosiderosis, should be used to refer to all other disorders leading to excessive iron loading.

Pathophysiology

Inappropriate absorption

Ingested iron is largely not absorbed and passes out of the gut. Iron absorption is normally controlled by the intestinal mucosal cells. These pass iron on into the portal blood if there is excess plasma-binding capacity. When stores are adequate most of the absorbed iron remains in the mucosal cells and is lost from the body when they exfoliate. Iron passing into the portal blood is transported on transferrin and taken up directly by cells requiring iron. Excess iron is stored in macrophages, initially as ferritin and longer-term as haemosiderin.

Inappropriate high absorption occurs in the following conditions:

Hereditary haemochromatosis. The precise biochemical abnormality associated with this disorder is not understood but iron continues to be actively absorbed even in the face of high transferrin saturations. The gene frequency for this condition appears to be very high. The disease occurs in homozygotes but is not always expressed due to the variable opportunity to accumulate excess iron in relation to diet and blood loss. It is thought that heterozygosity markedly increases the chances of developing iron overload when it is in association with other risk factors.

Where large amounts of readily absorbable iron are present in the diet. This is seen in Bantu siderosis and probably also accounts for the iron loading seen in other patients with high ethanol intakes.

Increased plasma iron turnover. This is usually associated with ineffective erythropoiesis or haemolysis. The thalassaemia syndromes account for the majority of such cases.

Iron overload appears to produce its toxic effects when the flux between storage and circulating iron pools is such that the plasma transferrin is highly saturated. This is thought to result in weakly bound, potentially toxic iron being present in solution. Several biochemical reactions are catalysed by 'free' iron and produce highly reactive superoxide and hydroxyl radicals. These probably produce tissue damage by lipid peroxidation. Ascorbate deficiency may also occur as it is oxidised to the inactive dihydroascorbate by 'free' iron. Vitamin C needs to be given with care to patients with iron overload as it markedly increases lipid peroxidation and can lead to increased cardiac dysfunction.

Toxicity occurs at different levels of iron stores in different patients and is probably related to plasma iron turnover.

Clinical features

The tissue damage produced by iron overload leads to increased pigmentation, hepatic cirrhosis, cardiac dysfunction, arthropathies and endocrine failure including diabetes mellitus. The presenting features will vary with the age at which the overload began and will be modified by pre-existing cardiac, hepatic or pancreatic dysfunction.

If iron overload is present prior to puberty, pituitary failure results in poor development of secondary sexual characteristics and a reduced or absent adolescent growth spurt.

Many of the features of iron overload are common in an elderly population and the diagnosis is probably frequently overlooked.

History

A careful family history needs to be taken, particularly for the conditions that occur secondary to iron overload. Enquiries should be made of the use of therapeutic iron and red cell transfusions. Alcohol intake should be assessed together with a careful dietary history. In females enquiry should be made of premature menopausal symptoms.

Examination

In children failure of puberty and growth should be assessed. In all patients pathological pigmentation should be sought together with evidence of cardiac arrhythmias and congestive cardiomyopathy. Hepatic size and texture should be assessed clinically and by ultrasound. In adult males testicular atrophy should be looked for. Joints should be examined for signs of arthropathy.

Investigation

A high level of clinical suspicion is necessary if the diagnosis is not to be missed. A good case can be made for screening all patients with maturity onset diabetes, cardiac arrhythmias (particularly if of early onset), congestive cardiomyopathy, early gonadal failure, pathological pigmentation, and unexplained hepatic dysfunction. The close relatives of patients with hereditary haemochromatosis should also be investigated. This is most important if the complications of iron overload are to be avoided, as treatment should be started at a pre-symptomatic stage.

Diagnostic tests

Serum iron and total iron-binding capacity are the most useful screening tests for iron overload and are essential when screening for hereditary haemochromatosis. In such patients a transferrin saturation of 50–70% usually indicates heterozygosity or an early case of homozygosity. Homozygotes usually have values in excess of 70% but this depends on their opportunity to have accumulated excess iron. Testing should be repeated in individuals at risk as a single value may give a misleading picture.

The serum ferritin test is useful in cases of transfusional siderosis where there is an excellent correlation with the amount of blood transfused. Falsely high levels are common in liver disease and falsely low levels in the early stages of iron accumulation in hereditary haemochromatosis.

Liver biopsy is helpful not only in providing evidence of hepatic damage but also in assessing the degree of iron overload by measuring the chemical iron content of part of the biopsy.

Desferrioxamine has been used to diagnose iron overload by observing the urinary iron excretion following a standardised test dose. The test does not, however, give quantitative results and its usefulness is probably limited.

Venesection can be used to assess mobilisable iron and provides the most accurate guide to the degree of iron overload in those patients in whom it can be used.

Management

Avoidance of excess iron

Patients at risk of iron overload should be carefully counselled to avoid medication containing iron unless it has been positively shown that this is required. Dietary advice can be given to reduce the amount of iron ingested and to increase the quantity of natural chelators present in the diet to reduce iron absorption. Transfusion therapy should be kept to the minimum necessary, remembering that in patients with conditions marked by gross ineffective haemopoiesis, iron absorption is reduced by maintaining the haemoglobin concentration at a high level through suppressing erythropoiesis and hence plasma iron turnover. In children, haemoglobin concentrations need to be maintained to ensure normal development. If hypersplenism increases transfusion requirements, splenectomy should be considered.

Venesection therapy

This is the most effective therapy in patients with iron overload and reserves of red cell production. The amount of blood removed should be dependent on the patient's size and ability to maintain their haemoglobin concentration. An otherwise fit adult male should tolerate the removal of 500 ml of blood weekly. Frequent measurements of plasma proteins should be made and if these are falling the patient's own plasma can be reinfused. A careful record of the total amount of iron removed should be kept. This can be calculated at each venesection from the following formula:

Hb concentration in grams/l × volume removed in litres × 3.5 = approximate quantity of iron removed in milligrams.

Venesection should be continued until body iron stores are depleted, as shown by falling red cell indices, inability to maintain the haemoglobin concentration, a low serum ferritin and transferrin saturation. The decision to recommence venesection should be based on the transferrin saturation and *not* on the ferritin concentration.

Chelation therapy

In patients who are not suitable for venesection, chelation therapy is the only alternative. At present the only effective therapy must be given parenterally and is expensive, hence precluding its widespread use in many countries where thalassaemic syndromes are common.

In patients in whom it can be predicted that iron overload and associated toxicity will occur, therapy should be commenced at the earliest practicable stage to avoid organ damage. Desferrioxamine is the most widely used chelating agent. It is most effective when given by infusion therapy, which for practical reasons is usually administered subcutaneously for 12 hours a day. It is important to follow the manufacturer's guidelines.

Course and prognosis

All forms of therapy for iron overload have poor patient acceptability and this still remains a major stumbling block in management. Compliance with chelation therapy may be particularly poor in teenagers with thalassaemia and careful counselling and support are essential. It would appear that rigorous adherence to a chelation regime in thalassaemia major markedly improves the prognosis.

In all forms of iron overload improvements in organ function are frequently seen following reduction of the iron load. This is, however, variable and unpredictable. Patients with cardiac and hepatic problems need to be counselled carefully with regard to alcohol use as it can lead to further deterioration in function. Hepatoma is a complication which can occur many years after otherwise successful therapy.

The only way to avoid irreversible organ damage is to commence therapy before there is significant iron overload. This makes family studies and appropriate genetic advice particularly important in patients with hereditary haemochromatosis.

Future developments

There has been considerable research in the development of oral iron chelators. Many highly effective substances have now been developed and the outcome of long-term toxicity studies is eagerly awaited.

The genetic basis of hereditary haemochromatosis is also under study and the availability of more specific genetic markers for the disorder will considerably help in diagnosis and counselling.

BIBLIOGRAPHY

Jacobs A Disorders of iron metabolism 1982 Clinics in Haematology II
Jacobs A 1982 Disorders of iron metabolism. Recent advances in haematology 3: 1–24. Churchill-Livingstone.
Pippard M J, Callender S T 1983 The management of iron chelation therapy. British Journal of Haematology 54: 503–507

14. Disorders of haem and porphyrin synthesis

D. S. Gillett

One might expect the clinical effects of disordered haem synthesis or porphyrin metabolism to be similar to those caused by the thalassaemias. Indeed, the sideroblastic anaemias are characterised by defective iron utilisation and haemoglobin production. Whereas in the thalassaemias globin chains accumulate and cause haemolysis, in the sideroblastic states iron accumulates but there is little effect on the red cell lifespan. The porphyrias are a group of hereditary disorders characterised by accumulation of intermediates of haem synthesis and the clinical manifestations depend on the exact biochemical defect involved. Most of the latter defects are now characterised. Although, perhaps surprisingly, only two subtypes of porphyria are associated with significant anaemia, these diseases are generally considered in the haematology texts as they throw considerable light on normal haem metabolism and on the acquired disorders of porphyrin metabolism which are associated with anaemia.

Haem and porphyrin metabolism

Haem consists of four linked pyrrole rings with a central iron atom co-ordinated to the four nitrogen atoms. The iron atom has two further ligand binding sites, one of which is bound to a globin histidine residue and the other binds reversibly to oxygen. Haem is synthesised mainly in the mitochondria of the erythroblast, although some steps take place in the cytoplasm (Fig 14.1). The initial and probably rate-limiting step is the fusion of succinyl-Co A with glycine mediated by ALA synthase to form δ-aminolaevulinic acid (ALA). This step also requires pyridoxal phosphate. Two molecules of ALA are fused to form porphobilinogen (PBG) by ALA dehydratase. A double enzymatic step is required to form uroporphyrinogen III which is decarboxylated to coproporphyrinogen III. At this point, the pathway re-enters the mitochondrium where protoporphyrin IX is formed by coproporphyrinogen oxidase. Finally, iron is inserted to form haem by ferrochetalase. End product

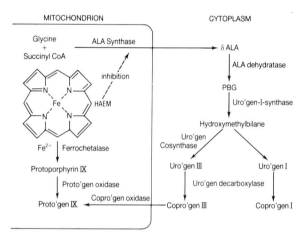

Fig. 14.1 Haem biosynthesis

inhibition of ALA synthetase controls the rate of haem synthesis.

A number of porphyrins are formed as byproducts or side reactions during the synthesis of porphyrin. Coproporphyrinogen I is also formed from porphobilinogen and this leads to a series of compounds with the porphyrin I structure which do not appear to be functional.

SIDEROBLASTIC ANAEMIAS

This is a diverse group of disorders (Table 14.1) characterised by the presence of ringed sideroblasts in the bone marrow. Large quantities of iron accumulate within the mitochondria which then degenerate, leading to a ring of coarse granules lying around the nucleus of the erythroblast which are visible with Perl's stain.

Hereditary sideroblastic anaemia

This is a rare disorder, mainly affecting males and

Table 14.1   Classification of sideroblastic anaemias

Hereditary
X-linked hypochromic microcytic anaemia due to defects of
heam pathway enzymes

Acquired
Primary acquired sideroblastic anaemia (RA-S)
Secondary (reversible)
    Abnormalities of pyridoxine metabolism. Antituberculous
    drugs, alcoholism, malabsorption
    Abnormal haem synthesis. Lead poisoning, alcohol,
    chloramphenicol, erythropoietic porphyria
    Other causes. Rheumatoid arthritis, megaloblastic anaemia

Associated with myeloproliferative disease
AML, myelofibrosis, primary proliferative polycythaemia,
MDS (subtypes other than RA-S)

presenting in youth or early adult life. Patients present
with a dimorphic anaemia and splenomegaly and may
be well compensated despite a low haemoglobin concentration. There may be an element of hypersplenism
resulting in leukopenia and thrombocytopenia. The
peripheral blood may also show basophilic stippling,
occasional siderocytes and nucleated red cells, and in
the marrow erythroblasts show cytoplasmic vacuoles.
Staining for iron shows that most of the late
erythroblasts are ringed sideroblasts. There is usually
increased iron absorption with a raised ferritin and
transferrin saturation even in the untransfused. The
differential diagnosis includes thalassaemia and congenital dyserythropoietic anaemia which can be excluded by
haemoglobin electrophoresis and by marrow appearances.

Primary acquired sideroblastic anaemia

This has been shown to be a clonal disorder resulting
from stem cell mutation and has now been reclassified
with the myelodysplastic syndromes (MDS) as refractory anaemia with ringed sideroblasts (RA-S). Like the
other MDS it is a disease of the elderly and cytogenetic
abnormalities may be observed but transformation to
AML is less common. The anaemia is usually
normochromic but macrocytic and occasional hypochromic cells are seen in addition to basophilic stippling. Other cytopenias not infrequently co-exist. The
bone marrow shows erythroid hyperplasia with dysplas-
tic and sometimes megaloblastic features mainly
affecting erythropoiesis. The majority of red cell precursors are abnormal ringed sideroblasts. The FAB
diagnostic criteria require more than 15% of the
erythroid precursors to be ringed sideroblasts.

Secondary sideroblastic anaemia

Pyridoxine deficiency

Reversible sideroblastic anaemia has been reported in
association with coeliac disease and haemolytic
anaemias, usually with co-existent folate deficiency.

Alcoholism

This is one of the most common causes of the
sideroblastic state, although the anaemia is multifactorial
in aetiology as such patients are generally malnourished.
Acute intoxication suppresses the haem synthetic enzymes ALA dehydratase and ferrochetalase and
increases ALA synthase in the bone marrow, and alcoholics have been noted to show excessive urinary
coproporphyrin excretion. Pyridoxine metabolism is also
abnormal. The anaemia is dimorphic and the marrow
is generally megaloblastic and sideroblastic. The changes remit rapidly following alcohol withdrawal and
pyridoxine supplements may be helpful.

Antituberculous drugs

A minority of patients treated with isoniazid, para-
aminosalicylic acid, cycloserine and pyrazinamide for
long periods develop sideroblastic anaemia.

Lead poisoning

Lead affects many of the haem synthetic enzymes and
chronic ingestion causes anaemia which is usually normochromic or mildly hypochromic. The mechanism is
probably due to chelation with enzymic sulphydryl
groups. There is a resulting accumulation of protoporphyrin in red cells with increased urinary excretion of
ALA, coproporphyrin and PBG. Inhibition of the enzyme pyrimidine-5'-nucleotidase causes precipitation of
reticulocyte RNA, leading to punctate basophilia which
is characteristic. The anaemia is partly due to a reduction in red cell lifespan due to denaturation of structural
proteins and partly due to inhibition of haemoglobin
synthesis. Plumbism generally used to occur in children
with pica who ingested flaking lead-based paints and
following industrial exposure to lead. It has now been
reported in Asians who have used lead-containing cosmetics or traditional medicines. Children with lead
poisoning are often iron-deficient as well. The clinical
features of lead poisoning are remarkably similar to
those of acute hepatic porphyria (abdominal pains,
neuropsychiatric symptoms) and are presumed to result
from disordered haem biosynthesis, although the
mechanism remains obscure.

Miscellaneous causes

Chloramphenicol causes a reversible sideroblastic anaemia in some patients, possibly by inhibition of mitochondrial protein synthesis with a secondary effect on haem synthesis. In erythropoietic porphyria there is reduced activity of ferrochetalase with resulting accumulation of iron in the mitochondria. The occasional observation of sideroblastic anaemia in association with rheumatoid arthritis, carcinoma, hypothyroidism, polyarteritis nodosa and other non-haematological conditions is difficult to explain. Sometimes there is co-existing folate deficiency and some may respond to pyridoxine therapy. Sideroblastic changes which are obscure in aetiology may also be observed in various haematological disorders, e.g. myelofibrosis, primary proliferative polycythaemia, AML, pernicious anaemia and in the other myelodysplastic syndromes. In the majority of cases such changes are minimal and they generally fail to respond to pyridoxine therapy.

Complications and management of sideroblastic anaemia

The major complication in primary sideroblastic anaemia, both hereditary and acquired, is that of iron overload due in part to increased absorption. Blood transfusion should be used sparingly since each 400 ml of blood adds 200 mg of iron to the body stores. Oral iron supplements must be prohibited and in the younger patient desferroxamine chelation should be considered, particularly if repeated transfusions are necessary. A variety of drugs has been used to treat sideroblastic anaemia but, in general, the response is disappointing. A minority of patients respond to combination treatment with pyridoxine 200 mg daily and folic acid 5 mg daily which should be given as a therapeutic trial for several months. Most patients with primary acquired sideroblastic anaemia require chronic transfusion support. The treatment of secondary sideroblastic states is the removal of the underlying cause. Symptomatic lead poisoning in children should always be treated energetically.

PORPHYRIAS

The porphyrias result from hereditary abnormalities of haem metabolism and are characterised by accumulation of haem synthetic pathway intermediates. They are all inborn errors of metabolism, perhaps with the exception of porphyria cutanea tarda where inheritance is not always demonstrable. The rest are inherited in an autosomal dominant manner with the exception of con-genital erythropoietic porphyria which is autosomal recessive.

Classification

Haem synthesis is most active in the bone marrow erythroblasts and in the hepatocytes where it is required for synthesis of a variety of enzymes. Thus, the porphyrias can be classified as erythropoietic (CEP, EPP) or hepatic (the rest) in type, depending on the major site of overproduction of porphyrins or their precursors. They can also be classified clinically into acute and non-acute forms. The acute porphyrias (AIP, HCP, PV) are characterised by neurovisceral symptoms; the non-acute porphyrias by cutaneous photosensitivity. Certain clinical features such as photosensitivity occur both in the erythropoietic and the hepatic porphyrias (except AIP) and therefore the above classification is not always very helpful. A more specific diagnosis should always be sought which should take account of clinical features, mode of inheritance, pattern of excretion of porphyrins and their precursors and, where necessary, determination of the specific enzyme deficiency. The enzyme uroporphyrinogen-I-synthase plays a pivotal role in determining the biochemical and clinical manifestations of the various porphyrias (Fig 14.1). In AIP, the activity is reduced, in HCP and VP it is normal and in the non-acute porphyrias it is increased.

Acute intermittent porphyria (AIP)

Clinical features

AIP is the most common type of porphyria and is inherited in an autosomal dominant fashion. The disease is more common in females and presents as an acute neuropsychiatric illness with a variable attack frequency. The first attack is usually in early adult life and any attack should be treated as potentially fatal. Most patients present with a constellation of symptoms including abdominal pain, anorexia, constipation, neuropathies, convulsions, acute psychosis, hypertension and tachycardia. Attacks are often precipitated by drugs (see below), alcohol, fasting and acute infections.

Diagnosis

The defect in uroporphyrinogen-I-synthase results in accumulation of ALA and PBG in blood and urine, particularly during attacks. Porphyrin excretion may be normal between attacks. Post-mortem studies show acute demyelination and axonal degeneration but the mechanism is unclear.

Management

The precipitating factors must be removed and adequate fluid, electrolyte and calorie intake instituted. Glucose can block the hepatic production of ALA which may help. A large number of drugs are contra-indicated, although the list in Table 14.2 is by no means exhaustive. Vomiting, severe abdominal pain, psychosis and hypertension may all require pharmacological control (see list of safe drugs). Intravenous haematin is often effective if given early during an attack (4 mg/kg over 20 min daily or 12-hourly). Patients generally recover completely between attacks but the neuropsychiatric symptoms may persist. Patients should be diligently counselled concerning the nature of their disease and the avoidance of precipitating factors and contra-indicated drugs. Relatives must be screened for occult or latent disease.

Table 14.2 Some indicated and contra-indicated drugs in acute porphyria

May precipitate condition	May be safe to use
Amitriptyline	Aspirin
Barbiturates	Atropine
Cytotoxics	Biguanides
Cimetidine	Cephalosporins
Dapsone	Chlorpromazine
Erythromycin	Codeine
Flufenamic Acid	Corticosteroids
Halothane	Diamorphine
Hydralazine	Fentanyl
Imipramine	Flurbiprofen
Isoniazid	Gentamicin
Ketoprofen	Heparin
Lignocaine	Ibuprofen
Methyldopa	Indomethacin
Metoclopramide	Methadone
Metronidazole	Morphine
Nitrazepam	Naproxen
Oral contraceptives	Paracetamol
Oestrogens	Penicillins
Pancuronium	Promethazine
Primidone	Propranolol
Pyrazinamide	Thiazides
Spironolactone	Trifluoperazine
Sulphonamides	
Sulphonylureas	
Tetracyclines	
Theophylline	
Tolbutamide	

Porphyria variegata (PV)

This type, which is the commonest in South Africa, presents with acute attacks as in AIP as well as photosensitive skin eruptions. Patients with PV may exhibit only dermatological symptoms or, conversely, only neurological disease but usually they occur simultaneously. The skin is fragile and sunlight induces vesicles or bullae with subsequent scarring, hyperpigmentation and hirsutism.

The biochemical defect is a deficiency of protoporphyrinogen oxidase and faecal excretion of protoporphyrin and coproporphyrin is increased. Urinary coproporphyrin is increased and, in the acute attack, ALA, PBG and uroporphyrin excretion increase as in AIP.

The treatment of the neurological manifestations of PV is the same as for AIP. Patients with skin disease should avoid sun exposure. Newer skin creams offer some protection but conventional UV barrier creams are of no use.

Hereditary coproporphyria (HCP)

This rare disease often remains latent and presents in a similar manner to PV. It is differentiated biochemically by demonstrating deficiency of coproporphyrinogen oxidase. Coproporphyrin III excretion is increased.

Cutaneous hepatic porphyria (CHP)

Also known as porphyria cutanea tarda, this disease which presents typically with photosensitive skin eruptions, particularly on the hands, is the commonest form of porphyria in Europe and North America. The appearances are similar to those seen in PV and there is usually an environmental precipitating factor. Most patients drink alcohol to excess or suffer from chronic liver disease and frequently in such cases no family history of PCT can be elicited. Liver biopsy usually shows hepatic siderosis. Hepatic porphyrin synthesis is increased and between attacks there is increased faecal excretion of coproporphyrin and proporphyrin. Activity of hepatic uroporphyrinogen decarboxylase is reduced.

Alcohol and a variety of chemicals must be avoided. Most patients have hepatic parenchymal iron overload and improvement in skin lesions and in liver function results from removal of iron by repeated venesection.

Congenital erythropoietic porphyria (CEP)

This is the rarest of the porphyrias and is transmitted

in an autosomal recessive manner. It presents in childhood with severe photosensitivity with bulla formation and scarring together with nail dystrophy and deformity of the fingers. Secondary infection of the skin is common and reddish discoloration of the teeth (erythrodontia) occurs. Hypertrichosis is often prominent and the urine is red in colour. These features are caused by excessive porphyrin production by the bone marrow. Most patients suffer from chronic haemolytic anaemia with marked splenomegaly which may result in other cytopenias. Ineffective erythropoiesis also contributes to the anaemia. The biochemical defect is a deficiency of uroporphyrinogen-III-cosynthase with increased porphyrin production by the erythron and increased urinary and faecal uroporphyrin-I excretion. The teeth, urine and bone marrow erythroblasts all fluoresce under UV light due to the presence of porphyrins.

Hypertransfusion (together with iron chelation with desferrioxamine) to maintain the PCV above 0.40 and suppress erythropoiesis has been shown to be effective. Splenectomy may be required. Exposure to sunlight must be avoided.

Erythropoietic protoporphyria (EPP)

Transmitted in an autosomal dominant manner, this disease can present at any age with photosensitivity and hepatic damage. Haemolysis is not a feature but there may be mild anaemia and liver damage is severe in a minority of patients. The defect appears to be a decreased activity of ferrochetalase resulting in overproduction of protopophyrin which is demonstrable in erythrocytes but urine porphyrins are normal, the excess being excreted in the bile. Cholestasis may occur and result in rapid hepatic porphyrin accumulation and consequent damage.

Cholestyramine may interfere with the enterohepatic circulation of protoporphyrin. Some workers have successfully used activated charcoal in a similar manner to increase faecal porphyrin excretion.

Other disorders associated with abnormal porphyrin metabolism

Porphyrinuria can occur in patients with liver disease or anaemia but is not associated with the clinical features of the diseases described above. Alcohol reduces the activity of most of the haem synthetic enzymes and changes the pattern of urinary porphyrin excretion. Ferrochetalase is particularly suppressed by alcohol and this may explain the occurrence of alcohol-induced sideroblastic anaemia. Porphyrin accumulation in erythrocytes is one of the first findings in iron deficiency before peripheral blood appearances alter. This can be used to differentiate iron deficiency from thalassaemia trait and it may also be useful in situations where the serum ferritin is misleading, for example, in chronic inflammatory states co-existing with iron deficiency.

BIBLIOGRAPHY

Goldberg A, Moore M R (eds) The porphyrias. Clinics in Haematology, vol 9. W B Saunders, London
Kappas A et al 1983 The porphyrias. In: Stanbury J B et al (eds) The metabolic basis of inherited disease, 5th edn. McGraw-Hill, New York
Moore M R Laboratory investigation of disturbances of porphyrin metabolism. Association of Clinical Pathologists broadsheet 109. British Medical Association, London
Piomelli S 1987 The diagnostic utility of measurements of erythrocyte porphyrias. Hematology and Oncology Clinics of North America 3: 419–30
The Porphyrias. Seminars in Haematology October 1988.

White cell disorders

15. Molecular and cytogenetic aspects of leukaemias and lymphomas

C. M. Steel

If the property of malignancy were not passed on to the progeny of a malignant cell, there would be no tumour. It is thus axiomatic that malignancy involves a permanent heritable change (i.e. a mutation) and hence that the seat of the disorder is in the DNA of the affected cells.

Leukaemias and lymphomas offer three lines of direct evidence in support of this theoretical conclusion. First, many animal leukaemias and lymphomas are caused by viruses, through a mechanism that involves synthesis of a DNA 'provirus' copy of the viral RNA, using reverse transcriptase, and insertion of that DNA in the host cell genome (Fig. 15.1).

Secondly, the monoclonal (or at most oligoclonal) origin of human leukaemias and lymphomas has been demonstrated repeatedly, initially by using the X-linked marker glucose-6-phosphate dehydrogenase (G6PD) which has two common alleles in Africans and black Americans. In female patients whose normal tissues are heterozygous for G6PD types A and B, leukaemias and lymphomas generally show only one G6PD type (either A or B) implying that in all the malignant cells the same X chromosome is inactivated and hence that they belong to a single clone. Clonality of B lymphoid neoplasms has been proved by demonstrating identity of the immunoglobulin synthesised by all the cells of the tumour. In recent years molecular analysis of rearrangements of immunoglobulin genes in the case of B cell malignancies and of T cell antigen receptor genes for T cell tumours has extended the same principle.

Thirdly, chromosome aberrations, often highly characteristic of specific histological types of malignancy, are relatively common and are more easily demonstrated in leukaemias and lymphomas than in most 'solid' tumours. Visible chromosome aberrations must imply some structural change in the DNA and the fact that the same abnormality can be found in all the cells of a given neoplasm serves to confirm their clonal origin.

Nowadays, the themes of viral oncogenesis, tumour monoclonality and chromosome aberration are tending to merge as awareness grows of their common relevance to the molecular basis of malignancy and, specifically, to the role of defined or putative oncogenes in leukaemia and lymphoma. An understanding of these issues requires, first, an outline of the principles of molecular biology and an introduction to some of the techniques applied in that expanding branch of science.

Basic molecular biology

Gene structure

The universal genetic code, in which each amino acid is specified by a triplet of nucleotides in one strand of the DNA helix, belongs to the realm of 'what every schoolboy knows'. Our understanding of gene structure at the next level of complexity, however, is still evolving.

It is clear that, for the great majority of genes, the 'text' in the DNA is broken up into discrete stretches. ('exons') interspersed with non-coding 'introns'. In the course of transcription from DNA to messenger RNA, the introns are bypassed so that exon transcripts appear contiguous in the nuclear mRNA. As a rule further trimming and splicing of the nuclear message takes place before the final version passes into the cytoplasm, en route for the ribosomes where it will be translated into the appropriate peptide (Fig. 15.2).

In addition to the structural component that encodes a particular sequence of amino acids, a gene requires certain elements for regulation of its expression. These include the sequence TATTAA, or something very similar, usually present 25 to 30 bases 'upstream' (i.e. in the 5' direction) of the start of the coding region. This 'TATA box' and a second highly conserved sequence, GGTCAATCT (the 'CAAT box') located a further 50 or so bases away, represent the fixed elements of the typical eukaryotic promoter region that extends for about 100 base pairs on the 5' side of most genes. The presence of a promoter implies that the level of gene expression can be varied, though the mechanics of

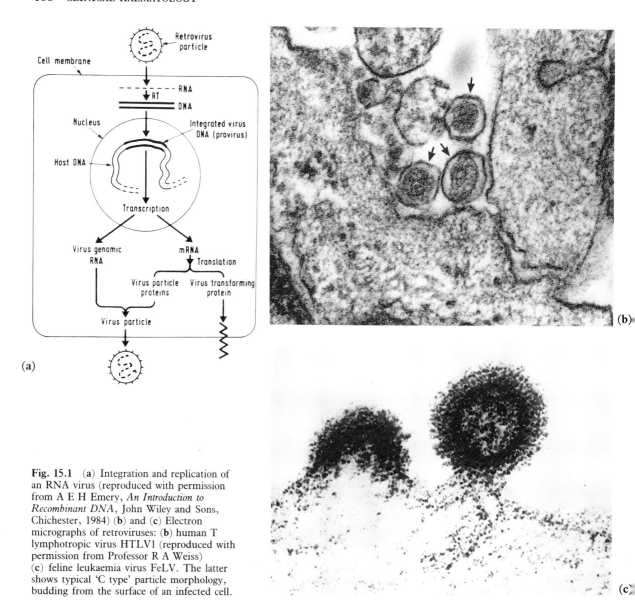

Fig. 15.1 (a) Integration and replication of an RNA virus (reproduced with permission from A E H Emery, *An Introduction to Recombinant DNA*, John Wiley and Sons, Chichester, 1984) (b) and (c) Electron micrographs of retroviruses: (b) human T lymphotropic virus HTLV1 (reproduced with permission from Professor R A Weiss) (c) feline leukaemia virus FeLV. The latter shows typical 'C type' particle morphology, budding from the surface of an infected cell.

the regulatory process are not yet fully understood. In some instances transcription is controlled at an additional level through the influence of 'enhancer' sequences which may be some distance away and either upstream or downstream of the structural gene (Fig. 15.3).

Genetic damage

It follows that a given gene may be affected in a variety of ways by structural change in the DNA. If the coding sequence is altered by deletion or substitution of one or more bases or by the insertion of new material, for example from a virus that has integrated itself into the DNA of the host cell, or by breakage and recombination with another part of the genome, as may happen in the course of a chromosome translocation, then the transcribed RNA message (and ultimately the translated protein product) will be abnormal. On the other hand, if similar damage occurs to one of the controlling elements, the gene product may be normal in itself but

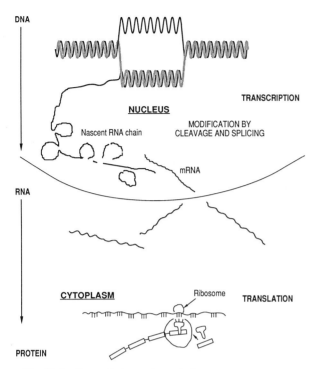

Fig. 15.2   Transcription and translation.

expressed in abnormal quantities or at an inappropriate phase of the cell's life history. There is evidence that all of these mechanisms may be implicated in human leukaemias and lymphomas. In addition, particular DNA sequences can be 'amplified' by the accumulation of multiple copies in the course of several cell divisions, though this may be a feature of tumour progression rather than an initiating event.

Analysis of genome structure

The entire edifice of molecular biology rests on the simple property that any given sequence of nucleotides can 'hybridise' (i.e. form a double helix, linked by hydrogen bonds) with its complementary sequence: adenine opposite thymidine, guanine opposite cytosine. Hence, if we have a single strand of DNA available in

the form of millions of identical copies, preferably (though not necessarily) of known sequence and labelled with a radionucleotide, this can be used to 'probe' a mass of 'unknown' DNA fragments, also in single strand form, to find any sequence or sequences complementary to it. This principle is most commonly applied in the technique known as 'Southern blotting' (after its originator, Dr E.M. Southern). In a typical experiment, DNA is extracted from a tissue specimen and cleaved into fragments averaging some thousands of kilobases long (1 kilobase = 1000 bases) by the use of a 'restriction' endonuclease. The term 'restriction' implies that the enzyme will cleave the DNA only where a specific sequence of bases, usually five or more in length, occurs. Different restriction endonucleases will recognise different cleavage sites. The DNA fragments are subjected to gel electrophoresis to separate them out by size; the smaller the fragment the further it travels in a given time. DNA is then transferred from the gel to an overlay of cellulose nitrate (this is the 'blotting' stage) where it becomes firmly bound. The strands of each fragment are separated by treating with alkali and any spare DNA-binding capacity of the cellulose nitrate sheet is taken up by dipping in an excess of irrelevant DNA, for example from salmon sperm. The sheet is then exposed to the radiolabelled 'probe' and, after washing, any specific binding, attributable to hybridisation between the probe and its complementary sequence, is revealed by autoradiography. By varying the conditions of washing (the 'stringency'), the exactness of fit between the probe and target sequence required for binding can be increased or decreased to meet the needs of the particular experiment. The position of the DNA fragment bearing the target sequence is a measure of its size and its intensity of binding is a measure of the number of copies of that fragment (Fig. 15.4). Either may be altered in DNA from malignant tissue if the probe is directed against a sequence that has been involved in structural rearrangement or amplification.

Analysis of RNA

If an alteration in the genome of a malignant cell is ac-

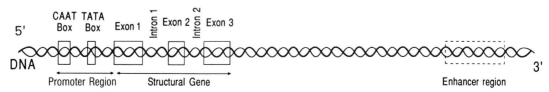

Fig. 15.3   The component elements of a 'typical' mammalian gene (reproduced with permission from *Current Medicine*, Gower Academic Journals, London, 1988).

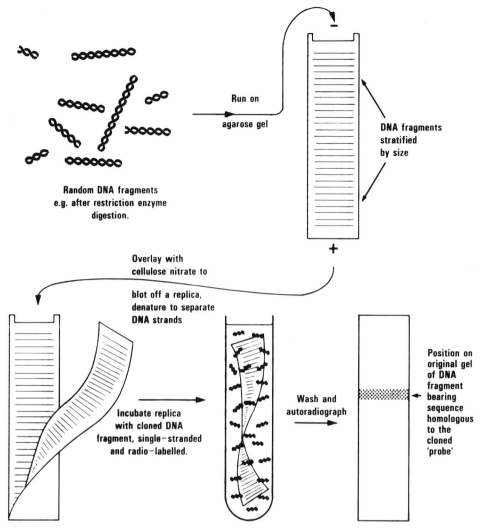

Fig. 15.4   The principles of Southern blotting (reproduced with permission from *The Lancet*, 1984)

tually contributing to the property of malignancy, rather than simply reflecting a secondary genetic instability, then it is likely that the abnormality will be expressed first in an RNA transcript and ultimately in a protein product. Because RNA and DNA have very similar structures, the principle of complementary sequence hybridisation applies to both. The technique of probing RNA extracted from a given tissue is termed 'Northern blotting', by analogy with its 'Southern' counterpart. Malignant cells can show increased levels of particular messenger RNA species or alterations in their molecular weights, depending on the nature of the underlying genomic lesions.

'In situ' probing

It is not, in fact, necessary to extract DNA or RNA from tissue in order to probe it. The chromosomal location of very many genes and of even more 'anonymous' DNA sequences have been established by hybridisation to metaphase spreads, followed by autoradiography and then scoring the distribution of silver grains over the chromosome set (Fig. 15.5a and b). The identification of genetic abnormalities in individual cells by in situ hybridisation presents some technical difficulties but where there is extraneous DNA in a subpopulation of cells as, for example, in cervical tissue infected with papilloma or *Herpes simplex* virus, these can be picked up quite readily (Fig. 15.5c). Similarly, where there is massive amplification of a cellular DNA sequence, this may be detectable by the use of appropriate labelled probes on tissue sections, smears, imprints or even in suspensions of cells to be assayed by flow cytometry. The potential power of approaches that can identify each malignant cell 'in a crowd' has led to a major investment of research effort, the fruits of which will certainly reach the diagnostic laboratory within the next few years. One of the first advances in this field has been the development of alternatives to radioactivity as a means of labelling probes. Chemical modification of probe DNA or tagging with biotin both allow subsequent visualisation of the bound probe with a fluorochrome or with an enzyme-linked antibody.

It is obvious that the techniques of molecular biology are beginning to overlap with those of immunology. With the appearance of a growing range of monoclonal antibodies directed against the products of genes that are altered or amplified in malignancy, the overlap promises to become a virtual merger.

SPECIFIC APPLICATIONS OF GENE PROBES

Ig and TCR gene rearrangements

Lymphoid cells are unique, so far as we know, in undergoing structural rearrangements of their DNA in the course of normal physiological development. B cell progenitors rearrange the regions of their genome that encode immunoglobulin heavy and light chains and in this way become committed to the synthesis of antibody whose amino acid sequence (and hence antigen-binding specificity) is faithfully reproduced in all the clonal descendants of each progenitor. The vast number of permutations available to these B cell progenitors in rearranging their immunoglobulin genes accounts for the normal immune system's huge repertoire of specific antibody responses. In a very similar fashion, T cell precursors rearrange their antigen-receptor (TCR) genes, of which there are 4, α β γ and δ. A close structural relationship indicates that Ig and TCR genes have evolved from a common ancestral DNA sequence. Rearrangement of the TCR genes generates clones of T cells, the members of a given clone interacting with the same antigenic determinant which is different from the determinant recognised by any other clone (Fig. 15.6).

As was pointed out above, the clonal origin of B cell malignancies can be demonstrated by showing that all the cells produce an identical immunoglobulin molecule.

The same information, however, can be obtained by showing, with a DNA probe, that they have all undergone an identical rearrangement of their immunoglobulin genes. The latter approach can also be applied to the TCR genes in the case of a T cell lymphoma or leukaemia. If DNA from normal lymphoid tissue is digested, run on a gel and Southern-blotted with a probe that hybridises to an appropriate part of the Ig or TCR gene complex, then a single autoradiographic band will appear, corresponding to the unrearranged ('germ-line') Ig or TCR DNA. This is present in non-lymphoid cells which will form a proportion of the tissue but, in addition, since a B or T cell expresses only *one* copy of its Ig or TCR genes (through a phenomenon known as allelic exclusion) the 'silent' homologue of the rearranged sequence will often be in the germ-line configuration and thus contribute to the distinct autoradiographic band. Conversely, the rearranged Ig or TCR genes will be different in structure for every clone and since normal lymphoid tissue comprises tens of thousands of such clones, the rearranged sequences will be distributed over a considerable length of the gel forming only a diffuse smear on probing. If, however, a single clone forms a substantial proportion of the total material, then the rearranged Ig or TCR genes from that clone may show up, on probing, as additional distinct bands. Under ideal conditions this technique may be sensitive enough to detect a malignant lymphoid clone that comprises as little as 1% of the cells in the tissue sampled (Fig. 15.7).

As far as we know, no normal lymphoid cell is capable of rearranging *both* Ig and TCR gene sets, since the rearrangements effectively define the mutually exclusive B and T cell lineages. A surprising finding from several studies of lymphoid malignancy, however, is that in a substantial minority of cases, clonal rearrangement of both types has occurred. The explanation is still uncertain. One possibility might be that in some cases of apparently monoclonal B cell lymphoma the actual malignant population is a numerically inconspicuous T cell clone which 'drives' the poliferation of a non-malignant B cell clone sharing specificity for the same antigen. Such a sequence of events is theoretically possible but where the majority of the cells from a lymphoma are chromosomally abnormal (as is often the case) the presumption must be that they have undergone malignant transformation and are not merely responding to a physiological growth signal. It seems more likely that in a proportion of lymphoid malignancies, rearrangement of both Ig and TCR genes has taken place in the same ancestral cell and that this aberration is one of the manifestations of malignancy.

Oncogenes

Nucleotide sequences responsible for (or contributing to) malignant transformation were first identified in oncogenic RNA viruses. These have been recognised in many species for over 30 years, although the first one unequivocally implicated in a human malignant disease was not discovered until 1981. This was HTLVI, the cause of a form of subacute adult T cell leukaemia found rather commonly in the south west of Kyushu Island, Japan, and in the Caribbean. These viruses are so small that they contain only three or four genes, most of which are required simply to ensure replication of the virus itself, while one, the 'onc' gene, induces malignant change in the infected cell. The functions of the different genes were established by studying the effects of mutations in viral RNA and the 'onc' genes or 'oncogenes' detected in this way were given names that reflect their viral origins (Table 15.1).

At first it caused something of a surprise when it was shown, by nucleic acid hybridisation, that sequences homologous to viral oncogenes are present in the DNA of many higher organisms, including man. Furthermore, in experiments that involved the transfection of DNA from human cancers into the living cells of a partially-transformed mouse epithelial line (3T3), it was

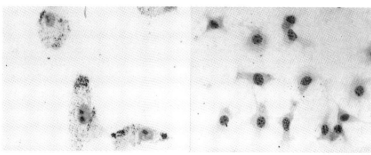

(a)

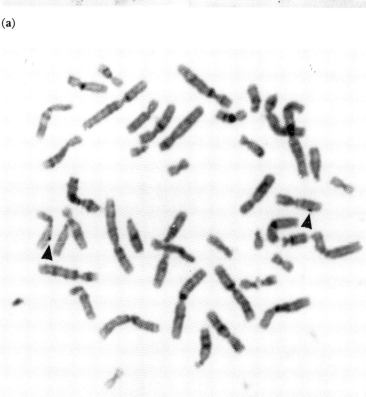

(b)

Fig. 15.5   In situ hybridisation: (a) Hybridisation of a viral probe to infected and non-infected cells. Note the autoradiographic grains over the cytoplasm of the infected cells on the left (reproduced with permission from Dr J. Gorden and Mr D. Rout) (b) On chromosomes: a 'G'-banded metaphase spread from a human cell has been probed with a radiolabelled probe recognising, in this example, the stromelysin gene. On autoradiography, silver grains (arrows) appear over the long arms of each of the chromosome 11 pair (reproduced with permission from Dr K. W. Jones) (c) The idiogram represents the cumulative distribution of grains from 25 metaphase spreads. Note the concentration over 11q, confirming localisation of the stromelysin gene to that region. The scatter of grains-elsewhere is largely due to background 'noise' though the occurrence of addition 'hot spots' raises the possibility of stromelysin-related sequences, for example on the tip of Xp.

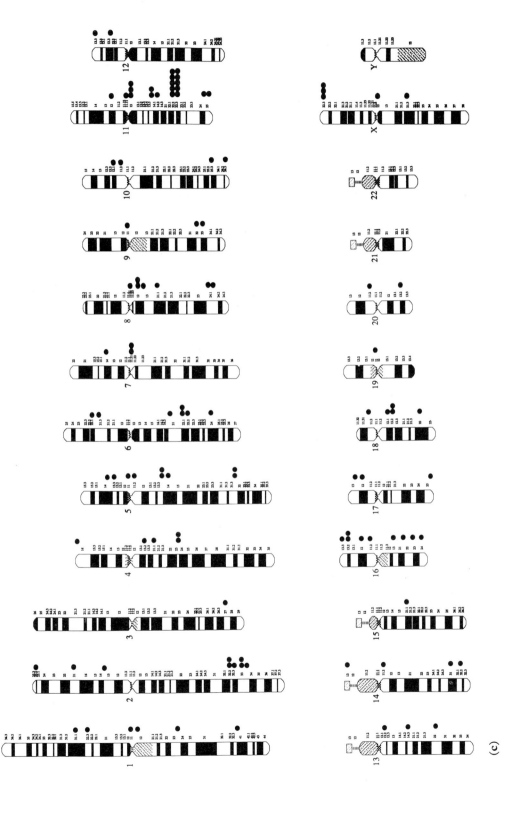

(c)

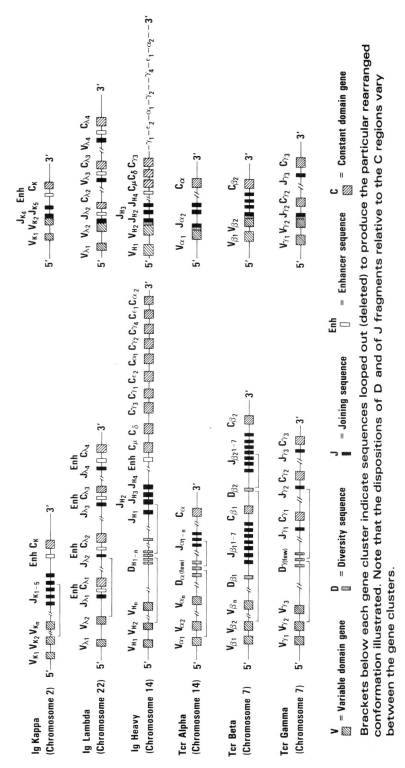

Fig. 15.6 Diagrammatic representation of the structural rearrangements that take place before immunoglobulin or T cell receptor genes become functional. The various component elements of each gene cluster are indicated in the key. Functional rearrangement essentially requires that a contiguous 'block' of DNA be formed from a V, D (if present) and J segment by excision of intervening DNA. The transcript of that V(D)J 'block' then encodes the complete variable domain of the Ig or Tcr chain to be expressed. Since the cell can 'choose' between several V, D and J segments and some addition or excision of bases is possible at the junctions between them, a vast repertoire of distinct variable regions can be constructed in different cells (reproduced with permission from I. Lauder and J. Habeshaw (eds) *Current Problems in Tumour Pathology: Malignant Lymphomas*, Churchill Livingstone, Edinburgh, 1988)

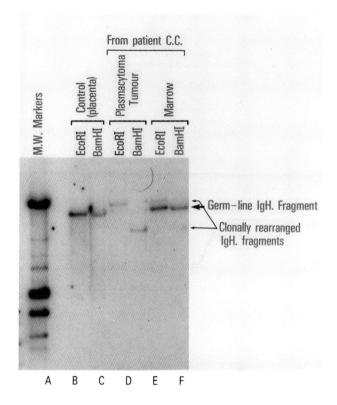

Fig. 15.7 Detection of clonal B cell malignancy by probing for rearranged Ig sequences. A young male presented with a localised bony deposit of myeloma. Histologically there was no marrow involvement but Southern blotting with a probe for the Ig heavy chain J region demonstrated that the clonal Ig rearrangement characteristic of the original tumour (lanes C, D) was also detectable in marrow DNA (lanes E, F) indicating that there was a significant component of myeloma in that tissue. Despite chemotherapy, the patient died from widespread myeloma.

found that in many cases a few completely transformed colonies grew out and that these had invariably incorporated some human DNA into their genome. When the human sequences associated with complete transformation of 3T3 cells were analysed, they almost invariably turned out to be the cellular homologues of viral oncogenes, usually belonging to the Ras family. Gradually the picture has become clearer and the position as currently understood can be summarised as follows.

The oncogenes found in RNA viruses have their origins as cellular DNA sequences. They have been 'picked up' by the viruses in the course of infection, transcribed into RNA as the virus replicates and usually modified to some extent as they have been incorporated into the viral genome. Oncogenic transformation by an RNA virus really amounts to a reverse of the above process. Viral RNA is reverse-transcribed (by 'reverse transcriptase') into a DNA 'provirus' copy including the 'proto-oncogene', i.e. the DNA version of the viral oncogene. There may be many hundreds of copies of the provirus in a given cell and some of those DNA sequences may become integrated, either at random or at specific sites, into the host cell genome. Once there, the viral oncogenes may be expressed, in which case their products are likely to differ from those of the normal

cellular homologue (the c-onc gene) in details of structure and in amount. Furthermore, transcription and translation of the viral oncogenes will be under different regulatory control, remaining active, for example, at phases of the cell cycle or under particular conditions of differentiation when the c-onc equivalent is 'silent'. In any or all of these ways, a viral derivative of what was once a normal component of cellular DNA can cause malignant transformation.

The c-onc genes generally appear to encode proteins that are involved in the generation or transduction of physiological growth and differentiation signals. Even in the absence of an oncogenic virus, it is possible for alterations to occur in the structure, copy number or regulation of c-onc genes and so to subvert their normal functions, leading to malignant change in the affected cell and its progeny. The causal event may be as apparently trivial as a single point mutation, substituting one amino acid for another in the protein product. This seems to be the most common means of oncogenic activation of the Ras family of genes, substitutions in codons 12, 31 or 61 being particularly dangerous. Other oncogenes, however, are activated by more substantial physical rearrangements of their DNA, sometimes involving visible chromosome aberrations. Two

Table 15.1 Some oncogenes identified in oncorRNAviruses

Gene	Virus of origin	Chromosomal localisation of human proto-oncogene*	Properties of gene product
Abl	Abelson mouse leukaemia	9q34	145kd protein with protein kinase activity
Ets 1	Avian leukaemia E26	11q	
Ets 2	Avian leukaemia E26	3q	
Erb A	Avian erythroblastosis	17	Cytoplasmic protein: homology with glucocorticoid receptor.
Erb B	Avian erythroblastosis	7	72kd membrane glycoprotein: truncated EGF receptor
Fes	Snyder-Theilen feline sarcoma	15q24–26	85kd glycoprotein: protein kinase
Fgr	Gardner-Rasheed feline sarcoma	1	72kd protein: protein kinase
Fms	McDonough feline sarcoma	5q34	180kd glycoprotein: CSF-1 receptor
Fos	FBJ murine osteosarcoma	14	DNA-binding
Mos	Moloney murine sarcoma	8q	40 kd protein. Serine/Thresmine kinase
Myb	Avian myeloblastosis	6q22–24	DNA- binding
Myc	MC29 avian myelocytomatosis	8q24	DNA-binding
Raf	Murine sarcoma 3611	3p25 and 4	78kd protein
H-ras	Harvey rat sarcoma	11p14	21Kd protein: GTP-binding
K-ras	Kirsten rat sarcoma	12q	21kd protein: GTP-binding
Rel	Avian reticulo-endotheliosis		
Ros	Rochester UR II Avian sarcoma	6q22	62kd protein: protein kinase
Sis	Simian sarcoma	22q11	28kd protein: PDGF homology
Ski	Avian sarcoma SkV770	1q	DNA-binding
Src	Rous sarcoma	20	60kd protein: protein kinase
Yes	Yamaguchi avian sarcoma		90 kd protein: protein kinase

* p = short arm
  q = long arm
Figures after the lower case letter refer to specific chromosome bands and sub-bands. In some instances the map locations are still tentative.

particularly clear examples of the mechanisms involved are afforded by the 9;22 translocation in chronic myeloid leukaemia and the 8;14 translocation in Burkitt's lymphoma.

The 9;22 translocation in CML

Although the 'Philadelphia chromosome' and its association with CML were recognised in 1960, it was not until 1973 that the origin of the abnormality was correctly ascribed to a reciprocal translocation, the commonest form designated, in standard cytogenetic notation 't(9;22) (q34;q11)'. This, being interpreted, means that breaks have occurred in the long arms of chromosomes 9 and 22, at bands 34 and 11 respectively, and the chromosome arms distal to the breakpoints have interchanged. It was obvious that the consistency of the association between translocation and disease was telling us something about the DNA sequences at one or both

breakpoints and in due course it was shown that a cellular oncogene 'c-abl' (so named because the v-onc equivalent was found in the Abelson mouse leukaemia virus) mapped to band q34 of chromosome 9. Another c-onc gene 'c-sis' (v-sis comes from the simian sarcoma virus) mapped to the long arm of chromosome 22 but this proved to be a red herring because it is some distance away from the breakpoint in cytogenetic terms, which means a very long way indeed in molecular terms. Blotting of DNA from CML cells with a c-abl probe showed that some structural rearrangement had taken place in the immediate vicinity of that gene and on Northern-blotting it was found that the abl gene mRNA transcript is abnormally large. What has, in fact, happened in the course of the 9;22 translocation (and indeed in some of the more complex CML translocations which do not result in an obvious Philadelphia chromosome) is a fusion between two functional genes, abl, normally on chromosome 9, and 'bcr' on chromosome 22. The hybrid bcr-abl gene is transcribed into mRNA and translated into a protein of MW 210 kd, compared with the normal abl-encoded protein of MW 145 kd. While there is some variation among individual cases of leukaemia in the exact positions of the breakpoints near the abl gene on chromosome 9 and within what is termed the 'break cluster region' ('bcr') on chromosome 22, splicing of the nuclear RNA transcript seems to eliminate this variation and leads to the synthesis of the same fusion-protein in every case. The c-abl product is a protein kinase and the chimeric bcr-abl protein appears to have enhanced enzymic activity. If confirmed, this will point the way to a real understanding of the mechanism whereby the translocation induces malignant proliferation of myeloid cells.

The 8;14 translocation in Burkitt's lymphoma

As in the previous case, this reciprocal translocation brings together two genes normally widely separated in the genome. As before, one of them is an oncogene, in this instance c-myc (the v-equivalent being carried by the avian myelocytomatosis virus). Gene mapping places c-myc on the long arm of chromosome 8 at band q24. The other breakpoint, on chromosome 14 at band 32, passes through the complex of gene segments that encode the immunoglobulin heavy chain. The consequence, however, is not a chimeric gene transcript nor even a change in the structure of the myc gene product but a dysregulation of its expression so that an apparently normal myc mRNA transcript and a myc protein are generated continuously when the process of cellular differentiation would require them to be switched off. It seems likely that myc dysregulation in B cells bearing the 8;14 translocation is directly related to the fact that they are synthesising immunoglobulin and hence that the Ig gene locus is active. However, that explanation is not entirely satisfactory since only one of the two heavy chain loci is expressed (allelic exclusion) and studies with hybrid cells have shown that it is normally the one on chromosome 14 *not* involved in the translocation. Nevertheless, juxtaposition of c-myc and an immunoglobulin gene is a recurring feature of B cell tumours in mice and rats as well as man. 'Variant' forms of the 8;14 translocation are recognised in Burkitt's lymphoma. The t8;22 version brings c-myc into contact with the λ light chain gene while in t2;8 the κ light chain gene is involved in the same way. Thus the very consistency of the association between c-myc and one of the Ig loci in B cell tumours is convincing evidence that it contributes in a fundamental way to the evolution of malignancy. It is now recognised that the same 8;14 translocation occurs in some cases of follicular lym-

phoma and in the L3 form of lymphatic leukaemia, in addition to 'classical' Burkitt's lymphoma in which it was first described and in which its occurrence is quite independent of the presence or absence of EB virus. The myc gene product is a DNA-binding protein which is normally expressed in many cell types (including normal lymphocytes) during activation and proliferation but which disappears before terminal differentiation. Increased expression of c-myc, for example when an artificial DNA construct of a myc gene with a powerful promotor is introduced into a recipient cultured cell, results in a more malignant growth pattern and experiments have been carried out with transgenic mice, in which a myc gene spliced to an immunoglobulin promoter sequence is incorporated into the cells of an early embryo, thereafter being expressed in most of B lymphoid cells. Such animals show abnormal proliferation of B cells in lymph nodes during the first few weeks of life and subsequently have a very high incidence of monoclonal B cell lymphomas.

These two examples of chromosome translocations accompanying haemopoietic malignancies illustrate quite different ways in which cellular genes may be converted to active oncogenes but they emphasise one common theme, namely that specific chromosome aberrations are associated with malignancy because of the underlying molecular rearrangements. It follows that careful analysis of the DNA sequences close to other recurring sites of chromosome breakage and recombination in leukaemias and lymphomas may reveal new genes contributing to the expression of malignancy.

Other recurring chromosome aberrations in leukaemia and lymphoma (Fig. 15.8)

In follicular lymphomas of small and medium cell type which, taken together, constitute the commonest B cell malignancy, there is almost always a reciprocal 14;18 translocation t(14;18)(q32;q21), while in a proportion of large cell lymphomas and occasionally in B-CLL an 11;14 translocation has been described, t(11;14)(q13;q32). In each case, the breakpoint on 14q passes through the Ig heavy chain gene complex and this has been exploited in the isolation and cloning of DNA fragments extending across the breakpoint into the region derived from the other chromosome. It transpires that in both situations the breaks are localised with great precision to sequences designated bcl 1(11q13) and bcl 2(18q21), both of which include coding regions. Juxtaposition of these sequences with the Ig heavy chain gene results in enhanced transcription of bcl 1 or 2 in the corresponding neoplastic cells. The functions of the bcl 1 and 2 genes are unknown but the report that bcl 2 shows some homology with a part of the EB virus

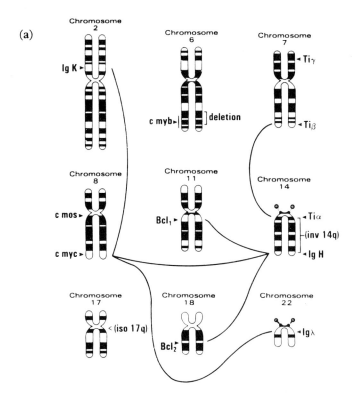

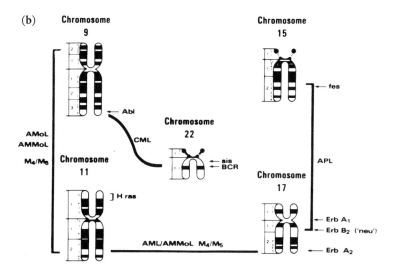

Fig. 15.8 Diagrammatic representation of structural chromosome aberrations frequently seen in (a) lymphoid, (b) myeloid malignancies. Lines connect breakpoints involved in reciprocal translocations. The locations of some oncogenes are indicated, though they have not all been implicated in the molecular events underlying visible chromosome aberrations, AMoL, acute monocytic leukaemia; AMMoL, acute myelomonocytic leukaemia; M_4/M_5, FAB classification of acute myeloid leukaemia; APL, acute prolymphocytic leukaemia.

genome is of interest since infection with that virus will induce human B lymphocytes to proliferate indefinitely in vitro.

Although T cell malignancies, being less common than their B cell counterparts, have been subject to less intensive cytogenetic analysis, characteristic recurring chromosome aberrations are recognised for them also. They appear to correspond very closely to those seen in B cell neoplasms with the gene complex encoding the α chain of the T cell receptor (at 14q11) substituting for the Ig heavy chain locus. Thus in a number of T cell leukaemias t(8;14)(q24;q11) has been found, bringing the TCR α constant region genes into close opposition with c-myc. In other translocations involving the TCR α locus the reciprocal breakpoints have not identified known genes. One of the regions affected is distal to the Ig heavy chain complex (the aberration is an inversion of almost the whole of the long arm of chromosome 14); another is on the short arm of chromosome 11, close to the centromere (11p13). If the precision of the break-points is confirmed, these loci may prove to be the sites of expressed genes important in the regulation of T cell growth and corresponding to bcl 1 and 2 in B cell tumours.

The origins of recurrent translocations in leukaemia/lymphoma

Since there is a 'background' level of DNA damage and repair detectable as chromosome damage in all dividing tissues and since many environmental factors (radiation, virus infections, drugs and chemicals) can add to the damage, inhibit the repair, or both, it might be thought that recurrent chromosome translocations in malignancy merely represent the emergence of chance rearrangements that give particular cells and their progeny a proliferative advantage. There does, however, appear to be more to the case than this. The physical rearrangement of Ig or TCR genes in the course of B or T lymphocyte ontogeny is brought about by an enzyme system, known as DNA recombinase, which uses specific DNA 'recognition' or 'signal' sequences, the heptamer CTGACAG and the nonamer ACAAGCCT separated by 12 bases and a different heptamer-nonamer combination, CAATGTG-GGTTTTTGT, separated by 23 bases, to identify the points of cleavage and re-joining of a DNA strand bearing the various Ig or TCR segments. It was found, on detailed sequencing of regions flanking bcl 1 and 2 that both contain heptamer-nonamer signal sequences with appropriate spacing to allow misidentification of these regions by the recombinase system. The same may be true of some translocations involving the TCR loci. Thus some, at

least, of the specific chromosome aberrations that characterise lymphoid tumours are thought to arise during the process of normal gene rearrangement through subversion of the enzymic machinery required to carry out that process.

Chromosome gains and losses

Gains and losses of whole chromosomes (trisomy or monosomy) are quite commonly observed in lymphomas and leukaemias. Trisomy 12 in B-CLL is perhaps the best documented example of an isolated chromosome gain characterising a particular neoplasm but it is found in only a minority of cases. In large series of unselected lymphoid tumours, gains of chromosomes 3, 8, 12 and 21 tend to predominate. Monosomy is less frequently observed, though loss of one of the number 7 pair is a recognised feature of Burkitt's and some other B cell lymphomas.

In most instances, these changes in chromosome number are seen as part of a generalised genomic instability, which includes additional breakage and recombination events as the tumour progresses. The term 'secondary' is applied to such changes, though this should not be taken to imply that they are merely effects of the malignant process. The fact that the changes are not totally random suggests that some, at least, contribute to the evolution of the malignancy including, perhaps, such properties as metastatic potential and resistance to therapy. An isochromosome for the long arm of number 17 is a typical feature of CML evolving towards blast crisis (an isochromosome is a 'mirror image' chromosome in which the long or short arm is duplicated about the centromere while the other arm is lost). Some, at least, of the late cytogenic changes seen in lymphoma and leukaemia are thought to be induced by the cytotoxic drugs used in treatment. Not surprisingly, the more potent combination chemotherapy regimes tend to cause most chromosome damage and virtually all cases of ANLL arising after treatment of lymphoma show multiple chromosome aberrations.

Loss of all or part of a chromosome ('deletion') is less easy to comprehend than the gain or structural alteration of an oncogene as a means of triggering malignant proliferation. Nevertheless specific deletions are very clearly associated with certain hereditary tumours, notably retinoblastoma (13q) and nephroblastoma (11p). The term 'anti-oncogene' has been coined to describe a DNA sequence the *absence* of which contributes to malignancy. It seems likely that these sequences act as regulators or repressors of true oncogenes. In leukaemia and lymphoma, recurring deletions of various parts of the chromosome set have been recognised. These include much of the long arm of chromosome 6, the short arms of chromosomes 2, 3 and 8 and a short segment of chromosome 13 (q13–14). The last-mentioned happens to be the site of the 'Rb' gene involved in retinoblastoma and there are early indications that mutations affecting the same gene may be implicated in some cases of myelodysplastic syndrome, lymphoma and CLL.

It should be borne in mind that chromosome analysis gives only the most crude indication of what may be happening at the molecular level and an apparently normal karyotype is entirely compatible with a highly malignant leukaemia or lymphoma in which there may be gross disturbances of oncogene structure and expression. Recurrent chromosome aberrations in malignancy are useful as clues to the likely location of oncogenes but even in a tumour which bears a distinctive cytogenetic abnormality there may be one or more activated oncogenes in chromosomal regions far removed from the visible aberrations. The evidence is now very strong that more than one oncogene requires to be activated before a cell (and its progeny) can become malignant. This is compatible with well-established observations on the multi-stage evolution of tumours in both experimental and clinical settings. The larger tumour viruses, such as polyoma and adenovirus, harbour at least two separate oncogenes in their genomes and it is possible to demonstrate positive interactions ('complementation') between individual oncogenes when these are used in transfection/transformation studies with normal cells as targets.

Future developments

Our current understanding of the molecular events that underlie the development of leukaemia and lymphomas depends upon a synthesis of cytogenetic observations, mainly in haemopoietic malignancies, and experimental work with oncogenes, especially in epithelial tumours. There are undoubtedly several (possibly many) new oncogenes still to be identified in lymphoma and leukaemia and almost certainly some surprises wait along the way.

One particularly desirable advance would be the development of transfection assays, comparable to the 3T3 epithelial cell system described in this chapter but using haemopoietic cells as targets and hence being more appropriate to the detection of oncogenes active in leukaemia and lymphoma. With the discovery of growing numbers of disease-specific molecular probes, we may reasonably expect further advances in the classification of leukaemia and lymphoma. The probes will also prove increasingly valuable for accurate assessments of the size of malignant cell populations as, for example, in following the response to therapy and early detection of relapse. Ultimately, however, the purpose of searching for the molecular basis of malignancy is to gain some insight into the normal regulation of cellular growth and differentiation, to discover precisely how these processes are disordered and so to develop specific therapy based on an understanding of the molecular pathology.

BIBLIOGRAPHY

Bishop J M 1988 The molecular genetics of cancer. Leukaemia 2: 199–208
Steel C M 1984 DNA in medicine: the tools. Parts 1 and 2. Lancet 2: 908–911 and 966–968
Steel C M 1988 Genes and chromosomes. In: Habeshaw J A, Lauder I (Eds) Current problems in tumour pathology: malignant lymphomas. Churchill Livingstone, Edinburgh, pp 89–126
Weatherall D J 1985 The new genetics and clinical practice, 2nd edition. Oxford University Press

16. Acute leukaemias

J. A. Whittaker   M. Judge

Understanding of the aetiology of the acute leukaemias is developing rapidly and recent observations have included the first real evidence for a viral aetiology (adult T-cell leukaemia) and the association of characteristic cytogenetic anomalies with specific subtypes of disease. However, other information, especially that from epidemiological studies, has been less clear and there is as yet no single causative factor that can explain the aetiology of these diseases.

EPIDEMIOLOGY

Incidence data for acute leukaemia are notoriously difficult to interpret, one major difficulty being that until recently there was no acceptable and reproducible classification of these diseases. Statistics from older studies must be judged against this background and a clear picture is unlikely to emerge until results from current studies are available. Analysis is further complicated by the difficulty of obtaining both incidence and mortality figures for the same population.

The majority of ALL* occurs in childhood with a sharp age peak at 3–4 years in industrialised societies, but not in data from some developing countries. Such a pattern must be due at least partly to changing socio-economic conditions and evidence is accumulating that the childhood peak is due to an increase in common ALL, the rarer T- and B-cell subtypes being found with the same incidence worldwide.

In adults, the great majority of leukaemia is AML which increases in incidence with age, although apparent childhood peaks have been seen in some tropical countries.

*Abbreviations: AML, Acute myeloid leukaemia; APL, Acute promyelocytic leukaemia; AMoL, Acute monocytic leukaemia; AMML, Acute myelo-monocytic leukaemia; ALL, Acute lymphoblastic leukaemia; CML, Chronic myeloid leukaemia; CLL, Chronic lymphatic leukaemia.

Overall age-adjusted death rates for leukaemia (including chronic leukaemia) vary from about 1–3 cases per 100 000 population in underdeveloped countries to 6–8.5 cases per 100 000 population in Western industrialised nations. The apparent deficit in the third world presumably at least partly reflects poor diagnostic facilities.

There has been a steady increase in leukaemia mortality in England and Wales throughout this century. Overall incidence trends for England and Wales show a steady increase in ALL incidence for the age range 0–14 for the years 1968–78 with constant or declining mortality reflecting treatment advances in this decade.

Several studies in different parts of the world have suggested a higher incidence of childhood leukaemia among families of higher social class which could reflect better diagnosis, but the higher mortality for both AML and ALL in patients of higher social class remains unexplained.

Interest in the possibility that leukaemia might be the result of an infectious agent has been stimulated by occasional descriptions of case aggregations or 'clusters'. For childhood ALL, modern epidemiological methods have demonstrated an excess in pairs of cases with the onset of the disease within two months resident within 1 km of each other. A number of other similar observations suggest that some cases of leukaemia occur in 'clusters', but the data are difficult to interpret and as yet no clear conclusions can be made.

AETIOLOGY

Radiation

There are several observations from large population studies that strongly support the role of ionising radiation as a major carcinogen, and data from atomic bomb survivors and from those exposed diagnostically, therapeutically and occupationally indicate a relationship principally with AML.

The Atomic Bomb Casualty Commission at Hiroshima and Nagasaki identified leukaemias as the first cancers reported in excess among survivors. Overall there was a 10–15-fold increase in the incidence of all leukaemias in exposed individuals, the first cases appearing after 12–18 months with a peak at 5–7 years and an increased incidence still present after 20 years. 83% of all radiation-induced leukaemias occurred between 5 and 21 years after exposure and generally the earlier the age of exposure, the shorter the latency, although in-utero exposure does not seem to have induced an excess of leukaemia.

The overall risk of developing leukaemia has been estimated at one case per million population per year per rad (cGy) exposure. Chronic myeloid leukaemia and ALL were seen most frequently with an absence of CLL. AML, acute 'undifferentiated' leukaemia and AMML occurred with an intermediate frequency. Curiously, all cases of AMoL were seen in people more than 1500 m from the epicentre of the explosion.

3072 (95.5%) of participants in the 1957 United States nuclear test ('Smoky') have been followed for more than 20 years and show an increase of leukaemia incidence with a mean latency period of 14 years. In addition, a five-fold excess of leukaemia has been demonstrated between 1958 and 1980 in Utah Mormons living downwind of the Nevada site.

Occupational exposure represents a definite risk of leukaemia and repeated low dose exposure over a number of years was associated with a 4.68% incidence in radiologists in the 1930s and 1940s compared with an incidence of 0.51% in doctors not exposed to radiation. The nature of the irradiation is critical, for example uranium miners who show a high incidence of non-haematological malignancies do not appear to have an increased incidence of leukaemia.

Therapeutic irradiation is also associated with an increased incidence of leukaemia and information is available for patients receiving radiotherapy for such benign conditions as ankylosing spondylitis, thymic enlargement, ringworm or tonsillitis. The classical Court-Brown and Doll study of over 14 000 British patients with ankylosing spondylitis treated with spinal irradiation detected 52 leukaemia deaths where only 5.48 were expected. All types of leukaemia were seen with the exception of CLL.

The effects of diagnostic irradiation remain controversial with some authors suggesting that a 'threshold' level of irradiation is important below which malignancy does not occur, while others believe that malignancy results from random gene damage which can occur at any level of irradiation. Pre-natal radiography has been linked with an increased incidence of acute leukaemia in early childhood and the risk has been shown to increase in proportion with the number of X-ray films taken. Women who received pelvic irradiation at doses below 19 Gy to induce artificial menopause have a two-to five-fold increased risk of leukaemia.

Questions have also been raised concerning the possibility that diagnostic non-ionising irradiation may cause leukaemia. Although a number of reports suggest that ultrasound may cause chromosomal damage, no increased leukaemia incidence was detected in a population of children exposed to diagnostic ultrasound in utero.

Several studies have suggested that occupations which require people to work in electrical or magnetic fields may increase the risk of leukaemia, but the data are unconvincing and complicated, particularly as these environments often also include exposure to solvents and to fumes from soldering, jointing and welding.

Chemicals

There are a number of reports suggesting that a variety of chemicals may cause leukaemia, but the only clearly established leukaemogen is benzene. Over 150 cases have been described and the risk of acute leukaemia for some occupations has been estimated at five-fold for all leukaemias and up to 20-fold for AML when compared with the risk for the general population. Shoe workers in Istanbul, chronically exposed to benzene, showed excesses of AML, AMoL, APL, CML and preleukaemia. The onset of leukaemia may be abrupt and can occur soon after exposure or be delayed by up to 15 years. Quite how benzene causes leukaemia is not clear, but many studies have shown an immunosuppressive effect on haemopoietic and reticulo-endothelial tissue and there is some evidence that these effects may act as a co-carcinogen for viruses or ionising radiation.

Other solvents and petrochemicals may be important aetiological agents and studies on workers in the rubber industry have suggested an increased risk for workers exposed to carbon tetrachloride and carbon disulphide. Unfortunately, the data are difficult to interpret as these workers are often exposed to coal tar-based solvents including benzene and xylene.

Some drugs may cause leukaemia and the risk is particularly high, possibly up to 50 times, for cytotoxic and immunosuppressive agents. Alkylating agents are the most leukaemogenic, accounting for three-quarters of reported cases, but vinca alkaloids, methotrexate, procarbazine, azathioprine and 5-fluorouracil have also been reported. Peak incidence is 3–5 years after treatment and the mechanism may relate either to chromosome damage or to the pronounced immunosuppression caused by many of these drugs.

Reports that phenylbutazone, which causes chromosomal damage, is associated with an increased incidence of leukaemia are difficult to interpret, particularly as patients have often received a variety of other drugs including immunosuppressive agents.

Viruses

It has long been known that RNA tumour viruses can induce neoplasia in experimental animals and they are probably responsible for the induction of a variety of leukaemias in some rodents, chickens, cats, cows and gibbon apes. The search for a human leukaemia virus has grown with the knowledge that type c retroviruses can cause leukaemia in animals and are widespread in primate species. There has been speculation that humans may be infected with animal viruses, but there is no conclusive evidence, although feline leukaemia virus (FeLV) has been shown to grow in human cell cultures. Another virus which may relate to human leukaemia is bovine leukaemia virus (BLV), a retrovirus causing a neoplasm, enzootic bovine leukosis (EBL), similar to some human lymphoreticular neoplasia in which both infection and tumour incidence are genetically controlled. Vector transmission by blood sucking flies accounts for most infections and in endemic regions nearly all cattle are affected. A positive correlation between its presence in dairy herds and human ALL has been demonstrated, but serological studies have failed to show a positive correlation between BLV antibodies and leukaemia in people exposed to EBL, suggesting that other factors may have been involved. In addition, exposure to FeLV is not associated with active infection in humans with or without leukaemia.

Several laboratories have isolated type c retroviruses from human cells including AML and ALL. These viruses are closely related to known primate retroviruses, but the findings are difficult to interpret, as human cells in vitro are permissive for the growth of a wide variety of mammalian retroviruses and cross-contamination cannot be excluded.

Recently, an unusual form of T-cell malignancy, adult T-cell leukaemia (ATL), has been described in Japan. Human T-cell leukaemia-lymphoma virus (HTLV1), which has a unique reverse transcriptase and lacks nucleic acid homology with other retroviruses, was first isolated in 1978 from a patient in the USA with cutaneous T-cell lymphoma and further studies demonstrated an association with clinical ATL pre-

viously described in Japan. Clustering of a similar HTLV1 positive disease since described in a number of separate populations, including those of Central and South America, some parts of West Africa, and in UK immigrants from the Caribbean, suggest that the virus is widespread. There appears to be an associated spectrum of clinical disease varying from typical non-Hodgkin's lymphoma to adult T-cell leukaemia and including T-cell cutaneous lymphoma. A sero-epidemiological survey of ATL in seven areas of southern Japan found ATL virus endemic and coincident with the areas in which clinical ATL was found. There was a lower prevalence in the young with a maximum of 30% sero-positivity at 40 years. A wider geographical study has since confirmed that 90% of HTLV1 positive cases are patients with T-cell malignancies. The remaining 10% were Japanese patients with myeloid leukaemias and lymphomas. Family studies on virus positive and negative subjects in endemic areas have shown that HTLV1 antibodies are found three or four times as commonly in relatives of ATL patients than in the general population, but subjects who are HTLV1 antibody negative may still be infected with HTLV1. These studies suggest that repeated close personal contact is needed for virus transmission. The presence of HTLV1 gives the most direct evidence yet of a viral cause for human leukaemia.

Other diseases

There is a frequent association between leukaemia and other types of cancer, although this relates chiefly to CLL and skin cancer. However, AML is increasingly reported following chemotherapy and/or radiotherapy for various tumours, especially Hodgkin's disease and multiple myeloma, but also for non-Hodgkin's lymphoma, CLL, ovarian cancer and breast cancer. The exact assessment of risk for these treatments is difficult because of small case numbers, lack of treatment data and the use of selected populations, but the risk appears potentiated when chemotherapy and radiotherapy are combined. The increased risk of AML in 440 000 patients treated at the USA National Cancer Institute between 1973 and 1980 has been estimated at 2.5 times for radiotherapy and 4.5 times for chemotherapy, but 7.5 times when both treatments were combined.

Patients with Down's syndrome have an increased risk of acute leukaemia, 70% of which is ALL, associated with an extra 21 chromosome. A number of instances of leukaemia in carriers of other congenital abnormalities of both somatic and sex chromosomes are also reported. Patients with Fanconi's anaemia, Bloom's

syndrome and ataxia telangiectasia also have a greatly
increased incidence of leukaemia associated with non-
random chromosomal abnormalities.

It has been estimated that the frequency of malignancy in patients with primary immunodeficiency is about
10 000 times greater than that for the general population. Each type of immunodeficiency appears to have an
associated specific spectrum of malignancy, for example
ALL with ataxia telangiectasia and infantile X-linked
agammaglobulinaemia. Generally lymphoreticular
tumours are most common (59%), but 12% of reported
malignancies are leukaemias.

HAEMATOLOGICAL FEATURES

Peripheral blood

Acute myeloid leukaemia

The appearances of the blood film (Plate 2) directly relate to marrow failure and to infiltration with leukaemic
cells. Red cell changes are unusual unless haemolysis or
disseminated intravascular coagulation is a feature. The
total leukocyte count may be increased, normal or
decreased, but most often reflects the number of blasts
present. Most patients show some degree of neutropenia
at presentation, which may be severe. Neutrophils are
often abnormal with few or absent granules and occasionally a Pelger-like abnormality of the nucleus.
These abnormal neutrophils are usually functionally and
metabolically abnormal with poor mobilisation and
phagocytic properties, decreased bactericidal activity,
decreased peroxidase and decreased terminal
deosynucleotidyl-transferase. This latter enzyme is
widely used as a help in differentiating AML and ALL.

Leukaemic blasts are present in varying number from
zero to counts exceeding $200 \times 10^9/l$ with a median
count of $15-20 \times 10^9/l$. There is a direct relationship
between blast counts in blood and bone marrow and
patients with high blood blast counts usually have almost complete replacement of the bone marrow by
leukaemic cells. However, quite frequently the blasts
seen in the blood differ in morphological characteristics
from those in the marrow, particularly in leukaemia
with a monocytoid component. Consequently, attempts
to classify leukaemia from the characteristics of blood
blasts should not be made.

Auer rods in leukaemic blasts (Plate 6), due to coales-
cence of primary granules, are pathognomonic of AML,
but are seen in less than 20% of patients. They are
usually more easily seen in marrow aspirates, but are
often detectable in blood blasts and rarely in neutrophil
granulocytes.

Acute lymphoblastic leukaemia

The blood count shows a variable degree of anaemia
which is usually normochromic and normocytic, a total
leukocyte count which may be normal or raised and a
platelet count which is usually reduced, although normal
in about 20% of patients. A leukocyte count above 100
$\times 10^9/l$ is seen in about 15% of patients.

There is usually an absolute neutropenia and
monocytopenia; myelocytes and metamyelocytes may be
present, but large numbers of these cells are suggestive
of Philadelphia positive (Ph +ve) ALL. The majority of
leukocytes are lymphocytes and blast cells and when
these are microlymphoblastic the distinction may be difficult. Blast cells may not be seen on the blood film
(so-called aleukaemic leukaemia), but in such cases
neutropenia is almost invariable.

Bone marrow

Acute lymphoblastic leukaemia

The French-American-British (FAB) classification sub-
divides ALL into L1, L2 and L3 subtypes. In L1, there
is typically a homogeneous proliferation of small blasts
from $10-20$ μ diameter with a large regular nucleus surrounded by a thin rim of basophilic cytoplasm. The
nuclear-cytoplasmic ratio (NC) is high with a delicate,
homogeneous nuclear chromatin and indistinct nucleoli.
This subtype is more frequently seen in children.

In the L2 subtype, there are pleomorphic blasts of
$15-25$ μ diameter and low NC ratio. The relatively
abundant cytoplasm is basophilic and rarely contains
negative peroxidase granules. The nucleus usually has a
regular shape, but occasionally is cleaved or folded. The
single or multiple nucleoli are easily seen. The L2 subtype is more frequently seen in adults.

There is no correlation between L1 and L2 morphology and immunological phenotype (Table 16.1). The
FAB group have defined a scoring system (Table 16.2)
to help differentiate the L1 and L2 subtypes based on

Table 16.1 Laboratory features of the main immunological
subtypes of ALL in children

	Common-ALL (%)	Null-ALL (%)	T-ALL (%)	B-ALL (%)
Frequency	70–75	10–15	10–25	1–3
L1	70	60	90	0–5
L2	30	40	10	0–5
L3	0	0	0	90–98
Normal WBC*	50–60	30	20	30–40
High WBC**	<10	10–20	50	0

* $<15 \times 10^9/l$
** $>100 \times 10^9/l$

Table 16.2 A scoring system to distinguish L1 and L2 in bone marrow aspirates

Increased NC ratio in 75% or more cells (Nucleus $\geqslant$ 80% of cell area)	= + 1
Decreased NC ratio in 25% or more cells (Cytoplasm $\geqslant$ 20% of cell area)	= − 1
Indistinct nucleoli (> 75% cells do not have visible nucleoli)	= + 1
Distinct nucleoli (> 25% cells have easily visible nucleolus)	= − 1
Regular nuclear membrane (> 75% cells have regular membrane)	= 0
Irregular nuclear membrane (> 25% cells have indented, cleft or convuluted membrane)	= − 1
Cell size (< 50% with diameter less than that of two small lymphocytes)	= − 1

L1 diagnosed for total scores of 0 to +2
L2 diagnosed for total scores of −1 to −4

(i) the NC ratio, (ii) visibility and number of nucleoli, (iii) regularity of the nuclear membrane, and (iv) cell size.

In L3 there is a homogeneous proliferation of large cells from 15 to 25 μ in diameter. The nucleus is round or oval with homogeneous, finely stippled chromatin and distinct nucleoli. Cytoplasm is abundant, deeply basophilic and usually contains one or more vacuoles. B-cell markers are almost always present on proliferating L3 cells.

Diagnostic difficulties in ALL. The morphological criteria described above are helpful in 90% of ALL, but the following problems are occasionally seen: (i) Hypocellular bone marrows may be difficult to analyse, requiring a bone marrow trephine which usually shows total bone marrow replacement by blast cells with an increased reticulin network. Myelofibrosis occurs in about 30% of ALL patients, although its prognostic significance is uncertain. (ii) Very occasionally, L2 may be confused with the M1 form of AML. It is important to remember that some normal myeloid cells may remain in patients with ALL and may also appear in the blood as part of a minimal leuko-erythroblastosis. Consequently, the presence of some myeloperoxidase positive cells does not mean that the whole blast cell proliferation is myeloblastic.

Acute myeloblastic leukaemia with maturation (M2)

(M2) is characterised by the presence of granulocytic maturation to or beyond the promyelocyte (Plate 5). Type I and type II blasts constitute 30–90% of the NEC. Type III blasts are present as well as myelocytes, metamyelocytes and polymorphonuclear neutrophils. Morphological features of dysgranulopoiesis and dyserythropoiesis are easily recognised and include degranulation, giant abnormal granules, a Pelger-Huet abnormality and micromegakaryocytes. Auer rods may be seen in all the cells of the granulocytic series.

Hypergranular promyelocytic leukaemia (M3)

Most cells are hypergranular blasts containing an oval or bilobed nucleus and numerous larger, abnormal azurophilic or dense purple granules in the cytoplasm (Plate 6). The small, fine azurophilic granules often seen in type II blasts are difficult to identify. Characteristically, the bone marrow cells contain multiple Auer rods often arranged in bundles or 'faggots' and these cells are sometimes seen in the blood. These abnormal cells may be disrupted leaving Auer rods free in the preparation.

A variant hypogranular form of M3 has been described with characteristic bilobed nuclei and frequently a higher total leukocyte count than in the standard form of M3 where leukopenia is common. A 15:17 chromosome translocation is invariably present in both types of M3.

Myelomonocytic leukaemia (M4)

The M4 subtype of AML may resemble M2 except for the presence of monocytes and monoblasts and its distinction requires care (Plate 7). In bone marrow, blast cells represent more than 30% of the NEC with more than 20% belonging to the monocytic series. In the blood, the monocytic component exceeds 5×10^9 cells per litre. The presence of monocytic cells may be confirmed by cytochemical methods and especially useful is the presence of naphthol ASD acetate esterase positivity, both with and without incubation with sodium fluoride. Several methods for 'combined' esterase allow the identification of cells from the monocyte and granulocyte series in the same preparation. In addition, the serum and urinary lysozyme is usually significantly increased when a monocytic component is present.

A few cases of M4 show a significant increase in eosinophils, at various stages of development, either in the blood or bone marrow. In the cytoplasm of these cells, normal and large abnormal eosinophilic granules co-exist. A variety of abnormalities of the number 16 chromosome, especially inversion, have been described in eosinophilic M4.

Acute monoblastic leukaemia (M5)

In the M5 subtype of AML, bone marrow and peripheral blood are invaded by a proliferation of monocytes or monoblasts (Plate 8). Two subtypes of M5 have been described: (i) A poorly differentiated form of M5 which is characterised by the presence of large blasts up to 30 μ in diameter with an abundant basophilic cytoplasm. The cell membrane is often irregular with pseudopodia or buds giving an appearance of a double membrane. The nucleus is round or oval and has a lacy chromatin pattern with large prominent nucleoli. (ii) The well-differentiated form of M5 includes monoblasts, promonocytes and abnormal monocytes. The latter cells are more easily observed in the blood. The cytoplasm is blue-grey with nuclei which are often oval or bean-shaped with inconspicuous nucleoli. These cells show strongly positive NASDA activity with significant inhibition by sodium fluoride (NASDA-F). The peroxidase reaction is negative or weakly positive. Serum and urinary lysozyme levels are significantly increased.

Erythroleukaemia (M6)

In the M6 subtype of AML, the erythroblastic component of the bone marrow represents more than 50% of all nucleated cells and the morphological features of dysmyelopoiesis are evident (Plate 9). The percentage of blast cells is variable, but represents more than 30% of NEC.

Acute megakaryoblastic leukaemia (AMkL) (M7)

The definition of this very unusual form of acute leukaemia is still a matter of controversy, but it seems possible to distinguish two forms: (i) A pure AMkL where the leukaemic proliferation appears relatively homogeneous. The blast cells are similar in size varying from 15 to 25 μ in diameter with an increased N/C ratio, sometimes greater than 80%. The nucleus is round with a delicate, fine chromatin pattern and one or two visible nucleoli. The cytoplasm is basophilic without granules. The peroxidase reaction is negative and the blasts look undifferentiated resembling L1 or L2 blasts. The presence of small cytoplasmic buds surrounded or not by a few platelets is very suggestive of the megakaryoblastic origin of the proliferation. Confirmation requires EM studies including the demonstration of a positive platelet peroxidase reaction (PPO). Monoclonal antibodies reacting with platelet glycoproteins or factor VIII-related antigen may also help in the identification of AMkL. (ii) A polymorphic proliferation of cells of the three myeloid series with a predominance of the megakaryoblastic proliferation which may be idiopathic or secondary to long-term chemotherapy. The blood usually shows a severe pancytopenia while the bone marrow aspirate is hypocellular because of the presence of a marked myelofibrosis. However, bone marrow biopsy is often hypercellular with numerous abnormal megakaryocytes, erythroblasts and immature cells of the granulocytic series. Precise identification requires EM studies. The prognosis is very poor with death due to bone marrow failure or associated with the development of an acute leukaemia characterised by a mixture of immature cells of the three myeloid series.

The cytochemistry of the acute leukaemias

As a routine, only a few techniques are necessary which include the peroxidase and/or Sudan Black B reactions, the NASDA-NASDA-F and acid phosphatase reactions. The PAS reaction has no specificity and should be abandoned. The peroxidase and/or Sudan Black B reactions are positive in all the cells of the granulocytic series from the earlier myeloblasts to more mature forms (Plate 4). These reactions are essential for distinguishing immature myeloblasts from lymphoblasts or megakaryoblasts. They are weakly positive or negative in monocytic cells.

The esterase reaction is positive with naphthol ASD acetate (NASDA) in the majority of acute myeloid leukaemias, but in the monoblasts, promonocytes and monocytes the reaction is more intense and completely inhibited by sodium fluoride (NASDA-F).

Cytogenetics

The incidence of cytogenetic abnormalities in AML is not yet exactly known and varies considerably in published series. However, it is clear that a number of specific anomalies are associated with the various FAB subtypes, while others are associated generally with AML.

The karyotypic changes associated with a particular AML subtype are shown in Table 16.3 and those changes without specific morphological changes are shown in Table 16.4.

(i) Specific karyotype changes

t(8;21)(q22;q22) – Occurs almost exclusively in young patients with M2 where it is the chief karyotype change. 80% have other changes, usually loss of a sex chromosome or 9q–. Morphologically, cells show ma-

Table 16.3 The main karyotype changes associated with AML morphology

Karyotype change	Morphology (FAB)	Probable frequency (%)
t(8;21)(q22;q2)	M2	12
t(15;17)(q22;12)	M3	10
t/del(11)(q23)	M5(M4)	6
inv/del(16)(q22)	M4 with eosinophilia	5
t(9;22)(q34;q11)	M1(M2)	3
t(6;9)(p21–22;q34)	M2/M4 with basophilia	1
inv(3)(q21;q26)	M1(M2, M4, M7) with thrombocytosis	1

inv = inversion; del = deletion; t = translocation

Table 16.4 The main characteristic karyotype changes not associated with a specific AML morphology

Karyotype change	Probable frequency (%)
+8	8
−7	4
7q−	3
5q−	3
−Y	1
+21	1

ture, often large, granules with thin Auer rods in blasts and maturing cells.

t(15;17)(q22;q12) – Seen in almost all M3 and in the M3 hypogranular variant. About one third of patients have an associated additional chromosome (+8).

t/del (11)(q23) – A group of various translocations, the commonest being t(9;11). All are characteristically associated with monocytic morphology.

inv/del (16)(q22) – A group showing various structural changes in chromosome 16, usually inversions and deletions, and associated with M4 with eosinophilia. Eosinophilic granules are characteristically large and numerous, often obscuring the cell nucleus. Many patients also have an additional chromosome 8.

t(9;22)(q34;q11) – The Philadelphia chromosome occurs rarely in AML where it is usually associated with M1 morphology.

t(6;9)(p21–22;q34) – Patients have M2 or M4 morphology often associated with basophilia and preceded by MDS in about 20% of cases.

inv(3)(q21;q26) – Is seen in various AML subtypes which are often preceded by MDS and often associated with thrombocytosis in the leukaemic phase.

Other changes. Small numbers of patients have been described with monocytic leukaemia (M5b) and t(8;16) with blast cells which characteristically show erythrophagocytosis. Changes in the short arm of

chromosome 12 described in patients with AML may be associated with basophilia in the M2 subtype. Trisomy 4 has been described in patients with M2 and M4 morphology.

(ii) Karyotypic changes not strictly associated with a particular AML morphology

Trisomy 8 – The commonest abnormality in AML occurs singly in 8% of patients usually with M1, M4 and M5 and in association with other changes in 11%, especially with M3 morphology.

Monosomy 7(−7), deletions of 7q(7q−) and 5q (5q−) – are usually associated with other karyotypic defects and often associated with a history of exposure to toxic agents.

−Y – This usually occurs as part of the process of aging in normal males. Its significance in AML is unknown.

The use of cell-surface marker analysis in leukaemia

A large number of monoclonal antibodies identify cell-surface antigens on leukaemic blasts and recent international workshops on leukocyte differentiation antigens have identified clusters of antibodies which can help to identify myeloid and lymphoid blasts (Table 16.5).

Correlation of FAB morphological subtypes with cell-surface immunophenotypes is not precise, but some associations have been established, the commonest being the expression of CD14 antigen with M4 and M5 and the absence of HLA-DR antigens in M3. In addition,

Table 16.5 Cluster designation of monoclonal antibodies useful in separating AML from ALL

Cluster designation	Antibodies
B-cell lineage	
CD 19	Anti-B4
CD 20	Anti-B1
T-cell lineage	
CD 2	Anti-T11, Leu 5, OKT11
CD 3	Anti-T3, Leu 4, OKT3
CD 5	Anti-T1, Leu 1, OKT 1
CD 7	3A1, WT-1, Anti-Leu 9
Myeloid lineage	
CD 11b	Anti- Mol, OKM1
CD 13	Anti-MCS-2, MY7
CD 14	Anti-MY4, Mo2, FMC17
CD 15	FMC10, VIM-D5
CD 33	Anti-MY9, L4F3

Table 16.6 Immunophenotyping and the separation of ALL and AML

	CD19	CD7	CD33	HLA-DR	TdT
B-cell lineage	+	−	−	+	+
T-cell lineage	−	+	−	−	+
AML	−	−/+	+	+	−

M1 may be differentiated from M2 where Leu M1 reactivity is negative.

Cell-markers are of much more practical use in separating B- and T-cell lineages from myeloid cell-lines and, when combined with measurement of the enzyme, terminal transferase (TdT) can provide a very valuable addition to morphological and cytogenetic information (Table 16.6).

CLINICAL FEATURES

Symptoms and signs

The presenting features of acute leukaemia are often directly related to bone marrow failure which may have been present from a few days to several months. This results in varying degrees of anaemia, granulocytopenia and thrombocytopenia, which are the direct or indirect cause of many of the symptoms and signs at presentation. In a minority of patients, the presenting clinical features may also be due to infiltration of tissues with leukaemic cells.

Bone marrow failure

Anaemia. Pallor and tiredness are the commonest symptoms of anaemia and occur in the majority of adult patients, of whom 80% have an initial haemoglobin concentration below 11 g/dl. The median haemoglobin concentration is 9 g/dl and in the elderly or when anaemia has been present for some time this may result in cardio-respiratory symptoms, particularly dyspnoea, tachycardia, syncope and angina. Apart from tachycardia, signs of anaemia are uncommon except in severely anaemic patients where pulmonary oedema and congestive cardiac failure can occur. Marrow failure is almost certainly mainly due to a direct reduction in stem cells and may be associated with ineffective erythropoiesis, especially in erythroleukaemia. Simple 'crowding-out' of erythroid tissue by leukaemic cells is unlikely to occur.

Anaemia due to marrow failure may be made worse by accelerated destruction of red cells and by blood loss. Marked haemolytic anaemia is rare, although a shortened red cell survival can be demonstrated in some patients. Reticulocytosis may occur and occasionally circulating nucleated red cells are seen in the blood of patients with erythroleukaemia.

Granulocytopenia. Fever occurs commonly at presentation and throughout the induction period. Infection, especially septicaemia, is the commonest cause of fever and must always be considered as likely, particularly in patients with granulocyte counts below 1.0 $\times$ 10^9/l. Although the median WBC in AML patients is 15–20 $\times$10^9/l, one third of patients are neutropenic at diagnosis with granulocyte counts of 0.5–1.9 $\times$ 10^9/l.

Fever without clinical or laboratory confirmation of infection occurs in about one third of febrile episodes and in a small proportion of patients may be related to widespread disease. In patients who have started treatment, infection is even more likely as a cause of fever, but in a few patients fever is due to reactions to drugs or to transfusion of blood products.

Thrombocytopenia. Bleeding occurs in 60% of AML patients at presentation and throughout the induction period, but is less frequently seen in children with ALL. It is almost always secondary to severe thrombocytopenia caused by marrow failure. There is a complex, poorly understood relationship between thrombocytopenia and bleeding, but the highest risk of bleeding is in patients with platelet counts less than 20 $\times$ 10^9/l, although many patients will not bleed at these and lower counts. Most patients do not bleed spontaneously at higher platelet counts, although bleeding is more frequent in patients with systemic infections or severe anaemia. Defects of platelet function, so frequently seen in myeloproliferative disorders, rarely occur in acute leukaemia.

The skin is the commonest site of bleeding with small petechial haemorrhages seen especially over the lower legs and feet. Bleeding from the gums is common, particularly in patients with poor dental hygiene and bleeding into the mucous membranes of the buccal cavity, tonsillar bed and pharynx is frequent. Epistaxis is less usual, although potentially much more troublesome and frank haematuria is rare, although microscopic haematuria is common and often undetected. Usually, blood loss from the gastrointestinal tract is microscopic, but may be severe and even life-threatening in patients with active peptic ulceration. In women, menorrhagia is common and it is probably wisest to suppress menstruation until remission is achieved.

Haemorrhage in the eye is most often seen in the retina, where it may occasionally cause visual disturbances, especially blind spots. Haemorrhage into the vitreous is even more serious, but fortunately rarely seen. Subconjunctival haemorrhage is not usually serious, although it will inevitably cause considerable concern to the patient.

Intracranial bleeding is extremely serious and often results in death. Fortunately, the general availability of platelet concentrates has reduced dramatically the number of deaths from this cause.

Leukaemia infiltration

Skin. Leukaemic skin deposits can occur occasionally in patients with any of the subtypes of AML, but are most frequently seen in acute monocytic leukaemia (FAB M5) and acute myelomonocytic leukaemia (FAB M4). They usually occur as small, rose-coloured or purple papular lesions which may be multiple and generalised or less commonly few in number. In a recent series, 18% of M4, 25% of well differentiated acute monocytic leukaemia (M5a) and 33% of poorly differentiated acute monocytic leukaemia (M5b) patients had skin infiltration. The ability of leukaemic monocytes to migrate to the skin has been demonstrated in skin windows and skin abrasion results in the migration of leukaemic cells in M5 patients, whereas only normal inflammatory cells migrate in AML. These findings may explain the high incidence of skin infiltration in M4 and M5 disease.

Mouth and gums. Gingival hypertrophy due to infiltration with leukaemic cells (Plate 10) occurs in 25% of patients with M5a, 50% of M5b and 50% of M4 disease, but in only 5–8% of other AML subtypes. Infiltration of the tongue, producing macroglossia and tonsillar infiltration, is seen rarely in M4 and M5 disease.

The testicle. Leukaemic infiltration of the testicle (Plate 11), which occurs in 10–20% of ALL patients, is rarely seen at presentation. Testicular relapse may occur during treatment, particularly in patients with high initial leukocyte counts, but most relapses occur within the first year after treatment stops. Although the disease may be clinically detected in one testicle only, the other testicle is frequently involved on biopsy.

The ovary. In contrast to testicular disease in male patients with ALL, ovarian involvement in females is rare, but occasionally occurs in girls in early puberty. Management of ovarian and testicular disease is discussed below.

The eye. All the parts of the eye have occasionally been affected by leukaemic deposits, but these disorders are less frequently seen in AML than in ALL, where choroidal and neural infiltrates frequently co-exist with meningeal leukaemia. However, retinal infiltrates probably occur with the same frequency in AML and ALL in childhood.

Liver, spleen and lymph nodes. Lymphadenopathy and hepatosplenomegaly occur more often in ALL, where some series report a 40% involvement. However, as with AML these signs are usually minimal and often clinically undetectable. When significant enlargement of liver, spleen and lymph nodes occurs, it may indicate an underlying alternative diagnosis, for example AML transformation secondary to chronic myeloid leukaemia.

Bone. Bone and joint pain is rare at presentation, but not uncommon terminally in patients with a rapidly increasing number of leukaemia cells. It may be caused by bone infarcts, by periosteal elevation due to leukaemic tissue, or by increased blood flow with raised marrow pressure. Bone pain is often associated with tenderness at major sites of marrow production, especially the sternum. Pain and tenderness over long bones, seen not infrequently in children with ALL, is rare in adults, but when present may be due to periosteal elevation, in which case the abnormality may be seen on X-ray.

The rapid disappearance of bone pain following successful cytoreduction indicates a possible relationship to leukaemia deposits.

Other organs. Infiltration occurs in other organs, but rarely causes clinical symptoms at presentation. The kidneys, lung and pleura, heart and pericardium, and gastrointestinal tract may be involved. Leukaemia in the lung and pleura have been associated with bleeding into the lung parenchyma and pleura, and deposits in the heart with pericardial bleeding and tamponade, but these syndromes are rare.

Other clinical features

Nonspecific skin lesions apparently unrelated to leukaemic infiltration include pruritus, urticaria, papules, vesicles and erythema multiforme. Painful indurated erythematous plaques have been reported.

Herpes simplex, although rare at diagnosis, is seen frequently during treatment. *Herpes zoster* is occasionally encountered (Fig. 16.1), but is much less common in AML than in patients with ALL, chronic lymphatic leukaemia and other lymphoid neoplasms. Varicella is rarely seen, but can be rapidly fatal in association with the severe immunosuppression usually found in leukaemia patients.

SPECIAL CLINICAL PROBLEMS

Acute monocytic leukaemia

Acute monocytic leukaemia is associated with a high frequency of extramedullary disease, particularly

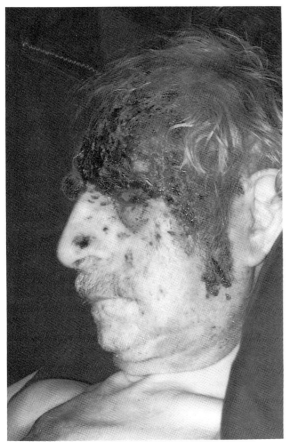

Fig. 16.1 *Herpes zoster* in first division of trigeminal nerve in a 75-year-old man with M1 AML. (Reproduced with permission from Whittaker J A 1986 Acute myeloid leukaemia in: Leukaemia. Blackwell, Oxford)

Table 16.7 Laboratory findings in patients with disseminated intravascular coagulation

Laboratory test	Severe DIC (with clinical disease)	Moderate DIC (often without clinical problems)	Mild DIC
Primary changes			
Plasma fibrinogen	<1 g/l	usually normal	usually normal
FDP	raised	raised	raised
Platelet count*	<50 × 10⁹/l	variable	variable
Thrombin time	very long⁺	variable	often normal
Secondary changes			
Prothrombin time	very long⁺	variable	normal
Partial thromboplastin time	very long⁺	variable	normal
Clotting time	very long⁺	variable	normal
Factors II, V, VIII	low	variable	normal
Plasminogen	low	low or normal	variable
Plasminogen activator	variable	variable	variable

* Low platelet count may be related to marrow failure and in isolation does not give reliable evidence of DIC in acute promyelocytic leukaemia
⁺ Blood often incoagulable

hepatosplenomegaly (50%), lymphadenopathy (42%), skin deposits (33%) and gum infiltration (25%). Less frequently, peri-anal deposits, gastrointestinal tract infiltration, bladder disease and deposits in lung and pleura are present. Patients have a poor prognosis largely due to a high incidence of central nervous system disease and the risk of leukaemic meningitis has been estimated to be five times greater than for other subtypes of AML. Renal failure and hypokalaemia occur frequently in association with increased levels of serum lysozyme, often in patients with high blood blast cell counts. The presence of excessive lysozyme in the glomerular filtrate in M5 disease produces renal tubular dysfunction resulting in the excretion of lysozyme in the urine.

Patients with M5 disease need careful clinical assessment, including examination of cerebrospinal fluid and assessment of renal function before treatment starts.

Potentially nephrotoxic antibiotics, for example aminoglycosides, if required, should be used with care, as they can cause a marked increase in the excretion of urinary lysozyme. Assessment of renal function before treatment is also worthwhile in patients with M4 disease, where many of the clinical features of M5 disease have been described. There is a high incidence of asymptomatic leukaemic infiltration in cerebrospinal fluid and some evidence for an association between the eosinophilic variant of M4, a chromosome abnormality, inv(16)(p13q22), and CNS disease.

Acute promyelocytic leukaemia

About 10–15 per cent of adult AML patients have acute promyelocytic leukaemia (M3) characterised by abnormal promyelocytes which constitute more than 50% of marrow cells containing distinctive large granules and multiple Auer rods and frequently showing a bilobed nucleus. Almost all cases are characterised by an abnormal karyotype with a 15:17 translocation. Patients with hypergranular M3 and those with the rarer variant may present with potentially fatal excessive bleeding which is often inappropriate to the degree of thrombocytopenia. Bleeding is due to disseminated intravascular coagulation (DIC) which occurs in 75% of

M3 patients accompanied by secondary fibrinolysis and is thought to be related to the release of procoagulants from the azurophilic granules in the leukaemic promyelocytes. These procoagulants are antigenically related to brain tissue factor. Occasionally DIC can complicate other subtypes of AML including acute monoblastic leukaemia. Initial granulocyte counts are below $10 \times 10^9/l$ in 80% of patients and above $30 \times 10^9/l$ in 10%. Somewhat surprisingly, there is no evidence to link the severity of DIC with the number of circulating promyelocytes, although often DIC appears to be precipitated by treatment, presumably by release of large amounts of procoagulant, when disruption of promyelocytes is maximal.

The laboratory features of DIC (Table 16.7) include a prolonged prothrombin time, a prolonged partial thromboplastin time, some reduction in platelet count, which is often severe, and reduction in plasma fibrinogen level. Depending on the severity of the DIC process, various combinations of these abnormalities are seen.

Associated with DIC, there is a high frequency of renal and respiratory failure which carry a poor prognosis and are probably related to deposition of microthrombi in the kidney and lungs. The acute respiratory distress syndrome (ARDS) is characterised by pulmonary platelet sequestration with frequent pulmonary haemorrhage and thrombosis. ARDS is unusual at presentation and is more commonly precipitated by cytotoxic treatment. In one large series, no patient with ARDS survived who required artificial ventilation. Renal failure is associated with renal cortical necrosis, but with renal dialysis many patients may survive.

The treatment of DIC in M3 disease is discussed below.

Leukostasis and hyperviscosity

10–15% of AML patients have a leukocyte count above $100 \times 10^9/l$ at presentation and these patients have a poor prognosis due to vascular infiltration of the central nervous system and lungs. A high incidence of fatal bleeding at presentation and during induction treatment is characteristic. About 50% of patients with AML and hyperleukocytosis have clinical or other evidence of leukostasis in the central nervous system or lungs and three-quarters of these patients have M4 or M5 disease.

Patients with hyperleukocytosis are usually protected from hyperviscosity by anaemia, but inappropriate transfusion may result in a clinical hyperviscosity syndrome with lethargy, unsteadiness of gait, visual disturbances and coma.

In patients with AML and hyperleukocytosis, large, relatively undeformable myeloblasts impede the microcirculation, causing plugging of the vessel lumen with leukocyte aggregates and thrombi. The vessels become distended and leaky leading to tissue infiltration by myeloblasts, occasionally associated with vascular rupture. The process is exacerbated by subsequent release of vasoactive peptides and nucleotides, which enhance stasis and cell aggregation. It is not clear whether vessels in the brain and lung are uniquely susceptible to leukostasis, or merely supply vital organs whose function is crucial to survival.

Success in reducing the WBC is an important predictor of survival in AML patients with hyperleukocytosis. Consequently, treatment must include early, intensive leukopheresis to reduce the leukocyte count significantly below $100 \times 10^9/l$ before anaemia is corrected.

Leukaemia in the central nervous system

Unless treatment is given to prevent its development, leukaemic infiltration of the central nervous system occurs in the majority of children and adults with ALL and appears to be increasing in incidence in AML as patients achieve longer survival. Most reports suggest an incidence of CNS disease in AML of about 10%, but leukaemic pleocytosis without overt clinical disease has been reported in over half the patients in a recent series, all of whom had the M4 subtype of the disease. Clinical studies have also indicated an increased incidence in M4 disease often associated with the eosinophilic variant of the disease and an abnormality of chromosome 16. 30–60% of CNS disease in AML patients is a focal abnormality, while this type of disorder is unusual in ALL.

The most frequent symptoms are those of raised intracranial pressure, headache, vomiting and papilloedema, while cranial nerve palsies (particularly of VI and VII) may occur as an isolated finding. Excessive appetite and weight gain are suggestive of hypothalamic infiltration, while hemiplegia or paraplegia occur infrequently. Convulsions and coma are rare and more suggestive of leuko-encephalopathy or viral encephalitis than leukaemic infiltration of the central nervous system.

The pathological features of CNS leukaemia have been well described and follow a characteristic pattern. Infiltration results from proliferation of cells in the walls of superficial arachnoid veins which presumably 'seed' at the time of presentation when there are large numbers of circulating blast cells. These cells, largely untouched by systemic chemotherapy, proliferate, sometimes very slowly, and destroy the arachnoid trabeculae with penetration of CSF channels. Thus CNS leukaemia is usually at first a meningeal disease and progressive parenchymal involvement only occurs at an advanced stage.

There have been attempts to define patients at high risk of leukaemic involvement of the CNS. Patients with a high leukocyte count and those with the rare B-cell ALL are at risk of early CNS relapse and it has been claimed that patients with a high platelet count are less likely to develop infiltration, but it is virtually impossible to define a group of patients who are not at risk of this complication.

The diagnosis of CNS infiltration should be confirmed by examination of a cytocentrifuged preparation of CSF which almost invariably shows leukaemic blast cells. There is usually a CSF pleocytosis but, particularly in cases with focal signs of cranial nerve or hypothalamic infiltration, the cell count may not be raised; the CSF protein may be raised and glucose decreased. The morphology of the leukaemic blast cell is usually apparent in a good preparation, but it can be difficult to distinguish leukaemic blasts from reactive mononuclear cells. Immunofluorescent stains for terminal deoxynucleotidyl transferase and monoclonal antibody studies may be of occasional help.

Purine metabolism

The lysis of leukaemic cells, which occurs spontaneously, or more usually in association with cytoreduction, liberates purines which are converted first to hypoxanthine and then to xanthine and uric acid by the enzyme xanthine oxidase. Uric acid may be deposited in various body tissues, but its clinical effects are seen almost exclusively in the kidneys and joints. Deposits of uric acid in the renal parenchyma, renal pelvis and ureters can result in acute renal failure. In most cases, serum uric acid is raised and urinary urate excretion is two to three times that seen in normal subjects.

Gouty arthropathy caused by deposit of uric acid crystals in large joints is rare prior to treatment, but not uncommon thereafter, especially in AML patients with high leukocyte counts. The pattern of joint involvement is 'secondary', nearly always single and most often affects the ankle or knee joints and less frequently the hip, wrist, elbow and shoulder. The small joints of the foot, most frequently involved in primary gout, are seldom affected.

The introduction of the xanthine oxidase inhibitor allopurinol has dramatically decreased the frequency of both urate nephropathy and arthropathy. The block in the conversion of hypoxanthine and xanthine to uric acid results in an increase of the serum levels of these substances and, although neither is appreciably more soluble than uric acid, their excretion occurs by a different mechanism so that they do not damage the kidneys, even if present in large quantities. However, large joint arthropathy caused by accumulation of xanthine crystals has been described, but is very rare.

Allopurinol, 300 mg daily, should be administered to all leukaemia patients receiving anthracyclines for remission induction. The breakdown of 6-mercaptopurine to thiouric acid is catalysed by xanthine oxidase, so that when this drug is used in AML treatment its dosage should be reduced to 25%. However, 6-thioguanine does not depend on xanthine oxidase for its breakdown, so that it can be given in normal dosage together with allopurinol.

Metabolic problems

Renal function. Renal function is often abnormal at presentation as a consequence of the disease (hyperuricaemia, hypokalaemia, renal infiltration) or of infection or its treatment. It is essential that uric acid production and electrolyte levels are corrected before treatment is started. Uric acid levels should be monitored throughout the induction period and prophylactic treatment with allopurinol is advisable as the initial WBC may not reflect the total body mass of leukaemic cells.

Hepatic function. Many cytotoxic drugs, especially the anthracycline antibiotics, are metabolised in the liver and are more toxic in the presence of liver cell damage. Consequently, it is essential that liver function should be assessed before treatment commences and again before subsequent treatments are given. An otherwise unexplained rise of serum bilirubin or an increase in levels of liver cell enzymes are indications to reduce or delay the administration of anthracyclines.

Cardiac function. The anthracycline antibiotics, used widely in remission induction treatments, show a cumulative cardiotoxicity which may be potentiated by hypokalaemia. The clinical features are those of congestive heart failure, the most striking characteristic being the rapidly progressive course. The condition may be controlled if diagnosed early and treated intensively, but the ECG, chest X-ray and measurement of cardiac enzymes are unhelpful in predicting its onset.

TREATMENT

Aims of treatment

Complete remission

(CR), defined as less than 5% of blasts in a normally cellular bone marrow in a patient with an essentially normal blood count, is the primary aim of treatment, without which long survival will not result.

Time to remission. The speed with which CR is achieved is important. When induction treatment is not intensive, multiple treatment courses are needed, resulting in a longer induction period and the exposure of the patient to a long period of potentially life-threatening neutropenia and thrombocytopenia. Modern management achieves early remissions by the rapid production of bone marrow hypoplasia with one or two courses of intensive treatment. This approach is possible largely because of improvements in supportive care.

Duration of remission and survival. There is little value in increasing the intensity of induction chemotherapy to improve the CR rate if the remissions produced are short-lived. Remission duration for ALL and AML has increased steadily during the past 10 or 15 years, but for AML it remains disappointingly short when considered against the background of the effort and cost of its achievement and the distress caused to the patient by modern treatments and their sequelae.

The prospect of cure. More than 50% of all children with ALL are now cured, with 80% (or better) cure rates for girls with common ALL. Results for ALL in adults are generally disappointing with few series reporting rates above 30% 5-year disease-free survival. In both adults and children with AML, although a small percentage of patients has survived in continuous complete remission even after non-intensive treatment, most patients are dead within 2 years. However, there are indications that more intensive treatments are increasing the percentage of long survivors.

The results of allogeneic bone marrow transplantation from matched sibling donors continue to improve, with several reports of 60–70% of AML and ALL patients surviving for more than 5 years. Unfortunately, at present this treatment is mostly available only to patients with a matched sibling donor less than 50 years old, although the use of unrelated and mis-matched donors is likely to extend its scope in the future.

Patient selection. It is important to identify which patients are suitable for intensive chemotherapy and which are not. Elderly patients do not tolerate intensive treatments and most, but not all, centres would not include patients over 70 years. On the other hand, in patients under about 55 years, results are satisfactory and, especially for AML, improving, so that almost all patients in this age group will be suitable for intensive regimens. Patients between about 55 years and 70 years cause most problems in selection. It seems obvious that elderly patients with a history of previous debilitating disease should be excluded, but otherwise selection is likely to vary according to local practice and the general condition of the individual patient.

Acute lymphoblastic leukaemia

Induction chemotherapy

The combination of oral prednisolone and weekly intravenous vincristine for 4–6 weeks induces remission in 80–90% of children with ALL and, with the addition of asparaginase, the rate rises to 93%. In adults, the two-drug combination is only effective in 40–50%, but remission rates rise to over 50% with the addition of L-asparaginase or an anthracycline and to about 80% if all four drugs are used. A similar high remission rate has been reported using a combination of prednisolone, vincristine, asparaginase and moderate-dose methotrexate. The addition of asparaginase to vincristine and prednisolone prolongs subsequent remission in childhood ALL and so there is sufficient evidence to warrant the use of at least three drugs for induction in children and four drugs for adults.

Failure to respond

If the blood count does not promptly improve following two or three induction treatments, it is essential to re-examine the bone marrow. Failure to respond is more common in adults, in patients with chromosomal abnormalities and in patients with high initial leukocyte counts. The addition of an anthracycline, epipodophyllotoxin with or without cytosine arabinoside, or anthracycline plus cytosine arabinoside may be effective, but failure to respond to initial induction treatment is a poor prognostic sign indicating a likely short survival.

Post-remission chemotherapy

It is essential that CNS prophylaxis is started as soon as possible and it is customary and convenient to introduce this as soon as patients enter remission. Because of the poorer prognosis in adults, it is not advisable to start CNS prophylaxis until remission has been confirmed.

Intensification therapy

It remains uncertain whether the use of additional drugs during induction or a period of post-remission intensification decreases the risk of subsequent bone marrow relapse. Haematological remission duration appears longest in protocols incorporating a third drug or a period of intensification, although the addition of daunorubicin to prednisolone, vincristine and asparaginase does not improve remission duration for adults with ALL.

Some results of studies of intensification treatment in childhood ALL are shown in Table 16.8, but unfor-

Table 16.8 Some studies of intensification treatment in childhood ALL

Induction	Intensification	Continuing treatment	Benefit of intensification	Year
PRED VCR± DNR	CY ARA- C	6MP MTX	No	1978
PRED VCR ASP	CY DOX	6MP MTX	No	1980
PRED VCR DNR ASP	CY ARA- C TG ASP DOX	6MP MTX	Yes	1981*
PRED VCR DNR	ASP early + late) ARA-C	6MP MTX	No	1984

PRED Prednisone; VCR Vincristine; ASP Asparaginase; DNR Daunorubicin; DOX Doxorubicin; MTX methotrexate; CY Cyclophosphamide; ARA-C Cytosine arabinoside; TG Thioguanine; 6MP 6 Mercaptopurine

* German study (see reference) but did not include randomised controls.

For sources of data see Table Referenes section at end of chapter.

tunately these studies have used either inadequate drug doses or historical controls. Undoubtedly among the best results reported are those from West Germany with a protocol incorporating a four-drug induction and a four-week period of post-remission intensification, and subsequently further intensification for patients at high risk of treatment failure. This intensive approach is not necessary for all children, since similar results in 'low risk' patients may be obtained with a less intensive protocol. The use of the similar protocol in adults has produced results which, though not as good, are better than others reported from multicentre trials. Results of some other adult studies are summarised in Table 16.9. While the use of additional drugs during induction has not always proved beneficial, the best reported results are from single centre studies using a complex intensification and maintenance schedule.

Further trials are needed in high-risk children and adults to clarify the value of early intensification therapy. Late intensification, as used in adult AML, has not been widely studied, but initial results have not indicated a major benefit.

Maintenance treatment

Older treatment schedules, which were used over periods of 15 to 65 weeks, were associated with a high rate of relapse, indicating the need for continuing treatment. However, the optimum type and duration of

Table 16.9 Induction treatment of adult ALL

Patient numbers	Induction	Remission rate (%)	Continuing treatment	CR (months)	3 year DFS (%)	Year
149	PRED VCR ASP DNR	72	Yes	15	30	1979
99	PRED VCR MTX	80	Yes	17	30	1980
72*	PRED VCR DOX	85	Yes	–	59	1983
170	PRED VCR ASP DNR	78	Yes	20	44	1984

DFS Disease-free survival; CR Complete remission; PRED Prednisone; VCR Vincristine; ASP Asparaginase; DNR Daunorubicin; DOX Doxorubicin; MTX Methotrexate

* Single centre study. Others are multi-centre.

For sources of data see Table References section at end of chapter.

continuing treatment for ALL are unknown and will probably vary according to the induction and intensification which has been used.

In patients receiving conventional induction treatment, continuation with one drug such as 6-mercaptopurine or methotrexate has been associated with a high relapse rate and consequently a combination of 6-mercaptopurine and methotrexate, with or without prednisolone and vincristine, is widely used for both children and adults. The use of additional drugs in a continuing schedule has increased toxicity without decreasing relapse rates. 6-mercaptopurine and methotrexate given intermittently at 3-weekly intervals is less immunosuppressive than continuous therapy, but this type of treatment is associated with a higher risk of marrow relapse.

The alternative approach of multiple drugs in an intermittent or rotating schedule does not appear to confer appreciable advantage and has the distinct disadvantage of being more complicated for both patient and doctor.

Bone marrow transplantation (BMT) for ALL in first remission

High dose chemo-radiotherapy followed by infusion of autologous or allogeneic bone marrow is an alternative to continuing chemotherapy in first remission. In view of the potential short- and long-term risks of this form of therapy, BMT in first remission should probably be reserved for patients with an unequivocally poor prognosis (for example, B-cell ALL, adult T-cell ALL, Ph +ve ALL).

Bone marrow transplantation should be considered in patients with ALL in the younger age group who achieve a second remission and have an HLA compatib sibling donor. Long-term follow-up of patients with refractory leukaemia who have achieved prolonged remissions following BMT indicates that this form of treatment may be curative for some patients. However, the number of potential recipients of BMT is in practice limited by lack of HLA-compatible siblings.

Duration of treatment

The optimal time for which treatment should continue is uncertain. Limited information from controlled trials suggests that treatment should continue for about 2 years. The MRC UK ALL I, II and III Trials showed that in girls treatment periods of 84 or 108 weeks were as effective as 3 years, but in boys 84 weeks was inferior to 2 or 3 years, with high rates of bone marrow and testicular relapse. The American Children's Cancer Study Group found that 5 years of treatment was not better than 3 years, and at St. Jude Children's Hospital treatment has usually been stopped after $2\frac{1}{2}$ years.

There are no comparable studies of treatment duration in adult ALL, but it seems highly unlikely that treatment for more than 2–3 years would increase overall disease-free survival. A policy of testicular biopsy before stopping treatment does not seem to have reduced the subsequent rate of bone marrow relapse off treatment, but the data are provisional and further observation is needed. Careful examination of the testes after treatment stops, with biopsy of any apparently abnormal testicle, is obviously essential and some clinicians will continue to biopsy the apparently normal testis.

Bone marrow relapse

The outlook for children and adults with ALL who develop a bone marrow relapse during treatment is extremely poor and further relapses are almost inevitable. A second remission can usually be achieved with vincristine, prednisolone, L-asparaginase and an anthracycline and other regimens which have proved effective include VM26 in combination with cytosine arabinoside or with vincristine and prednisolone, while the combination of an anthracycline with a ten-day infusion of cytosine arabinoside has induced remission in 60–70% of adults with refractory ALL. The major problem is maintenance of remission and drug combinations used include cytosine arabinoside and methotrexate, or methotrexate with L-asparaginase. If prolonged second remissions are achieved, the patients are at risk of CNS relapse, but it is debatable whether further CNS prophylaxis should be given or is indeed possible for all patients.

Patients who relapse on treatment or within 6 months of stopping treatment have a poor prognosis. However, patients who relapse after a prolonged unmaintained remission may achieve long second remissions, but whether such patients are curable with conventional chemotherapy remains uncertain. Further central nervous system prophylaxis is essential because of the high risk of CNS relapse and effective re-prophylaxis has been reported with intrathecal methotrexate and cytosine arabinoside in combination, but not with methotrexate alone.

CNS leukaemia

Prevention

Disease in the CNS is difficult to eradicate and almost impossible to cure. Its association with an increased rate of bone marrow relapse limits life expectancy and therefore treatment to prevent leukaemic infiltration of the CNS is an essential part of the management of both children and adults. While CNS leukaemia is not prevented by prophylactic craniospinal irradiation of 12 Gy, it can be prevented by 24 Gy to the whole neuraxis or by cranial irradiation at that dose and a course of intrathecal methotrexate injections. Craniospinal irradiation is marginally more effective than cranial irradiation and intrathecal methotrexate in prevention of CNS relapse, but is myelosuppressive and immunosuppressive and carries a greater risk of marrow relapse, particularly in high risk patients. These considerations have led to the use of cranial irradiation and intrathecal MTX as the standard in both children and adults with ALL. Concern about the late effects of cranial irradiation, particularly in the young child, have prompted investigation of slightly lower doses of radiation. Reduction from 24 Gy to 18 Gy has proved equally effective and alteration of MTX dose from one based on surface area to a dose based on CSF volume has produced a significant decrease in CNS relapse rate.

It remains uncertain whether cranial irradiation is an essential part of CNS prophylaxis and long-term follow-up of patients who have stopped therapy is needed to determine whether CNS leukaemia has been prevented or just deferred.

Intermediate dose methotrexate infusions (500 mg/m^2) (IDMTX) have been used for CNS prophylaxis in the belief that the drug crosses the blood – brain barrier at this dosage. IDMTX gives better protection against marrow and testicular relapse, while cranial irradiation is more effective in prevention of CNS relapse. It may be unwise to assume that IDMTX is less toxic than cranial irradiation, since CT scan appearances were abnormal in some children receiving this form of prophylaxis. Other studies in childhood ALL have confirmed that IDMTX provides effective CNS prophylaxis and a retrospective review of adult ALL demonstrated an equal effect for prophylaxis with regular intrathecal MTX compared with short term MTX with cranial irradiation.

Critical observation must continue in order to find the best method of CNS prophylaxis. At present, the best standard regimen is probably intrathecal MTX with 18 Gy cranial irradiation in children and 24 Gy in children with high leukocyte counts, adolescents and adults. Cranial irradiation in children under 2 years should be deferred because of its late effects, but intensive intrathecal or intravenous therapy may be required, particularly in infants under 1 year who tend to have high leukocyte counts at presentation and a high incidence of CNS leukaemia.

Treatment

CSF blasts are detectable in 1–2% of patients at presentation and a further 5–10% develop CNS leukaemia despite conventional prophylaxis. Patients with CNS disease at diagnosis should receive cranial irradiation and continuous weekly intrathecal MTX. It is possible to obtain CNS remission, even when standard CNS prophylaxis has failed, using weekly intrathecal MTX, but unless further treatment is given, relapse is rapid. Long-term intrathecal chemotherapy alone may achieve prolonged CNS remissions, but does not eradicate the disease. More prolonged remissions may be achieved with intraventricular therapy via an Omaya reservoir, but this carries a greater risk of encephalopathy. Cytosine arabinoside given intrathecally or in high doses systemically may be effective in patients refractory to MTX.

Because of the high risk of marrow relapse, treatment for patients with a CNS relapse should include reinduction and intensification with systemic chemotherapy. Those patients who re-enter CNS and marrow remission should be considered for allogeneic BMT.

The testicle

In ALL testicular relapse, presenting as a painless swelling of one or both testes, occurs in about 10% of male patients within a year of completing treatment. Patients with apparent unilateral disease often have histological change in the clinically unaffected testis, but involvement of bone marrow and CSF is variable.

Orchidectomy or radiotherapy are equally effective, but because of the risk of disease in an apparently uninvolved testis, bilateral radiotherapy is preferable. Subsequent haematological and CNS relapse may be avoided by an additional two-year treatment including both systemic and intrathecal drugs.

In patients with clinically normal testes, bilateral wedge biopsies should be obtained before treatment is discontinued, although regrettably negative biopsy does not preclude subsequent testicular relapse and some clinicians recommend repeat biopsies at 6 months and 1 year. The alternative, which is gaining wider acceptance, is to give 'prophylactic' bilateral testicular radiotherapy to all males, but preliminary results are conflicting with one American study showing no advantage, while the MRC UK ALL VI and VII trials have shown a reduced frequency of testicular disease, but not of bone marrow relapse.

The use of immunological markers, for example the identification of TdT-positive cells in testicular biopsies, may have potential for the future, but the prevention of testicular disease may require improved systemic chemotherapy.

The ovary

Ovarian involvement is rare, but is occasionally seen in girls in early puberty. Disease can usually be detected by examination with ultrasound or computerised tomography, but biopsy is necessary unless disease is evident in bone marrow. Bilateral oophorectomy followed by a further two-year programme of systemic and intrathecal chemotherapy may provide successful treatment, but little information is available for treatments which include radiotherapy.

The eye

Ocular relapse may occur in patients with multiple relapses and CNS involvement, but may also present with an iridocyclitis in patients otherwise in remission and off treatment. Local irradiation followed by further intrathecal and systemic chemotherapy should be given, but the prognosis for these patients is poor.

Other extramedullary sites

Other sites at which disease may occasionally occur in remission patients include the pleura and kidneys, but splenomegaly persisting during treatment is more likely to be due to portal fibrosis or viral infection than to leukaemic infiltration. Prognosis is poor in these cases, but the bone marrow should be examined, chemotherapy revised and local radiotherapy considered.

Complications of treatment

Infective complications. Prolonged intensive chemotherapy results for at least some of all patients treated in severe lymphopenia and immunosuppression associated with serious infections including *Pneumocystis carinii*, pneumonitis and *Varicella zoster*. In unvaccinated children, a high incidence of measles may be expected.

Neuropsychological. A variety of neurological complications may be seen during treatment, especially arachnoiditis following intrathecal chemotherapy and post-radiation somnolence. Patients receiving prolonged intrathecal chemotherapy or repeated radiotherapy may suffer convulsions and dementia associated with a necrotising leukoencephalopathy. Such florid disease is rare, but the increasing incidence of learning problems in young children who have received prophylactic CNS radiotherapy is worrying. Children who receive cranial radiotherapy under 3 years of age generally have lower than average IQs and tend to be backward in reading and arithmetic. These problems are often heightened by poor school attendance and associated social and psychological stresses in the family. As a result, many centres now empirically delay radiotherapy or reduce dosage for infants, but progress may depend on identifying alternative methods of CNS prophylaxis.

Growth. There is no doubt that prolonged continuous treatment results in retardation of growth, and most centres restrict treatment to 18 months or 2 years and, as growth is normal for children off treatment, the resulting loss of height is minimal. Puberty appears normal in both boys and girls.

Fertility. Although abnormal gonadal histology has been seen in both sexes, there are many examples of girls who have given birth to normal infants following successful chemotherapy for ALL and at present there is no evidence that these children have an increased risk of malignancy or congenital abnormality.

Prophylactic or therapeutic testicular irradiation will cause male infertility and prepubertal boys show delayed or altered puberty.

Other organs. Other organ damage is rare. Anthracycline-induced cardiac damage, often seen in AML patients, is less usual in ALL because of lower total drug dosages. Transient abnormalities of liver function are common during treatment, but rarely associated with chronic disease.

Acute myeloid leukaemia

Induction chemotherapy

Single agents. Attempts at remission induction with one drug alone now have little place in AML treatment and no place in first remission induction therapy. This is because there are few reports of CR rates above 40% and also because of the higher risk of producing drug resistance when agents are used singly. Results from a number of selected trials are shown in Table 16.10.

Table 16.10 The use of single agents in the treatment of AML

Drug	Dosage	No. of patients	CR (%)
Daunorubicin	60 mg/m²/d × 3d	22	50
	60 mg/m²/d × 3d		49
	60 mg/m²/d × 3d	46[+]	29
Rubidazone	4 mg/kg/d × 5d	66[+]	56
Cytosine arabinoside	800 mg/m² × 48h (iv inf)	79	20
	1000 mg/m² × 120 h (iv inf)	85	38
	4 mg/kg × 8h (iv inf)	31	46
	100 mg/m² × 1h (iv inf)*	49	14
	200 mg/m²/d × 5d	57	49

CR Complete remission; iv inf intravenous infusion
* Repeated until marrow hypoplasia produced
[+] Includes some children

Table 16.11 The use of newer agents used singly in the treatment of adult AML

Drug	No. of patients	CR (%)	Year of publication
Aclacinomycin	38[+]	34	1984
	44	18	1984
Amsacrine	30*	30	1980 1982
(AMSA)	18	17	1981
	38	8	1984
5-Azacytidine	45	24	1976
4-Demethoxy-	18	17	1985
daunorubicin	28	19	1985
Etopside	20*	10	1976
	12*	33	1973
Homoharringtonine	28	25	1985
Mitoxantrone	38(26)[+]	26(40)[+]	1984
	13	31	1985

Except where otherwise stated, all studies are in relapsed or refractory patients.
CR Complete remission
* Previously untreated patients
[+] Relapsed patients only
For sources of data see Table References section at end of chapter.

However, Ara C used in very high dosage has given very encouraging results in the treatment of relapsed and resistant AML. Its use is considered separately (see below).

Some older agents which give even less good results have been excluded from the Table. For example, mercaptopurine and methotrexate when used alone give a CR rate below 10%.

A number of newer agents have been used singly to treat patients with relapsed or resistant disease (Table 16.11) and several of the more promising drugs are now being incorporated into multiple drug treatments.

Combination chemotherapy. The chief aims of combination chemotherapy are the rapid production of early CR and the reduction of the risk of the emergence of disease resistance. Modern treatments result in rapid marrow hypoplasia requiring a period of haematological support until marrow recovery occurs.

Combinations of an anthracycline and cytosine arabinoside. Combinations of an anthracycline antibiotic and Ara C with or without 6-thioguanine (6TG) are the most frequently used AML induction regimens (Table 16.12) and can be expected to give CR rates of 60–80% in patients under 60 years of age. The combination of a 7-day continuous infusion of Ara C with daily doses of an anthracycline antibiotic for 3 days

provides an effective induction regimen. A 10-day Ara C infusion does not increase CR rate, but does increase gastrointestinal and other toxicity. Possibly remission rates may be higher when 6TG is included in the treatment, but regrettably most series which include this drug are small and may reflect understandably better results in initial studies in a single centre.

Continuous infusion of Ara C and intermittent intravenous injection probably give comparable results.

Much has been made of minor differences in CR rate for patients treated with DNR or doxorubicin (DXR), but the evidence is conflicting and it seems likely that the two drugs give very similar results when used in equivalent doses.

Remission rates do not improve, but toxicity increases when higher anthracycline doses are used and, since both DXR and DNR are associated with clinical cardiotoxicity in up to one third of patients at cumulative doses exceeding 500 mg/m^2, schedules which limit dosages are to be preferred.

Induction combinations including vincristine. Combinations of vincristine and prednisone with intravenous infusions of Ara C for 5 or 10 days give CR rates which are slightly lower than those for combinations of Ara C and anthracyclines. The addition of vincristine and prednisone to combinations of Ara C and anthracyclines does not increase CR rates and is not warranted in adult practice.

Induction combinations including amsacrine. Amsacrine (AMSA), an acridine derivative which has proved useful as a single agent, when combined with Ara C or 5-azacytidine has given encouraging results in the treatment of relapsed or resistant AML, and drug combinations which include amsacrine are now under study as initial AML induction tratments (Table 16.13).

Remission duration

Comparison of the lengths of remission produced by the induction treatments outlined in Table 16.12 is difficult, as almost all regimes include additional treatment during remission (see below). However, the remission duration associated with most induction treatments is disappointingly short, although better results are emerging, particularly from some treatment trials in children.

Consolidation and maintenance of remission

A further major objective in leukaemia treatment is the prevention of disease recurrence once remission has been established. Most patients subsequently relapse, presumably because their induction treatment did not completely abolish the leukaemia, but unfortunately as

Table 16.12 Some combinations of cytosine arabinoside and an anthracycline for initial treatment of adult AML

Dosages	No. of patients	Age	CR (%)	CR (%) patients <60 yr	MRD (months)	Year of publication
ARA-C 100 mg/m²/d × 7d (iv inf) DNR 45 mg/m²/d on d 1–3(iv)	226	A★	58	72	12	1982
or DNR 30 mg/m²/d on d 1–3 (iv)	117	A★	55	59	12	
or DXR 30 mg/m²/d on d 1–3(iv)	105	A★	50	58	12	
ARA-C 100 mg/m²/12h on d 1–7 + 22–26(iv) DNR 60 mg/m²/d on d 1–3 + d 22,23(iv) 6TG 100 mg/m²/d on d 1–7 + d 22–26 (oral)	50	A★	68	–	13	1985
ARA-C 100 mg/m²/d × 7d (iv inf) DNR 45 mg/m²/d on d 1–3 (iv)	508	A	66	–	9–17	1984
ARA-C 100 mg/m²/d × 7d(iv inf) DXR 30 mg/m²/d on d 1–3(iv) or DNR 45 mg/m²/d on d 1–3(iv)	40	<70★	60	68(80)[+]	12.5	1979
ARA-C 100 mg/m²/d × 10d(iv inf) DXR 30 mg/m²/d on d 1–3 (iv)	46	<70★	88[++]	–	–	1979
ARA-C 100 mg/m²/d × 7d(iv) DNR 60 mg/m²/d × 3d(iv) 6TG 100 mg/m²/12h × 7d (oral)	28	A	79	71	9	1977
ARA-C 100 mg/m²/d × 5d(iv) DNR 50 mg/m²/d on d 1 (iv) 6TG 100 mg/m²/d × 5d (oral)	20	A	85	–	11	1977

★ Includes some children; [+] 80% in previously untreated patients; [++] under 50 yr; A Adults of all ages; CR Complete remission; MRD Mean remission duration; ARA-C Cytosine arabinoside; DNR Daunorubicin; DXR Doxorubicin; 6TG 6-Thioguanine

For sources of data see Table References section at end of chapter.

Table 16.13 Amsacrine in combination schedules for the treatment of relapsed or refractory AML

Amsacrine dosage per treatment	Other agents	No. of patients	CR (%)	Year of publication
30 mg/m²/d × 7d	Ara-C 70 mg/m²/d × 7d VCR 2 mg/d × 1d (iv) Pred 100 mg/d × 5d (oral)	56	46	1981
75–100 mg/m²/d × 3d (Days 7–9)	Ara-C 3000 mg/m²/12h × 12	40	70	1984
200–225 mg/m²/d × 3d or 175–185 mg/m²/d × 4d	Ara-C 200 mg/m²/d × 5d 6TG 100 mg/m²/12h × 5d	25	32	1981
75–150 mg/m²/d × 4d (Days 5–8)	5-Aza 112–200 mg/m²/d × 4d (Days 1–4)	80	16	1985
150 mg/m²/d × 5d	5-Aza 150 mg/m²/d × 5d	12	58	1983

CR Complete remission
ARA-C Cytosine arabinoside; VCR Vincristine; Pred Prednisone; 6TG 6-Thioguanine; 5-Aza 5-Azacytidine

For sources of data see Table References section at end of chapter.

Table 16.14   Controlled trials of maintenance chemotherapy in adult AML

Induction treatment	Maintenance		CR (%)	Total patients	MRD** (months)	Year of publication
1. DNR ARA-C 6TG (DAT)	ARA-C 6TG	Cycle 1	72	48	18	1984
	ARA-C VCR PRED versus Nil	Cycle 2		26	18	
2. DNR ARA-C 6TG (DAT)	ARA-C 6TG versus	(repeated weekly × 2 years)	65	69	8	1984
	ARA-C DAT × 2 6TG	(repeated weekly × 2 years)		77	10	
3. DNR ARA-C 6TG (DAT)	ARA-C 6TG versus Nil		63	13	10.3	1977
				13	6.7	
4. DNR*	6MP MTX versus ARA-C Methyl GAG		16–43	129	5	1973

* Complicated three-way randomisation in two protocols at six dosages
** Studies 1, 2, 4 no significant difference. Study 3 p = 0.05. CR Complete remission; MRD Medium remission duration; DNR Daunorubicin; ARA-C Cytosine arabinoside; 6TG 6-Thioguanine; VCR Vincristine; PRED Prednisone; MTX Methotrexate; Methyl GAG Methylglyoxal-bisguanylhydrazone; 6MP 6-Mercaptopurine
For sources of data see Table References section at end of chapter.

yet there are no reliable methods of detecting minimal residual disease. The persistence of leukaemia cells is supported by the presence of abnormal marrow culture patterns during remission.

The place of both consolidation and maintenance treatment is controversial and, while it seems logical to use some further treatment after the induction of remission, there are no clear indications as to what that treatment should be. Furthermore, results from the few available controlled trials are conflicting (Table 16.14), but suggest that occasional low dose maintenance treatment confers no advantage. However, as residual leukaemia cells will probably begin to multiply as soon as induction chemotherapy ceases, it is customary to give further treatment to patients in remission in the hope that this will delay or prevent leukaemic relapse.

Many regimes include one or more courses of treatment at high doses, usually with the same drugs for the induction of remission. This type of treatment is usually termed consolidation to distinguish it from maintenance chemotherapy, in which lower doses of the same or additional drugs are given at intervals over a prolonged period of time.

Intensification therapy

In an attempt to eradicate residual leukaemic cells and to prevent the emergence of drug-resistant leukaemic cell-lines, additional intensive chemotherapy has recently been incorporated into some treatment regimes. Either 'early' or 'late' in remission, patients receive combinations of drugs which were not part of their induction treatment. Consolidation treatment differs from early intensification in that it is given immediately following remission, usually with the same drugs, and is often simply an additional course of induction treatment. Late intensification is further high-dose treatment with new drugs given to patients who have been in con-

Table 16.15 High-dose cytosine arabinoside in the treatment of AML

Ara-C dosage	Other agents	No. of patients	CR (%)	Year of publication
3 g/m^2/12h × 12 (iv)	–	16	25	1984
up to 3 g/m^2/12h × 12 (iv)	–	37	.51	1983
3 g/m^2/12h × 4 (iv)	Asp (im)	13	70	1984
3 g/m^2/12h × 8 (iv)	–	8	20	1985
2 g/m^2/12h × 12 (iv)	DXR Ara-C 6TG	12*	75	1985
1 g/m^2/12h × 12 (iv)	Amsa Days 5–7	6	83	1985
2 g/m^2/12h × 12 (iv)	Amsa Days 5–7	21	47	
3 g/m^2/12h × 4 (iv)	Amsa Days 1–5	26	46	
3 g/m^2/12h × 12 (iv)	Amsa Days 7–9	40	70	1984
3 g/m^2/12h × 12 (iv)	–	19	63	1985
3 g/m^2/12h × 12 (iv)	DXR⎫ or DNR⎭	17	65	

Except where otherwise stated, all studies are in relapsed or refractory patients.
* Previously untreated patients; CR Complete remission; Ara-C Cytosine arabinoside; Asp Asparaginase; DXR Doxorubicin; 6TG 6-Thioguanine; Amsa Amsacrine

For sources of data see Table References section at end of chapter.

tinuous remission for varying periods of time, usually in excess of 9 months. Both types of intensification differ from maintenance treatment, which generally uses low doses of drugs.

The results of these studies are often difficult to compare with conventional treatments, as they are uncontrolled trials in patients who have already achieved remission. However, current results suggest that both types of intensification increase the duration of CR and hence survival.

Treatment of patients with relapsed or resistant disease

The majority of patients with AML in remission will eventually relapse, so that treatment of the relapsed patient is a major problem.

Up to 50% of patients with relapsed disease may re-enter remission when retreated with an anthracycline antibiotic and Ara C in a similar fashion to first remission induction treatment. However, second remissions are disappointingly short at about 4 months and almost always shorter than the first remission for any given patient. As might be expected, the incidence of drug-resistant disease is much higher in relapsed patients and death due to inability to tolerate repeated intensive treatments is common. Several observers have reported higher rates of second remission in patients whose previous treatment has included immunotherapy.

Patients with disease which proves resistant to treatment with an anthracycline antibiotic and Ara C (Type I and Type II failure, Table 16.16) have a particularly

poor outlook. However, during the past few years preliminary results of treatment with high dose Ara C have shown promising results (see below and Table 16.15).

High dose cytosine arabinoside (HD-Ara C)

Recently, cytosine arabinoside, has been used in AML treatment at dosages which are 30-fold higher than those usually employed (3 g/m^2 vs 100–200 mg/m^2). The reason for the use of HD-Ara C is the concept that resistance to Ara C is due to inadequate cellular uptake which can be circumvented by the use of high dosages. At low drug concentrations, Ara C uptake is limited by facilitated diffusion, while at high dosage Ara C enters cells by passive diffusion. A number of recently published results of the use of HD-Ara C either alone or in combination with other agents are shown in Table 16.15. These results are encouraging, as they principally relate to the treatment of relapsed or resistant disease. In consequence, HD-Ara C is now being incorporated into trials of initial induction chemotherapy. However, although haemopoietic toxicity is similar to that produced by standard combination chemotherapy, other toxicities occur which necessitate extra care and limit the use of HD-Ara C to younger patients. The most distressing problem which occurs in 10–15% of patients is cerebellar toxicity, from a mild tremor to irreversible cerebellar damage. This may be a cumulative effect as it occurs particularly in patients receiving more than one treatment, but it also occurs in the elderly, alcoholics

Table 16.16 Causes of induction failure in AML

I	Major drug resistance	Failure to produce significant marrow hypoplasia. Patient surviving for > 7 days after chemotherapy finishes.
II	Relative drug resistance	(i) Chemotherapy produces hypoplasia. Leukaemic cells repopulate marrow in < 40 days.
		(ii) As for (i), but with repopulation by some normal cells
III	Regeneration failure	Marrow severely hypoplastic for > 40 days after chemotherapy finishes
IV	Hypoplastic death	Patient dies during severe marrow hypoplasia*
V	Inadequate trial	Patient dies > 7 days after chemotherapy with a cellular bone marrow
IV	Extramedullary persistence	Patient enters complete haematological remission, but leukaemic cells persist in extramedullary sites (principally CSF, liver or spleen)

* Classified as regeneration failure if death occurs > 40 days after chemotherapy

and those treated previously with radiation to the central nervous system. Patients who have recovered from severe cerebellar toxicity may show a recurrence if treated with Ara C at conventional dosage. Up to 50% of patients suffer a severe conjunctivitis, which is preventable by the prophylactic use of steroid-containing eye drops and a severe respiratory distress syndrome has been associated with continuous infusion. Other toxicity includes somnolence, liver damage, diarrhoea, skin rashes and skin hyperpigmentation. Major toxicities appear to correlate with total dosage of HD-Ara C.

Reasons for failure of induction chemotherapy

In spite of recent improvements in remission rates, a significant number of AML patients still fail to reach CR. It has long been obvious that some patients die from septicaemia and other infections associated with severe neutropenia resulting from intensive chemotherapy and, although improvements in supportive care have reduced the number of these deaths, they continue to be a problem. About two thirds of those dying after the third week of induction treatment, before which remission is rare, have marrow hypoplasia and these patients might enter remission with better supportive care. Infection accounts for about 70% of deaths during the first four courses of treatment (30%

Table 16.17 Prolonged disease-free survival in AML

Remission induction	CR (%)	Other treatment	Total no. of patients	MRD (months)	Continuous disease-free survival		Year of publication
DNR Ara-C 6TG	65	Ara-C 6TG + DAT × 2 (weekly maintenance)	77	9	28%	2 yr +	1984
DNR Ara-C	60	DNR Ara-C (consolidation × 1)	28	29	44%	3 yr	1984
DNR Ara-C	66	Ara-C 6TG (Intensive, 3-monthly to hypoplasia)	115	18	25%	4 yr +	1984
DNR Ara-C Or Ara- C DNR or Pred	58	Ara-C 6TG (weekly maintenance)	45	17	31%	5yr +	1981

MRD median remission duration; DNR Daunorubicin; Ara-C Cytosine arabinoside; 6TG 6-Thioguanine; CR Complete remission; Pred Prednisone; DAT Daunorubicin, Ara C, 6TG
For sources of data see Table References section at end of chapter.

were bacterial alone, 15% fungal alone and 10% due to a combination of bacterial and fungal infection). It is important to distinguish these deaths from those related to failure to eradicate leukaemia after an adequate trial of chemotherapy (Table 16.16). The majority of treatment failures are due to drug resistance (Types I and II) or early death of the patient with Type IV or Type V failure.

Prospects for prolonged disease-free survival

High remission rates in AML patients aged less than 60 years have been associated with a disappointingly short median duration of remission. However, some recent studies have reported a median duration of remission of about 18 months or more and for about one fifth of patients a disease-free survival of 3 years of more. Some of these studies (Table 16.17) suggest that these rates of disease-free survival are likely to continue for 4 or 5 years and the possibility arises that at least some of these patients are cured. The reason for this improvement is uncertain, although it may relate to much more intensive induction and consolidation treatment in recent years. However, there is no doubt that long survival and possibly cure can occur with minimal therapy. Several retrospective reports describe disease-free survival in AML patients treated many years previously and often without any form of consolidation or maintenance. Whether these patients represent a more sensitive variety of AML, or whether their survival is due to chance, is not clear.

Special problems in AML treatment

Treatment of AML in the elderly

Remission rates and survival duration for AML patients are closely related to age, with elderly patients faring badly. Intensive modern induction treatments achieve high remission rates, which are often confined to patients of less than 50 or 55 years, possibly because the elderly are less well able to tolerate the septicaemia frequently associated with severe neutropenia. In consequence, any less intensive treatment likely to produce reasonable CR rates is worthy of consideration for older patients. Induction treatment with an anthracycline antibiotic and Ara C are best tolerated at lower than normal dosages. Results are related to age with satisfactory CR rates for patients aged 50–70 years, but lower rates for those over 70 years.

Recent results of low dose Ara C therapy indicate that this treatment should be considered for patients over 65 years at dosages of 10 mg/m^2 every 12 hours for 2–3

weeks. Treatment is well tolerated, and toxicity is low with few treatment-related deaths, although some reports stress profound neutropenia and thrombocytopenia requiring intensive support. Early investigators related the benefit of low dose Ara C to the production of differentiation in myeloid leukaemic cells, but others have recently questioned this view, and suggest a conventional effect of Ara C by cumulative cytotoxicity on cells in S phase. Low dose Ara C treatment seems to be most beneficial in patients with a low to moderate leukaemic cell mass, that is those with early AML, hypoplastic myeloid leukaemia or refractory anaemia with excess of myeloblasts in transformation. The bone marrow blast cell count may be helpful in predicting response, with little or no effect when blast cell counts exceed 85%. These conclusions are based on several small studies and await the confirmation which may come from wider usage.

Childhood AML

Until recently, treatment results in childhood AML differed little from those in adults and the infrequent occurrence of the disease made for slow progress. However, the use of intensive induction, consolidation and maintenance treatments, often similar in design to those used in ALL, has resulted in high remission rates and in the prolongation of survival. Some modern protocols and their results are summarised in Table 16.18. These treatments are possibly even more intensive than those described above for adults and can only be contemplated in centres equipped with the full range of support facilities.

Induction treatment using a combination of Ara C and an anthracycline with or without the addition of vincristine and prednisone gives CR rates of 70–80%. Several studies have demonstrated that disease-free survival for up to 5 years is possible for a high proportion of children, but the need for intensive maintenance treatment remains uncertain.

Central nervous system disease

Compared with adult AML, the haematological relapse rate is lower in children, but CNS relapses, which are unusual in adults, occur more frequently with an incidence of about 20%. In a series of 111 adult AML relapses, only six were in the CNS, but in a recent study which included adults and children without CNS prophylaxis, CNS disease in the adults was uncommon, but relatively frequent in the children.

Studies in childhood AML which have included CNS prophylaxis indicate a significantly lower CNS relapse

Table 16.18 Some chemotherapy protocols for the treatment of childhood AML

Induction treatment	Consolidation or maintenance treatment	Total patients	CR (%)	Survival[+]	Year of publication

(VAPA 10)
VCR
DXR
Pred
Ara-C
	Rotating14-month sequence each of
	12–16 weeks
	  (i) DXR
	     Ara-C
	  (ii) DXR
	     5-Aza
	  (iii) VCR
	     Methyl Pred
	     6MP
	     MTX
	  (iv) Ara-C
	     No specific CNS prophylaxis
		45*	74	5 yr 44%	1983

0-28 d VCR DXR Pred 6TG Ara-C	Two-monthly cycles for 2 yr Ara- C DXR 6TG (DXR stopped at cumulative dose of 300 mg/m^2)	151*	79	5 yr 45%	1985
DNR 5- Aza Ara-C Pred VCR	Monthly cycle for 2 yr TG 5-Aza Ara- C VCR MTX IT	163	71.8	30 mo 20.4%	1984
	or Same cycle *plus* Cyclo	166	72	30 mo 31.5%	

* Age 0–17 yr; [+] Life table estimate; CR Complete remission; CNS Central nervous system; VCR Vincristine;
DXR Doxorubicin; Pred Prednisone, Ara-C Cytosine arabinoside; 6TG 6-Thioguanine; 5-Aza 5-Azacytidine;
MTX Methotrexate; 6MP 6-Mercaptopurine; Cyclo Cyclophosphamide; iv intravenous; iv inf intravenous infusion;
sc subcutaneous; IT intrathecal

For sources of data see Table References section at end of chapter.

rate and confirm the need for CNS prophylaxis in children. Intrathecal methotrexate with or without cranial irradiation has also proved effective in CNS prophylaxis, but the exact value of these treatments is not fully known, as none of these studies has included a true control group. As with adults, children with myelomonocytic (M4) or monocytic (M5) disease have the highest risk of CNS leukaemia.

Treatment of acute promyelocytic leukaemia

Until relatively recently, patients with M3 disease had a poor prognosis with an early high death rate usually related to bleeding from disseminated intravascular coagulation, often precipitated by induction treatment. Previously, death from bleeding has occurred in over 50% of patients and has been a particular problem in patients over the age of 30–35 years. Early death is related closely to intracerebral haemorrhage and is significantly related to the appearance of large retinal haemorrhages. However, with improved management of DIC-related bleeding, remission rates in M3 have

steadily improved and current CR rates of 60–80 per cent have led to the demonstration of generally better survival rates than for patients with other subtypes of AML. In these reports, induction chemotherapy has been similar to that for other subtypes of AML and has usually included Ara C and an anthracycline with or without 6-thioguanine.

Disseminated intravascular coagulation (DIC)

There remains controversy about the place of heparin treatment in M3 and there is no doubt that the most important aspect of treatment is the rapid reduction of the leukaemic cell mass. However, where DIC has been demonstrated, patients may be given 7.5–15 U of heparin/kg/hour by continuous intravenous infusion, although lower doses appear to have been successful. There may even be merit in heparin treatment for all patients with M3 because of the risk of procoagulant release from hypergranular promyelocytes following cytotoxic treatment.

Table 16.19   Controlled trials of bone marrow transplantation vs chemotherapy alone for adult AML in first remission

Centre	Bone marrow transplantation			Chemotherapy			P value* (relapse %)	Year of publication
	No. of patients	Relapse (%)	Survival (%)	No. of patients	Relapse (%)	Survival (%)		
University of California, Los Angeles	23	40	40	44	71	27	0.01	1985
Seattle	33	–	48**	46	–	20**	–	1984
Royal Marsden Hospital, London	22	35	67	28	90	35	0.005	1980 1982

* In all three trials, P values showed no significant difference in long-term survival % between BMT patients and chemotherapy patients.
** Disease-free survival

For sources of data see Table References section at end of chapter.

Heparin treatment has been shown to reduce the incidence of bleeding in M3 during induction treatment. During treatment, prothrombin time, partial thromboplastin time and serum fibrinogen levels should be carefully monitored every six hours. Decreasing values of serum fibrinogen, sometimes accompanied by increased bleeding, indicate the need to increase heparin dosage.

Some authors have suggested the recurrent use of multiple platelet transfusions to maintain a count of at least $60 \times 10^9/L$ before and during heparin treatment. In addition, fresh frozen plasma should be used freely to replace coagulation factors consumed by DIC. General support with packed red cell transfusion and fluid and electrolyte replacement is important, particularly initially in patients showing signs of shock.

Clinical and laboratory evidence of DIC usually resolves rapidly once marrow hypoplasia is achieved and in one recent series it was not necessary to continue heparin beyond the fifth day.

Additional methods of treatment in AML

Allogeneic bone marrow transplantation

The basic principles and results of bone marrow transplantation (BMT) for leukaemia are fully discussed in Chapter 21. Recent reports from several chemotherapy trials show that about 20% of all adults with AML in first remission have remained disease-free for 5 years or longer and these results have generated debate about the place of BMT in AML. Although initial results appear better for BMT than for chemotherapy, with more than 50% of long-term survivors, the comparisons are retrospective and may mislead, as most series of BMT patients are under 45 years,

although many intensive chemotherapy programmes accept patients up to the age of 60 years. Several controlled trials have compared chemotherapy with BMT in adult AML, and the results of three of these trials are outlined in Table 16.19. Larger studies, with a longer period of observation, are needed, but these reports suggest that BMT confers definite advantage for adult patients with AML in first remission.

Autologous bone marrow transplantation

Allogeneic BMT leads to a longer leukaemia-free survival than chemotherapy alone, but death and high rates of morbidity often result from transplant-related problems, particularly infections and graft-versus-host disease (GVHD). Most AML patients are not suitable for allogeneic BMT, which is generally available only to about one in four patients with an HLA matched donor, and is rarely successful for patients over 40 years.

Autologous remission bone marrow is a potential source of stem cells and avoids many of the problems of an allograft. Its major theoretical disadvantage is the possible reinfusion of residual leukaemic cells and the basis for the technique is the hope that any such cells will be in a resting phase not available to marrow aspiration. In addition, no graft-versus leukaemia effect is possible in the absence of GVHD.

Promising initial results have been reported with a predicted 3 year leukaemia-free survival in one study of 58%. Both purged and unpurged marrow has been used, but as yet no advantage for marrow purging has been demonstrated, although experimental approaches in ALL have included the treatment of bone marrow in vitro with antileukaemic antiserum or monoclonal antibodies. The procedure appears to be well tolerated and successful for patients aged up to about 60 years.

PROGNOSTIC FACTORS

Acute lymphoblastic leukaemia (Table 16.20)

Table 16.20 Prognostic factors in childhood ALL

	Good prognosis	Poor prognosis
Age (years)	2–10	<1 >10
Sex	Female	Male*
Hb (g/dl)	> 10.0	< 7.5
WBC ($\times 10^9$/l)	< 10.0	> 100
Platelets ($\times 10^9$/l)	> 100	<50
Lymphadenopathy	Nil	Present
Splenomegaly	Nil	Present
Liver	Nil	Present
CSF blasts	Nil	Present

* Probably reflects the occurrence of late testicular disease

Immediately following marrow harvest, patients are treated with conditioning similar to that used in allogeneic BMT to ablate residual bone marrow and the harvest is then reinfused after an interval of up to 72 hours.

It is too early to assess these preliminary studies and clinical trials on larger numbers of patients are needed. It is possible that the effect of autologous transplantation may simply be that of intensification therapy.

Prediction of long remission and cure

Patients surviving in complete remission, off treatment for more than 5 years, are probably cured and a number of attempts have been made to define presentation factors which will predict remission duration and consequently length of survival. These studies aim to identify patients with high risk of relapse who might benefit from more intensive treatment, but they are applicable only to children. Care is needed when analysing results because of the possible association of individual prognostic factors with others which are already well defined (for example, high leukocyte count). In consequence, multivariate analysis is needed to determine which factors are of independent prognostic significance. In addition, it is clear that most adverse prognostic factors lose significance after about two years in remission, except male sex, which probably continues to reflect the late occurrence of testicular disease.

Clinical and haematological features

The most important prognostic factor both for children and adults is initial extent of disease which correlates well with total blood leukocytes or blood blast cells, counts about 100×10^9/l being particularly unfavourable. Extent of disease is also reflected by enlargement of lymph nodes (including mediastinal enlargement), liver and spleen.

Age at diagnosis is also important, with patients aged 2–10 years doing much better than others. Other adverse factors include low platelet counts ($< 50 \times 10^9$/L), early CNS disease, low levels of immunoglobulin, slow response to induction treatment and Negro race.

Since use of the FAB classification and scoring system (see above), which allows accurate subtyping of ALL, has become widespread, it is clear that L1 ALL has a more favourable prognosis than L2 disease, but patients who present with L1 ALL may revert to L2 at relapse.

The great majority of childhood studies show that prognosis is better for girls. This difference has also been reported for adults and appears to be due to the late occurrence of testicular disease in males and a higher rate of bone marrow relapse, although it is uncertain whether these two features occur independently or are associated with each other. The sex difference in prognosis is not explained by the higher incidence of T-cell disease in males, as the difference also occurs in children with common ALL.

Immunological features

The application of cell markers has revealed a number of interesting observations, some of which have clinical significance (Table 16.1). There is a predominance of common ALL in childhood and an increased frequency of 'Null'-ALL in infancy and adult life, which partly explains the age difference for prognosis.

T-ALL, which is seen more frequently in males, is often associated with a high initial leukocyte count and a mediastinal mass. There is evidence from adult studies that prognosis is not as good as that for common ALL. Recent childhood studies indicate that the apparent poor prognosis may not be an independent feature. However, the adverse effects of high leukocyte count and T-ALL markers are lost after 2 or 3 years.

B-ALL occurs in only 3–5% of patients and has a characteristic L3 morphology and a karyotypic abnormality (t8:14). It has a poor prognosis with a low remission rate, early haematological relapse and a high incidence of CNS disease.

There is insufficient information to determine the exact prognostic significance of 'Null'-ALL, but in adults survival is shorter than for T-ALL and common-ALL. It has also been suggested that the Pre-B subtype has a less favourable prognosis, but among children the remission rate is comparable to that for common ALL.

Other features

Cell kinetics. Recent results for blood and bone marrow suggest a correlation between high proliferative activity and short remission duration and confirm that in B-ALL and T-ALL a higher proportion of cells are in S phase, probably indicating a more active disease process.

Cytogenetics. Indicators of a poor prognosis include the Ph anomaly, t4:11 and t8:14. Marked hyperdiploidy (greater than 50 chromosomes) is a favourable prognostic factor which in children is associated with a low initial leukocyte count and the presence of the common-ALL antigen.

Acute myeloid leukaemia

There are few clear indicators of prognosis for AML patients which can be identified at presentation. The age of the patient is closely related to the chance of obtaining complete remission, with children and teenagers showing the best results. Similarly, age is related to survival, but this is partly an effect of complete remission.

Various studies have demonstrated a positive correlation with a number of other factors, but the results have not always been supported by re-examination. Factors said to be favourably related to the possibility of obtaining complete remission include low total blood white cell count, low total blood blast cell count, FAB subtype (M1 unfavourable; M2 favourable), normal platelet count, presence of Auer rods in blast cells and colony growth pattern.

BIBLIOGRAPHY

Bennett J M, Catovsky D, Daniel M-T et al 1976 Proposals for the classification of the leukaemias. British Journal of Haematology 33: 451–458

Bloomfield C D 1984 Acute lymphoblastic leukaemia: clinical and biological features. In: Goldman J M, Preisler H D (eds) Leukemias. Butterworth, London, pp 163–189

Boros L, Bennett J M 1984 The acute leukemias. In: Goldman J M, Preislar H D (eds) Leukaemias. Butterworth, London, pp 104–135. (Excellent description of morphology and cytochemistry of AML)

Cartwright R A, Bernard S M 1987 Epidemiology of the leukaemias. In: Whittaker J A, Delamore I W (eds) Leukaemia. Blackwell, Oxford

Chessels J 1987 The acute lymphoid leukaemias. In: Whittaker J A, Delamore I W (eds) Leukaemia. Blackwell, Oxford

Foon K A, Gale R P 1987 Principles of leukaemia treatment. In: Whittaker J A, Delamore I W (eds) Leukaemia. Blackwell, Oxford

Franchini G, Gallo R C 1985 Viruses, onc genes and leukaemia. In: Hoffbrand A V (ed) Recent advances in haematology, 4th edn. Churchill Livingstone, Edinburgh, pp 221–237

Gunz F W, Henderson E S 1983 Leukemia, 4th edn. Grune & Stratton, New York (Reference text containing much detailed information)

Jacobs A D, Gale R P 1984 Recent advances in the biology and treatment of acute lymphoblastic leukemia in adults. New England Journal of Medicine 311: 1219–1231

Jarrett O, Onions D E 1984 Retroviruses in leukaemia of animals and man. In: Goldman J M, Preisler H D (eds) Leukaemias. Butterworth, London pp 1–34

Whittaker J A 1987 Acute myeloid leukaemia – clinical features and management. In: Whittaker J A, Delamore I W (eds) Leukaemia. Blackwell, Oxford

Wiernik P H 1982 Acute leukemias of adults. In: de Vita V T, Hellman S, Rosenberg S A (eds) Cancer principles and practice of oncology. Lippincot, Philadelphia, pp 1402–1426

TABLE REFERENCES

Table 16.8
Sackman-Muriel F, Svarch E, Eppinger-Helft M et al 1978 Cancer 42: 1730–1740

Camitta B M, Pinkel, Thatcher L G et al 1980 Medical and Pediatric Oncology 8: 383–389

Henze G, Langermann H-J, Ritter J et al 1981 In: Neth et al (eds) Modern trends in human leukaemia IV. Springer, Heidelberg, pp 87–93

Pui G H, Aur R J A, Bowman W P et al 1984 Cancer Research 44: 3593–3598

Table 16.9
Henderson E S, Scharlau C, Cooper M R et al 1979 Leukaemia Research 3: 395–407

Omura G A, Moffitt S, Vogler W R et al 1980 Blood 55: 199–204

Schauer P, Arlin Z A, Mertelsman R et al 1983 Journal of Clinical Oncology 1: 462–470

Hoelzer D, Thiel E, Loffler H et al 1984 Blood 64: 38–47

Table 16.11
Carella A M, Santini G, Martinengo M et al 1985 4-Demethoxy-daunorubicin (Idarubicin) in refractory or relapsed acute leukemias. Cancer 55: 1452–1454

Cassileth P A, Lyman G H, Bennett J M 1984 High dose Amsacrine (AMSA) therapy of relapsed and refractory adult acute nonlymphocytic leukemia: a phase II study. American Journal of Clinical Oncology 7: 361–363

Dagnestani A N, Arlin Z A, Leyland Jones B et al 1985 Phase I and II clinical and pharmacological study of 4-Demethoxydaunorubidin (Idarubicin) in adult patients with acute leukemia. Cancer Research 45: 1408–1412

Ehninger G, Ho A D, Meyer P et al 1985 Mitoxantrone in the treatment of relapsed and refractory acute leukemia. Onkologie 8: 146–148

European Organization for Research on the Treatment of Cancer 1973 Epipodophyllotoxin VP16213 in treatment of acute leukaemias, haematosarcomas, and solid tumours. British Medical Journal iii 199–202

Legha S S, Keating M J, McCredie K B et al 1982
Evaluation of AMSA in previously treated patients with
acute leukemia: results of therapy in 109 adults. Blood
60: 484–490

Machover D, Gastiaburu J, Delgado M et al 1984 Phase
I–II study of aclaribicin for treatment of acute myeloid
leukemia. Cancer Treatment Reports 68: 881–886

Moore J O, Olsen G A 1984 Mitoxantrone in the treatment
of relapsed and refractory acute leukemia. Seminars in
Oncology II (Suppl): 41–46

Pedersen-Bjergaard J, Brincker J, Ellegaard J et al 1984
Aclarubicin in the treatment of acute non-lymphocytic
leukemia refractory to treatment with daunorubicin and
cytarabine: a phase II trial. Cancer Treatment Reports
68: 1233–1238

Slevin M L, Shannon M S, Prentice H G et al 1981 A phase
I and II study of m-AMSA in acute leukemia. Cancer
Chemotherapy and Pharmacology 6: 137–140

Smith I E, Gerken M E, Clink H MacD et al 1976
VP 16–213 in acute myelogenous leukaemia. Post-graduate
Medical Journal 52: 66–70

Vogler W R, Miller D S, Keller J W 1976 5-Azacytidine
(NSC 102876): a new drug for the treatment of
myeloblastic leukemia. Blood 48: 331–337

Warrell R P, Coonley C J, Gee T S 1985
Homoharringtonine: an effective new drug for remission
induction in refractory nonlymphocytic leukemia. Journal
of Clinical Oncology 3: 617–621

Table 16.12

Yates J, Glidewell O, Wiernik P et al 1982 Blood
60: 454–462

Link H, Frauer H M, Ostendorf P et al 1985 Blut 51: 49–57

Vogler W R, Winton E F, Gordon D S et al 1984 Blood
63: 1039–1045

Preisler H D, Rustum Y, Henderson E S et al 1979 Blood
53: 455–464

Preisler H D, Bjornsson S, Hendersn E S et al 1979 Medical
and Pediatric Oncology 7: 269–275

Gale R P, Cline M J 1977 Lancet i: 497–499

Rees J K H, Sandler R M, Challener J et al 1977 British
Journal of Cancer 36: 770–776

Table 16.13

McCredie K B, Keating M J, Estey E H et al 1981
Proceedings of the American Association for Cancer
Research and the American Society for Clinical Oncology
22: 479

Hines J D, Oken M M, Mazza J J et al 1984 Journal of
Clinical Oncology 2: 545–549

Arlin Z A, Flomenburg B, Gee T S et al 1981 Cancer
Clinical Trials 4: 317–321

Winton F E, Hearn E B, Martelo O et al 1985 Cancer
Treatment Reports 69: 807–811

Kahn S B, Sklaroff R, Lebedda J et al 1983 American
Journal of Clinical Oncology 6: 493–502

Table 16.14

Sauter C, Berchtold W, Fopp M et al 1984 Lancet
i: 379–382

Cassileth P A, Begg C B, Bennett J M et al 1984 Blood
63: 843–847

Embury S H, Elias L, Heller P H et al 1977 Western
Journal of Medicine 126: 267–272

Neil M, Glidewell O J, Jacquillat C et al 1973 Cancer
Research 33: 921–928

Table 16.15

Cantin G, Brennan J K 1984 American Journal of
Hematology 16: 59–66

Herzig R H, Wolff S N, Lazarus H M et al 1983 Blood
62: 361–369

Capizzi R L, Poole M, Cooper M R et al 1984 Blood
63: 694–700

Zittoun R, Marie J P, Zittoun J et al 1985 Seminars in
Oncology 12 (Suppl): 139–143

Barnett M J, Waxman J H, Richards M A et al 1985
Seminars in Oncology 12 (Suppl): 133–138

Hines J D, Oken M M, Mazza J J et al 1984 Journal of
Clinical Oncology 2: 545–549

Herzig R H, Lazarus H M, Wolff S N et al 1985 Journal of
Clinical Oncology 3: 992–997

Table 16.17

Cassileth P A, Begg C B, Bennett J M et al 1984 Blood
63: 843–847

Vaughan W P, Karp J E, Burke P J 1984 Blood 64: 975–980

Wiernik P H 1984 Seminars in Oncology 11 (Suppl): 12–14

Peterson B A, Bloomfield C D 1981 Blood 57: 1144–1147

Table 16.18

Weinstein H J, Mayer R J, Rosenthal D S et al 1983 Blood
62: 315–319

Creutzig U, Ritter J, Riehm H et al 1985 Blood 65: 298–304

Baehner R L, Bernstein I D, Sather H et al 1984 Cancer
Treatment Reports 68: 1269–1272

Table 16.19

Champlin R E, Ho W G, Gale R P et al 1985 Annals of
Internal Medicine 102: 285–290

Applebaum F R, Dahlberg S, Thomas E D et al 1984
Annals of Internal Medicine 101: 581–855

Powles R L, Morgenstern G, Clink H M et al 1980 Lancet
i: 1047–1050

Powles R L, Watson J G, Morgenstern G R et al 1982
Lancet i: 336–337

17. Chronic leukaemias

M. Judge   J. A. Whittaker

Chronic leukaemia is a progressive malignancy of blood-forming tissue resulting in the accumulation of abnormal white cells in the marrow. This eventually causes disruption of normal marrow activity, and results in the infiltration into blood and other tissues of the abnormal white cell clone. Chronic leukaemic processes differ from acute leukaemia in time scale (being more insidious in onset) and in the greater maturity of the target cell. With their longer natural history, resistance to eradication and less severe effect on patient well-being, treatment is less intensive.

Classification is based on cell type, the major types being chronic lymphocytic leukaemia and chronic myeloid leukaemia (chronic granulocytic leukaemia). Hairy cell leukaemia is a sub-variety included in the chronic leukaemias, but chronic myelomonocytic leukaemia is now usually classified with the myelodysplastic syndromes (see Ch. 25). Occasionally, a blood picture resembling that of a chronic leukaemia results from a severe systemic disease. This is termed a leukaemoid reactions.

Epidemiology

Chronic lymphocytic leukaemia (CLL) is the most common type of leukaemia in Europe and North America, accounting for 25–30% of leukaemia deaths, with an incidence of 3 per 100 000. The incidence in these areas seems to be rising, but it remains an uncommon condition in Japan and China. It is more common in males and increases in incidence with age over 40 years, the median age at diagnosis being 60, with an incidence approaching 1/1000 at age 70.

There have been several reports of familial CLL and a characteristic chromosomal abnormality, Ch', (Ch' chromosome = Christchurch anomaly, a p deletion of chromosome 22) has been described in some kinships. In addition, a significantly increased incidence of leukaemia has been observed in the relatives of patients with CLL.

Chronic myeloid leukaemia (CML) accounts for 15% or so of leukaemias and does not show either the marked geographic variation of CLL or its slowly increasing incidence with age. It has equal sex distribution and occurs mainly in young and middle-aged adults, the median age of onset being approximately 45. Its incidence approaches 1/25 000 at age 70. The increased incidence of CML (in addition to the acute leukaemias) following the atomic bomb at Hiroshima and following therapeutic irradiation, as for ankylosing spondylitis, implicates ionising radiation as a causative factor in CML.

CHRONIC LYMPHOCYTIC LEUKAEMIA

CLL is a lymphoproliferative disorder resulting from the neoplastic proliferation of moderately mature lymphocytes in the marrow and blood and, to a lesser extent, in nodes, spleen and liver. It differs from well-differentiated lymphocytic lymphoma only in the distribution of disease at diagnosis.

Classification

CLL results from a monoclonal transformation usually of B lymphocytes, less than 5% of cases showing a T-cell phenotype. T-cell CLL usually displays specific clinical and morphological features not seen in B-cell CLL (see Table 17.1).

A small number of patients displaying more immature lymphocyte morphology and surface markers with either B-cell or T-cell phenotype are labelled prolymphocytic leukaemia (Plate 12). These generally show more extreme clinical and laboratory features and a more aggressive course with a less satisfactory response to chemotherapy.

Waldenstrom's macroglobulinaemia, often classified with multiple myeloma in the paraproteinaemias (see Ch. 20), represents the monoclonal transformation of a more functionally mature B lymphocyte, showing plasmacytoid features with both surface and cytoplasmic IgM and secretion of a monoclonal IgM protein.

Table 17.1   Clinical and laboratory features of chronic lymphocytic leukaemia

	Median age at diagnosis	M:F	WCC ($\times 10^9$)	Clinical	Biochemical
B-CLL	60	2:1	10–200	Adenopathy Splenomegaly	Autoimmune haemolysis Hypogammaglobulinaemia
T-CLL	60	M>F	20–200 convoluted nuclei	Adenopathy Hepatosplenomegaly Skin lesions 10% Poor response to chemotherapy Tendency to neurologic infiltration	
Prolymphocytic leukaemia	65	4:1	100->500 Large lymphocytes	Marked splenomegaly Poor response to treatment	
Waldenstrom's macroglobulinaemia	50	1:1	4–50 Plasmacytoid features	Moderate hepatosplenomegaly and adenopathy	IgM paraproteinaemia Hyperviscosity
Hairy cell leukaemia	50	5:1	<1–100 Hairy lymphocytes	Pancytopenia Marked splenomegaly	Tartarate-resistant cytoplasmic acid phosphatase

Hairy cell leukaemia, another type of chronic B cell lympho-proliferative disease, is characterised by multiple cytoplasmic projections on the neoplastic clone.

Some patients with non-Hodgkin's lymphoma manifest a leukaemic phase following bone marrow infiltration, either at diagnosis or more usually late in the course of the disease. Even in the low grade follicular or small cleaved cell lymphomas, the morphology and immunologic features should enable their differentiation from typical CLL.

Recently, a low grade lymphoproliferative disorder characterised by the presence in the circulation of large granular lymphocytes and neutropenia has been described. The finding of T-cell surface markers has led to the condition being termed chronic T gamma lymphocytosis.

Aetiology and pathogenesis

The monoclonal nature of CLL is established by the finding of surface, cytoplasmic and occasionally serum immunoglobulins restricted to one light and heavy chain class. The variable region of the immunoglobulin heavy chain shows idiotype specificity. The clonal expansion of immunologically immature B-cells results from transformation of a target early or intermediate B-cell which has acquired surface membrane Ig following Ig gene rearrangement, but cannot yet secrete Ig on antigenic

stimulation. These long-lived cells have a low proliferative capacity, but doubling time shortens with disease progression. The target cell in prolymphocytic leukaemia is paradoxically a more differentiated B-lymphocyte.

Chromosomal studies

The occurrence of familial cases of CLL, some with specific chromosomal defects, suggests a genetic aetiology in these patients. Chromosomal analysis is hampered by limited in vitro proliferation of B-cells, but some reports have listed abnormalities occurring in 50% of patients. The most common defects are trisomy 12, 14qt, del 14 (especially in T-cell CLL), and t(11,14). The more common chromosomal abnormalities occurring in CLL affect the chromosomes responsible for either heavy chain (chromosome 14) or light chain (chromosomes 2, 22) synthesis, or those which contain oncogenes (chromosomes 8, 11, 12).

Progressive disease and resistance to therapy may be associated with the finding of additional chromosomal defects reflecting clonal evolution.

Oncogenes

Recent studies, in which DNA transfection from tumour cells has caused malignant transformation of cultured cell lines, have led to the identification of cellular oncogenes in many tumours, including Burkitt's lymphoma, AML and CML. Some of these cellular oncogenes resemble viral oncogenes identified in RNA tumour viruses and others are sited at the exact chromosomal breakpoints of translocations frequently found in certain tumours, e.g. c myc oncogene on chromosome 8 (q24) in the t(8:14) of Burkitt's lymphoma.

A gene probe for chromosome 11 has detected DNA rearrangement on 14qt chromosome in a CLL patient with t(11:14) and the postulated transforming oncogene on chromosome 11 has been labelled Bcl-1 (B-cell leukaemic lymphoma 1).

Viruses

Most forms of animal leukaemia and lymphomas have been associated with the finding of viruses, most often RNA tumour viruses (retroviruses), occasionally DNA viruses such as *Herpes simplex* in neoplastic cells. A retrovirus first isolated from human T-cell lymphoma (*Mycosis fungoides*) and T-cell leukaemia in 1981 has been labelled HTLV1 (Human T-cell leukaemia virus 1). In subsequent studies of endemic adult T-cell leukaemia in Japan and the Caribbean using DNA analysis, the HTLV1 pro-viral sequence was detected in all patients, indicating the monoclonal derivation from a single infected cell. Specific gene probes to detect DNA rearrangements have indicated that HTLV1 viral sequence does not have a common integration site in the leukaemic cell genome and so cannot activate an adjacent cellular oncogene to mediate leukaemogenesis. It is postulated that the viral genome may code for proteins which activate other genes.

Evidence of viral mediation in B-cell CLL, in the form of reverse transcriptase activity and isolation of viral particles that cross react with HTLV1 monoclonal antibody, has been published.

Immune function

The neoplastic cell population in CLL arises from a transformed immature B-cell which is 'fixed' and cannot differentiate further. These are long-lived cells with low proliferative capacity and, though they may secrete a monoclonal immunoglobulin, they are functionally incompetent. They possess receptors for mouse red blood cells, the Ia, B_1, B_2 and B_4, surface antigens, and display IgM and sometimes IgD surface membrane immunoglobulins. These cells have lost the pre-B-cell characteristics of CALLA surface positivity and of Tdt expression. They show defective response to B-cell mitogens in vitro, but the membrane defect which

blocks activation is unknown. B-CLL lymphocytes from different tissues display varying densities of surface markers, reflecting some maturation in spleen and nodes. Recent attention has focused on T-cell changes in B-cell CLL. The absolute number of T-cells is usually increased at the time of diagnosis, and their levels fluctuate with disease activity and treatment, but tend to fall with progressive disease. Most patients have inverted T-helper: T-suppressor ratios and in some reports an inverse relationship between T-suppressor numbers and immunoglobulin levels has been noted. T-cells from patients with B-cell CLL are functionally normal in vitro when tested against standard T-cell mitogens, but they show impaired reactivity to cultured B-cells and cytotoxicity is reduced reflecting defective natural killer lymphocyte function. Some T-cell defects are improved by interferon therapy and splenectomy.

Hypogammaglobulinaemia occurs in 50% or more of patients with B-CLL and involves all immunoglobulin subclasses. Bacterial infections, especially due to pneumococcal organisms, are particularly common in these patients and with disease progression fungal and viral infections also occur. The impaired B-cell function may be secondary to T-cell changes. Rarely, a monoclonal immunoglobulin spike occurs, usually an IgM, rarely IgG or IgA, but these seldom cause clinical problems. Also rarely, allergic hypersensitivity reactions to insect stings may occur.

Autoimmune reactions directed against haemopoietic cells occur in 15% of patients with CLL, leading to autoimmune haemolysis, or immune thrombocytopenia. Neutropenic T-cell CLL may be associated with pure red cell aplasia.

Although autoimmunity against non-haemopoietic tissue is no more common than in normal populations, there is an increased incidence of autoimmune conditions in the relatives of CLL patients. In families where more than one member has had CLL, abnormalities of T-cell function in vitro and reduced immunoglobulin levels have been found. These findings indicate that inherited defects in immune responsiveness may predispose certain families to develop lymphoproliferative disorders, possibly by increasing susceptibility to leukaemogenic viruses.

Clinical features (Table 17.1)

In most patients with CLL, the symptoms are insidious in onset with progressive fatigue, weakness and breathlessness on exertion. Enlarged superficial glands may be detected by the patient and, in more advanced cases, infective or bleeding problems may lead to the diagnosis. Anorexia, weight loss and night sweats occur late in the course of the disease and unusual complications of enlargement of mediastinal, retroperitoneal and mesenteric nodes may occur. Up to 25% of patients with CLL are asymptomatic and are detected on routine testing or when being investigated for other conditions.

Physical examination usually reveals moderate superficial adenopathy in the cervical, axillary or inguinal areas, the nodes being symmetrical, firm, non-tender, discrete, and fixed to deep structures but not to skin. Mild or moderate splenomegaly and later hepatomegaly develop and the presence of jaundice may reflect periportal node enlargement or associated haemolytic anaemia. As the disease progresses, anaemia and bruising are apparent, weight loss occurs and the nodes may become greatly enlarged and cause pressure effects related to position. The tonsils may be enlarged at some stage and node enlargement in the scalp, conjunctiva, orbit, pleura, gastrointestinal tract and central nervous system has been recorded. Skin infiltration, especially in T-cell CLL, may appear as dark red or brown nodules and, if widespread, may lead to generalised eczema and desquamation known as l'homme rouge. T-cell leukaemia and lymphomas also have a predilection for CNS infiltration. Respiratory tract infections are very common in CLL, especially when hypogammaglobulinaemia exists or when steroid therapy is used. Other common sites of infection are middle ear, sinuses, urinary tract and skin, while fungal infection of the mouth and skin and viral infections such as oral *Herpes simplex* and atypical or severe *Herpes zoster* may complicate the condition.

In prolymphocytic leukaemia, gross splenomegaly is an early feature, while adenopathy is rarely significant. With hyperleukocytosis, especially in prolymphocytic leukaemias, hyperviscosity syndromes may occur and pseudohyperkalaemia may result from lymphocytic fragility and lysis in a venesected sample.

Investigation

The diagnosis rests on the finding of a persisting lymphocytosis of $>15 \times 10^9/l$ lymphocytes. The overall white cell count varies from $20–200 \times 10^9/l$ with 70–95% lymphocytes. The neutrophil proportion is usually markedly reduced, but absolute counts may be normal in the early stages at least. In the blood film, normal mature-looking lymphocytes may be present, but CLL lymphocytes are slightly larger with scant light blue agranular cytoplasm, clumped chromatin and rarely nucleoli (Plate 12). They seem more fragile than normal lymphocytes and may rupture on smearing, leading to the appearance of so-called smudge cells. T-cell CLL lymphocytes usually contain azurophilic cytoplasmic granules, and may have

lobulated or even folded nuclei, though there is often morphological variation in these cases. The granules of T-cell CLL lymphocytes are tartarate sensitive acid-phosphatase positive. In prolymphocytic leukaemia (Plate 13) of either B or T-cell type, the lymphocytes are larger with clear pale-blue cytoplasm, condensed chromatin, and a large, single nucleolus. Acid phosphatase dot positivity and focal or diffuse acid α naphthyl acetate esterase positivity indicate their T-cell origin. The white cell count in these patients may reach $1000 \times 10^9/l$ and smudge cells on the blood film are uncommon. Anaemia, which may not be present in the early stages, worsens with advancing disease and is usually normochromic normocytic in type. It may result from reduced erythroid activity due to increasing marrow infiltration, reduced red cell survival, especially when splenomegaly is prominent, and occasionally as a result of autoimmune haemolysis, which affects 10–15% of patients with CLL. The latter condition will be associated with a variable reticulocytosis, spherocytosis and erythroid hyperplasia in addition to a positive direct Coomb's test, and it may arise at any stage of the disease process. Thrombocytopenia due to marrow replacement, or rarely auto-antibody production, is a feature of advanced CLL.

The marrow aspirate and trephine biopsy shows a lymphocytic infiltrate of 10% or more with associated hypercellularity and a reduction in normal haemopoietic elements. Initially, there may be a nodular or paratrabecular distribution of lymphocytes, later becoming diffuse, and in T-cell CLL the degree of marrow involvement may be less than expected for the existing blood lymphocytosis.

The surface marker studies show receptors for mouse erythrocytes (mouse red cells form rosettes around B-CLL lymphocytes), small amounts of surface membrane immunoglobulin of IgM or IgA subclass, and receptors for the C3d portion of complement. Another characteristic finding is reduced receptor capping on exposure to fluorescent concanavalin A, a B-cell mitogen.

In prolymphocytic leukaemia, the lymphocytes have lost the ability to form rosettes with sheep red blood cells and have an increased density of surface immunoglobulin.

T-cell CLL lymphocytes, apart from their distinctive morphology, possess sheep red cell receptors and show a typical pattern of T-cell monoclonal positivity reflecting T-suppressor lineage.

In advanced B-cell CLL, increasing pleomorphism with the appearance of nucleoli in the lymphocytes may suggest prolymphocytic transformation, but these cells still retain characteristic B-CLL markers.

Serum immunoglobulin estimation and protein electrophoresis may reveal hypogammaglobulinaemia and a monoclonal paraprotein spike as already discussed. Monoclonal light chain excretion is rarely found. If a node biopsy is done in a patient with CLL, the histology resembles that of diffuse well-differentiated lymphocytic lymphoma. Chest X-ray may reveal mediastinal adenopathy and the rare occurrence of a leukaemoid reaction in tuberculosis should not be forgotten.

Staging and prognosis

The natural course of untreated B-cell CLL is variable and survival from diagnosis varies between 1 and 20 years with an average of 3–5 years. A more benign course tends to occur in older patients with minimal clinical evidence of disease and, in these, it is often an incidental diagnosis. These patients may require no specific therapy.

Various staging systems have been proposed and these help to identify those patients with more active disease who require early treatment. One such staging system is that proposed by Rai in 1975 (Table 17.2).

Table 17.2 Rai staging for chronic lymphatic leukaemia

Stage	Feature
0	lymphocytosis $>15 \times 10^9/l$ marrow lymphocytosis $>40\%$
1	+ adenopathy
2	+ splenomegaly and/or hepatomegaly
3	+ Hb < 11 g/dl
4	+ platelet count $<100 \times 10^9/l$

The median survival for each group ranges from 15 years in Stage 0 to between 1 and 3 years for Stage 4. A newer staging system, devised by Binet in 1980, using statistical methods to identify major prognostic factors is now used widely in distinguishing good and poor risk groups (Table 17.3).

Table 17.3 Binet classification for chronic lymphatic leukaemia

Group	Prognosis	Features
A	Good	Hb >10 g/dl Platelets $>100 \times 10^9/l$ <3 sites of organomegaly
B	Intermediate	As above Plus ≥ 3 sites of organomegaly
C	Poor	Hb <10 g/dl Platelets $<100 \times 10^9/l$

While these systems provide a useful measure of the stage of the disease, they do not indicate the speed of progression and even with poor prognostic features it may be thought unnecessary to treat a particular patient unless there is deterioration in clinical or haematological parameters. Progressive or end-stage CLL may evolve into a morphologically less-differentiated type resembling prolymphocytic leukaemia or transform into a diffuse lymphoma (Richter's syndrome) or even an acute lymphoblastic leukaemia L2 type blast crisis.

Treatment of CLL

By applying standard criteria for staging and clinical response, various trials have shed some light on the usefulness of different treatment schedules which include chemotherapy, radiotherapy and steroids. CLL is not curable, but patients who are sensitive to treatment survive longer and some experts recommend ongoing treatment from diagnosis. Others have found no evidence of any benefit in patients with Stage I–II disease treated from diagnosis.

A complete remission is defined as disappearance of abnormal lymphocytes from blood and marrow and normalisation of blood counts, immunoglobulins and light chain λ (kappa : lambda) ratio. Reversal of the immunoglobulin gene rearrangement is a more sensitive indicator, but this technique is not widely available.

A partial response is a 50–75% reduction in lymphocytosis and 50% reduction in adenopathy and splenomegaly with a haemoglobin > 11 g/dl and platelets $> 100 \times 10^9/l$.

Chemotherapy

The alkylating agents chlorambucil and cyclophosphamide are the most effective agents in CLL. Chlorambucil was introduced in the 1950s and is still the drug of first choice. It alkylates the guanine moiety of DNA, causing cross-linkage and preventing replication. It is given by mouth in a dose range of 0.1 to 0.2 mg/kg daily and may be continued until a response is evident, at which time the dose is reduced. Complete remissions of clinical disease occur in 10% of patients and partial remissions in a further 50% and prolonged treatment up to 2 years may be required before maximum response is reached. The addition of steroids has increased the partial remission rate to 67% at the risk of increased susceptibility to infection.

High dose intermittent chlorambucil, 0.4 mgs to 0.6 mgs/kg, given daily for 3 days every 2–4 weeks appears to be as effective as low dose daily treatment and less toxic. This is being assessed in the current MRC

Trial, which also includes steroid treatment as an option. Steroids, although lympholytic, should not be used alone in the long-term treatment of uncomplicated CLL. They may be useful as priming treatment in advanced disease before the addition of chlorambucil, but may cause a rapid rise in lymphocytosis. Steroids are effective in controlling the autoimmune complications of CLL (haemolysis and thrombocytopenia) and are given in doses of 40–80 mg of prednisolone daily, tailing off rapidly when a good response occurs.

Cyclophosphamide is a useful alternative to chlorambucil and does not show cross-resistance. It can be given orally either continuously or intermittently or as regular intravenous boluses. It causes less suppression of megakaryocytes and so is more useful in thrombocytopenic patients.

Busulphan is rarely used, being less effective and more myelotoxic.

The addition of vincristine to an alkylating agent and prednisolone in treating advanced disease has produced a higher complete remission rate of 33–44% in some studies, but others have found no advantage over chlorambucil and prednisolone.

Studies of more aggressive combination chemotherapy have yielded little evidence of extra benefit over conventional treatment regimens, and drugs such as melphalan, carmustine and doxorubicin are best reserved for resistant advanced CLL.

Side effects of chemotherapy. Myelosuppression due to chlorambucil and cyclophosphamide is rarely a problem and improves 1–2 weeks after stopping the drug. Nausea and upper gastrointestinal symptoms are usually mild and may respond to reduced doses. A serious late effect of continued alkylating therapy is the development of acute myeloid leukaemia in up to 8% of patients. This usually occurs 5–10 years after commencement of treatment and is a highly resistant form of AML. This is the major argument against maintenance chemotherapy in CLL. The additional use of radiotherapy undoubtedly enhances the leukaemogenic effect of chemotherapy and the intrinsic immune suppression of CLL known to increase the risk of second malignancies.

Radiotherapy

Total body irradiation was used to treat advanced CLL in the 1960s and high response rates were reported after doses of 10–40 Gy over 20 weeks or so. Severe marrow toxicity was common and this approach is seldom used now. Spaced splenic irradiation may be useful in controlling advanced disease, as it damages both resident and transit lymphocytes. It provides useful palliation of painful splenomegaly and hypersplenism and, rarely,

has induced complete remission in predominant splenic disease.

Extracorporeal blood irradiation theoretically achieves the same degree of control of lymphocytosis without marrow toxicity, but in principle is no more effective than splenic irradiation.

Local radiotherapy to bulky node masses or nodes interfering with organ function, e.g. bile duct obstruction, is effective and induces rapid relief in most cases. Lytic bone lesions complicating T-cell CLL also respond to local irradiation also.

Other treatments

Patients presenting with very high white cell counts, as in prolymphocytic leukaemia, may require leukopheresis to reduce the tumour load until chemotherapy induces a response. Patients with T-cell CLL who respond poorly to chemotherapy may be maintained for long periods on regular pheresis. It may also be the only available measure in patients who are hypersensitive to chemotherapy.

Splenectomy is reserved for those patients who have hypersplenism or steroid-resistant immune mediated cytopenias (even if Coomb's negative). High dose immunoglobulin may produce transient elevation of red cell and platelet counts in preparation for surgery. The therapeutic use of monoclonal antibodies has been disappointing. Even in T-cell CLL, T-cell monoclonal antibodies such as T101 have produced only transient reductions in peripheral lymphocytosis without influencing sites of bulk disease.

α interferon has proven largely ineffective in halting disease progress, with a response rate of only 10% in a pilot study of 19 patients.

Regardless of which treatment is used, adequate hydration and allopurinol are necessary to prevent hyperuricaemia when cell lysis commences. Symptomatic and supportive treatments of anaemia, infection due to leukopenia and hypogammaglobulinaemia and bleeding due to low platelets are as described elsewhere. An additional supportive measure in CLL patients with recurrent and opportunistic infection is the regular administration of intramuscular or intravenous gammaglobulin. Even in patients with a good response to therapy Ig levels rarely improve.

Treatment of prolymphocytic leukaemia

The response to conventional CLL chemotherapy in patients with PLL is less satisfactory and sustained. Since it is a more aggressive disease, combination chemotherapy including anthracyclines may be justified from the outset. Splenic irradiation and splenectomy have an important role in short term control and leukopheresis may maintain control for some years.

Future trends in CLL

B-cell CLL lymphocytes express a T-cell marker antigen identified by T101 or anti-LEU I. Normal B-cells can be induced to express this antigen by exposure to tumour promoters. However, the monoclonal T101 has not been effective in treatment, since the antigen's expression may change and vary from patient to patient and free circulating antigen may mop up the antibody before it reaches the cell membrane.

Monoclonal antibodies specific for CLL lymphocytes may be tagged with cytotoxic drugs which could increase their delivery to target cells while reducing toxicity to normal tissues.

Anti-idiotype monoclonal antibody specific for a patient's B-cell surface immunoglobulin has produced transient responses in a number of patients but not in others, and its application is limited.

The value of clinical staging in prognosis is enhanced by defining specific chromosomal abnormalities such as trisomy 12 or multi-chromosomal defects.

Studies of the ratios of certain complement receptors on B-cells, the type of surface Ig or the presence of steroid receptors may lead to more accurate prognostic grouping and therapeutic manipulation.

HAIRY CELL LEUKAEMIA

This condition was first described as leukaemic reticuloendotheliosis in 1958 when it was recognised as a distinct lympho-proliferative disease. Its modern name derives from the characteristic neoplastic lymphocytes which possess wisplike cytoplasmic projections and the specific disease entity usually includes pancytopenia and isolated splenomegaly.

Epidemiology

Hairy cell leukaemia (HCL) accounts for approximately 2% of haematologic malignancy and occurs worldwide. It is more common in males and the mean age at diagnosis is 51 years. There are few clues as to the aetiology, but a few reports suggest a link with chronic low dose radiation exposure and a small number of families with various haematologic malignancies and HCL have been reported.

Immunologic features

Hairy cells generally display B-cell characteristics, al-

though in some cases T-cell surface antigens and monocytic features may occur. Rarely, they resemble null cells.

They carry surface IgG with restricted light chain type, form mouse red cell rosettes, react with B-cell specific monoclonal antibody and show heavy and light chain gene rearrangement typical of B cell lineage. Hairy cells also possess the IL2 surface antigen which is a marker of activated B-cells, but so far they have not been shown to mature into plasma cells in vitro. T-cell function and subset ratios are usually normal and immunoglobulin levels are maintained. Rarely, an IgG paraprotein has been detected and the co-existence of HCL and typical multiple myeloma has been recorded. Monocytopenia is very common in HCL, although fixed tissue macrophages are normal in marrow and spleen sections.

Clinical features

The main presenting symptoms relate to splenomegaly, causing abdominal discomfort, and/or pancytopenia, leading to fatigue, infections and bruising. Rarely, the disease may be diagnosed by chance; the spleen may not be palpable or the liver and superficial nodes may be enlarged. HCL is particularly associated with mycobacterial infections and Legionnaire's disease also seems more common, perhaps as a result of reduced monocytic activity. More common, however, are bacterial pneumonias caused by *Pseudomonas* and *E. coli* and, in advanced cases, systemic fungal infections due to *Candida*, *Aspergillus* and *Cryptococcus*. Such is the risk of serious opportunistic infection in these patients that prompt and intensive investigation of any fever and early aggressive antimicrobial chemotherapy is warranted. The low yield of positive cultures in mycobacterial infections may be augmented by early lung, liver or node biopsy and early introduction of anti-tuberculous treatment should follow.

Investigations

A moderate normocytic normochromic anaemia is very common, but macrocytosis without megaloblastic change also occurs. The white cell count is usually less than $4 \times 10^9/l$ with 20% or so being hairy lymphocytes. In those with high white counts, the majority are hairy cells. Severe neutropenia and monocytopenia occur in up to 80% of cases and moderate to severe thrombocytopenia in a similar percentage. The LAP score is raised. Hairy cells are larger than normal lymphocytes with a moderate amount of pale-blue cytoplasm, an eccentric nucleus with fine lacy chromatin and a fringe of filamentous microvilli or hairs. These cytoplasmic projections are more obvious in a thick spread film or under phase contrast, but even so are not present on all abnormal mononuclear cells.

Scanning electron microscopy may show surface ruffles even when microvilli are absent. Cytoplasmic vacuoles and azurophilic granules may be seen.

Cytochemical stains show characteristic tartarate-resistant acid phosphatase positivity (TRAP) due to the predominance of isoenzyme 5 in hairy cells. Intensity of staining varies and some patients have a proportion of negative cells. Non-specific esterase positivity not inhibited by fluoride occurs in most cases.

Marrow aspirate may be non-productive or yield hypocellular smears which show a diffuse lymphocytic infiltrate ranging from 10 to 90% and myeloid hypoplasia.

A marrow trephine should always be performed and will confirm a mononuclear infiltrate with inconspicuous hairy projections and increased reticulin. Splenic histology, when available, also shows hairy cell infiltration and marked congestion, though a patient with typical HCL did not have splenic involvement. The single most important prognostic factor at diagnosis is the degree of marrow impairment.

Immunoglobulin levels may show a polyclonal IgG rise and rarely a monoclonal peak. A few patients with co-existent myeloma have been described.

Immune surface marker profile and a specific anti-HC monoclonal antibody have helped to distinguish HCL from the occasional atypical splenic forms of non-Hodgkin's lymphoma with hairy cells and weak TRAP positivity.

Bony lesions do not occur but minor intra-abdominal adenopathy can be detected on CT scans in some patients.

The main differential diagnoses are Waldenstrom's macroglobulinaemia, early myelofibrosis and hypoplastic anaemia.

Treatment

In the early phase of HCL, no specific treatment is required, but with advancing disease pancytopenia and splenomegaly may cause clinical problems. Both hypersplenism and increasing marrow infiltration contribute to the pancytopenia, but splenectomy is the usual first line treatment in those with adequate marrow reserves who are fit for surgery. This often induces prolonged recovery of blood counts lasting some years, but 10% of patients will not respond and some deteriorate post-splenectomy.

Interferon has proven effective in most patients who are unfit or unsuitable for splenectomy and now it is used as first line treatment with splenectomy. It is usually started in a dose of 2–3 mega units sc and continued daily for some months until maximum response is achieved. Apart from flu-like symptoms early on in treatment, it is well tolerated and can be continued in a low maintenance dose.

Alkylating agents, especially chlorambucil, have been used with limited effect in the past and steroids are not generally useful and increase the risk of opportunistic infection. Other forms of treatment including marrow transplantation have met with minimal success.

Supportive therapy for infective and bleeding complications follows the same principles as in the management of acute leukaemic patients, with the additional precaution of early antituberculous therapy in patients with persisting unexplained fever.

Future trends

Further studies to clarify the origin and natural counterpart of hairy cells are in progress. Marked fluctuations in disease activity and the occasional clinical remission are paralleled in some patients by changes in peripheral lymphocyte populations with increased expression of T-cell markers. The development of specific monoclonal antibodies may allow therapeutic manipulation of these subsets.

The remarkable success of interferon in some patients should lead to increased knowledge of the role of retroviruses in the pathogenesis of HCL.

CHRONIC MYELOID LEUKAEMIA

CML is classified as a myeloproliferative disease and results from a clonal stem cell proliferation. A characteristic cytogenetic abnormality, the Philadelphia chromosome, occurs in most cases and was the first chromosomal marker of malignant disease to be discovered. A minority 15% of patients with features of CML are Philadelphia negative and may differ in their natural course and response to treatment. CML is usually taken to mean chronic granulocytic leukaemia, which is the commonest manifestation, but rare cases of chronic eosinophilic, basophilic or neutrophilic leukaemia also occur and juvenile CML appears to be a different disease. Chronic myelomonocytic leukaemia is now included in the myelodysplastic syndrome, but may resemble atypical CML and often blends with acute myelomonocytic leukaemia. The recognised subtypes of CML are listed in Table 17.4.

Typical CML is a slowly evolving condition with unrestricted overgrowth of myeloid cells and, to a lesser

Table 17.4 Clinical and laboratory features of chronic myeloid leukaemia

CML Subtype	Age	Laboratory features	Clinical features
Chronic granulocytic leukaemia (>90% Ph'+)	20–70	WCC >100 × 10⁹/l (usually) Low LAP Leuko-erythroblastic blood film Basophilia	Splenomegaly Hyperviscosity syndrome Bone tenderness Predictable course
Atypical CML (>90% Ph'−)	30–70	WCC 50–100 × 10⁹/l Low to normal LAP Monocytosis	Mild splenomegaly Poor response Rapid course
Juvenile CML (Ph'−)	<5 yrs usually <2 yrs	WCC 20–100 × 10⁹/l Monocytosis Raised Hb F	Hepatospleno-megaly Adenopathy Infections, especially of skin Poor response Rapid course
Chronic neutrophilic leukaemia (Ph'−)	>50 Rare	WCC 20–100 × 10⁹/l >80% mature neutrophils High LAP ± coagulopathy	Mild splenomegaly Resistant Survival 1–5 years Low rate of transformation
Chronic eosinophilic leukaemia (mainly Ph'−)	>30 M > F Rare	Eosinophilia (Left shift) Pancytopenia Low LAP Marrow fibrosis	Fever, CNS lesions Hepatosple-nomegaly Cardiac failure Pulmonary infiltrates Variable response
Chronic basophilic leukaemia (mainly Ph'+)	>30 very rare	Basophilia + + + High LAP PAS positivity	Hepatosple-nomegaly Histamine release Bleeding, DIC Bone lesions Poor response

extent, megakaryocytic and erythroid cells in marrow with overspill into the circulation. A leuko-erythroblastic blood picture is characteristic and, apart from karyotypic changes, the marrow changes are not diagnostic. After a chronic phase lasting 3–7 years, the disease evolves into an accelerated resistant phase or transforms to acute leukaemia or myelofibrosis. Chemotherapy, while it helps to control myeloproliferation in the chronic phase, is not curative and recently allogeneic bone marrow transplantation has given the best hope of long-term survival.

Aetiology

In the majority of cases of CML, no definite aetiological factors can be identified. However, radiation exposure is the major factor about which much data exists, both as a result of the atomic bombs exploded in Japan in 1945 and the use of diagnostic and therapeutic radiation since the early 1900s.

Radiation

Reports of a greatly increased incidence of solid tumours, especially osteosarcoma in workers exposed to radioactive paints, appeared in the 1930s and the occupational exposure to X-rays of radiologists and physicians who subsequently developed leukaemia was noted in the 1940s.

Following the single high dose exposure to neutron radiation suffered by the survivors of the Hiroshima atomic explosion in 1945, there was a dramatic increase in leukaemias, especially CML, 3–10 years later. This incidence peaked 7 years after exposure, with a 50-fold rise in those who received the highest radiation doses. Follow-up of patients with alkylosing spondylitis who were given spinal irradiation, in some cases up to 12 000 rads over some years, revealed a 10-fold increase in leukaemias. A large proportion were CML with a latent period averaging 6 years.

A small increase in leukaemia risk (not statistically significant) has been noted in children exposed to low dose irradiation for tinea capitis or thymic enlargement. The influence of radioactive phosphorus in the control of primary proliferative polycythaemia (PPP) in the causation of leukaemia is unclear. The intrinsic predisposition to transformation in PPP clouds the issue in the latter.

In spite of these and other reports indicating a causal link between radiation and CML, the majority of patients show no discernible excessive exposure. The role of background radiation in these cases is unclear, since an accurate assessment of radiation dosage and timing in a large population is impossible to determine.

Chemicals

Such is the range of chemicals, drugs and toxins to which some individuals are exposed that it is almost impossible to identify a strong association in the few who develop leukaemia. The solvent benzene is most closely linked to aplasia and AML, but may be responsible for a small number of cases of CML.

Viruses

The range of retroviruses isolated from animal species who develop leukaemias and lymphoma continues to increase. The gibbon ape leukaemia virus was isolated from some captive gibbons with CML and induced CML when injected into young animals. It is likely that species-specific genetic susceptibility plays a role in the evolution of leukaemia in these primates.

Cytogenetics of CML

In 1960, the occurrence was reported in CML of the characteristic chromosomal defect later to be called the Philadelphia chromosome after the city of its discovery. This exists in 95% of patients with features of CML and in most consists of reciprocal translocation of half of the long arm of one of the chromosome 22 pair to one of the chromosome 9 pair, t(9t;22q–). Special banding techniques identified the translocation, which originally was thought to be a deletion and loss of chromatid material. In 50% of Philadelphia positive (Ph′+) patients the translocation is to another chromosome, sometimes many sharing the translocated material, and these patients behave in a similar way to the more typical Philadelphia positive cases. This is an acquired defect and the first recognisable abnormality in evolving CML. It is present in myeloid, monocytic, erythroid and megakaryocytic cell lines at diagnosis, but spares the lymphocyte and fibroblast marrow lines. It has been found in peripheral B-lymphocytes. It persists during clinical remission and only allogeneic marrow transplantation with supralethal pretreatment eradicates the Philadelphia positive clone.

Additional chromosomal abnormalities precede acute transformation of chronic phase CML to acute leukaemia or myelofibrosis in up to 80% of patients. The most common are duplication of the chromosome 22 translocation, trisomy 8, and isochromosome of the long arm of chromosome 17.

Philadelphia negative (Ph′–) CML patients usually show a more rapid deterioration and are more resistant to the usual chemotherapy agents. It is likely that some of these patients have smaller chromosomal translocations not yet detected. A small proportion of male patients with CML have lost the Y chromosome and they may have a more favourable outcome. Approximately 2% of otherwise typical cases of childhood ALL are Ph′+ and in adult ALL the percentage is higher. Most of these apparently arise de novo and are not a stage in the evolution of CML. Their prognosis is similar to that of usual ALL at the relevant age.

Oncogenes

Recent developments in the understanding of oncogenes in the pathogenesis of malignancy have clarified the association between the Philadelphia translocation and the evolution of CML. The exchange of genetic material between chromosome 9 and 22 involves translocation of proto-oncogenes C-abl and C-sis. It appears that C-abl derived from chromosome 9 links with the residual DNA of the long arm of chromosome 22 to form a hybrid gene and altered expression. An RNA product and specific abl-related protein have been identified in Ph′+ cells from CML patients and these may be mediators in the proliferative advantage of these cells over Ph′– clones. The oncogene activation may render the Ph′+ cells more susceptible to further genetic change preceding transformation to blast crisis.

Genetic factors

There is no definite evidence of a genetic predisposition to CML from family studies of patients. However, a small number of twin pairs with CML have been reported, usually in young children, which rather than confirming a genetic factor may imply a prenatal event which favoured growth of a leukaemic utreine event which favoured growth of a leukaemic clone. This is also suggested by the fact that the authors know of a female sibling-pair who developed CML within years of each other.

Pathogenesis and clonality

Acquisition of the Philadelphia chromosome by a pluripotent haemopoietic stem cell is the first event in the natural course of CML in most patients and may precede haematological changes by many years. This potentially malignant clone has a growth advantage over normal haemopoietic stem cells, but has to overcome a differentiation block before giving rise to a rapidly proliferating myeloid line. The Ph′+ stem cell is presumed to be pre-lymphoid pre-myeloid, since malignant transformation can give rise to myeloid or lymphoid blast cell crisis and the erythroid and megakaryocytic lines also possess the Ph′ chromosome. The occurrence of additional chromosomal abnormalities at blast crisis marks the selective progression of a truly malignant subclone of the original premalignant Ph′+ clone.

Additional evidence of the monoclonality of CML is provided by studies on heterozygote G6PD carriers who had CML. In these patients, only one type of G6PD was found in myeloid cells, whereas other tissues contained both enzyme types.

When symptoms eventually occur and lead to diagnosis, most of the myeloid cells in the marrow are Ph'+ and the myeloid compartment is grossly hyperplastic. Extramedullary myelopoiesis is established and there is variable expansion of erythroid and platelet production.

Immature myeloid cells are released prematurely and total white cell count rises exponentially. Splenomegaly is palpable when the white cell count exceeds $100 \times 10^9/l$. The neutrophil circulation time is increased and neutrophil function as measured in vitro declines with increasing white cell count and normalises with effective treatment of the disease. Neutrophil morphology is unremarkable and, though LAP is reduced, other enzyme levels are near normal. Monocyte numbers are relatively low and their normal regulatory influence on neutrophil production via colony stimulating factor (CSF) is lost. The number of CFU-GM (stem cells producing granulocyte and monocyte colonies in culture) is greatly increased in the marrow and blood of CML patients and their normal self-inhibitory feedback activity is depressed. Erythroid stem cells giving rise to BFU-E in vitro are also increased in the early stages, as are the multipotential progenitor cells CFU-GEMM.

But as normal marrow elements are crowded out, anaemia and thrombocytopenia develop in accelerated CML. The onset of blast cell crisis 1–5 years after diagnosis results from loss of myeloid differentiation and the evolution to myelofibrosis is due to collagen deposition.

The rare conversion of Ph'− CML to Ph'+ disease after some years of treatment may be due to the effects of chemotherapy or may suggest that the Philadelphia chromosome is in fact secondary to some other precipitating factor.

Clinical features

The most common presenting symptoms are those of anaemia, tiredness, dyspnoea on exertion, lightheadedness and palpitations. Anxiety, sweating and weight loss may suggest hyperthyroidism, but are due related to the raised metabolic rate associated with hyperleukocytosis. Abdominal distension and discomfort may result from splenomegaly and bone tenderness, especially in axial bones, reflects myeloid hyperplasia.

Bruising is common, but overt bleeding and infective complications are unusual, although fever may be present. Hyperviscosity syndrome with headache, dizziness, acral cyanosis, priapism, retinal haemorrhages,

blurred vision due to dyspnoea and congestive cardiac failure may occur when the white cell count exceeds 400×10^9.

Rare symptoms at diagnosis include pruritus and the effects of gouty arthropathy and pleural effusion. A few patients are identified on routine blood testing or karyotype analysis in the early stage and are asymptomatic.

Prominent signs at diagnosis are pallor, fever, sternal tenderness and moderate splenomegaly. The liver may be enlarged and, apart from bruising, retinal haemorrhages may be found.

The minority of patients who present in the transformation phase show more florid signs with bruising, bleeding, wasting, widespread or localised bone pain at sites of blast cell tumours, skin nodules due to myeloblast infiltration, adenopathy and rapidly enlarging splenomegaly. Splenic infarcts cause localised pain and sometimes a rub and ascites may occur with advancing disease.

In Ph'− CML, the spleen may remain impalpable and the white cell and platelet counts are usually lower. Some experts prefer to label this as 'atypical myeloproliferative syndrome'.

Investigations

At diagnosis, most patients have a white cell count in excess of $50 \times 10^9/l$, many over $100 \times 10^9/l$. A large percentage are myelocytes (up to 20%) and metamyelocytes (up to 40%) and small numbers of promyelocyte blasts (up to 4%) are seen on the film (Plate 14). The remainder are mature normal-looking neutrophils, eosinophils and basophils, both relatively increased, and monocytes which may be raised, particularly in Ph'− CML. Lymphocytes are inconspicuous, but numerically appropriate and nucleated red cells may account for a low percentage of nucleated cells.

A moderate normochromic anaemia – the haemoglobin is rarely less than 9 g/dl – and modest thrombocytosis are common at this stage. Giant platelets or megakaryocyte fragments may be seen on the blood film and there is no reticulocyte increase.

In early CML, a concurrent stress such as infection or surgery may induce a leukoerythroblastic response which disappears on recovery, only to recur later as the disease progresses.

A marked erythrocytosis and increased red cell mass may lead to a diagnosis of primary proliferative polycythaemia before the more typical features of CML appear.

The marrow aspirate shows marked hypercellularity confirmed on trephine with absence of fat spaces due to myeloid hyperplasia. The myeloid series is left-shifted and eosinophil and basophil myelocytes are usually increased. Mitotic figures are prominent, minor megaloblastic changes may occur in the erythroid series and increased numbers of micro-megakaryocytes are common.

Marrow morphology in itself does not make the diagnosis of CML, which depends on the identification of the Philadelphia chromosome in either marrow or blood in a patient with a typical blood picture.

Leukocyte alkaline phosphatase is greatly reduced in the neutrophils of CML patients in contrast to the leukocytosis associated with infection, pregnancy (used as a positive control) and other myeloproliferative disorders. The only exceptions are some $Ph'-$ CML patients, treated or post-splenectomy CML, and intercurrent stresses which may lead to elevation of the LAP to the normal range.

Biochemical studies usually show a raised uric acid due to rapid cell turnover. Impaired renal function due to some other factor or secondary to hyperuricaemia increases the risk of complications such as gouty arthritis and nephropathy and special precautions (allopurinol and high fluid intake) are important when cytotoxic therapy is being planned.

Rarely, pseudohyperkalaemia may result from cell lysis following phlebotomy in patients with very high white cell counts, but in these cases the ECG will not reveal hyperkalaemia.

Serum Vitamin B_{12} is markedly elevated in CML, even following successful treatment. This is a result of B_{12} binding by leukocytes (due to their high content of transcobalamin 1 (a B_{12} binding protein).

Differential diagnosis

The leuko-erythroblastic blood film that occurs in myelofibrosis and malignant marrow infiltrations may resemble that of CML. However, in myelofibrosis tear drop erythrocytes are characteristic, the splenomegaly is more prominent, there is no Philadelphia chromosome and pronounced marrow fibrosis is the hallmark. With malignant marrow infiltrates, there may be clinical evidence of a primary carcinoma or lymphoma and marrow biopsy usually makes the diagnosis. In these patients, circulating immature cells are small in number.

Primary thrombocythaemia may mimic early CML with thrombocytosis, but there is minimal myeloid hyperplasia with prominent platelet clouds and abnormal megakaryocytes in the former.

Some patients with septicaemia, advanced tuberculosis or solid tumours without marrow infiltration have white cell counts in excess of 30×10^9 with a small percentage of myelocytes and metamyelocytes, often with monocytosis. These are termed leukaemoid reactions and the marrow is less hyperactive with a normal karyotype.

Treatment of CML

Treatment of typical chronic myeloid leukaemia at diagnosis is relatively simple and uncomplicated by the severe infection and haemorrhage that often mars induction treatment of the acute leukaemias. It has not altered much over the past 35 years and, while it is easy to control CML during its chronic phase, induction and maintenance treatment never leads to complete remission and probably does not alter the natural progression or tendency to transform. The differential drug sensitivity of the $Ph'+$ clone and normal haemopoietic precursors is very slight and it is impossible to eradicate the CML clone without permanent marrow damage. The rare patient with early CML detected in the presymptomatic phase requires no active treatment. Progressive and symptomatic disease is usually treated with busulphan alone or busulphan with an antimetabolite such as thioguanine or mercaptopurine.

Chemotherapy

Busulphan, the cornerstone of treatment of chronic phase CML, is an alkylating agent derived from butane. It is myelotoxic and in CML induces a delayed reduction in the white cell count in almost all patients, an effect which may continue for 2–3 weeks after cessation of treatment. The white cell count, differential count and, later on, spleen size return to normal and symptoms resolve. It probably exerts its effect at progenitor stem cell level and in a few sensitive patients may cause severe prolonged hypoplasia lasting several weeks.

The usual induction dose is 4 mg daily (half that if used in combination) and this is continued until the white cell count drops to $20 \times 10^9/l$, when busulphan should be stopped. The maintenance dose, if required, to keep the white cell count $\leq 10 \times 10^9/l$ varies from 1–2 mg daily for 5 days weekly, or 4 mg a day from 1–5 days weekly, depending on counts and other cytotoxic drugs used. There is no advantage in using intermittent high dose busulphan and it remains controversial whether or not continuing maintenance busulphan in patients in stable chronic phase offers any long-term advantage in delaying disease progression. Infrequent toxic effects of busulphan are hyperpigmentation and interstitial pulmonary fibrosis, the incidence of each increasing with duration of treatment. Nausea and anorexia may occur and rarely progressive weakness and muscle wasting may follow prolonged busulphan therapy.

Patients who present with hyperleukocytosis (white cell count $> 250 \times 10^9/l$) may develop complications secondary to hyperviscosity and rapid reduction in white cell count is best achieved by leukopheresis or high dose hydroxyurea at a dose of 4 g daily for 3 days. Hydroxyurea inhibits ribonucleotide reductose, so interfering with DNA synthesis in rapidly proliferating tissues. Its major advantages are its rapid effect and lack of prolonged marrow depression on stopping treatment. It is preferred in Ph′− patients and in those with thrombocytopenia. A maintenance dose of 500 mg to 1500mg daily is usually sufficient in chronic phase CML. Regular blood counts are needed to ensure effective treatment. Chlorambucil, melphalan, dibromannitol and cyclophosphamide are rarely used, but sometimes effective in CML.

Recently, human leukocyte interferon has been used with some success in both chronic phase and busulphan-resistant CML and seems to exert an inhibitory effect on CML progenitor cells.

Allopurinol and a high fluid intake should prevent hyperuricaemia during induction treatment, but allopurinol and mercaptopurine should not be used together. No chemotherapy regimen has yet succeeded in clearing the Ph′ + clone and indeed some experts feel that busulphan may promote transformation to acute leukaemia which is highly resistant to further chemotherapy.

Satisfactory control can be maintained for 2–6 years, at which point the disease enters its second phase of either progressive resistance to even intensive therapy or abrupt blast crisis.

Splenic irradiation

In the past, splenic irradiation was used in newly diagnosed patients and was effective in normalising blood counts and reducing splenomegaly for some months. It is not as effective as busulphan in long-term control and leukopheresis is safer and more effective in rapid reduction of high white cell and platelet counts. Extracorporeal irradiation of blood is no more effective and is rarely used now.

Splenectomy

Elective splenectomy early in chronic phase CML was thought to prolong survival by delaying progression or transformation to blast crisis, but controlled trials over the past 10 years do not show any advantage in splenectomised patients.

Bone marrow transplantation (BMT) in CML (see Ch. 21)

In an effort to eradicate the malignant Ph′+ clone, syngeneic marrow transplantation after ablative chemoradiotherapy was first carried out by the Seattle group in 1976. They used high dose cyclophosphamide and total body irradiation of 1000 rads and by infusing normal twin marrow avoided the complication of graft versus host disease (GVHD). All patients became Ph′− after transplant and after 3 years only one of 12 had relapsed. Further experience has shown that syngeneic BMT in chronic phase CML prolongs survival in most patients and may be curative in some. In contrast, the results in accelerated or blastic-phase CML have been disappointing.

The next logical step was to use ablative treatment and rescue with HLA identical sibling marrow in young patients with chronic phase CML (allogeneic BMT). Prophylaxis against GVHD using either cyclosporin and/or T-cell depletion of donor marrow is standard practice.

A report in 1984 from the International Registry, which analyses results from many centres, shows that while transplant-related mortality averages 30% in patients in chronic phase, their rate of relapse in the first 2 years post-transplant is 5–10%. Actuarial survival of 72% at 2 years remains static up to 4 years and results are slightly better for younger patients (<30). There is an inverse relationship between duration of chronic phase disease and length of survival after BMT, and the risk of relapse is much higher in patients transplanted in the accelerated phases. Splenectomy in these patients does not seem to influence survival and T-cell depletion of donor marrow, while it may reduce the incidence and severity of GVHD, may also increase the risk of marrow failure.

The prospect of long-term cure of chronic phase CML by allogeneic BMT makes this disease the prime indication for BMT in patients <50 years of age with an HLA-identical sibling. Unrelated HLA-identical donors may also be used, but the incidence and severity of GVHD is greater.

For older patients and those without a suitable marrow donor, autologous BMT after conventional ablative therapy may restore chronic phase disease in patients with accelerating or transformed CML.

Autotransplant is achieved by collecting and cryopreserving, at diagnosis or in chronic phase, marrow or blood buffy coat containing pluripotential haemopoietic stem cells. This can be stored for years and in most cases its engraftment results in Ph′+ haemopoiesis and stable chronic phase disease. Some patients have a percentage of Ph′− marrow and treatment with 4-hydroperoxycyclophosphamide may selectively deplete Ph′+ progenitor cells, allowing repopulation by Ph′− stem cells. This technique is still in the experimental stage.

Autografting patients with blast transformation has not substantially prolonged survival and graft failure occurs in up to 50% of these patients.

The role of autologous BMT in chronic phase CML is not yet clear, but progress in the area of in vitro manipulation of chronic phase marrow may improve the clinical outcome in patients who cannot receive allogeneic BMT.

Complications of CML

Reference has been made to the occurrence of hyperviscosity syndrome and hyperuricaemia at diagnosis. Splenomegaly in advancing CML may be complicated by splenic infarcts, thrombocytopenia and transfusion-dependent anaemia. At this stage, when the disease is drug-resistant, splenectomy, while it is hazardous, may relieve pain and hypersplenism. Splenic irradiation or local intra-arterial cytotoxic infusion are less satisfactory options.

Platelet function defects are not uncommon in patients with CML, even in those with thrombocytosis. Invasive procedures may need to be performed with infusion of normal platelets.

Transformation of CML chronic phase is almost inevitable and may be gradual and insidious (approximately 80%) or abrupt and catastrophic. It may be apparent at initial presentation, but the interval between CML diagnosis and transformation usually varies from 1–6 years. In most patients, the first indication is increasing resistance to chemotherapy, followed by symptoms of fever, weight loss and bone pains. Adenopathy and increasing splenomegaly occur and over the following months a larger percentage of the increasing white cell count is made up of myelocytes, atypical granulocytes, eosinophils and basophils. Thrombocytopenia and transfusion-dependent anaemia ensue. Additional chromosomal abnormalities are common at this stage and increasing numbers of blast cells occur in the marrow. In 20% or more of these 'chronic transformations' myelofibrosis occurs, with lytic bone lesions occurring in some.

In acute transformation, blast crisis supervenes in apparently well controlled chronic phase CML. Extramedullary blast cell tumours of the skin,

mucosal surfaces, pleura, bone or nodes may rarely be the only sign of blast transformation in otherwise stable chronic phase disease. Spread to, or multicentric transformation in, marrow quickly follows and the solid tumours are radioresistant. If transformation is suspected, busulphan should be stopped and supportive treatment instituted while a decision on further treatment is made.

Most blast transformations result in myeloblastic acute leukaemia with a small proportion showing features of M6 and M7 subtypes. A further 20% are lymphoblastic, having a similar immunologic phenotype and TdT positivity as in common ALL. The rest have features of both myeloid and lymphoid blast derivation.

Myeloid blast crisis rarely responds to conventional AML chemotherapy regimes, marrow hypoplasia is prolonged and remissions are short-lived.

Lymphoid blast crisis is generally more chemosensitive and many patients enter remission with residual Ph′+ chronic phase marrow. Vincristine and prednisolone are the first line drugs for remission induction and conventional ALL maintenance regimes may extend remission for up to 1 year. In a few patients, the lymphoid blasts appear to overwhelm the Ph′+ clone which disappears and, if marrow hypoplasia results in eradication of the blasts, attempts at allogeneic BMT in patients with frank blast crisis have been fruitless. But if a second chronic phase can be established, the procedure may succeed in prolonging survival in 50% of cases.

Accelerated disease, even before features of blast crisis occur, can rarely be controlled by allogeneic transplantation. Recent results from the Hammersmith Hospital show only one long-term survivor (40 months) and a significantly higher incidence of fatal GVHD and pneumonitis in patients transplanted in the accelerated phase.

Ph′− myelopoiesis may ensue, though this phase is usually transient. Further lymphoid blast crisis or mixed lymphoid myeloid blast crisis occurs and meningeal infiltration complicates the picture in 40% of these patients.

Prognosis in CML

Presenting features such as age, spleen size, percentage blasts in marrow and platelet count may give some idea of long-term outlook, but there are few clues in early CML to the eventual outcome. Typical Ph′+ CML has a more favourable course than Ph′− CML; the presence of basophilia and myelofibrosis at diagnosis represents a prognostic advantage; female patients are said to do better; and the maintenance of a white cell count $< 10 \times 10^9/l$ in chronic phase prolongs the course of events.

Bad prognostic features include a high percentage of Ph' + cells, additional chromosomal abnormalities, poor response to induction therapy and short remissions. A cumulative dose of busulphan in excess of 300 mg in the first year may also indicate a poor outlook. Features which herald probable transformation, such as fever, bone lesions, increasing eosinophilia and basophilia, and late thrombocytosis obviously indicate bad prognosis, but the rare occurrence of hypodiploidy in transformation is said to increase the chance of remission. Serial cytogenetic analyses may detect transformation before other features develop.

Variants of chronic myeloid leukaemia

Philadelphia negative CML

This represents about 5% of CML and is sometimes difficult to separate clinically from Ph'+ve CML. Basophilia is unusual, monocytosis is common and immature granulocytes are seen in the blood. Prognosis is less good than for the Ph'+ve disease, with poor response to busulpan and a median survival of only 18 months.

Juvenile CML

This is a very rare variant of CML which occurs in children of 1–5 years. It resembles subacute CMML or adult atypical Ph'− CML and usually runs a rapidly progressive course. Common presenting features are anaemia, infections of respiratory tract and skin, rashes, hepatosplenomegaly and adenopathy. The white cell count rarely exceeds $50 \times 10^9/l$ at presentation and a leuko-erythroblastic picture occurs, often with an accompanying monocytosis. A characteristic feature is a rise in fetal haemoglobin and it is likely that the malignant clone arises during fetal development.

Typical Ph'+ CML may rarely occur in children over 5 years old and follows a similar course in most. Response to cytotoxic drugs is poor and survival is short.

Chronic eosinophilic leukaemia

This is a very rare Ph'− condition arising in middle life. Eosinophils are produced in large numbers and typically contain masses of large eosinophilic granules. Differential diagnosis includes classical CML with marked eosinophil component (almost always Ph'+) and reactive eosinophilia which is usually self-limiting. Patients often have splenomegaly and may show the cardiac and pulmonary lesions of the hypereosinophilic syndrome. Prognosis is variable, but usually similar to classical CML. Some patients show a terminal blast-cell phase.

Chronic basophilic leukaemia

This is another very rare Ph'− condition of middle life, which should be distinguished from classical CML, with excess basophil production.

The disease is characterised by hyperhistaminaemia with excess 5-hydroxytryptamine production. Hyperhistamine symptoms respond to cyproheptadine or adrenaline. The disease may run a variable course over several years.

Chronic myelomonocytic leukaemia

CMML is an atypical myeloproliferative condition, though recently it has been included in the myelodysplastic syndromes as defined by the FAB group. It may be detected coincidentally in its early stages, when the only abnormality is a monocytosis (monocytes $> 1 \times 10^9/l$), sometimes with atypical monocytoid cells (Plate 15). It progresses slowly, with increasing white cell counts and monocytosics, normochromic anaemia, thrombocytopenia and symptoms of pancytopenia. Moderate hepatosplenomegaly occurs in some patients and the leukocytosis does not tend to rise to the levels seen in CML. The marrow shows myeloid hyperplasia with predominance of myelocytes and a proportion of ($\geqslant 20\%$) monocytoid cells which show increasingly malignant features as transformation to acute myelomonocytic leukaemia occurs. Serum lysozyme levels are markedly elevated and the Ph' chromosome is absent, though other cytogenetic markers of AML may occur.

Most patients are over 60 and, since disease progression is often slow and response to chemotherapy disappointing, supportive treatment is the best policy. Hydroxyurea or mercaptopurine are the most effective drugs in controlling progressive disease without serious toxicity.

Future trends

Recent studies in the role of oncogenes in CML suggest a central role for the C-abl proto-oncogene sited on chromosome 9. It is activated by translocation to chromosome 22 and a CML-specific protein is thought to be the resulting product. The development of a monoclonal antibody to this protein might prove useful in treatment or in purging autologous marrow or blood prior to autograft in chronic phase CML.

Studies of stem cell culture in chronic phase CML have shown that, in contrast to the proliferative advantage enjoyed by the Ph'+ clone in vivo, long-term culture of marrow selectively favours growth of the Ph'− normal progenitor stem cells with repression of Ph'+ clone. This technique has been used in autotransplanting a patient in first AML relapse and should be applicable to CML patients also.

The disappointing facts of the management of CML are

(i) that it cannot be cured by conventional treatment
(ii) that palliation does not postpone tranformation
(iii) that transformation is unpredictable and
(iv) that no treatment significantly prolongs survival after transformation.

It is now widely accepted that allogeneic BMT from identical sibling donors offers the best chance of cure when carried out in chronic phase. Recent reports emphasise the importance of proceeding to BMT as early as possible in the chronic phase, preferably within the first year from diagnosis. Prognostic factors may identify those patients who will do badly and warrant early BMT, but with the increasing availability of BMT at regional level and reduction in transplant-related mortality, this option should be available to all newly diagnosed patients who have a suitable donor.

BIBLIOGRAPHY

Cawley J C 1985 Hairy cell leukaemia. British Journal of Haematology 60: 213–218
Cawley J C 1987 Hairy cell leukaemia. In: Whittaker J A, Delamore I W (Eds) Leukaemia. Blackwell, Oxford
Gale R P, Foon K A 1985 Chronic lymphocytic leukemia. Recent advances in biology and treatment. Annals of Internal Medicine 103: 101–120
Galton D A G 1982 The chronic leukaemias. In: Hardisty R M, Weatherall D J (Eds) Blood and its disorders. Blackwell, Oxford, pp 877–917
Gunz F W, Henderson E S 1983 Leukemia, 4th Edn. Grune and Stratton, New York

Koeffler, Golde 1981 Chronic myeloid leukemia: new concepts. New England Journal of Medicine 304: 1201–1209 and 1269–1274
Sawitsky A, Rai K 1987 The chronic lymphoid leukaemias. In: J A, Delamore I W (Eds) Leukaemia. Blackwell, Oxford
Spiers A S D 1987 The chronic myeloid leukaemias. In: Whittaker J A, Delamore I W (Eds) Leukaemia. Blackwell, Oxford.

18. Hodgkin's disease

T. Sheehan   A. C. Parker

Malignant lymphomas are a heterogeneous group of neoplasms which originate from cells of the immune system. Traditionally they have been divided into two broad categories: Hodgkin's disease and the non-Hodgkin's lymphomas. Taken as a whole, the incidence of malignant lymphomas is approximately equal to that of acute and chronic leukaemias combined, and a sound understanding of the immunological and histological principles involved is essential for any clinician responsible for the management of patients with these disorders.

Paradoxically, while there is now almost complete agreement on the histological classification of Hodgkin's disease and a considerable consensus of opinion regarding appropriate investigation and management, our understanding of the biology of this disease is limited, and indeed the normal counterpart of the malignant cell remains a hotly contested issue. The numerous proposed classifications of non-Hodgkin's lymphomas, on the other hand, have caused a great deal of confusion among clinicians but, thanks to recent advances in immunology and the sophisticated investigative techniques now available to the histopathologist, our understanding of the biology of these disorders has become much clearer.

The normal immune system is highly complex and comprises T or thymus-derived and B or Bursa-derived lymphocytes which are programmed to respond to specific antigens and circulate widely throughout the body, 'homing' preferentially to specific T- and B-cell areas within lymph nodes, spleen and other organs. (Fig. 18.1). They are concerned with cell-mediated and humoral immunity respectively. In addition, T-cells can be further subdivided into suppressor and helper subtypes according to their role in regulating humoral and cell-mediated immune responses. Cells of the monocyte-macrophage system perform important accessory functions including antigen presentation and regulation of immune responses, and there are specialised macro-

a) Lymph Node
Both B and T lymphocytes exit from blood vessels in the paracortical area. B cells then migrate further to their own specific region where they are found grouped together in follicles

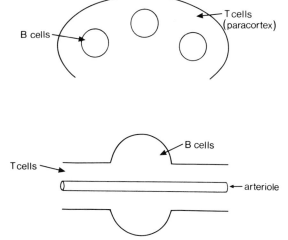

b) Spleen
Central arteriole surrounded by a sheath of lymphoid tissue (white pulp) containing mostly T cells. At irregular intervals along this sheath nodular projections of lymphoid tissue consisting of B cells are found

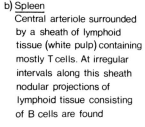

Fig. 18.1 Lymphocyte homing patterns.

phage-derived cells present in lymphoid tissue which interact specifically with T- or B-lymphocytes. Although far from complete, our knowledge of lymphocyte maturation and transformation has increased in recent years and the recognition that in many acute and chronic lymphocytic leukaemias and non-Hodgkin's lymphomas the malignant cells mirror their normal counterparts in terms of antigen expression, 'homing' patterns and kinetic behaviour has not only facilitated our understanding of these disorders but has important implications for treatment.

Since the first description of Hodgkin's disease in 1832, by Thomas Hodgkin, considerable progress has been made in terms of histological classification, investigation and management, but many fundamental questions remain unanswered. On the basis of clinical behaviour and cytogenetic features, Hodgkin's disease appears to be a neoplastic process, but there is no entirely specific marker available for the malignant cell, nor is there general agreement about the normal cell counterpart. Conflicting evidence has been produced over the years supporting a lymphocytic or histiocytic origin, and since the diagnosis is still essentially based on the histological demonstration of Reed-Sternberg cells and Reed-Sternberg-like variants in an appropriate cellular background, it is possible that Hodgkin's disease may not be one entity but a group of disorders sharing a common morphological phenotype. The cellular background in Hodgkin's tissue has traditionally been regarded as reactive. In particular, the lymphocytes present have been thought to exert an anti-tumour effect. Although there is a correlation between the lymphocytic component as defined by the histological type and the stage of disease (and therefore prognosis) the nature of the interaction between lymphocytes and Reed-Sternberg cells remains unclear. Hodgkin's disease is associated with defects in cell-mediated immunity, the degree of which correlates with disease stage. This immune defect, which remains imperfectly understood, is responsible for some of the complications suffered by patients, and may yet shed important light on the nature of the disease.

Epidemiology and aetiology

In advanced countries Hodgkin's disease is rare in childhood and shows a bimodal pattern of incidence with a sharp peak in early adult life and a second gradual increase after the age of 45 years. Overall the disease is slightly more common in males but the nodular sclerosis subtype is more common in young females and has a predilection for mediastinal involvement.

Abdominal presentation is more common in the older age groups and tends to be associated with the mixed cellularity or lymphocyte-depleted histological subtypes. In developing countries, however, the disease is much more common in childhood, with the lymphocyte-depleted subtype, which is rare in advanced countries, accounting for a significant proportion of cases. The frequency of the lymphocyte-depleted subtype in countries where immunosuppression secondary to malnutrition and other factors is rife is interpreted by some as supportive evidence for the concept that the lymphocytes in Hodgkin's disease may represent an anti-tumour response on the part of the host.

The hypothesis that Hodgkin's disease may be caused by a virus, the oncogenic potential of which may be related to the age and immunocompetency of the host at the time of first exposure, has received considerable attention. In advanced countries there is an association between Hodgkin's disease and higher socio-economic status, small family size and, possibly, tonsillectomy in childhood. There have also been several controversial reports of 'clustering' of cases within populations and of an increased incidence in physicians and teachers exposed to patients with the disease.

However, despite these reports and the demonstration of reverse transcriptase in Hodgkin's tissue in some cases, the evidence for a viral aetiology is at present unconvincing. Recent reports of atypical Hodgkin's disease complicating the acquired immunodeficiency syndrome (AIDS) have aroused considerable interest but there is no convincing evidence that the incidence of Hodgkin's disease is actually increased in patients with AIDS.

Clinical features

Lymphadenopathy

Approximately 70% of patients present with superficial lymphadenopathy involving, in order of frequency, cervical, axillary or inguinal regions. The glandular enlargement is usually painless and progressive, although there may be some waxing and waning in the early stages. The nodes are usually non-tender, discrete and of a firm, rubbery consistency, although in the nodular sclerosis subtype the fibrosis may be so marked that the glands have a hard consistency suggestive of metastatic carcinoma. The oft-quoted pain induced in Hodgkin's nodes by alcohol ingestion is rare, of no prognostic significance and entirely non-specific, being found with equal frequency in non-Hodgkin's lymphomas and metastatic carcinoma.

Mediastinal lymphadenopathy is usually associated

with supraclavicular involvement, but abdominal presentations of disease can be more difficult to diagnose; in these cases the lymphadenopathy may reach massive proportions before becoming clinically apparent. Such patients may present with obstructive symptoms such as lower limb oedema, or with 'B' symptoms, which are present in over one quarter of all patients with Hodgkin's disease and may be the presenting feature in patients with occult abdominal disease.

'B' symptoms (see Table 18.1)

These comprise unexplained weight loss of more than 10% of total body weight over the 6 months prior to diagnosis, night sweats and unexplained fever with temperature above 38°C. The so-called 'classic' Pel-Ebstein pattern of fever is very rare. The pathogenesis of 'B' symptoms is unknown but their presence is of major prognostic importance.

Table 18.1 'B' symptoms

Unexplained night sweats
Unexplained fever (>38°C)
Unexplained weight loss (i.e. > 10% of normal body weight in 6 months prior to diagnosis)

Pruritus occurs in 10% of patients and may be the first manifestation of occult disease but, unlike 'B' symptoms, is of no prognostic importance.

Splenomegaly

This is uncommon and does not necessarily imply infiltration with Hodgkin's disease; conversely the majority of spleens which are infiltrated with Hodgkin's disease are not clinically enlarged.

Hepatomegaly

This and other clinically overt extralymphatic disease is rare at presentation and usually implies advanced disease. It should be emphasised that, unlike non-Hodgkin's lymphomas, a genuine extranodal presentation of Hodgkin's disease is extremely rare and such a diagnosis should be made with great caution.

Histological classification

The Rye classification (Fig. 18.2) recognises four main histological types of Hodgkin's disease: lymphocyte-pre-

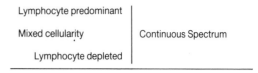

Fig. 18.2 Rye classification

dominant, mixed cellularity, lymphocyte-depleted and nodular sclerosis. This classification is based on both the type of malignant cell present in a given case and the nature of the 'reactive' component. The sine qua non of Hodgkin's disease is the Reed-Sternberg cell, a large, binucleate cell with prominent large eosinophilic nucleoli. Similar cells can be seen in a variety of other disorders and the diagnosis of Hodgkin's disease rests on the demonstration of these cells and variants thereof in an appropriate cellular background. Lymph node involvement may be total or partial; when partial the infiltrate is usually confined to the interfollicular or T-cell areas with preservation of normal germinal centres.

Therapy may induce changes in the histological appearances, commonly producing a lymphocyte-depleted pattern. Accurate subclassification is therefore only possible prior to therapy.

The natural history of untreated Hodgkin's disease is one of progression to more unfavourable histological subtypes, leading eventually to lymphocyte depletion, but nodular sclerosis is an entirely separate category with no overlap with other histological subtypes.

Lymphocyte-predominant

Both nodular and diffuse patterns exist, but are grouped together in the Rye classification. In this type classic Reed-Sternberg cells are few in number and the predominant malignant cell is a distinctive variant with a large, solitary, irregularly shaped nucleus with an open chromatin pattern and one or two small, indistinct nucleoli. (Plate 16). While occasional neutrophils, eosinophils and plasma cells may be found, the 'reactive' component comprises mainly small lymphocytes which are often slightly irregular in shape. Histiocytes may also be present, either scattered singly throughout the node or grouped together in compact epithelioid granulomas. This subtype is commonly associated with limited (Stage I and II) disease and therefore tends to have a favourable prognosis.

Mixed cellularity

In this subtype classic Reed-Sternberg cells and morphologically similar mononuclear cells are found in large numbers and the 'reactive' cellular background consists of a variable mixture of lymphocytes, histiocytes, neutrophils, eosinophils and plasma cells. (Plate 17). This subtype is more often associated with advanced (Stage III or IV) disease and is therefore prognostically less favourable.

Lymphocyte-depleted

Two distinct histological patterns may be recognised within this subtype. In the reticular pattern the vast majority of cells present in the lymph node are classic Reed-Sternberg cells, and pleomorphic, multinucleated variants. In the diffuse fibrosis category the process appears to have 'burnt out' and the lymph node architecture is replaced by a fine diffuse fibrosis with few residual cells. The lymphocyte-depleted subtype tends to be the most aggressive and is usually regarded as particularly prognostically unfavourable.

Nodular sclerosis

In this subtype nodules of pathological cells are separated from each other by wide bands of collagen. (Plate 18). Classic Reed-Sternberg cells may be few or numerous and the hallmark of this type of Hodgkin's disease is the lacunar cell, a multinucleated cell which in formalin-fixed tissue appears to sit in a lacuna or empty space. This is an artefact induced by fixation and in tissues fixed with mercuric-based fixatives lacunae are not seen but the cell retains its other distinctive cytological features. The nuclear lobes are numerous, small and characteristically resemble a cluster of grapes. Nucleoli are indistinct or absent. The lacunar cell is so distinctive that the diagnosis of 'cellular phase' nodular sclerosis can be made at a stage before fibrosis has developed.

The reactive component varies from predominantly lymphocytic through varying degrees of lymphocyte depletion. It now appears that subclassifying nodular sclerosis according to the degree of lymphocyte predominance or depletion may be of prognostic importance.

Investigation

The two pieces of information required before embarking on therapy in Hodgkin's disease are the histological type and stage or extent of disease. In all suspected cases a histological diagnosis is mandatory. As with all lymphomas accurate classification depends on the provision of good quality material to the histopathologist.

Lymph node biopsy

The largest lymph node that can safely be removed should be taken; macroscopically unimpressive nodes have a disconcerting habit of proving histologically unimpressive and may not be involved in the pathological process. The node should be removed in its entirety and surgical trauma kept to the minimum. Fresh unfixed material should be made available for the sophisticated immunohistochemical investigations which may be required to achieve an accurate diagnosis.

Staging

Having established the histological type of Hodgkin's disease, the next step is to determine the stage of the disease according to the Ann Arbor staging system (Table 18.2). Careful clinical examination of the lymphoreticular system is essential. In Hodgkin's disease, unlike the non-Hodgkin's lymphomas, involvement of Waldeyer's ring is unusual and ENT examination rarely indicated. Well-penetrated chest X-rays, tomograms or CT scan are essential to exclude mediastinal, hilar or parenchymal lung involvement. If mediastinal involvement is present, its extent should be determined and documented, since the bulk of disease may have important implications for treatment.

Abdominal disease may be investigated either by lymphangiography or CT scan. An illustration of these two modes of investigation is shown in (Fig. 18.3). At present computerised tomographic scanning is most commonly used as the primary investigative technique

Table 18.2   Ann Arbor staging system

Stage I	Involvement of single lymph node region (I) or single extralymphatic site (I_E)
Stage II	Involvement of two or more lymph node regions on the same side of the diaphragm (II), which may also include spleen (II_S), localised extralymphatic involvement (II_E) or both (II_{SE}) if confined to the same side of the diaghragm
Stage III	Involvement of lymph node regions on both sides of the diaphragm (III), which may also include spleen (III_S), localised extralymphatic involvement (III_E) or both (III_{SE})
Stage IV	Diffuse or disseminated involvement of extra-lymphatic sites (e.g. lung, liver, bone marrow)

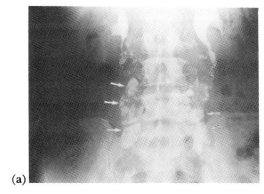
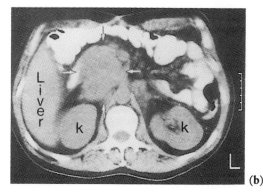

(a)   (b)

Fig. 18.3 Lymphangiogram (a) demonstrates multiple enlarged abnormal and abdominal lymph nodes. CT scan (b) shows large abdominal mass which consists of marked pathological lymph nodes.

to assess abdominal and, when necessary, intra-thoracic involvement. This technique does not reliably assess splenic or hepatic disease. The use of lymphangiography as a first-line approach is limited to centres in which there is special expertise both in its performance and interpretation. In occasional patients ultrasound detects hepatic and splenic involvement, when CT scanning has failed to do so. Modified CT scanning using etheiodised oils to increase detection rate is presently being evaluated. Ultrasound is a very useful method of detecting intra-abdominal lymphadenopathy, is non-invasive and economical, but is heavily dependent on the skill of the operator.

Trephine biopsy of bone has in the past been performed routinely but as bone marrow involvement is found in only 5% of cases at presentation, its use is decreasing. Although the non-invasive investigative techniques currently available cannot reliably exclude splenic involvement, staging laparotomy with its associated morbidity and small mortality risk is now rarely performed.

It is clear from the above that the presence or absence of splenic involvement is not reliably excluded by present radiological techniques. A definitive answer can only be obtained by performing staging laparotomy, of which splenectomy has been an integral part when used in Hodgkin's disease. Staging laparotomy involves a formal abdominal exploratory operation in which representative lymph nodes are removed for examination, liver biopsies are taken and finally splenectomy performed. Over recent years the use of splenectomy and staging laparotomy for diagnostic and staging purposes has declined significantly. The major reason for such change is that morbidity and long-term risks of this procedure are not balanced by clear benefit for patients in terms of survival, although if relapse does occur treatment with chemotherapy in the majority of cases is successful.

Laboratory features

A wide range of entirely non-specific laboratory abnormalities may be found at presentation. The ESR is commonly elevated, particularly if the patient has 'B' symptoms, and there may be a diffuse increase in gammaglobulins. Anaemia is present in 10% of cases at presentation and is usually normochromic normocytic in nature and mild in degree. There may be a neutrophilia, eosinophilia or monocytosis but leukopenia is rarely seen prior to therapy. Lymphopenia is present in one-third of cases and tends to correlate with disease stage and possibly with response to therapy. Anergy is common but humoral immunity is usually well preserved. Autoimmune thrombocytopenia or haemolytic anaemia are uncommon complications of Hodgkin's disease.

Treatment

The choice of treatment in Hodgkin's disease depends mainly on the extent or stage of the disease and to a lesser extent on the histological type.

Localised disease

Localised, asymptomatic Hodgkin's disease is best treated by radiotherapy. While there is no clear-cut evidence that extending the field of radiotherapy beyond the site of obvious disease results in improved survival, in most centres such 'extended field' high dose supervoltage therapy is the preferred approach. Limited stage supradiaphragmatic disease is treated by the 'mantle'

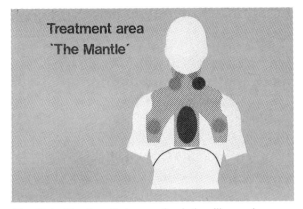

Fig. 18.4 Mantle radiotherapy. Cervical, axillary and mediastinal regions are included in the treatment field.

technique, which involves irradiating the cervical and axillary regions on both sides, the mediastinum and, in some cases, the upper para-aortic region (Fig. 18.4). A total of 35–40 GY is usually administered over a 3–6-week period and key organs may be shielded to minimise toxicity. Nausea and vomiting are common but unmanageable side effects and major complications are unusual. Radiation pneumonitis of variable degree occurs in 6–20% of patients receiving 'mantle' radiotherapy, while radiation-induced myo- or pericarditis is uncommon. Hypothyroidism may occur as a late complication and may require lifelong hormone replacement therapy. Provided the disease is accurately staged and the treatment properly administered, the prospects for 'cure' in localised Hodgkin's disease are excellent, with 5-year disease-free survivals in excess of 80%.

Disseminated disease

There is general agreement that the treatment of choice for Stage IV or Stage IIIB disease is chemotherapy, but the approach to Stage IIIA or limited, symptomatic disease (Stage IB or IIB) varies according to the expertise and preference of the centre concerned. Stage IB is rarely seen in clinical practice. Most authorities would consider radiotherapy alone insufficient treatment for patients with Stage IIB disease, for whom chemotherapy, or combined modality therapy if there is bulk disease, is the preferred approach. Approximately 50% of patients with advanced Hodgkin's disease can expect to be 'cured' by conventional combination chemotherapy.

It should be emphasised from the outset that there is no place for single agent chemotherapy in the management of Hodgkin's disease except as a purely palliative measure in patients who are unfit for aggressive therapy

Table 18.3 MOPP

Mustine	6 mg/m^2 IV days 1 and 8
Vincristine	1.4 mg/m^2 IV days 1 and 8 (max 2 mg)
Procarbazine	100 mg/m^2 oral days 1–14 inclusive
Prednisolone	40 mg/m^2 oral days 1–14 inclusive

Minimum of 6 cycles (complete remission plus 2) with 2-week intervals between cycles

or for some reason are regarded as incurable. Not only is single agent chemotherapy incapable of achieving 'cure' in Hodgkin's disease, such treatment also seriously compromises the later response to combination chemotherapy. The yardstick against which all other regimens have to be judged remains MOPP, (Table 18.3) developed by De Vita and co-workers in the late 1960s. Mustine is commonly associated with nausea and alopecia and most patients experience some degree of neurotoxicity from the vincristine, but in general the regimen is safe and well tolerated and can nearly always be administered on an outpatient basis. Patients should receive at least six cycles of treatment, including two complete cycles after clinical remission has been achieved. Maintenance treatment is of no proven value in Hodgkin's disease. Complete remission is achieved with this protocol in 80% of cases, one third of whom will subsequently relapse, usually within the first two years. Patients who relapse within the first year of stopping treatment are almost invariably MOPP-resistant and require some form of second-line therapy, but the prospects for 'cure' in this group are poor, with fewer than 25% long-term survivors. Patients who relapse after a lengthy first remission, however, may respond to conventional therapy. In the latter group it seems likely that a small amount of chemosensitive residual disease escaped detection after apparently successful treatment, while in the former group there are likely to have been chemoresistant sub-clones present from the outset.

Prognostic features

Approximately half of patients with advanced Hodgkin's currently die of their disease. Although it is not possible accurately to predict outcome in individual cases, certain factors, including 'B' symptoms, stage, bulk disease, high erythrocyte sedimentation rate, degree of anaemia, extent of splenic involvement, lymphocytopenia and prior single agent chemotherapy appear to be prognostically unfavourable. The patient's age and the histological type of disease may also be prognostically important. Relapse is more likely in nodular sclerosis, perhaps because the dense fibrosis prevents adequate penetration of drugs. Despite this, presumably because of the generally more indolent nature of this disease, the survival compares well with other histological types. Within the nodular sclerosis type, lymphocyte-depleted histology may also be associated with a higher relapse rate and a propensity for local invasion. Many authorities feel that lymphocyte-depleted Hodgkin's disease is biologically unusually aggressive and would treat all patients aggressively (e.g. with radiotherapy and chemotherapy) irrespective of stage.

Prior radiotherapy appears to be associated with a better prognosis, perhaps because the fact that the disease was initially localised implies a less rapidly progressive type of disease. An alternative explanation is that relapse is likely to be detected at a relatively early stage, since these patients are reviewed and examined regularly after receiving radiotherapy.

Various strategies have been employed in attempts either to reduce the toxicity of conventional chemotherapy or to improve the overall 'cure rate'. Substituting oral chlorambucil for mustine in the MOPP protocol (ChLVPP) (Table 18.4), reduces nausea and vomiting and the long-term results appear to be equivalent to those achieved with MOPP. In an attempt to improve the 'cure' rate, Bonadonna has treated patients with alternating cycles of MOPP and ABVD (Table 18.5), a non-cross-resistant regimen developed as a salvage protocol. It is hoped that this approach will minimise the problem of drug resistance, and indeed initial results are encouraging.

Other workers have subjected high-risk patients to combined modality therapy which as yet has not proved clearly superior to conventional chemotherapy. Furthermore, the use of chemotherapy and radiation increases

Table 18.4 CHLVPP

Chlorambucil	6 mg/m² oral days 1–14 inclusive (max 10 mg)
Vinblastine	6 mg/m² IV days 1 and 8
Procarbazine	100 mg/m² oral days 1–14 inclusive
Prednisolone	40 mg oral days 1–14 inclusive

Minimum of 6 cycles (complete remission plus 2) with 2-week intervals between cycles

Table 18.5 ABVD

Adriamycin	25 mg/m² IV days 1 and 14
Bleomycin	25 mg/m² IV days 1 and 14
Vinblastine	6 mg/m² IV days 1 and 14
DTIC	375 mg/m² IV days 1 and 14

Minimum of 6 cycles (complete remission plus 2) with 2-week intervals between cycles

the risk of inducing secondary acute non-lymphocytic leukaemia, which is usually refractory to treatment. Since the incidence of bone marrow involvement in Hodgkin's disease is very low, the possibility of treating high-risk patients with supralethal chemo-radiotherapy and autologous bone marrow 'rescue' is an attractive proposition and is currently being studied. Certain particularly poor prognosis groups, such as patients with bulky mediastinal disease and 'B' symptoms or patients with early relapses, might benefit from more aggressive therapy than has been traditionally employed.

Complications

Patients with Hodgkin's disease are liable to complications both as a direct result of their disease and as a result of treatment. Although extranodal presentations are rare, extranodal involvement is common in advanced disease and virtually any organ may be involved at post-mortem. It is also not uncommon for relapsed Hodgkin's disease to present in an extranodal fashion. Diagnosis can be particularly difficult in these patients, who may present with unexplained fever, pancytopenia or respiratory symptoms and may have infiltration of lung parenchyma, liver or bone marrow in the absence of lymphadenopathy. Extradural infiltration is an uncommon but important complication of Hodgkin's disease and may present with sensory or motor symptoms, sphincter disturbances, spinal cord compression or an eruption of varicella zoster in the appropriate dermatome. Prompt treatment with radiotherapy or surgery is essential in these circumstances if major neurological sequelae are to be avoided.

Even in the absence of therapy, patients with Hodgkin's disease have a defect in cell-mediated immunity. Following successful treatment, this defect may persist for many years so that infective complications may occur. Tuberculosis is less common than formerly but should still be considered in any patient with persistent cough, night sweats or fevers which are otherwise unexplained. Varicella zoster is common, may occur when the patient is in complete remission, and should be promptly treated with antiviral agents, since dissemination occurs readily in the immunocompromised host. Chemotherapy renders these patients even more vulnerable to a whole range of viral, fungal, protozoan and bacterial infections as a result of neutropenia or the immunosuppressive qualities of the drugs involved, particularly steroids. The risk of overwhelming pneumococcal septicaemia following splenectomy performed as part of a staging laparotomy may be reduced by prophylactic pneumococcal vaccine and long-term prophylactic antibiotics.

The majority of males treated with combinations such as MOPP can expect to be rendered sterile and must be warned of this possibility in advance and offered the opportunity of having sperm cryopreserved prior to treatment. Only half of female patients are rendered sterile by combinations containing alkylating agents. One of the attractive features of the ABVD protocol is that the risk to fertility is minimal.

Second malignancies, either acute myeloid leukaemia or high grade non-Hodgkin's lymphomas, have caused considerable concern. The risk of developing such malignancies is greater for patients treated with radiotherapy and chemotherapy than for those patients treated with either modality alone. Potentially curative treatment should certainly not be withheld because of this potential complication, but of course there is great interest in protocols such as ABVD which appear to be much less leukaemogenic.

BIBLIOGRAPY

De Vita V T, Simon R M, Hubbard S M et al 1980 Curability of advanced Hodgkin's disease with chemotherapy. Annals of Internal Medicine 92: 587–595

Dady P J, McElwain T J, Austin D E, Barrett A, Peckham M J 1982 Five years' experience with ChlVPP: effective low-toxicity chemotherapy for Hodgkin's disease. British Journal of Cancer 45: 851–859.

Santoro A, Bonadonna G, Bonfante V, Valagussa P 1982 Alternating drug combinations in the treatment of advanced Hodgkin's disease. New England Journal of Medicine 306: 770–775

Straus D J 1986 Strategies in the treatment of Hodgkin's disease. Seminars in Oncology 13, no. 4, Supplement No. 5: 26–34

19. Non-Hodgkin's lymphomas

T. Sheehan   A. C. Parker

Non-Hodgkin's lymphomas are a heterogeneous group of neoplasms derived from the immune system. They are heterogeneous in terms of histogenesis, natural history and response to treatment, and their optimal management requires close co-operation between various medical disciplines. The surgeon is charged with the task of providing the pathology laboratory with appropriate tissue in a condition suitable for histological and immunological studies. In all cases the largest node which can be excised safely should be removed intact with a minimum of surgical trauma and delivered promptly, without fixative, to the laboratory, so that optimal processing and sophisticated immunological studies can be performed. The histopathologist, who is expected to provide accurate and reproducible histological diagnoses in one of the most difficult and challenging areas of pathology, requires to have special experience in this field and a familiarity with the immunophenotyping methods currently in use. The radiologist has a critical role to play in staging the patients, the methods chosen depending mainly on the facilities and expertise available in the institution concerned. The clinician responsible for the care of patients with non-Hodgkin's lymphomas may be primarily a haematologist, oncologist or radiotherapist by training; whatever his background he requires a sound understanding of the biology of these fascinating neoplasms if he is to manage them successfully.

Aetiology of non-Hodgkin's lymphomas

Viruses

Although many animal lymphomas are of viral origin, viral involvement has been convincingly demonstrated in only a few human lymphomas. The exact role of Epstein Barr virus (EBV) in the development of Burkitt's lymphoma and the relationship to co-existent immune suppression requires further clarification. EBV has also been implicated in B-cell lymphomas oc-

curring after renal or cardiac transplantation. These post-transplant lymphomas are often confined to the central nervous system, and in some instances are polyclonal.

Aggressive central nervous system lymphomas are also being recognised with increasing frequency in patients with HIV infection, but the aetiology has not been fully elucidated. The association of HTLV I infection with the exceptionally aggressive adult T-cell lymphoma-leukaemia is now well established. The disease is endemic in the Caribbean and some areas of Japan but sporadic cases occur world-wide.

Pre-existing immune disorder

There is an increased incidence of non-Hodgkin's lymphomas in a variety of congenital immune deficiency syndromes, including X-linked agammaglobulinaemia, severe combined immune deficiency, Wiskott-Aldrich syndrome, common variable immune deficiency and ataxia telangiectasia. Whether the lymphomas simply reflect an intrinsically abnormal and perhaps genetically unstable immune system or are related to opportunistic infections with oncogenic viruses is not clear.

Acquired autoimmune disorders such as Sjogren's syndrome, systemic lumps erythematosus and rheumatoid arthritis also predispose to the development of non-Hodgkin's lymphomas.

Chemo-radiotherapy

Non-Hodgkin's lymphomas have been reported following radiation and chemotherapy administered for a variety of malignant disorders, particularly Hodgkin's disease.

Cytogenetics

The vast majority of cases of non-Hodgkin's lymphomas appear to have clonal cytogenetic abnormalities when analysed with sensitive techniques. Furthermore, characteristic abnormalities have been associated with certain histological types.

Translocations involving chromosome 8 and chromosomes bearing the genes which code for immunoglobin chain production [t(2;8), t(8;14), t(8;22)] have been consistently demonstrated in Burkitt's lymphoma (Ch. 15). The localisation of the cellular oncogene c-myc to chromosome 8 has aroused considerable interest and speculation regarding the pathogenetic mechanism of B-cell proliferation in this neoplasm.

The majority of follicular lymphomas (centroblastic/centrocytic follicular) are associated with a distinctive translocation [t(14;18)]. When transformation to a more aggressive malignancy occurs in this disease, additional chromosomal abnormalities involving chromosomes 6 and 7 are often found.

Our knowledge of cytogenetics in lymphomas is still at an embryonic stage. Additional disease-specific abnormalities which might prove to be useful diagnostic aids may be identified in the future. The consistent involvement of oncogenes in various translocations may be of major pathogenetic significance and could lead to exciting new developments in therapy, possibly involving monoclonal antibodies directed against oncogene products.

Classification

The large number of pathological classifications of non-Hodgkin's lymphomas currently in use has understandably added to the confusion of clinicians. The Rappaport system remains popular with many, largely because of its simplicity (Table 19.1). Essentially only three decisions are required of the pathologist who uses this classification: Do the neoplastic cells resemble lymphocytes or histiocytes? If lymphoid in appearance do they resemble small mature lymphocytes (well-differentiated) or not (poorly differentiated)? Is the pattern of growth nodular or diffuse?

Using these simple criteria it is possible to subclassify non-Hodgkin's lymphomas into prognostically useful

Table 19.1 Rappaport classification

Nodular	Lymphocytic well-differentiated
	Lymphocytic poorly-differentiated
	Mixed
	Histiocytic
Diffuse	Lymphocytic well-differentiated
	Lymphocytic poorly-differentiated
	Mixed
	Histiocytic
	Undifferentiated

categories. There are, however, serious objections to this classification; firstly, it is now recognised that the majority of so-called histiocytic lymphomas are not derived from histiocytes at all, but rather from transformed lymphocytes; secondly, the concept of differentiation, implying an irreversible change in the maturational state of a cell, is inappropriate in the context of the lymphocyte's ability to undergo dramatic but reversible transformation upon contact with antigen; thirdly some of the categories are heterogeneous and contain several biologically distinct disease entities with important differences in natural history and prognosis.

Nowadays clinicians specialising in the management of malignant lymphomas must acquire familiarity with at least one of the more modern immunologically-based classifications which attempt to relate the morphological, immunological and kinetic features of lymphoma cells to those of their normal cell counterparts within the immune system. The two most widely used immunologically-based classifications are the Kiel (see

Table 19.2 Kiel classification

Low-grade malignancy	Lymphocytic, chronic lymphocytic leukaemia
	Lymphocytic, other
	Lymphoplasmacytoid
	Centrocytic
	Centroblastic – centrocytic follicular
	Centroblastic – centrocytic diffuse
High-grade malignancy	Centroblastic
	Immunoblastic
	Lymphoblastic, Burkitt's type*
	Lymphoblastic, convoluted cell type

* In fact the malignant cell in Burkitt's lymphoma appears to be a centroblast.

Table 19.3 Lukes-Collins classification

Undefined cell type
T-cell, small lymphocytic
T-cell, Sezary – mycosis fungoides (cerebriform)
T-cell, convoluted lymphocytic
T-cell, immunoblastic sarcoma

B-cell, small lymphocytic
B-cell, plasmacytoid lymphocytic
Follicular centre cell, small cleaved
Follicular centre cell, large cleaved
Follicular centre cell, small non-cleaved
Follicular centre cell, large non-cleaved
B-cell, immunoblastic sarcoma
Histiocytic
Unclassified

Each type of follicular centre cell lymphoma is subclassified according to growth pattern (i.e. follicular, diffuse or follicular and diffuse) and the presence or absence of sclerosis.

Table 19.2) and Lukes-Collins (see Table 19.3) systems; while differing in terminology, they are in fact in broad agreement regarding the categorisation of lymphomas and are for practical purposes virtually interchangeable. In an attempt to make translation from one classification to another easier, the National Cancer Institute has produced a working formulation which it is hoped will 'facilitate clinical comparisons of case reports and therapeutic trials' but is not intended to be used as yet another histological classification. In this chapter the major lymphoma subtypes will be described where possible according to the Kiel system. It must be realised, however, that no single classification is devoid of defects or difficulties and that recent advances in our understanding of T-cell lymphomas has made classification of this group of diseases especially problematical.

75% of malignant lymphomas are of B-cell, 20% of T-cell and 5% of undetermined origin. It has become increasingly clear in recent years that true histiocytic lymphomas are extremely rare. Non-Hodgkin's lymphomas vary greatly in terms of their aggression and chemosensitivity but for clinical purposes can usefully be grouped into neoplasms of low, intermediate and high grade malignancy (see Table 19.4).

Table 19.4 Clinical classification of non- Hodgkin's lymphomas

	Low grade	Intermediate grade	High grade
Cell type	Small	Variable	Large
Stage	Usually extensive	Variable	Occasionally localised
Growth rate	Slow	Moderate	Rapid
Survival	Prolonged	Intermediate	Short
Curability	Incurable	Probably curable	Curable
Treatment	None or mild	Probably aggressive	Aggressive

Low grade lymphomas are generally widely disseminated at presentation, are compatible with prolonged survival but are currently incurable.

High grade lymphomas may present with localised or widespread disease and are potentially curable but in the absence of effective treatment will usually result in death in a relatively short period of time. Intermediate grade lymphomas, as might be expected, occupy an intermediate place in the spectrum.

Lymphomas of low grade malignancy may transform into high grade lymphomas at some stage in their natural history, the frequency of such transformation

varying for each histological type. The phenomenon of two different histological patterns of lymphoma existing simultaneously in one patient is sometimes referred to as a composite lymphoma. The immunological classifications attempt to relate the surface marker, recirculatory and kinetic characteristics of the various lymphoma subtypes to those of the normal cell counterpart within the immune system, and in addition to being more clinically valuable than the other classifications, render the differences in behaviour and response to treatment more understandable.

Non-Hodgkin's lymphomas of B-cell origin

Diffuse lymphocytic lymphoma

This is the tissue equivalent of B-cell chronic lymphocytic leukaemia (CLL) as recognised by the haematologist. The neoplastic cell, a small mature lymphocyte with clumped nuclear chromatin, a scanty rim of basophilic cytoplasm and a small amount of membrane-bound immunoglobulin, is morphologically and immunologically indistinguishable from the B-cell CLL cell. It remains possible that the two neoplasms originate in distinct subpopulations of B-lymphocytes, with preferential homing patterns involving either lymph nodes or blood and bone marrow, but at present the distinction is based entirely on the presence or absence of recognisable neoplastic cells in the peripheral blood. In a proportion of cases of diffuse lymphocytic lymphoma leukaemia eventually supervenes and the disease is then completely indistinguishable from CLL.

Presentation. Patients usually present in middle age or beyond with progressive, painless lymphadenopathy. Splenomegaly may be present. As in CLL, autoimmune complications (haemolysis or thrombocytopenia) may occur and there may be 'B' symptoms. Detectable paraprotein secretion is rare, but a proportion of patients are hypogammaglobulinaemic and susceptible to bacterial infections. The histological features of diffuse lymphocytic lymphoma are indistinguishable from those of CLL. The normal lymph node architecture is replaced by a diffuse proliferation of small mature lymphocytes with occasional foci of larger cells with open nuclear chromatin and prominent nucleoli. These larger cells tend to be grouped together in so-called 'proliferation centres'. Mitoses are infrequent and virtually confined to proliferation centres.

Therapy. As in all cases of non-Hodgkin's lymphoma an accurate tissue diagnosis is mandatory but staging investigations can be limited to identifying lymphadenopathy located in strategically important sites (e.g. near bile ducts or ureters) which may require specific treatment, either local radiotherapy or chemotherapy. Cosmetically unacceptable lymphadenopathy can be treated in similar fashion.

Chemotherapy is required in the presence of 'B' symptoms, but autoimmune complications should if possible be controlled with steroids first before cytotoxics are introduced. In many cases asymptomatic patients can be managed successfully for prolonged periods without specific therapy.

When required, chemotherapy should initially comprise oral chlorambucil (approximately 5–10 mg daily for 5 to 7 days out of each month) with or without steroids, since in most circumstances there is no evidence that more aggressive approaches result in improved survival. Combination chemotherapy may be required, however, if the tumour proves resistant to single agent cytotoxic therapy and may possibly be advantageous in the presence of bone marrow impairment.

Splenectomy should be considered if hypersplenism leads to serious cytopenias, and contributing causes of bone marrow impairment, such as folate deficiency, should not be forgotten.

As with CLL survival is usually prolonged and transformation to a high grade lymphoma rare.

Lymphoplasmacytoid

This neoplasm may consist of a mixture of small mature lymphocytes and plasma cells or cells with typical lymphocytic nuclei but variably increased amounts of basophilic cytoplasma, the so-called plasmacytoid lymphocyte. Paraprotein secretion is common, and most often IgM, although IgA or IgG secretion are by no means rare. This is the histological type of lymphoma most commonly associated with the clinical syndrome of Waldenstrom's macroglobulinaemia, although the syndrome can occur in any B-cell neoplasm associated with substantial paraprotein production. This hyperviscosity syndrome is manifest by a variety of signs and symptoms including transient visual upsets or cerebral ischaemic attacks, abnormal bruising or bleeding due to platelet dysfunction resulting from paraprotein coating of the platelet surface, and engorged tortuous retinal veins (p. 199). These signs and symptoms are an indication for urgent plasmapheresis, which is particularly effective when the paraprotein is IgM in type and therefore largely confined to the intravascular compartment.

The disease may involve lymph nodes and spleen or, in some cases, may apparently be confined to the bone marrow. The clinical distinction between lymphoplasmacytoid lymphoma and myeloma is not always easy, some patients presenting with bone pain, lytic lesions and marrow impairment.

Therapy. The disease is of low grade malignancy and should be managed according to the same principles as for diffuse lymphocytic lymphoma. If treatment is required, plasmapheresis alone or single agent chemotherapy may suffice, with local radiotherapy playing a valuable role in terms of control of bone pain or strategically sited lymphadenopathy. Prompt treatment of infections is an important component of management, as a proportion of patients are hypogammaglobulinaemic. In general, survival is prolonged and transformation to a high grade lymphoma uncommon but less rare than with diffuse lymphocytic lymphoma.

Lymphomas of follicular centre cell origin

Depending mainly on the predominant follicular centre cell type involved and to a lesser extent on the pattern of growth (nodular or diffuse), lymphomas arising from germinal centre cells may be of low, intermediate or high grade malignancy.

Centroblastic/centrocytic follicular

The standard 'follicular lymphoma' is the commonest histological type of non-Hodgkin's lymphoma seen in clinical practice. The presence or absence of sclerosis within the tumour is of doubtful clinical relevance, and partial loss of nodular architecture with areas of diffuse growth pattern does not adversely affect prognosis. Involved lymph nodes show complete architectural effacement by a nodular proliferation of lymphoid cells, predominantly centrocytes, with an admixture of smaller numbers of centroblasts (Plate 19). The centrocyte is slightly larger than a small mature lymphocyte and has a deep nuclear cleft which is readily apparent on blood films and smears but is less easily identified in tissue sections. Also present within the neoplastic follicles are B-cell-specific stromal cells (dendritic reticulum cells) and small numbers of T-lymphocytes which may play some role in regulating tumour proliferation.

Distinction from reactive follicular hyperplasia can sometimes be difficult, but generally neoplastic follicles are more uniform in size and shape with a poorly defined corona or mantle zone and much fewer mitoses or tingible-body macrophages than reactive germinal centres, reflecting their lower proliferation rate.

Presentation. Patients usually present in middle age with slowly progressive, painless lymphadenopathy, but some waxing and waning of lymph node size is by no means uncommon. Spontaneous regression of disease (which may appear complete but is temporary) is commonest in this histological type of lymphoma and occurs in more than 20% of cases. Splenomegaly may be a feature and can lead to significant hypersplenism.

'B' symptoms may be present but when prominent should raise clinical suspicions that the disease may have transformed in some site to a high grade malignancy. Rapid enlargement of nodes would also suggest transformation, which occurs at some stage in over 40% of cases, and may be difficult to demonstrate histologically unless the transformation includes the particular node biopsied.

Hypogammaglobulinaemia, autoimmune complications and paraprotein secretion are all rare. The disease is usually widespread at presentation, with bone marrow involvement in approximately 80% of cases, and staging is aimed primarily at identifying lymphadenopathy in strategically important sites which may have a bearing on management. In a small proportion of cases recognisable lymphoma cells may be present in the peripheral blood; the presence of such 'exfoliation' in this histological type of lymphoma does not adversely affect the prognosis.

Therapy. Follicular lymphomas are of low grade malignancy with a median survival in excess of seven years, but they are incurable and at the present time patients invariably ultimately succumb to their disease. Many patients have now been followed up untreated for prolonged periods without apparent detriment to their survival. Strategically important or cosmetically unacceptable lymphadenopathy may be managed with chemotherapy or radiotherapy, while the presence of 'B' symptoms necessitates the use of chemotherapy. Splenectomy may be of value where hypersplenism is a problem. When required, chemotherapy should initially take the form of oral chlorambucil with or without steroids. Combination chemotherapy may result in a quicker response, but does not improve the duration of response, and has never been shown to be superior to single agent cytotoxic therapy in terms of overall survival. Relapse is virtually inevitable after so-called complete remission and cure does not at present appear to be possible.

Centroblastic/centrocytic diffuse

The predominant cell is the centrocyte with a variable admixture of centroblasts. All semblance of a follicular or nodular architecture has been lost and the growth pattern is entirely diffuse. The disease is of intermediate malignancy, is commoner in males and has a tendency to involve the gastrointestinal tract and Waldeyer's ring in addition to peripheral lymph nodes. There is some evidence from survival curves that 'cure' may be possible in some instances, and more aggressive treatment may therefore be warranted than is generally the case with low grade lymphomas.

Centrocytic diffuse

Monomorphic or 'pure' proliferations of centrocytes (small or large) are rarely seen in the USA but have been well documented by European pathologists. A distinctive hyaline thickening of blood vessels is sometimes seen in these neoplasms, which have a predilection for the retroperitoneal area but otherwise behave in a similar fashion to diffuse centroblastic/centrocytic lymphomas. It is felt by some pathologists that neoplasms of large centrocytes are associated with a poorer prognosis than small centrocytic lymphomas. Conversely, the presence of sclerosis may be associated with a slightly better prognosis.

Centroblastic (follicular or diffuse)

This is an aggressive or high grade non-Hodgkin's lymphoma in which the centroblast (small or large) is the sole or predominant malignant cell. The pattern of growth (follicular or diffuse) appears to be of little prognostic significance. The centroblast is classically round in shape with open nuclear chromatin, a scanty rim of basophilic cytoplasm and multiple small nucleoli adjacent to the nuclear membrane. In practice, however, it is often impossible to distinguish histologically between centroblastic and immunoblastic lymphomas. The presence of a 'starry sky' appearance within involved nodes in some cases attests to this tumour's propensity for rapid growth. African and non-African Burkitt's lymphomas are examples of centroblastic lymphomas. The association of the former with Epstein Barr virus infection is well known. Centroblastic lymphomas may arise de novo or, less commonly, may evolve from a preexisting low grade non-Hodgkin's lymphoma. They may occasionally be localised at presentation and theoretically amenable to curative surgery or radiotherapy, but are usually more widespread.

Single agent chemotherapy is of little value in these highly aggressive diseases, except as a palliative measure in patients who are unable to tolerate more aggressive treatment. Combination chemotherapy protocols such as 'CHOP' (see Table 19.5) can be expected to 'cure' only 20–30% of patients with advanced high grade lymphomas (centroblastic or immunoblastic). 'Cure' is more likely with centroblastic histology, de novo presentation

Table 19.5 CHOP

Cyclophosphamide	750 mg/m^2 IV day 1
Adriamycin	50 mg/m^2 IV day 1
Vincristine	1.4 mg/m^2 IV day 1 (max 2 mg)
Prednisolone	40–100 mg oral days 1–5

Minimum of 6 cycles (complete remission plus 2) with 2–3 week intervals between cycles.

and an absence of 'B' symptoms or extralymphoid (Stage IV) disease.

Immunoblastic lymphoma

Classically the B-immunoblast is a large cell with open nuclear chromatin, a large, solitary, central nucleolus and moderately abundant basophilic cytoplasm, although in practice the histological distinction between centroblastic and immunoblastic lymphomas is sometimes impossible. Immunoblastic lymphomas usually arise de novo but can evolve from a pre-existing low grade lymphoma. When transformation occurs in follicular lymphoma, the high grade lymphoma which supervenes is usually immunoblastic rather than centroblastic. The association of high grade lymphomas, usually immunoblastic, with disorders such as Sjogren's, SLE and immunoblastic lymphadenopathy, and their occurrence in AIDS patients, cardiac and renal transplant recipients and patients treated for Hodgkin's disease is of interest with regard to possible pathogenesis. Clinically the disease is usually indistinguishable from centroblastic lymphoma and should be managed according to the same principles, although it is felt by some workers that immunoblastic lymphomas may be particularly aggressive.

Therapy. There is clearly a need to develop new treatment strategies for the majority of patients with high grade lymphomas. Some recent protocols, e.g. Pro-Mace MOPP (Table 19.6) and MACOP-B (Table 19.7), appear to show some promise, particularly in patients with adverse prognostic factors. These more aggressive regimens usually involve either the use of multiple agents (as in ProMace MOPP) in order to minimise the development of drug resistance or the addition of non-myelotoxic drugs in mid-cycle when the blood counts are too low to safely permit treatment with myelosuppressive agents (as in MACOP-B).

Table 19.6   ProMace MOPP

ProMace	VP-16 120 mg/m^2 IV days 1 and 8
	Cyclophosphamide 650 mg/m^2 IV days 1 and 8
	Adriamycin 25 mg/m^2 IV days 1 and 8
	Methotrexate 1.5 g/m^2 IV day 14
	With leucovorim 50 mg/m^2 6-hourly for 5 doses
	Prednisolone 60 mg/m^2 oral days 1–14 inclusive
	No treatment days 15–28

Initially ProMace until complete response (CR) plus one course or decreasing response, then MOPP (same number of cycles if in CR after ProMace; if not, until CR + 1). Late intensification with ProMace (same number of cycles as MOPP) with 56-day intervals between cycles.

Table 19.7   MACOP- B

Methotrexate	400 mg/m^2 – weeks 2, 6, 10
Doxorubicin	50 mg/m^2 – weeks 1, 3, 5, 7, 9, 11
Cyclophosphamide	350 mg/m^2 – weeks 1, 3, 5, 7, 9, 11
Vincristine	1.4 mg/m^2 – weeks 2, 4, 6, 8, 10, 12
Bleomycin	10 units/m^2 – weeks 4, 8, 12
Prednisolone	75 mg daily throughout, tapering over last 15 days
Co-trimoxazole	Two tablets twice-daily throughout

T-cell lymphomas

Neoplasms of T-cells originate in primitive, precursor cells or mature, 'peripheral' lymphocytes. Neoplastic proliferations of T-cell precursors arise in the bone marrow or thymus, are highly aggressive diseases and occur predominantly in childhood or early adult life. Mature T-cell neoplasms represent a group of diseases with a wide spectrum of malignancy and are virtually confined to adults.

T-cell lymphoblastic lymphoma

This disease occurs mainly in young males and may present with superficial lymphadenopathy, most commonly in the cervical or supraclavicular regions, or with signs and symptoms related to mediastinal lymphadenopathy, which is present in the vast majority of cases. The natural history is one of rapid progression to frank leukaemia, the disease being then indistinguishable from T-cell ALL. Although not necessarily intrinsically more aggressive than 'common' ALL, the T-cell subtype is often associated with adverse features, such as a very high blast count or central nervous system involvement, and therefore a poorer prognosis. The blast cell in T-cell ALL or T-cell lymphoblastic lymphoma classically has an irregular, convoluted nucleus, and the vast majority of cases exhibit a characteristic focal acid phosphatase positivity localised to the Golgi zone (Plate 20). In the absence of leukaemic manifestations the clinician has the option of treating these patients with a combination chemotherapy protocol suitable for high grade non-Hodgkin's lymphoma or with anti-ALL therapy. The management of T-cell ALL is largely dependent on the presence or absence of adverse prognostic features at presentation, and is dealt with in detail elsewhere (Ch. 16).

Adult T-cell lymphoma-leukaemia

This highly aggressive lymphoma is associated with

HTLV1 infection and is endemic in Japan and the Caribbean, although rare sporadic cases occur throughout the world. In almost all cases studied the malignant cell expresses surface markers normally associated with the T-helper subtype. Despite these immunological markers the cell functions as a suppressor cell and may in fact originate in a specific subset of CD4 suppressor cells. The morphological features are variable but characteristically the malignant cell is large with an irregular nucleus which can at times be indistinguishable from that of the Sezary cell. Hypercalcaemia and frank leukaemia are common complications and the prognosis is very poor.

T-cell CLL

Clinical, morphological and immunological features distinguish this disease, which accounts for 1% of cases of CLL in the Western hemisphere, from classical B-cell CLL. Affected patients are younger, with an average age of under 50 years, splenomegaly and cutaneous involvement are common, and lymphadenopathy is conspicuous by its absence. The lymphocytosis is usually mild, with total white cell counts rarely exceeding $15 \times 10^9/l$. The neoplastic cell is usually a large lymphocyte with condensed nuclear chromatin and abundant cytoplasm containing azurophil granules. Acid phosphatase positivity is virtually invariable and the neoplastic cell marks as a T-suppressor cell.

In some cases natural killer cell activity has been demonstrated. Anaemia and neutropenia are common accompaniments and may be related in some way to the T-suppressor cell's normal role in regulating haematopoiesis. The disease is usually indolent and compatible with prolonged survival, and management is largely symptomatic. Prompt treatment of the recurrent infections which are a prominent feature of this disorder is particularly important. The response to chemotherapy is variable; if treatment is required, single agent alkylating therapy should be tried initially.

T-zone lymphoma

This uncommon lymphoma is characterised by an infiltrate of T-helper cells which is confined to the interfollicular areas, with sparing of normal germinal centres. The infiltrate comprises a mixture of small, medium-sized and large lymphoid cells and is commonly associated with a striking increase in non-branching epithelioid venules. Patients usually present with generalised lymphadenopathy and may have a polyclonal hypergammaglobulinaemia. Prognosis is poor with a median survival of 6 months in advanced disease.

Lympho-epithelioid cell lymphoma (Lennert's lymphoma)

This uncommon neoplasm of T-helper cells is characterised by an infiltrate of small, irregularly-shaped lymphoid cells associated with large numbers of macrophages, which in areas form small, compact epithelioid granulomata. Eosinophils are sometimes also prominent. A very similar histological picture can at times be seen in Hodgkin's disease and non-malignant conditions such as angio-immunoblastic lymphadenopathy. The presence of macrophages within involved lymph nodes may be related to lymphokine production by the malignant T-cells.

T-cell immunoblastic sarcoma

In many cases distinction from B-cell immunoblastic sarcoma is not possible on purely morphological grounds. In a minority of cases, however, the malignant T-immunoblast has a characteristic appearance with abundant clear staining cytoplasm reminiscent of renal carcinoma cells.

This disease is a high grade lymphoma and should be managed accordingly. It is felt by some that T-cell immunoblastic sarcoma is intrinsically more aggressive than its B-cell counterpart.

Mycosis fungoides and Sezary's syndrome

Mycosis fungoides is a curious disorder in which a monoclonal proliferation of morphologically distinctive T-helper cells, which may be frankly malignant or possibly pre-neoplastic, appears largely confined to the skin. (In fact occasional abnormal cells can often be identified in carefully scrutinised peripheral blood films.)

In the early stages the clinical manifestations may resemble benign dermatological disorders such as dermatitis or psoriasis. Plaque and tumour formation occur as the disease progresses. The generalised, erythrodermatous form of the disease with associated frank leukaemia is known as Sezary's syndrome.

Distinctive, large lymphoid cells with highly irregular, 'cerebriform' nuclei are identified in tissue sections and characteristically are found within intra-epidermal Pautrier micro-abscesses. (Fig 19.1). It should be noted, however, that similar cells can be seen in reactive skin disorders and the histological diagnosis of mycosis fungoides can be extremely difficult in the early stages.

While confined to the skin, local treatment such as ultraviolet radiation, radiotherapy and topical or whole body applications of nitrogen mustard are usually effective. Although it is an unpleasant and disfiguring

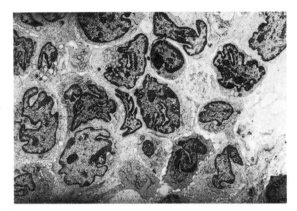

Fig. 19.1 Sezary's syndrome. Electron micrograph — cerebriform nuclei.

disease, patients with mycosis fungoides may survive for many years while the disease remains localised to the skin. Once spread to lymph nodes occurs, however, the prognosis is bleak. Although some success has been achieved with aggressive combination chemotherapy and monoclonal antibodies, the average survival is around 2 years.

Extranodal lymphomas

20% of cases of non-Hodgkin's lymphomas originate in extranodal tissue. Favoured sites include stomach, small bowel, testis, brain and thyroid. Genuine extranodal presentations of disease should be distinguished from extranodal involvement; in advanced disease lymphomas may infiltrate almost any organ or tissue in the body. Management is dictated by stage and histological type and may thus involve surgery, local radiotherapy, and single agent or combination chemotherapy.

The occurrence of small bowel lymphomas of T-cell or histiocytic type in coeliac disease is well known.

The incidence of primary lymphomas of brain (usually of B-cell immunoblastic type) in organ transplant recipients and patients with AIDS is of interest with regard to pathogenetic mechanisms.

Histiocytic lymphomas

In the past many large cell lymphomas were thought to be of histiocytic origin, largely on the basis of the morphological resemblance of the neoplastic cells to histiocytes or macrophages. With the advent of sophisticated immunohistochemical techniques, however, it has become apparent that the vast majority of such neoplasms in fact arise from transformed lymphocytes, either of T- or B-cell type. The possible histiocytic origin of some intestinal lymphomas remained in doubt

until more recently, partly because of technical difficulties in obtaining material suitable for study. This issue has now largely been resolved: it seems clear that so-called 'malignant histiocytosis of the intestine' is, in the majority of cases, a T-cell malignancy.

Lymphomas of genuine histiocytic origin are thus exceedingly rare and insufficient data have been accumulated to build up an accurate picture of their natural history or optimal management. It is beyond the scope of this chapter to discuss non-lymphomatous disorders of histiocytes or related cells such as monocytic leukaemias, 'histiocytosis X' or the various haemophagocytic syndromes, including histiocytic medullary reticulosis.

Angio-immunoblastic lymphadenopathy

In this rare disorder, which mainly affects elderly patients, generalised lymphadenopathy and hepatosplenomegaly occurs following drug therapy, viral infection or, most often, without any identifiable antecedent cause. Polyclonal hypergammaglobulinaemia and a positive direct Coomb's test are common accompaniments and there may be a considerable degree of systemic upset.

Lymph node biopsy shows a striking proliferation of arborising blood vessels and a pleomorphic lymphoid infiltrate ranging from small 'mature' lymphocytes to large immunoblasts and plasma cells.

In most, but not all, cases so far studied a monoclonal proliferation of T-cells has been demonstrated in involved nodes. A small proportion of cases may regress spontaneously or after steroid therapy but in the majority of cases the disease pursues an inexorable downhill course with progressive immune failure and, ultimately, death from infection. In approximately one-third of cases a frank immunoblastic sarcoma develops at some stage during the illness.

Future developments

The role of autologous and allogeneic bone marrow transplantation in non-Hodgkin's lymphomas, particularly in poor prognostic groups, is currently being assessed. In future it may be possible to selectively remove lymphoma cells from bone marrow prior to autologous transplantation. It also appears that apparently normal stem cells are transiently found in the peripheral blood following chemotherapy for Burkitt's lymphoma, in numbers sufficient to be used as an alternative to bone marrow harvesting in autologous transplantation. Such an approach may obviate the need for purging of the bone marrow.

There is also increasing interest in the use of various biological response modifiers, particularly in non-Hodgkin's lymphomas of low grade malignancies. As our knowledge of lymphomas and various growth factors develops, the possibilities for this sort of approach may increase dramatically.

NON-MALIGNANT DISORDERS CAUSING SPLENOMEGALY

Storage disorders

Splenomegaly occurs in a variety of inherited lysosomal enzyme defects. All are rare and many are exceedingly rare. Only two will be discussed in some detail, Gaucher's disease and Nieman-Pick disease.

Gaucher's disease

In Gaucher's disease there is an inborn deficiency of the enzyme glucocerebrosidase with high levels of glucocerebroside in red cells and plasma. Three types are recognised. Type I is particularly common in Ashkenazi Jews and may present at any age. Splenomegaly is a prominent feature and cytopenias due to marrow dysfunction or hypersplenism are common. Brownish pigmentation of the skin and curious radiolucent lesions in the lower femur are characteristic. Typical Gaucher cells may be identified in bone marrow or spleen. These cells are macrophages containing large quantities of glucocerebroside, giving rise to a foamy, often distinctly laminated or 'onion skin' appearance. The clinical course is variable but usually slowly progressive.

Splenectomy may benefit patients with hypersplenism or recurrent painful splenic infarction, while the role of enzyme replacement therapy is currently being evaluated.

In types II and III, in addition to hepatosplenomegaly, neurological damage is a prominent feature.

Niemann-Pick disease

Five clinical variants of Niemann-Pick disease or sphingomyelinase deficiency has been described. Lipid-laden 'foamy' macrophages are common to all. The most common variety (Type A) is associated with hepatosplenomegaly, lymphadenopathy and severe neurological damage, with death usually occurring during infancy or early childhood. Treatment is at present unsatisfactory and splenectomy in particular is rarely beneficial.

BIBLIOGRAPHY

Armitage J O, Dick F R, Corder M P, Garnean S C, Platz C E, Slymen D J 1982 Predicting therapeutic outcome in patients with diffuse histiocytic lymphoma treated with cytophosphamides, adriemycin, vincristine and prednisolone (CHOP). Cancer 50: 1695–1702

Bonadonna G 1985 Chemotherapy of malignant lymphomas. Seminars in Oncology vol XII, no 4, Supplement no 6: 1–14

Fisher R I, De Vita J R, Hubbard S M et al 1983 Diffuse aggressive lymphomas: increased survival after alternating flexible sequences of ProMace and MOPP chemotherapy. Annals of Internal Medicine 98: 304–309

Klimo P, Connors J M 1985 MACOP-B chemotherapy for the treatment of diffuse large cell lymphoma. Annals of Internal Medicine 102: 596–602

Shipp M A, Harington D P, Klatt M M et al 1986 Identification of major prognostic sub-groups of patients with large cell lymphoma treated with m-BACOD or M-BACOD. Annals of Internal Medicine 104: 757–765

20. Myeloma and related disorders

S. A. Schey   D. C. Linch

The presence of a paraprotein is indirect evidence for an underlying proliferation of B-cells. Only mature plasma cells secrete significant quantities of immunoglobulin, the immunoglobulin molecules being predominantly bound to the cell membrane or present in the cytoplasm at earlier stages of differentiation. Multiple myeloma is a neoplastic condition due to the uncontrolled and progressive proliferation of mature and immature plasma cells. Other B-lymphoproliferative disorders represent the uncontrolled growth of B-lymphocytes at earlier stages of development with a 'block' at different stages of development. Thus, in chronic lymphocytic lymphoma, a 'hiatus' at an early stage of development results in the bulk of the cells being of the small lymphocyte type, while in non-Hodgkin's lymphoma the block is at a different stage of differentiation (often later) and the bulk of cells are of a larger cell type.

The paraprotein in these conditions can be of any subclass but tends to be representative of that subclass secreted normally at a comparative stage of differentiation. A neoplastic clone of cells usually produces both light and heavy chains which are assembled in the cytoplasm into complete immunoglobulin before being secreted into the plasma. On occasions, however, the malignant clone is incapable either of producing one or other of the immunoglobulin chains or of assembling or secreting them, leading to failure of immunoglobulin production.

BENIGN MONOCLONAL GAMMOPATHY

The term 'benign monoclonal gammopathy' (BMG) refers to any condition that gives rise to a monoclonal paraprotein in the absence of a detectable B-cell tumour. The term was originally used by Waldenstrom but many other synonyms have been used to describe this condition.

Clinical associations

There appear to be two distinct categories of BMG:

Transient paraproteinaemia

A proportion of patients will develop a paraprotein in a setting which suggests that restricted antigenic stimulation has resulted in the production of the paraprotein. Hence, a number of patients may develop a paraprotein during the course of acute viral hepatitis, cytomegalovirus or leptospirosis, in autoimmune disease such as rheumatoid arthritis or, more interestingly, in association with non-B-cell tumours. When the underlying cause is removed the paraprotein will often disappear. These observations suggest the host's immune system is being stimulated to produce an immunoglobulin against specific antigenic determinants and that the stimulated clone remains under the control of normal regulatory mechanisms. Only in rare instances, e.g. mycoplasma pneumonia infections, has paraprotein specificity been identified. However, certain tumours that have been associated with a BMG have been found, on histological examination, to be infiltrated by plasma cells which may well be the source of immunoglobulin and might represent a host immune response against the tumour. It should be noted that the majority of paraproteins associated with non-B-cell tumours do not regress on removal of the tumour, indicating that the presence of the paraprotein was probably coincidental.

Stable benign paraproteinaemia

This second group represents those patients whose paraprotein remains unchanged for many years. Approximately 5–15% will progress to become overtly malignant with the features of plasma-cell myeloma and the question arises whether these cases represent a premyelomatous state, with all patients progressing to a malignant state if they would live long enough. In animals there is much evidence to suggest that chronic antigenic stimulation can cause plasma cell tumours but such an association in man is far from proven. The chronic skin condition lichen myxoedematosus has, however, consistently been found to be associated with a paraprotein of IgG lambda type. In addition, immunofluorescence studies have shown this same immunoglobulin to be localised in the skin, suggesting a causal relationship.

Hereditary factors may also be of importance. Certain strains of mice have been shown to have a high incidence of spontaneous benign paraproteins and a number of authors have suggested an increased incidence of paraproteinaemias in family members of affected individuals.

Incidence. Many studies have been performed which clearly show an increasing incidence with age. In patients of less than 60 years the incidence is less than 1% rising in some studies to 3% in patients over the age of 70 years and even higher in the over-90 year age group.

Clinical

By definition, these patients do not have an underlying B-cell neoplasm and do not have symptoms related to the paraprotein. Consequently, they present with symptoms of the associated non-lymphoid neoplasm or inflammatory condition or the paraprotein is found coincidentally and the patient is asymptomatic.

Investigations

Investigations should be directed to the identification of an underlying cause such as non-B-cell malignancies, chronic sepsis, autoimmune disease and in particular to the presence of a B-cell lymphoproliferative disorder. A number of features pertaining to the paraprotein itself should be assessed as an indication of the benign nature of the paraprotein. Although not an absolute indicator, the level of paraprotein has been found to be a valuable discriminatory factor between benign and malignant paraproteins. Over 90% of patients with malignancy have an initial paraprotein level of >10 g/l, whilst 85% of patients considered to have a benign paraproteinaemia present with levels less than 10 g/l. Each case must, however, be assessed individually and all patients with a paraprotein need to be followed regularly to ensure there is no progressive increase in the concentration of the abnormal protein.

Bence-Jones protein can occasionally be detected in normal urine at low levels (<0.25 mg/100 ml) if the urine

is concentrated. Bence-Jones proteinuria is also uncommon in BMG and, if present, is detectable only at low concentrations. Normal immunoglobulin production is not suppressed in BMG (cf. myeloma) and, in contrast to the findings in multiple myeloma, no imbalance of T-cell subpopulations can be demonstrated in the peripheral blood.

Management and prognosis

Having ruled out a secondary cause of a paraproteinaemia it is most important to follow up patients to ensure both the clinical picture and the paraprotein level remain stable with time. As the condition is, by definition, not associated with marrow failure, immune suppression or lytic bone lesions, no specific therapy is indicated. In a study of 241 cases, Kyle identified 37% of patients who remained stable over 10 years, 5% of the cases had a >50% rise in monoclonal protein or subsequently developed Bence-Jones proteinuria (BJP) and 11% developed overt myeloma, although the time lag from presentation to development of malignancy varied greatly from 2 to 15 years. 45% of those patients progressing over 5 years with a rise in monoclonal protein of >50% developed myeloma in the ensuing 5 years. Patients who present with 'idiopathic' BJP also appear to have a high risk of progression to overt myeloma and should be followed up closely.

PLASMACYTOMA

A plasmacytoma represents a localised plasma cell tumour and occurs either in bone or in a variety of extramedullary sites. It is an unusual condition accounting for approximately 7% of plasma cell tumours.

Clinical features

1. Solitary myeloma of bone is defined by the following criteria:

a) Solitary osteolytic lesion on radiological examination
b) Histological evidence of plasma cell tumour on biopsy
c) Normal bone marrow aspirate and trephine from remote sites.

There is a 2:1 M:F ratio with a peak incidence at 50–60 years of age. Approximately 50% of cases will have an M-protein in the circulation or urine. In a large study of 114 patients, IgG was identified as the most common type of monoclonal component (68%) and light chain only the next most frequent (19.6%). The M-protein was always present in low concentations. The commonest sites of involvement are spine, pelvis and femur.

2. Extramedullary plasmacytoma refers to plasma cell tumours arising primarily at an extra-osseous site and excludes those patients who have bone marrow spread due to extension through the cortex to form an associated soft tissue mass. It occurs mainly in males (3:1 ratio) with a peak incidence age at 50–70 years. These tumours occur most commonly in the upper respiratory tract where they may be multiple and become polypoid or pedunculated and may ulcerate. In a much smaller number of patients the tumour may initially present in the gastrointestinal tract, lower respiratory tract or lung, lymph nodes, spleen, skin or thyroid. Spread to non-haemopoietic bone is common at both local and remote sites producing large osteolytic lesions which are often clinically 'silent'.

Investigations

Radiological investigation demonstrates the bone lesions either as well-defined lytic lesions, usually situated in the spine, or as a multi-loculated, 'soap-bubble' lesion seen most commonly in the limbs or ilium.

Bone marrow aspiration should by definition be normal but serial studies may show evidence of a diffuse plasma cell infiltration in the presence of other evidence of dissemination.

Protein studies may demonstrate a paraprotein at presentation but this should disappear after adequate local therapy of the tumour. Persistence of the M-protein is highly suggestive of occult multiple myeloma.

Management

Treatment of solitary plasmacytoma is somewhat controversial. Surgical curettage or excision should be performed where possible and radiotherapy given as follow-up. The dose of radiation has varied in different series but numerous authors have now emphasised the importance of giving high-dose irradiation (approximately 5000 cGy) in order to obtain control of the disease. Local control can be achieved in solitary myeloma of bone in 90% of patients but only 15% remain relapse-free at 10 years. In an attempt to improve these figures and prevent progression of disease it has been suggested that adjuvant chemotherapy may be of value but results of prospective trials are not as yet forthcoming.

The prognosis of both forms of plasmacytoma is better than for multiple myeloma, the median survival for solitary myeloma of bone being 10 years whilst that for extramedullary plasmacytoma may be even longer.

MULTIPLE MYELOMA

Myeloma is a neoplastic disease of plasma cells at differing stages of maturation. The level of malignant transformation has not been well defined but may be at a stage more primitive than the plasma cell. Limited cytogenetic studies have been reported and the commonest abnormalities are of chromosomes 1, 11 and 14. The incidence is approximately 3/100 000, a figure comparable to that seen for Hodgkin's disease and chronic lymphocytic leukaemia. It does occur in persons under 40 years but it tends to be a disease of older age groups with a median age at diagnosis between 60 and 65 years of age. The male to female ratio approaches unity but in the United States the incidence amongst blacks appears to be twice that seen in Caucasians.

Clinical features

The clinical features resulting from plasma cell myeloma can be directly attributed to the uncontrolled growth of plasma cells in the bone marrow and the production of an abnormal paraprotein. The pathogenic consequences can be summarised thus:

1. Bone marrow failure due to infiltration of marrow spaces by plasma cells (Plate 21), resulting in anaemia, thrombocytopenia and neutropenia. The cytopenias, especially anaemia, are often more severe than might be expected from the degree of infiltration seen on a trephine biopsy. This may in part be due to an increase in plasma volume associated with a large paraprotein, but additionally there may be suppression of normal haemopoiesis by the malignant clone.

2. Localised lytic bone lesions due to both mechanical erosion of the cortex by plasma cell infiltrates and resorption secondary to plasma cell products released locally that stimulate osteoclast activity. It has been variously suggested that one such product, known as osteoclast activating factor (OAF), may be identical to interleukin Iβ or TNF β. This process of erosion and resorption frequently leads to hypercalcaemia.

3. Immunodeficiency due to suppression of normal immunoglobulin synthesis and cellular abnormalities of both the B- and T-cell series. The susceptibility to infection may be further increased by the presence of neutropenia.

4. Physiochemical properties of the M-protein may result in clinical problems. These include hyperviscosity (Plate 22) and cold precipitation which are discussed in Chapter 5.

5. Renal failure secondary to a variety of complex factors, including infection, hypercalcaemia, amyloidosis and, most commonly, light chain-induced proximal tubular dysfunction.

6. Neurological problems resulting from direct compression by tumour, or peripheral neuropathies due to amyloidosis, or as an ill-defined non-metastatic manifestation of malignancy.

Haematological abnormalities

Anaemia

In myeloma the anaemia is due to a diverse number of factors and undoubtedly is a contributing factor to the non-specific symptoms of ill-health described by myeloma patients. It may be due to a number of mechanisms including bone marrow suppression or bleeding secondary to the coagulation defects that are frequently seen.

Infection

The myeloma patient is highly susceptible to infection which is the immediate cause of death in 70% of patients. The causative organisms are similar to those seen in other haematological malignancies and immuno-compromised persons with gram negative organisms particularly common. Cutaneous eruptions due to herpes simplex and varicella zoster are seen but not as frequently as in some other haematological malignancies. The immune impairment appears to be due to a variety of defects, both humoral and cellular. The pathogenesis of the humoral defect is obscure but there appears to be a deficiency of mature B-cells with an impaired ability to mount a primary immune response. The ratio of CD4 (helper/inducer) to CD8 (suppressor/cytotoxic) T-cells is often inverted, suggesting that there may be an increase in functional suppressor cells. It has also been reported that plasma cells are capable of secreting a substance (plasmacytoma-induced macrophage substance) which stimulates macrophages to produce a factor that suppresses antibody production, probably indirectly by action upon accessory cells. Granulocytopenia is a common finding in myeloma secondary either to bone marrow infiltration or, more commonly, to cytotoxic drugs used for treatment. In addition to this quantitative abnormality, numerous reports have demonstrated a variety of functional abnormalities in the normal circulating granulocytes which also contribute to the impaired host defence.

Haemostatic defects

Haemorrhagic complications occur in approximately 10% of patients with myeloma but are usually mild. In-vitro tests are, more commonly abnormal but correlate poorly with clinical bleeding. Qualitative abnormalities of platelets and complexing of the paraprotein with coagulation factors II, V, VII and VIII have all been described. The thrombin time is the test most often described as being abnormal and is due to inhibition of fibrin monomer aggregation.

Skeletal abnormalities (Fig. 20.1)

Bone pain is the most common symptom of myeloma and must not be overlooked in patients presenting with non-specific symptomatology. In myeloma (unlike metastatic disease) the pathogenetic mechanisms resulting in bone erosion are painless and only when the weakened bone is stressed does pain develop. Hence, patients with bone destruction secondary to myeloma are usually pain-free at night when not weight-bearing, rarely have pain in non-stressed areas such as the skull vault and arms and may often develop pain abruptly if the bone undergoes sudden deformation, infraction or fracture.

Fractures occur frequently in this condition and can prove very troublesome as a pre-terminal event occurring with minimal trauma such as combing the hair. Not uncommonly the fractures involve the trunk, and multiple rib fractures may result in a 'fluid' chest with respiratory embarrassment and pulmonary complications. Such fractures may be mistaken for pleurisy or root pain. Compression fractures of the vertebrae often result in nerve compression and significant loss of stature.

In contrast to the generalised demineralisation that is seen most commonly in myeloma, a small percentage of patients (<1%), have been described with osteosclerotic changes. Such patients often present with other unusual features such as polyneuropathy and extramedullary plasmacytomas.

Renal failure

Renal failure is the second most common cause of death in multiple myeloma, with up to 50% of patients demonstrating some evidence of acute or chronic renal failure at some stage of the disease. Acute renal failure is most often precipitated by dehydration and any procedure which exacerbates dehydration, such as intravenous pyelography, should be avoided unless an

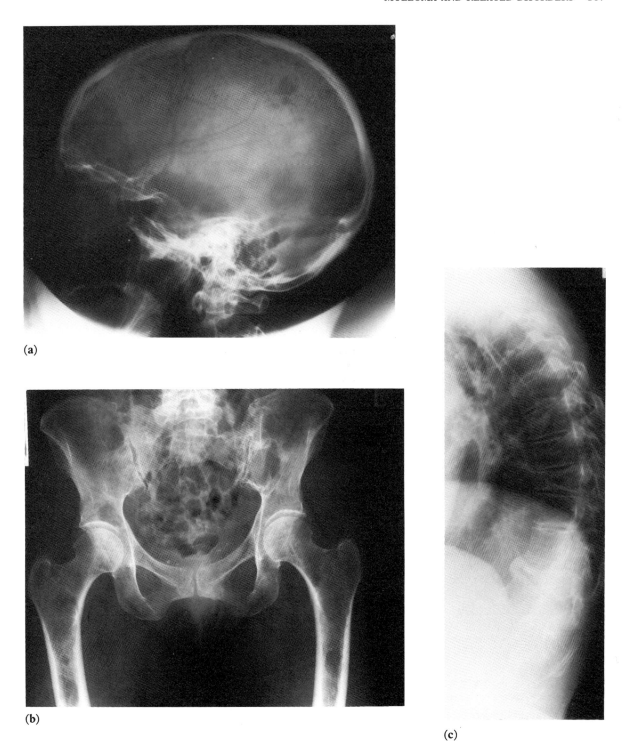

Fig. 20.1 Osteolytic lesions in skull (**a**), pelvis and femora (**b**) and vertebral bodies (**c**) where generalised osteoporosis and collapse of two vertebrae can be seen.

adequate urinary flow can be assured. Other causes of acute renal failure include hypercalcaemia, hyperuricaemia, hypotension and the administration of nephrotoxic drugs for treatment of infectious complications. The chronic renal insufficiency so commonly seen as a feature of this condition is most often accredited to the deposition of light chains in the tubular cells (myeloma kidney). This produces bilateral uniform enlargement of the renal outline on radiological investigation. Bence-Jones protein is secreted not only by patients with Bence-Jones myeloma but also in approximately 70% of patients whose myeloma cells secrete much complete immunoglobulin. This is probably due to an imbalance between the production and assembly of light and heavy chains. In the first Medical Research Council therapeutic trial, λ chains were found to be secreted higher concentrations than κ chains, with the highest concentration being in λ-Bence-Jones myeloma. A more unusual cause of chronic renal failure is the development of amyloid nephrosis or renal vein thrombosis.

Neurological complications

The most common neurological complications arise as a result of the anatomical relationships between the nervous tissue and bony structures.

Root symptoms may result from compression fractures but the potentially more serious problem of cord compression and paralysis may result from vertebral collapse or extension extradurally of myeloma tissue from the vertebral body. Patients presenting with signs of paralysis, sensory disturbance or loss of sphincter control must be treated as a medical emergency, and examination and investigation instigated to identify the level of compression. Immediate intervention with surgical decompression and local radiotherapy is indicated.

Peripheral neuropathy has been described as a complication in a smaller number of patients. In most of these cases the pathogenetic mechanisms operating are obscure but a number of factors have been well described, including paraprotein epiphenomena and amyloid deposition. Of interest is the fact that peripheral neuropathy occurs in only 1% of myeloma patients but appears to be much more common in particular sub-sets of this disease. Thus, there is an association between this complication and osteosclerotic disease, which is associated with a young age of onset, a high incidence of solitary plasmacytomas, organomegaly, endocrinopathy and cutaneous lesions (POEMS). Why the association exists is not known but the signs and symptoms often resolve on treatment of the plasmacytoma. Peripheral

neuropathy is not uncommonly seen following treatment of myeloma with second-line chemotherapy regimes, which often contain vinca-alkaloids and frequently give rise to this complication.

An encephalopathic clinical picture is a more dramatic manifestation which can be caused by a number of complications, the most common of which is hypercalcaemia. Initially, hypercalcaemia will cause weakness, fatigue and malaise but as it progresses confusion, delirium or coma may ensue. Common associated symptoms include nausea, vomiting, constipation and dehydration. There is not, however, a direct relationship between the severity of symptoms and the degree of hypercalcaemia. The hyperviscosity syndrome may also present with localised CNS signs and symptoms or with encephalopathic features (see Ch. 5). Thirdly, the metabolic consequences of renal failure, which is a major cause of early death, often result in confusion and delirium.

Diagnostic criteria

At presentation, investigations should be aimed at confirming a diagnosis and secondly the assessment of prognostic factors. There are three major criteria in the diagnosis of myeloma, but none of these are specific, as they may occur in many other conditions (Table 20.1). At least two criteria need to be present to confirm a diagnosis of plasma cell myeloma.

Bone marrow plasmacytosis

The normal bone marrow contains <5% plasma cells but an increase to greater than 20% is necessary to support a diagnosis of plasma cell myeloma (Plate 21). Some centres accept a lower value (>10%) especially if monoclonality has been demonstrated. Many other conditions can also produce a marked plasmacytosis, including liver disease, acute serum sickness and chronic infections (especially tuberculosis where plasma cell concentrations >60% have been reported), and these conditions need to be excluded. The absence of a plasmacytosis does not rule out myeloma and aspirates from other sites and trephine biopsies should be performed to exclude patchy infiltration if the index of suspicion is high.

Monoclonal paraprotein in serum or urine, or both

An M-component may be seen in a variety of benign and malignant conditions which need to be excluded by characterisation of the abnormal protein. The com-

Table 20.1 Differential diagnosis of paraproteinaemia, marrow plasmacytosis and osteolytic lesions

Paraproteinaemia	Benign monoclonal gammopathies	
	Malignant lymphoproliferative disorder	
	Reactive	infections
		autoimmune disease
		liver disease
		non-lymphoid tumours
Bone marrow plasmacytosis	Chronic infections	
	Chronic inflammatory disorders	
	Liver disease	
	Other tumours	
Lytic lesions	Multiple metastases	
	'Spotty osteoporosis'	
	Multiple eosinophilic granulomas	
	Hyperparathyroidism	
	Primary amyloid	
	Hydatid disease	
	Fibrous dysplasia	

monest cause of an anomalous serum protein is benign monoclonal gammopathy, the characteristics of which have been discussed above. Other conditions that should be excluded include other lymphoproliferative disorders, a number of rare dermatological conditions and, also rare, tumours of non-lymphocytic origin (see Ch. 5).

Bone lesions

Lytic lesions due to myeloma are most readily identified by plain skeletal X-rays. They occur in bones containing haemopoietic marrow and are most commonly well demonstrated 'punched out' lesions. Diffuse demineralisation frequently occurs and may be present in the absence of lytic lesions. In less than 1% of patients osteosclerosis may develop but such lesions should raise the suspicion of coincident Paget's disease or metastatic carcinoma. CT scanning may detect lytic lesions in the ribs or axial skeleton which are not visible on routine X-rays. The osteolytic lesions do not incite any osteoblastic activity and hence radio-isotope studies, which localise in areas of new bone formation, are rarely of value in the investigation of myeloma.

If lytic bone lesions cannot be demonstrated or a bone marrow plasmacytosis is not seen in the presence of high levels of paraprotein, a careful search should be made for an extramedullary plasmacytoma, paying particular attention to the nose, paranasal sinuses, oral pharynx, skin, bronchi, lymph nodes and intestinal mucosa.

In uncertain cases some centres include minor diagnostic criteria such as hypercalcaemia and a raised ESR,

but where there is doubt about the diagnosis it is usually advisable to wait and reassess later.

Prognostic features

Staging is important in multiple myelomas as a guide to prognosis and treatment. Because the vast majority of patients present with disseminated disease, distribution of disease is of no value in this process but a number of other features have been reported to be of unfavourable prognostic significance (Table 20.2).

Table 20.2 Poor prognostic features in multiple myeloma

Severe anaemia
Hypoalbuminaemia
Poor performance rating
Renal failure
Hypercalcaemia
Lambda light chain disease
Extensive osteolytic lesions
High monoclonal component
High serum B_2 microglobulin
High mitotic index of plasma cells
Expression of CD10 on plasma cells

The total body myeloma cell mass can be estimated in the laboratory by measuring the paraprotein synthesis rate and patient survival is closely correlated to this parameter. The total myeloma mass can be related to certain pretreatment clinical features, which allows for a more practical staging system. The British MRC trials have identified three major prognostic factors: the pretreatment Hb, the post-hydration urea concentration and the Karnovsky score. On the basis of these parameters, patients can be divided into good, intermediate and poor categories (Table 20.3). Although renal failure at presentation is a poor prognostic feature, it has little significance once the patient has survived for one year. In the MRC studies hypercalcaemia and hypoalbuminaemia had little independent prognostic significance. Some studies have suggested that patients with light chain only or the rare IgD disease have a more aggressive course.

In 1968 Berggard and Bern isolated and characterised from the serum a low molecular weight protein (MW 12 000) which they called serum B_2-microglobulin. This is now known to be present on the surface of all nucleated cells. It is coded on chromosome 15 and it is associated, with the Class I MHC antigens. Serum levels of B_2-microglobulin protein are elevated in the elderly, in

Table 20.3 Staging systems in multiple myeloma

	Measurement of tumour mass	Clinical and simple laboratory criteria	
		Curie & Salmon	British MRC
I/good	$<0.6 \times 10^{12}$ cells/m^2	Hb >10.5 g/dl Normal calcium IgG <50 g/l IgA <30 g/l Normal X-rays or solitary plasmacytoma Urine light chains <4 g/24 h	Hb >10 gd/l Post-hydration urea <8 mmol/l No, or few, symptoms
II/Inter-mediate	$0.6–1.2 \times 10^{12}$ cells/m^2	Values Intermediate between I & III	Intermediate between good and poor
III/Poor	$>1.2 \times 10^{12}$ cells/m^2	Hb <8.5 g/dl Calcium >2.7 mmol/l IgG >70 g/l IgA >50 g/l Extensive bone lesions on X-ray Urine light chains >12 g/24 h	Hb <7.5 g/dl + restricted activity *Or* Post-hydration urea >10 mmol/l + restricted activity

renal failure and in certain malignancies, in particular B-cell lymphoproliferative disorders.

Numerous studies have now shown that the level of serum B$_2$-microglobulin at presentation is one of the most powerful prognostic indicators in myeloma. In part this is because of the influence of renal failure, but even the values corrected for the level of urea or creatinine provide good discriminatory information.

In vitro techniques to determine the number of myeloma cells synthesising DNA may identify a subgroup of patients with a high labelling index and a very poor prognosis. The expression of the CD10 antigen (CALLA) on the myeloma cells may also be a poor prognostic feature.

Following the initial establishment of total tumour burden, the serial estimation of cell mass can be estimated by measurement of the M-component. An increase in tumour mass is reflected by a similar increase in paraprotein. Two situations may occur however, when this rule does not apply. In the presence of deteriorating renal function, immunoglobulin may be lost in the urine giving the false impression that the tumour is regressing in size, and secondly myeloma sub-

clones may occasionally develop with altered secretory properties.

Treatment

Prior to the advent of the alkylating agents median survival of patients with myeloma was 6–12 months. Now with the use of currently available drug regimens the median survival is 2–3 years with some patients showing prolonged survival. At presentation patients may be in any one of a number of clinical phases and it is important to ascertain whether the patient is in an active phase requiring chemotherapy or in a quiescent stage requiring no active therapy or supportive measures only. Some patients will be diagnosed as multiple myeloma whilst under investigation for an unrelated condition. Thus, although they exhibit features of multiple myeloma (i.e. increased plasma cells in the bone marrow, serum M-component, depression of normal immunoglobulins and monoclonal protein in the urine), they can be distinguished from those with 'active disease' by the lack of anaemia, azotaemia, hypercalcaemia, lytic bone lesions and a low DNA labelling index. Such patients are considered to have 'smouldering' multiple myeloma, and account for approximately 4% of cases. Most such patients, if properly staged, remain stable for long periods without chemotherapy. This should be withheld to avoid the effects of marrow toxicity, increased risk of second malignancies and the selection of drug-resistant clones. Progressive disease is identified by serial electrophoresis during the first year of follow-up, although Alexanian has suggested that the presence of an IgA M-protein or the presence of >200 mg/day of BJP are indications for early treatment.

Supportive therapy

Analgesia

The most common symptom in myelomatosis is pain and every effort should be made to relieve pain in order to ensure that patients remain ambulatory. Pain may be the result of a localised osteolytic lesion and the treatment of choice, if a localised site can be identified, is radiotherapy. This is usually given 800–2000 rads in divided doses. If delivered to medullary bone (e.g. spine), it is myelosuppressive and care must be taken if systemic chemotherapy is being given at the same time. Inactivity promotes bone resorption and can exacerbate the demineralisation and osteoporosis seen in multiple myeloma, so patients should be encouraged to remain as active as possible. The pain due to osteoporosis and vertebral collapse is rarely relieved by radiotherapy.

Fluids

Maintenance of an adequate plasma volume and good urine output serves to ensure good clearance of light chains, calcium and urate and hence minimises renal damage. A fluid intake of three litres per day should be aimed for. This is particularly important in patients with some degree of renal impairment who can readily become dehydrated. Their ideal weight should be determined and followed carefully in the clinic as a measure of hydration status; lying and standing blood pressure measurements should also be made at each visit as postural hypotension may be a sensitive indication of hypovolaemia.

Treatment of sepsis

Because of the immunosuppression seen in patients with myelomatosis they are at increased risk of infections. These are usually bacterial but repeated episodes of herpes zoster have been reported. The most common organisms are gram negative infections of the urinary tract but pneumonia secondary to *S.pneumoniae* and septicaemia due to gram positive organisms are all seen with increased frequency. Patients presenting with signs or symptoms of infection should therefore be investigated promptly and treated vigorously with broad spectrum antibiotics in the first instance until an organism is isolated. The use of prophylactic broad spectrum gammaglobulin in patients with suppression of immunoglobulin is at present under investigation and has been advocated for those patients with recurrent infections. It is, however, expensive.

Management of hypercalcaemia

Hypercalcaemia occurs in approximately 60% of patients at some time during the course of their disease and must be sought in any patient presenting with polyuria, polydipsia, nausea, vomiting, constipation, drowsiness, confusion or coma. At presentation, hypercalcaemic patients are often dehydrated and the first step is to replace extracellular fluid by rehydration with at least 3 litres of normal saline per day. This will ensure an adequate glomerular filtration rate which in turn increases the calcium load filtered by the kidney. Rehydration should be combined with a 'loop diuretic', either frusemide or ethacrynic acid which also increase urinary calcium excretion. The effects of rehydration and diuretics is rapid but both are associated with hypokalaemia and hypomagnesaemia. In addition, saline infusions can cause fluid overload and hyponatraemia, which is of special significance in the management of elderly patients.

Inorganic phosphate at a dose of 1.5 g iv stat has been used to rapidly lower serum calcium but metastatic calcification (deposition of calcium phosphate), particularly in the renal parenchyma, is a frequent complication. This approach should, therefore, be avoided. Oral phosphates, 1–3 gm daily in divided doses, are safer, and probably bind calcium in the gut, so reducing its absorption. It is frequently associated, however, with nausea and diarrhoea, and its effect is slow in onset so it is more suitable for the management of chronic hypercalcaemia rather than in the acute setting.

In patients resistant to the above therapy or who have markedly elevated serum calcium (>3.0 mmol/l) or who are symptomatic, hydrocortisone 200–300 mg i.v. daily or prednisolone 40–60 mg daily should be used. Steroids may act in a number of ways, including inhibition of osteoclast-activating factor, a cytotoxic effect on tumour cells, an increased urinary Ca^{++} excretion and a delayed effect on gut absorption of Ca^{++} due to its antagonistic action against 1-25 dihydroxycholecalciferol. Glucocorticoids are particularly effective in renal insufficiency but their major effect is delayed for 2–3 days.

Second-line therapy should be reserved for severe or resistant cases. Calcitonin acts as an inhibitor of parathormone and therefore decreases bone resorption. It is available as salmon or porcine calcitonin and needs to be given as a s.c. or i.m. injection of 8 units/kg 6–8 hourly. It must not be used with glass equipment because it is absorbed.

Side effects are uncommon although hypersensitivity has been reported. Tachyphylaxis limits its long-term use and antibody formation has been reported with the use of porcine calcitonin. Its effect has been disappointing with high serum calcium levels but because of its rapid onset of action and lack of side effects it is worthy of trial in resistant cases.

Oral diphosphonates, which as pyrophosphate analogues become incorporated into bone crystals, are reported to inhibit bone resorption. They may be of value prophylactically in myeloma to minimise bony destruction and the development of hypercalcaemia. Clinical trials are in progress.

Management of hyperviscosity

As an emergency or short-term measure, plasma exchange can be performed to rapidly lower plasma viscosity. A number of automated machines are available to carry out continuous or intermittent plasmapheresis but, in an emergency, if such machinery is not available, then plasmapheresis can be performed at the bedside by venesecting one unit of whole blood and then either allowing sedimentation to occur, or centrifuging the blood to accelerate the process, re-infusing the red cell layer diluted with saline and discarding the patient's plasma. This is, however, a tedious and time-consuming procedure, as 4–6 units must be exchanged. IgM paraproteinaemias respond best to this form of therapy because 80% of the total protein load is confined to the intravascular space. Because of the exponential relationship between protein concentration and plasma viscosity, a small reduction in serum protein will result in a disproportionate reduction in plasma viscosity. If an automated plasmapheresis machine is available, an exchange of 3–4 litres should be performed. In practice, viscosity should be measured before and after plasmapheresis. In general, symptoms will not occur unless the relative viscosity of the plasma is above 6 cps, and the aim of therapy therefore is to maintain the plasma viscosity below this level. As stated, plasmapheresis should only be considered a temporising measure and at the time of commencing such treatment more specific therapy should be given as appropriate to the underlying cause to prevent recurrence.

Cryoglobulinaemia

The management of patients with cryoglobulinaemia remains very problematic. General measures such as avoidance of cold cannot be over-stressed: however, in practical terms this is often easier said than done. Similarly, bed-rest is often effective for the treatment of skin ulceration, and aspirin and non-steroidal anti-inflammatory drugs have proven of benefit in some patients with arthralgia. Plasmapheresis may be of real benefit in these patients, although no controlled trials exist to show such a benefit. Great care must be exercised to prevent the cryoglobulins precipitating out in the extra-corporeal circulation during the procedures where the protein has a high thermal activity. Cytotoxic drugs and steroids may be indicated for the treatment of any underlying malignant condition. In the absence of any predisposing condition they may also have a role for the treatment of progressive renal or neurological disease and for disabling skin manifestations. Despite such measures, however, this condition will very often remain resistant to therapeutic intervention and conservative management remains the backbone of treatment.

Specific therapy

Most patients with myeloma will present with symptoms attributable to bone marrow suppression or the complications of their disease and will require specific anti-tumour therapy.

Chemotherapy

The comparison of response rates in different studies using various chemotherapy regimens has been hampered by the lack of universally accepted criteria of response. Until recently, few complete remissions had been reported so varying degrees of tumour regression have been taken as evidence of a response. Most groups accept a >50% reduction of tumour as such evidence.

Before the introduction of melphalan in 1958 the median survival of patients with plasma cell neoplasia was less than 12 months and at least one large study showed median survival from diagnosis as short as 3.5 months. With the use of melphalan or cyclophosphamide in varying dosages, however, the median survival can be doubled to approximately 24 months, with a median survival for responders of approximately 40 months (range 2–6+ years).

The choice between melphalan or cyclophosphamide lies with their toxicities, cyclophosphamide having less myelotoxic effect, although it may cause haemorrhagic cystitis even at low dose, if used over a long period of time. Interestingly cross-resistance between these two agents cannot be predicted and patients resistant to one may subsequently be shown to be sensitive to the other if therapy is changed. The optimum dose schedule has been investigated by numerous groups and although there is no difference between continuous or intermittent therapy in terms of survival, intermittent treatment causes less myelotoxicity and is at present the schedule of choice. Melphalan is typically given at a dose of 7 mg/m^2/day for 4 days every 3 weeks but it should be noted that absorption of melphalan from the gastrointestinal tract is unpredictable and the dose may need to be increased until haematological toxicity or tumour response is observed. Similarly, the dose should be reduced if neutrophils fall below 0.5×10^9/l or platelets to less than 50×10^9/l. Dosage reductions are also necessary for renal impairment. Cyclophosphamide may be given as a daily oral regime (100 mg/m^2), weekly intravenously (300 mg/m^2) or at higher doses intravenously (600–1000 mg/m^2) at 2–4-weekly intervals.

With intermittent regimes, failure of neutrophils to

reach $2.0 \times 10^9/l$ or platelets to reach $100 \times 10^9/l$ prior to the next course may be an indication to delay the next course for 1–2 weeks, or reduce the drug dosages.

By the late 1960s Salmon and Alexanian had been able to demonstrate an anti-tumour effect of prednisolone and, in an attempt to improve survival, combinations of an alkylating agent and prednisolone began to be used in clinical trials. It has been found, however, that the addition of prednisone in moderate doses to an alkylating agent does not affect the overall survival. Prednisone is an effective treatment for hypercalcaemia, however, and will initially make some patients feel better non-specifically.

Other chemotherapeutic agents have also been added to melphalan with variable results. Although some studies have shown an advantage for the addition of vincristine, this has not been upheld in other large trials. Recent studies suggest that a combination of adriamycin, BCNU, cyclophosphamide and melphalan may be superior to the use of melphalan alone, although it is clearly more toxic. This regime takes advantage of the supposed synergy between adriamycin and BCNU.

In an attempt to induce complete remissions and prolong the interval to relapse that inevitably occurs with conventional chemotherapy, McElwain and colleagues pioneered the use of very large doses of melphalan. Preliminary analysis has shown a comparable 2-year survival rate with conventional dose chemotherapy of 59% but 33% of patients entered a complete serological and haematological remission, with only 7% relapsing at up to 16 months from treatment. These improved results have been attained at the expense of an increased treatment-related mortality due to drug-induced bone marrow failure. To further evaluate this treatment high dose melphalan, with or without methyl prednisolone, is now being tested as part of the VIth MRC Myelomatosis Study.

Overall, approximately 70% of patients will respond with a >50% fall in M-protein to reach a stable, lower value and/or disappearance of light chain proteinuria. In 'good responders' this plateau phase usually represents a 1–2 log cell kill and represents a kinetically quiescent phase of the disease. Other serological evidence of plateau phase includes a low serum B_2 microglobulin level (NR 2–4 µg/ml) and light chain isotype suppression on peripheral blood lymphocytes. In addition to the serological parameters, patients in plateau phase should have minimal symptoms attributable to active myelomatosis and a stable Hb without requirement for transfusion. The IVth MRC Myelomatosis Study showed that continuing treatment during plateau phase confirmed no survival advantage. Furthermore, continuous therapy may lead to myelosuppression and an increased incidence of acute leukaemia or refractory anaemia, with an attendant increase in morbidity and mortality.

Patients failing to attain the above criteria or exhibiting evidence of increasing M-protein whilst on therapy are classified as non-responders. If patients fail to achieve >50% fall but remain with stable M-protein and no other evidence of disease, then treatment should be stopped and the patients closely followed up. Patients who exhibit progressive disease constitute a poor prognosis group for whom second-line therapy needs to be considered.

Second-line chemotherapy

Patients who relapse several months after ceasing therapy with first-line drugs mostly respond to repeat courses, although the length of responses becomes progressively shorter. Patients who relapse whilst receiving therapy should be given alternate therapy and a 15–30% response can be expected. For primary refractory cases this figure falls to 5–15%.

Multiple agent chemotherapy. A number of multiple agent regimens have been used in relapsing patients with varying results. The choice of regimens depends on the first-line treatment used. For patients treated initially with melphalan a combination of adriamycin, BCNU and vincristine is widely used. Bourlogie et al have recently described encouraging results using a continuous infusion of vinca alkaloid and doxorubicin over 4 days, plus high dose intermittent dexamethasone (VAD). They were able to show, by using this regime, a rapid and marked reduction (>75%) of tumour mass in 70% of previously resistant patients with myelomatosis. Such an approach requires the placement of a central line to facilitate administration of the drugs and is associated with a number of complications. The most common side effect is gastrointestinal upset due to dexamethasone, which may need to be omitted. The risk of infection using this regime is high despite the relatively mild neutropenia induced. Several centres are now evaluating the VAD regime as first-line therapy.

High/medium dose cyclophosphamide. Cyclophosphamide may be of value in patients who have failed on melphalan, and high/medium dose cyclophosphamide may induce a respone in patients failing on low dose cyclophosphamide. The ECOG have used intermediate dose intravenous cyclophosphamide and have obtained a 38% response rate in patients previously treated with lower dose cyclophosphamide. Bone marrow failure was, however, a major complication with death due to aplasia a significant risk.

High dose pulsed prednisolone. Alexanian and others have noted a 25% response rate in patients with advanced and refractory disease treated with frequent large doses of prednisolone with or without the addition of a vinca alkaloid. Although remission durations were short, the quality of life during remission was reported to be excellent. It is particularly of value for patients with pancytopenia or as systemic treatment for patients undergoing palliative radiotherapy. A course of therapy consisted of prednisolone 60 mg/m^2/day for 5 days at 8 intervals for 3 pulses with a 3-week break prior to the next course. Such treatment is associated with significant complications such as gastrointestinal bleeding, perforation of the gut, fungal and pyogenic infections and glucose intolerance.

α Interferon. α$_2$rIFN has now been used in a number of studies as a single agent for patients with relapsed or refractory multiple myeloma. CR rates (>50% reduction in tumour mass) between different studies have been remarkably consistent at 11–14%, with a similar number showing a partial response. Side effects from IFN include mild to moderate leukopenia and thrombocytopenia which is rarely dose-limiting. Occasional elevation of the alanine transaminase occurs but it rapidly returns to normal on cessation of treatment. Virtually all patients develop a 'flu-like' illness which has on occasion necessitated stopping treatment. Less commonly patients complain of somnolence and confusion and a number of patients have had to stop therapy after developing numbness and parasthesiae of the extremities, all of which are reversible. Alopecia, xerostomia, anorexia, nausea and vomiting are other side effects of minor severity which tend to be non-dose-dependent.

In an attempt to increase response rates, studies are now under way to assess the value of using IFN and other chemotherapeutic drugs in combination.

Deoxycoformycin. A number of workers have noted that plasma cells contain adenosine deaminase and that if inhibited with the purine nucleotide analogue deoxycoformycin, cell death will result. Consequently a number of studies are now underway to evaluate the response of non-responding patients to the use of deoxycoformycin and initial phase II studies have shown promising results. A recent study by Belcher et al showed that of 7 evaluable patients, 2 had a greater than 50% reduction in paraprotein and improvement of bone pain, while another 2 showed marked reduction in soft tissue mass but no reduction in monoclonal protein. Toxicity from deoxycoformcyin, even in the low doses

used in this trial, posed a significant problem. Anorexia and nausea occur in all patients receiving the drug. Myelotoxicity was not significant, although the lymphocyte count dropped routinely to approximately 40% by the fourth or fifth day. Mild confusion and disorientation was seen in 3 patients and appeared to be related to therapy.

Bone marrow transplantation. Allogeneic bone marrow transplantation following chemo-radiotherapy is available only for those few young people with an HLA-matched sibling donor. Only a small number of patients have yet been treated by this modality but early results offer some encouragement.

Autologous bone marrow transplantation in myeloma is being tried in several centres, although there is the major problem of malignant contamination of the marrow.

Role of irradiation

Myeloma tumour cells are exquisitely sensitive to X-rays and radiation therapy has been a mainstay in the treatment of localised plasma cell neoplasms and fractures (Fig. 20.2). Approximately 50% of myeloma presenting as solitary plasmacytomas of bone subsequently become generalised but in the other 50% that are truly localised high dose radiotherapy is curative.

Less than 5% of myelomas will present with disease at an extramedullary site, most commonly around the oro-nasopharynx. These tumours are best treated by local radiotherapy, in divided doses. However, the tumour not infrequently fails to shrink completely and if an M-protein is present it also may not disappear completely. In these patients surgical removal usually results in complete resolution of all signs of disease. In a few patients recurrence has been seen in the cervical chain and irradiation of these areas has been advocated for this reason. The treatment of painful localised lytic bone lesions with radiotherapy relieves pain in the majority of patients and, similarly, pathological fractures are best treated by irradiation, preceded if necessary by intramedullary pinning.

Spinal cord compression due to extradural plasma cell deposits constitutes a medical emergency. Lermittes sign (girdle pain aggravated by raised intracranial pressure due to coughing or sneezing) is an early warning symptom of impending compression and must never be ignored. A myelogram will demonstrate any cord compression and where obstruction to the subarachnoid space is complete a follow-up myelogram should be performed after therapy to ensure there is no lesion higher up. Treatment is with 20 Gy over 5 days and should be

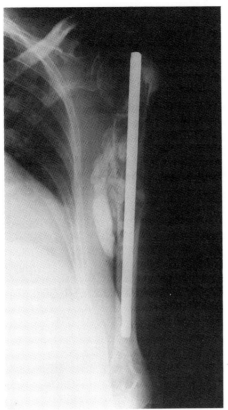

Fig.20.2 Fracture through shaft of humerus treated by insertion of stabilising pin and radiotherapy; callous formation is readily evident.

carried out as an emergency to prevent permanent damage.

In 1971 Bergsagel proposed using systemic irradiation for the management of patients with multiple myeloma. Because of the severe myelosuppressive toxicity caused by this form of therapy, hemibody or sequential hemibody irradiation has been performed in a number of clinical trials. Virtually all patients treated to date have had advanced myeloma and the majority have failed first-line therapy. Median survival figures compare favourably with other second-line treatment modalities and symptomatic improvement or resolution of bone pain occurs within 24 to 48 hours in the majority of patients. Toxicity, however, has frequently been severe in those patients receiving sequential hemibody irradiation. Although myelosuppression is the most common and severe problem, gastrointestinal dysfunction and stomatitis have been reported in a significant number of patients. Pneumonitis has been reported but is rare in patients receiving less than 800 rads in one dose to the upper half.

HEAVY CHAIN DISEASE

Heavy chain disease comprises a group of disorders characterised by the presence in the serum and/or urine of a protein related to the Fc fragment of normal immunoglobulins. These proteins can be identified immunologically as incomplete heavy polypeptide chains that are devoid of light chains. Biochemical analysis shows them to have been terminated either at the hinge region or between the variable and constant regions of the heavy chain. It has been well established that these proteins are synthesised and not the result of biological degradation of intact immunoglobulin. Since the light and heavy chains are coded for on separate chromosomes, it would suggest either that there are two separate genetic abnormalities or that the abnormal protein is incapable of combining with light chains or in some way exerts a negative feedback inhibition on light chain production, the latter being the most likely explanation.

The first member of this group to be described was the 'gamma heavy chain disease' in 1964 by Franklin et al and since that time heavy chain diseases related to all the other immunoglobulin classes have been described.

γ-Heavy chain disease

Although the first of this group of disorders to be described, it is not as common as α-chain disease. The clinical features are distinctive but careful immunological assessment is required to confirm the diagnosis, as histological features are variable and non-specific. The condition is seen only rarely under the age of 40 years and there has been a preponderance of males in the cases reported. The onset of symptoms is generally insidious with weakness, malaise and low grade fever often associated with infection. Lymphadenopathy occurs frequently, is usually generalised and frequently waxes and wanes in size. Another characteristic feature of the condition is the presence of palatal erythema and oedema which in severe cases may give rise to respiratory obstruction. Hepatosplenomegaly is commonly found but bony involvement is rare.

Investigations

Haematological findings are non-specific. Anaemia, leukopenia and thrombocytopenia often occur and are frequently associated with eosinophilia and the presence of atypical lymphocytes and plasma cells. Plasma cell leukaemia has been reported terminally in a number of cases. In addition the ESR and urate levels are often elevated. Bone marrow aspiration usually demonstrates an abnormal lymphocyte infiltration with a spectrum of morphological features and, not infrequently, eosinophilia.

Histological findings are variable, non-specific and not usually of help. Most often a lymphoplasmacytoid infiltrate is seen, usually in association with an eosinophilia.

Careful serological investigations are essential to make the diagnosis. In some patients no 'peak' has been identifiable on cellulose acetate electrophoresis, the abnormal protein being present as a broad, heterogeneous band. The most common feature on serum electrophoresis is hypogammaglobulinaemia. The paraprotein is more easily picked up in the urine where it is often excreted in high concentration.

Management

Most patients pursue a relentless downhill course and usually die of infection, although a few patients survive beyond 5 years. Treatment is unsatisfactory and various chemotherapeutic agents have been used either singly or in combination. Prednisolone and vinblastine, steroids plus alkylating agents or combination chemotherapy such as the CHOP regime may also produce responses in some patients. Radiotherapy has only produced transient effects and is not routinely used.

α-Heavy chain disease

The first patient with this condition was an Arab woman with abdominal lymphoma and malabsorption reported by Seligmann in 1968. Since that time many other cases have been described, predominantly in patients from North Africa, Southern Europe and the Middle East. Clinically patients present at a young age (<45 years) with a characteristic symptom complex of abdominal pain, diarrhoea, steatorrhoea, finger-clubbing and hypocalcaemia. Weight loss is common and this disease is often mistaken for coeliac disease. These patients do not respond, however, to a gluten-free diet. Hepatosplenomegaly and peripheral lymphadenopathy are rare but abdominal masses are frequently palpable. Pathologically there is diffuse lymphomatous involvement of long loops of upper small intestine and mesenteric nodes, with sparing of the other lymph nodes and extralymphatic organs. Rarely, patients have been reported with involvement limited to the respiratory tract and mediastinal lymph nodes.

Investigations

The diagnosis, if suspected, must be confirmed by the demonstration on serum electrophoresis of an α-like heavy chain travelling in the $\alpha_2 B_1$ position but lacking a κ or λ-light chain with an associated decrease in albumin and gammaglobulin. Occasionally, if the paraprotein level is low, simple electrophoresis may produce a normal pattern and immuno-electrophoresis is necessary to demonstrate the abnormal protein. The abnormal protein may be found in other secretions including urine. Histopathological assessment of the intestine is non-diagnostic showing a non-specific lymphoplasmacytoid infiltrate occasionally extending down to the muscularis propria of upper jejunum or duodenum.

Immunocytological techniques may identify α-heavy chains in the cell cytoplasm. The bone marrow is characteristically spared and consequently abnormalities of the peripheral blood are uncommon. However, biochemical and coagulation abnormalities may often be identified secondary to the malabsorptive state that is induced.

Radiological investigations are of help, showing hypertrophic folds and pseudopolyp formation in the duodenum and jejunum, with areas of distention and narrowing often with fluid levels. There is epidemiological data to suggest that the α-heavy chain disease occurs secondarily to chronic, low grade gastrointestinal infection. However, repeated attempts have failed to identify a causative agent. The evidence supporting the role of microorganisms in the pathogenesis of this disease is further strengthened by the fact that occasional patients have entered complete and lasting remissions with the use of antibiotics alone.

A number of workers have noted the striking similarity between this condition and Mediterranean lymphoma. The clinical manifestations of the two conditions are identical but histologically the latter is composed of large, frequently binucleate immunoblasts. Occasional rare patients have also been described whose sera contains the α-heavy chain protein. It is now felt that these two conditions represent either end of a spectrum of a single disease entity which has been called immunoproliferative small intestinal disease (IPSID).

Management and prognosis

The clinical course is variable with spontaneous remissions, usually of short duration, being not uncommon. Because of the association of the condition with a high incidence of intestinal parasitaemia, tetracycline as a single agent has been used for treatment with many reports of clinical histological and immunological remission. In addition, prednisone and cyclophosphamide in continuous low dose as single agents have also been reported to induce remissions. More durable remissions have been obtained with combination chemotherapy with or without tetracycline, although cachectic patients with advanced disease do not tolerate aggressive therapy well. Although prolonged remissions have been reported the disease tends to relapse and follow a progressive downhill course with a 5-year survival in one series of only 22.7%.

μ-Heavy chain disease

This is the rarest of the heavy chain diseases. The condition has, without single exception, been associated with a lymphoproliferative type condition, most commonly CLL. Whilst hepatosplenomegaly is common, peripheral lymphadenopathy has been reported in a minority of patients and some patients have no increase in lymphocyte counts, although immunological analysis has demonstrated an abnormal clone of μ-bearing lymphocytes in the circulation. Lytic bone lesions and amyloidosis have been reported but are rare.

Investigations

Unless suspected clinically this condition may be missed on electrophoresis as a peak in the α_2 region is usually absent and only hypogammaglobulinaemia is demonstrated. Any abnormal component should be identified by immuno-electrophoresis plus ultracentrifugation or gelfiltration to document the absence of light chains. The μ-heavy chain is rarely excreted in the urine. In addition, in contrast to the other heavy chain disorders, Bence-Jones protein has been identified in the urine of two thirds of these patients. It appears that both components are secreted by the same clone of cells but that due to an internal genetic deletion they are unable to be joined to form a complete macroglobulin.

AMYLOIDOSIS

Amyloid was first described by Virchow in 1853 as a 'waxy eosinophilic' material which, because of its staining properties, was thought to be derived from starch or polysaccharides. It has become clear, however, that amyloid is composed of protein fibrils which on X-ray diffraction analysis can be seen to be arranged in a unique, spiral β-pleated sheet arrangement. The nature of the protein was difficult to ascertain because of its insolubility and resistance to enzymatic degradation. This problem has been overcome and amyloid can be shown to be derived from either immunoglobulin proteins or

from a diverse class of proteins having a common N-terminal amino acid sequence.

Classification

The early classification of amyloidosis into primary and secondary was based upon clinico-pathological criteria dependent upon the distribution of amyloid in different organs and by distinguishing systemic from localised disease. This proved unsatisfactory because of the marked overlap in the distribution of deposits between the two types.

Biochemical and immunochemical analysis of amyloid fibrils from different forms of amyloidosis have clearly shown that they are distinct from one another and this forms a useful basis for the classification of the amyloidoses (Table 20.4).

'Primary' amyloid. In this form of the disease the major component consists of material homologous to

Table 20.4 Aetiology of amyloidoses

Acquired systemic

Immunocyte-related (Primary):
  Plasma cell myeloma
  Waldenstrom's macroglobulinaemia
  Heavy chain disease
  Non-Hodgkin's lymphoma

Reactive systemic

Chronic inflammatory disease (Secondary):
  Rheumatoid arthritis – Adult
                       – Juvenile
  Ankylosing spondylitis
  Reiter's disease
  Psoriatic arthropathy
  Chronic rheumatic heart disease
  Scleroderma
  Dermatomyositis
  Behcet's disease
  Systemic lupus

Chronic infections:
  Tuberculosis
  Leprosy
  Syphilis
  Bronchiectasis
  Osteomyelitis
  Paraplegia with decubitus ulcers
  Chronically infected burns

Tumour-forming

Localised masses, e.g. Endocrine neoplasms

Organ-limited, e.g. Cardiac

Heredofamilial

Familial Mediterranean fever

Familial Portuguese polyneuropathy

part of the immunoglobulin light chain (AL). It may consist of intact immunoglobulin light chain, an N-terminal fragment of a light chain corresponding to the variable region, or a mixture of the two. Interestingly the proportion of patients with 'light-chain disease' who develop amyloidosis is low, suggesting some amyloidogenic peculiarity of certain light chains. To date, no uniform property or abnormality has been detected. A strong body of evidence supports the suggestion that primary amyloidosis is secondary to the proliferation of an abnormal clone of immunocytes, even though in a proportion of patients no monoclonal serum or urinary protein can be detected.

Secondary amyloid. This form of the disease, sometimes called the reactive systemic form is very often associated with a chronic inflammatory or infective process, but its presence is not essential to the diagnosis and its absence does not exclude the diagnosis. The amyloid fibrils in this condition are heterogeneous in composition but are identical in their N-terminal amino acid sequences. They are called AA protein. The cell of origin is unknown, but an acute phase serum component approximately 180 000 daltons in size has been identified which is immunologically related to the amyloid fibrils and is known as serum amyloid associated protein (SAA).

Clinical features

Primary amyloid

The main clinical features of the acquired systemic or

Table 20.5   Clinical features of primary amyloidosis

Organ	Disorder
1. Heart	Restrictive cardiomyopathy Constrictive pericarditis Conduction defects
2. Gut	Macroglossia Intestinal motility disorders
3. Nervous system	Autonomic neuropathy Sensory neuropathy Carpal tunnel syndrome
4. Joints	Polyarthropathy Subcutaneous nodules
5. Skin	Cutaneous nodules 'Purpura' Scleroderma-like lesions Alopecia
6. Liver	Hepatomegaly
7. Kidneys	Nephrotic syndrome
8. Lungs	Infiltration

primary form of amyloidosis are shown in Table 20.5. The major organs involved are cardiac and gastrointestinal.

1. Cardiac involvement is manifest as congestive cardiac failure, usually with a normal cardiac contour on plain chest X-ray, angina, unresponsive to vasodilators and ECG abnormalities. The latter usually take the form of varying degrees of heart block or changes consistent with infarction which occur in the absence of other findings of myocardial damage. Cardiac disease accounts for approximately 50% of deaths in primary amyloid, the majority of which (60%) are secondary to acute arrhythmias. Care must be taken in administering digitalis to patients with amyloidosis as they are exquisitely sensitive and sudden deaths due to dysrhythmias have been reported.

2. Renal manifestations usually arise insidiously with the development of proteinuria and azotaemia leading to the nephrotic syndrome and chronic renal failure as a late event. Less commonly patients may present with acute renal failure due to renal vein thrombosis. Involvement of the lower renal tract has been reported.

3. Gastrointestinal amyloidosis can involve all levels of the gastrointestinal tract but the most distinctive feature is macroglossia which presents with a large stiff tongue. Occasionally this can be so gross as to interfere with deglutition and respiration. The oesophagus is usually spared, although microscopic involvement has been demonstrated. Involvement of the lower gastrointestinal tract is a result of vascular infiltration which manifests clinically as diarrhoea, malabsorption or rarely as an obstructive lesion.

5. Peripheral neuropathy may be the presenting feature in acquired systemic amyloidosis. Sensory abnormalities occur early with a 'glove and stocking' sensory impairment but an autoimmune disturbance resembling diabetic neuropathy has also been described early in the disease, with dyshidrosis, orthostatic hypotension and impotence being prominent features. Motor disturbances occur later in the course and median nerve palsy due to entrapment in the carpal tunnel and weight loss are frequent associations.

6. Polyarthropathy of amyloidosis is typically symmetrical involving mainly the larger joints, wrists and interphalangeal joints. Affected joints are often associated with subcutaneous nodules of amyloid deposits. These features closely mimic those of rheumatoid arthritis but differ from it by occurring in an older age group, being unassociated with tenderness or inflammation and lacking any fever. Massive deposition of periarticular amyloid around the shoulder joint may produce a pathognomonic 'shoulder-pad' sign.

7. Skin. Amyloid is often deposited extensively in the

dermis where it produces hyaline deposits found characteristically in skin folds which are often palpable and are non-pruritic. Purpura may result either from deposition of amyloid in the wall of small vessels in the skin and mucous membrane or from a haemostatic defect due to absorption of factor X by the amyloid material. Purpura are characteristically seen in a periorbital distribution and may be precipitated by vomiting, coughing or post-sigmoidoscopy.

Secondary amyloid

The incidence of secondary or reactive systemic amyloidosis is highly variable but has been reported by one study as occurring in 61% of patients with rheumatoid arthritis, although most studies report an incidence of 10–25%. The average duration of the underlying disease was approximately 15 years. Amyloidosis has also been reported in other chronic inflammatory diseases including juvenile rheumatoid arthritis, inflammatory bowel disease, Reiter's syndrome, dermatomyositis, scleroderma and Beçhet's syndrome, in which it accounts for 20–30% of deaths. In addition there is a long list of infectious causes commonly cited as predisposing to amyloidosis but in the UK tuberculosis, bronchiectasis, osteomyelitis and chronically infected burns are the most common.

Clinically these patients usually present with the insidious development of proteinuria leading to the nephrotic syndrome. This is followed later by hepatosplenomegaly due to infiltration by amyloid material and passive congestion. Cardiac involvement is very common on histological examination but is rarely clinically significant, mortality in this group being attributable mainly to uraemia or the nephrotic syndrome.

Senile amyloidosis increases with age. Amyloid confined to the heart has an overall incidence of approximately 2% but over the age of 90 years this rises to 50%. It may produce symptoms identical to those seen in acquired systemic amyloidosis.

In the central nervous system congophilic vascular lesions have been described in pre-senile dementia (Alzheimer's disease and Crutzfeld-Jacobs' syndrome) and in normal brains of elderly persons. It has been suggested by some that these amyloid deposits may predispose to cerebral haemorrhage in the elderly.

Investigations

Biopsy

An essential step to making the diagnosis of amyloidosis is to obtain tissue from an organ suspected of being involved and demonstrating amyloid deposition. This can be done by a number of methods, none of which is specific, but the birefringence seen under polarised light with congo-red staining allows amyloid to be distinguished from the other causes of this tinctorial reaction (i.e. cellulose fibres and chitin) by morphological criteria. Immunochemical reactions may be valuable but must be interpreted with extreme caution, as both false-negative and false-positive results have been reported.

If a specimen cannot be obtained from a suspected organ for some reason, then rectal, renal, gingival or skin biopsies have been reported as giving a high yield of positive results in systemic disease provided an adequate biopsy is obtained. Care must be taken in obtaining liver biopsies, as fatal bleeding has occurred post biopsy and a coagulation screen to detect a bleeding diathesis is mandatory.

Non-invasive procedures

Examination of peripheral blood is generally unhelpful although anaemia may be seen in a proportion of patients. If amyloid occurs secondary to myeloma or macroglobulinaemia then typical abnormalities may be found in the blood and bone marrow.

Serum immunoglobulin levels may be helpful showing a polyclonal elevation if there is underlying infection or inflammation and occasionally suppression in primary acquired amyloid reflecting immunosuppression secondary to proliferation of an immunocyte clone.

WALDENSTROM'S MACROGLOBULINAEMIA

Macroglobulinaemia is the term first used by Waldenstrom in 1944 to describe a condition characterised by the presence of a circulating monoclonal IgM paraprotein in association with generalised tissue infiltration consisting of abnormal plasma cells, lymphocytes and intermediate cell forms. These histological appearances are referred to as lymphocytic lymphoma with plasmacytoid differentiation and may be found in a variety of clinical settings, in association with IgG, IgA or light chain only paraproteins as well as the classical IgM production. Occasionally the tumour may fail to produce any immunoglobulin component. Such tumours should not strictly be referred to as Waldenstrom's macroglobulinaemia, although hyperviscosity (especially with IgA-producing tumours) may occur giving rise to a very similar clinical picture.

Clinical manifestations

Macroglobulinaemia is approximately 10 times less frequent in the population than myeloma. There is a 2:1 male to female frequency, with the average age at presentation of 60 years. It is rare below 40 years of age.

The most common presenting feature is weakness and fatigue which is out of proportion to the anaemia that is commonly associated. Haemorrhage, usually in the absence of thrombocytopenia, is also a common manifestation, presenting as epistaxis, purpura and gastrointestinal haemorrhage. It is most usually due to coating of platelets with IgM and interaction of the paraprotein with labile coagulation factors. Other non-specific features include weight loss and low grade fever.

The more specific clinical features seen in this condition are the result either of the physico-chemical properties of the circulating immunoglobulin or of tumour bulk. Hyperviscosity is common in Waldenstrom's macroglobulinaemia and the clinical features are discussed above (p. 27).

Such patients often present with neurological symptoms such as the Bing-Neal syndrome (i.e. progressive peripheral neuropathy associated with hyperviscosity or cryoprecipitation in the vasa nervorum), cardiovascular abnormalities or visual disturbances. Other paraprotein effects include: cold haemagglutinin syndrome, cryoglobulinaemia and amyloidosis. Raynaud's phenomenon has been reported in 3% of patients. Bence-Jones proteinuria has been described in up to 25% of patients but in far lower concentrations than seen in classical multiple myeloma. Probably as a result of this, renal insufficiency is an uncommon finding but amyloidosis is not an infrequent association.

The abnormal lymphocytic infiltrate most commonly involves the extramedullary lymphocytic tissue causing hepatosplenomegaly and lymphadenopathy. Atypical sites of involvement are occasionally seen, however, with involvement of the gastrointestinal tract producing a malabsorption syndrome or upper gastrointestinal tract haemorrhage. Involvement of the respiratory tract is manifested as specific infiltrates of the parenchymal tissue or bronchial tree, effusions or pseudo-tumours.

Skeletal lesions are not a prominent feature. Lytic lesions have been reported in 2–5% of cases of macroglobulinaemia implying that some of these tumours have the ability to secrete an osteoclast-activating factor and further emphasising the spectrum of disease that this group of disorders represents. Osteoporosis is not uncommon but is not a dominant feature.

Investigations

A full blood count demonstrates anaemia in up to 90% of patients at presentation. It is normochromic, normocytic anaemia due to a variety of factors including haemodilution secondary to the paraprotein effect and bone marrow infiltration, and in some cases a decreased RBC survival has been demonstrated. Rouleaux are often present but not as commonly as with multiple myeloma. Leukopenia is seen in a small number of patients but a moderate 'atypical' lymphocytosis is more common, the cells showing a spectrum of morphological features ranging from small lymphocytes to plasmacytoid lymphocytes. Thrombocytopenia has been reported in up to 6% of patients. The ESR is characteristically elevated but a more useful measurement is the serum viscosity which is elevated in approximately 50% of cases.

Bone marrow biopsy shows a diffuse lymphoplasmacytoid infiltrate, many of which contain PAS positive, intranuclear globules. A mild eosinophilia is often present and mast cells are characteristically increased. EM demonstrates an abundant endoplasmic reticulum in the lymphocytes of the bone marrow.

Pathological examination of lymph nodes reveals destruction of the normal architecture with a diffuse replacement by lymphocytes with significant numbers of plasmacytoid cells, thus distinguishing this condition histologically from well differentiated lymphocytic leukaemia.

Immunological investigations should be performed in all lymphoproliferative disorders to detect the presence of a circulating paraprotein. Screening tests for cryoglobulins, cold-reacting antibodies and Bence-Jones protein should also be performed.

Management

The clinical course of the disorder varies markedly from patient to patient. Patients will usually present with symptoms and will therefore require therapy. Chemotherapy has formed the cornerstone of treatment, most usually in the form of single agent alkylating agents such as chlorambucil, cyclophosphamide or melphalan, with or without steroids. Supportive therapy for infections may be indicated. However, despite the impaired antibody response to foreign antigens, infection is far less common in this condition than in multiple myeloma. Hyperviscosity is a common presenting symptom and plasmapheresis is indicated for this condition. Plasmapheresis has also been advocated for the treatment of cryoglobulinaemia but technical difficulties in handling the protein ex vivo may limit the usefulness of this procedure. Patients responding to treatment have a median survival of 49 months, whilst median survival for non-responders is only 24 months, the causes of death being haemorrhage, infection, cold-precipitation syndromes and severe anaemia.

PARAPROTEINS IN LYMPHOMAS AND LEUKAEMIAS

In a large study by Alexanian of 1150 patients with a variety of lymphomas defined by Rappaport criteria, he found a four-fold increase in the incidence of IgG paraproteins in patients with diffuse lymphocytic lymphoma and a one hundred-fold increase in incidence of IgM paraproteinaemia. The index of suspension for Waldenstrom's macroglobulinaemia or a lymphoma must therefore be high when an IgM paraprotein is detected in the serum.

Acute leukaemia represents an abnormality of haemopoietic cells at an early stage of development and consequently paraproteinaemia is an exceedingly rare event. Chronic lymphocytic leukaemia is composed of a more mature cell population and a variety of dysgammaglobulinaemias have been reported, including paraproteinaemias, most commonly of IgM type.

CRYOGLOBULINAEMIA

Cryoglobulins are proteins, mostly immunglobulins, which possess the ability to precipitate out of solution at temperatures below 37°C. Cryoglobulins tend to be composed of three types of protein: either an isolated monoclonal immunoglobulin (Type I), a mixed cryo-globulin composed of a monoclonal immunoglobulin with polyclonal IgG (Type II), or a mixed polyclonal cryoglobulin consisting of one or more classes of polyclonal immunoglobulin (Type III). In Type III the cryoglobulins are usually present as immune complexes. It has been suggested that different types of cryoglobulin produce different clinical features but the overlap between them is too great to be of diagnostic importance. However, there is a strong association of Type I disease with Waldenstrom's macroglobulinaemia and multiple myeloma and the mixed types II and III with a variety of connective tissue disorders and vasculitides. Type III cryoglobulins may also be found (often transiently) in association with a variety of infections.

The most common clinical feature of the disease is vascular purpura which curiously does not seem to be related to the ambient temperature. Other cutaneous manifestations include urticaria, distal necrosis and livedo reticularis. Early in the disease arthralgia is common which may progress later to frank arthritis and deformity of the joint.

Glomerulonephritis occurs in approximately 50% of patients, and may prove fatal. Gastrointestinal involvement and neurological lesions are seen in a smaller percentage of patients, as are endocrine, cardiac and hepatic involvement, all of which reflect an underlying diffuse vasculitis.

The treatment of cryoglobulinaemia has been discussed in the preceding chapter.

BIBLIOGRAPHY

Delamore I W, Yin 1986 Multiple myeloma and other paraproteinaemias. Churchill Livingstone, Edinburgh
Durie B G 1988 Staging and kinetics in multiple myeloma. Seminars in Oncology 13: 300–309
Galton D A, Brito-Babapulle F 1987 The management of myelomatosis. European Journal of Haematology 39: 385–398
Jacobson D R et al 1986 Immunosuppression and infection in multiple myeloma. Seminars in Oncology 13: 282–290
Osserman E F, Merlini G, Butler V P 1987. Multiple myeloma and related plasma cell dyscrasias. Journal of the American Medical Association 258: 2930–2937
Somer T 1987 Rheology of paraproteinaemias and hyperviscosity syndrome. Bailliere's Clinical Haematology 1: 695–724

21. Bone marrow transplantation

M. J. Mackie

In the late 1940s and early 50s it became apparent that animals could be protected from the marrow toxic effects of irradiation by the subsequent infusion of bone marrow. The protection was due to the population of the host by donor marrow cells. The survival of the animals in these early experiments was limited by what is now recognised as graft versus host disease. The feasibility of marrow infusions in man was demonstrated in the late 50s in Seattle and Paris; early results in terms of survival were disappointing, as patients with advanced disease who were often in poor condition were used and marrow was obtained from donors who were frequently inadequately matched.

However, by the late 1960s and early 1970s the determinants of histocompatibility has been described and a systematic approach could be adopted to select compatible bone marrow donors.

Terminology

Following from the above early work two major approaches to transplantation are employed. Allogeneic bone marrow transplantation involves the transfer of marrow from one individual to another; a syngeneic transplant involves twins. Autologous transplantation is performed using the patient's own marrow; attempts may be made to remove any abnormal cells from the marrow before it is infused (purging). This latter approach will be discussed more fully at the end of the chapter.

ALLOGENEIC BONE MARROW TRANSPLANTATION (ALLO BMT)

Patient selection

The main current indications for allo BMT are given in Table 21.1.

As can be seen, the trend is to transplant early in the disease. Patients who have relapsed and remitted on a

Table 21.1 The main indications for allo BMT

Disease	Disease status
1. Acute non-lymphoblastic leukaemia	First remission
2. Acute lymphoblastic leukaemia	
Children	Second remission
Adults – standard risk*	Second/first remission
Adults – high risk	? First remission
3. Chronic myeloid leukaemia	Chronic phase
4. Aplastic anaemia	Severe
5. Miscellaneous	
Severe combined immunodeficiency syndrome (SCID)	

* standard risk = common ALL antigen positive, low white count at presentation.

number of occasions do not survive as long as patients transplanted in first or second remission; the problem in multi-relapsed patients is recurrent leukaemia after the transplant.

It is also clear that not all patients in the same remission category do equally well after transplantation. Patients with acute lymphoblastic leukaemia presenting with a high white count and/or a non-common ALL antigen phenotype do relatively badly with chemotherapy; even if these patients attain a remission they tend to relapse early and a second remission may be particularly difficult to obtain. This has led several centres to transplant patients with these 'high risk' features early in the course of their disease. The detailed influence of remission status and stage of disease will be discussed later in the section on survival after transplantation.

A further important consideration at present is the age of the patient. Experience has shown that survival after transplantation varies with the age of the patient. In acute non-lymphoblastic leukaemia patients under 20 years of age have a 60% 2-year survival compared to 30% in patients under 30. The reason for this difference relates to the increased mortality from graft versus host disease in older patients. The exact cause for this is not fully understood, although it is felt that the involution of the thymus that accompanies aging may be important: however, attempts at thymic replacement have not been particularly successful. This consideration has led most centres to impose an age limit of 45 years.

Donor selection

A 'sine qua non' of allo BMT is the availability of a donor. The best results are obtained using a sibling who is fully matched at the HLA loci and non-reactive in mixed lymphocyte culture. Unfortunately the chance of a patient having such a sibling is only 1 in 3. If a patient is fortunate enough to have a choice of donors it is best to use the person who is the same sex and has a compatible ABO group. Transplantation between patients of opposite sexes is associated with a higher incidence of graft versus host disease. ABO blood group incompatibility between donor and recipient is not a barrier to successful transplantation. The patient can be plasmapheresed prior to transplant to lower the titre of antibody, or probably more conveniently the donor marrow can be depleted in vitro of its red cells by sedimentation techniques before infusion into the recipient.

The use of mismatched family members or matched non-family donors seems, at first sight, an attractive alternative for patients who lack a compatible sibling. As far as non-family members are concerned, there are two major registers in the UK (in London and Bristol) of individuals willing to donate marrow. The patients have been HLA, A & B typed but may not be DR typed; this means that once any potential compatible donors have been found, further testing (DR typing and eventually mixed lymphocyte culture) has to be carried out. The whole process is time-consuming and, if a large number of potential donors is screened, very expensive. Results from IOWA and Seattle indicate a 25% survival; at present it must be concluded that the use of non-family members for transplantation is not routine.

Two studies at least have evaluated transplantation using mismatched family members. In a series from the Marsden, Powles showed that only one-third of patients survived more than 6 months. Most patients experienced severe graft versus host disease and a number pulmonary oedema. By contrast the group from Seattle have recently reported similar survival for patients transplanted with mismatched family donors who were compared with a series of allogeneic transplants. However the Seattle patients were in the main only mismatched at one locus, whereas Powles patients were often mismatched at three loci. Furthermore, the survival of the allogeneic group to which the mismatched

Seattle patients were compared was rather short in comparison to other published data. Again it must be concluded that at present transplantation using other than HLA-identical donors should be considered experimental.

Pre-transplant procedures

Family interview

It is essential to interview the family and patient, usually on several occasions, to explain the procedure and in particular the hazards of BMT. This should be done in ample time before the BMT to allow the patient, donor and family to consider all the implications and allow clarification of any misunderstandings. As far as the donor is concerned the main risk is that of an anaesthetic and the family should be reassured that pre-transplant checks will be made on the donor to ensure he is fit for anaesthesia. Time in hospital is usually short (approximately 48 hours) and uncomplicated. The family should be told that the donor will quickly make up the donated marrow but it is common practice to venesect the donor one week before transplant so that he can be safely transfused at the time of donation with his own blood.

Some of the hazards of BMT will be well known to the majority of patients, in particular those associated with marrow hypoplasia. However, the problem of graft versus host disease must be discussed. Other parts of the procedure requiring mention are the insertion of a central line, the isolation policy, and the expected duration of in-patient stay (approximately 4 weeks). If radiotherapy is used as part of the conditioning the patient will lose his hair; a wig can be supplied and the patient reassured that his hair will regrow. The deleterious effect of the conditioning regimen on fertility should be explained. Obviously the complications of BMT must be put in the context of the potential benefit to the patient; those with chronic phase chronic myeloid leukaemia often have difficulty in understanding the seriousness of their situation, especially as clinically they may never have felt very ill. A further problem in this disease is the timing of the transplant: the best results are obtained when the patient is in chronic phase. Most centres therefore advise transplantation to be carried out as soon as is practical after the patient's white count has been brought under control.

Investigations

Following a full medical history and examination of the donor, pre transplant investigations are carried out as in

Table 21.2   Donor pre-transplant investigations

Full blood count
Biochemistry profile
Virology (CMV, HSV, HVZ titres)
HBs Ag
HIV serology
Blood group including genotype
Chest X-ray
ECG

Table 21.2. The purpose of these checks is to ensure the donor is fit for anaesthesia and to exclude a haematological abnormality or infection risk in the donor. If both donor and recipient do not have elevated titres to cytomegalovirus, then blood products should be given to the recipient from cytomegalovirus-negative donors.

Preparation of patient for transplantation

In the week prior to the patient receiving donor marrow several events occur

1. Remission status is checked by performing a bone marrow count and examination of the CSF
2. Measures to guard against infection are instituted (see Ch. 35)
3. A central line is inserted if one is not already in place
4. Chemotherapy is given with a view to immune suppression and cytotoxicity.
5. Total body irradiation is usually administered.

Conditioning regimens

For patients with acute leukaemia these constitute the treatment given to the patient prior to marrow infusion to ensure immunosuppression to allow graft acceptance and eradication of residual leukaemia. This treatment usually involves chemotherapy and radiotherapy (see Table 21.3). The most commonly used chemotherapeutic agent has been cyclophosphamide. This has been most frequently given in two doses at a dose of 60 mg/kg. In view of potential bladder toxicity of this regimen, intravenous fluids (2 l/m^2 per 24 h) must be given to ensure a good urine output. An accurate fluid and input and output chart must be established and the patient weighed 24-hourly. The urine is examined for red cells and the urea and electrolytes monitored every 12 hours. In addition, 2-mercaptoethane sulphonite sodium (mesnum) is given; this binds the toxic metabolite, acrolein, responsible for haemorrhagic cystitis. The dose for adults is 20% of the

Table 21.3   Examples of regimens used for cytoreduction in patients with leukaemias and lymphomas prior to BMT (auto or allo)

Regimen	Agents	Dosage
	Cyclophosphamide	60 mg/kg × 2
CY + TBI	Total body irradiation	
	a) Unfractionated	7.5–10 Gy
	b) Fractionated	10–12 Gy
BuCY	Busulphan	4 mg/m^2 × 4
	Cyclophosphamide	50 mg/m^2 × 4
HDM	Melphalan	120–175 mg/m^2 × 1
BEAM	Carmustine	300 mg/m^2 × 1
	VP16	75 mg/m^2 × 4
	Cytosine	200 mg/m^2 × 4
	Melphalan	140 mg/m^2 × 1 (day 4)
TACC	Thioguanine	200 mg/m^2 × 4
	Cytosine	200 mg/m^2 × 4
	Cyclophosphamide	45 mg/m^2 × 4
	Lomustine	200 mg × 1 (day 2)

cyclophosphamide given at 0, 4 and 8 hours. Children appear to eliminate mesnum more rapidly than adults; thus 40% of the cyclophosphamide dose should be given at the times indicated for adults.

Approximately 48 hours after the cyclophosphamide has been given the patient who is being transplanted for leukaemia receives radiotherapy. This can either be given as a single dose or fractionated over a number of days. If given as a single dose the radiation is either administered at a relatively fast rate (4–25 cGy/min) to a dose of 7.5–8 Gy or at a slower rate to a higher total dose (10 Gy). Fractionated treatment is given to a total dose of 12–14 Gy by doses per fraction varying from 200–600 cGy and fractionation intervals from 3 to 24 hours. This form of administration was introduced to reduce toxicity, in particular to the lung, and also to increase leukaemic cell kill. However, studies to date have not demonstrated a reduced incidence of leukaemic relapse in patients given fractionated radiotherapy; nor has a significant reduction in the frequency of interstitial pneumonitis been consistently seen, although radiation is only one of the factors aetiological in producing this complication (vide infra). Fractionated radiotherapy may, however, be generally better tolerated by the patients in terms of severity of mucositis, diarrhoea and parotitis. Long-term side effects of irradiation are infertility, which is universal, and cataract formation, which is correctable by surgery. The potential hazard of second malignancies in patients exposed to high dose chemoradiotherapy has not, as yet, been a significant problem.

Radiation in the form of total lymphoid irradiation is one of the techniques which has ensured engraftment in patients with aplastic anaemia who have been previously transfused. This may also be employed in the conditioning of patients who received marrow which has been T-cell-depleted (vide infra); marrows subjected to this treatment have a significant incidence of failure to engraft.

Patients with acute leukaemia have been conditioned with chemotherapy only; successful regimens have included the combination of busulpan (4 mg/kg daily for 4 days) and cyclophosphamide (50 mg/kg daily for 4 days) and the use of high dose melphalan (see Table 21.3).

Patients with aplastic anaemia undergoing transplantation do not require total body irradiation but should receive conditioning with 2 days of cyclophosphamide; further measures are required in multitransfused patients (vide infra).

Table 21.4   Preparation of patient for BMT using single dose total body irradiation

Day	Procedure
−5	Admission. Assessment of remission status – marrow, lumbar puncture
−4	Insertion of central line
−3	Isolation policy commenced; antimicrobials, antifungals, acyclovir begun
−2	Chemotherapy: cyclophosphamide and mesnum
−1	Chemotherapy: cyclophosphamide and mesnum
0	Total body irradiation Marrow infusion

The schedule of events in the week prior to transplant is shown in Table 21.4. A central line is inserted, if not already in situ, following which the isolation policy and other prophylactic measures against infection are commenced (Ch. 35). Chemotherapy and radiotherapy are then administered as shown in Table 21.4. The exact scheduling of the treatment is dependent on the conditioning regimen selected. Marrow is harvested from the donor on the day radiotherapy is completed; the donor is anaesthetised and heparinised and marrow is taken via multiple puncture sites from anterior and posterior iliac crests bilaterally. The aim is to collect 2–6 $\times 10^8$ cells/kg for infusion into the recipient. In the average adult donor this will entail removing 500–800 ml of marrow; this can then be infused directly into the donor. However, if there is an ABO incompatibility between donor and recipient, the red cells must be removed by centrifugation or sedimentation; similarly a mononuclear fraction would have to be separated if any

form of purging (e.g. T-cell depletion) was to be performed.

Complications following BMT

Early complications following BMT are conventionally those which occur during the first 100 days after infusion of the marrow and are listed in Table 21.5.

Table 21.5   Early (<100 days) complications of BMT

1. Cytopenia-related
2. Acute graft-versus-host disease (acute GVHD)
3. Interstitial pneumonitis
4. Non-engraftment

Cytopenia-related

Infections related to neutropenia are discussed in Chapter 4. The median time to reach a neutrophil count of >0.5 × 10⁹/l is 20 days in patients given methotrexate for GVHD prophylaxis and 14 days in those receiving cyclosporin. When the neutrophils are sustained at >0.5 × 10⁹/l the isolation policy can be discontinued.

Patients are supported with red cell and platelet transfusions. The value of prophylactic versus administration of platelets only when a thrombocytopenic patient bleeds is still controversial; however, most units give platelets prophylactically. Platelets, like red cell transfusions, should be irradiated (1500 rad) prior to their administration to prevent contaminating lymphocytes from causing GVHD. If the patient is cytomegalovirus-negative the blood products he receives should be from donors who are negative. The median time to reach a platelet count of >70 × 10⁹/l is 44 days in patients given methotrexate for GVHD prophylaxis and 29 days in those receiving cyclosporin. Consideration may have to be given to the use of HLA-matched platelets in donors who are bleeding and fail to have an increment to platelet infusion.

Acute GVHD

This syndrome represents the clinical manifestations of the interaction of immunocompetent donor cells with histocompatibility antigens of an immunosuppressed host; it occurs in 30–60% of patients undergoing BMT and is fatal in approximately 25% of these. Although its exact pathogenesis is not fully understood, T-cells from the donor are thought to play a crucial role; these may, by secreting lymphokines, recruit and activate other cells (e.g. natural killer cells). Predisposing factors are donor-recipient incompatibility, recipient age (increased incidence with greater age) and donor-recipient sex mismatch. In particular a male recipient of marrow from a female donor who has been transfused or has been pregnant is an especially high risk situation.

Acute GVHD can affect the skin, liver and gut, and usually commences sometime after the first week following transplant. The skin rash is macular and erythematous and often has a predilection for the palms and soles. It may disappear spontaneously or spread to involve the whole body and become a severe desquamative erythrodermia. Concomitant with or following the skin lesions, liver function abnormalities may occur; these take the form of hyperbilirubinaemia and cholestasis. Gut involvement consists of abdominal pain, nausea and diarrhoea. The diagnosis of acute GVHD can be confirmed by appropriate biopsy as characteristic changes are described. However, the histological appearances may be confounded by the influence of factors such as irradiation, infections and drug therapy. A further disorder that may affect the liver within the first month after BMT is veno-occlusive disease. This results in jaundice, ascites and eventually hepatic failure and is probably caused by high dose chemoradiotherapy. Histologically it should be distinguished from GVHD. The more severe forms of GVHD (Grade III and IV) are usually associated with intercurrent infections: the GVHD delays haematological reconstitution predisposing to infection.

The severe grades of GVHD require treatment with intravenous high dose methyl prednisolone. This should be given over one hour at a dose of 20 mg/kg every 12 hours for 48 hours and then the dose should be halved every 48 hours with clinical improvement. Vigorous antacid therapy should be given and the patient observed for the well known side effects of steroids (see Ch. 23), in particular hyperglycaemia. The response is good for the skin manifestations of GVHD with complete resolution in about half the cases; however gut and particularly liver GVHD respond much less satisfactorily. For those who fail on high dose steroids the outlook is poor; early encouraging reports of success with antithymocyte globulin have not been substantiated by more recent studies. A most important aspect of the management of a patient with severe acute GVHD is support; parenteral nutrition will often be required and infections are common and are the usual cause of mortality.

A number of methods have been introduced to try and prevent GVHD. Methotrexate was shown to be effective in dogs and has been widely used in the human BMT situation. Various regimens have been used, some including daily prednisolone during the first 3 months. The Seattle schedule uses 15 mg/m^2 iv. on day 1 and 10 mg/m^2 on days 3, 6, 11, 18 and 25 and then every 2 weeks until day 95. In a variant the methotrexate is given weekly. However, despite the use of methotrexate the incidence of acute GVHD is 50% in studies performed in Seattle and Minnesota. Indeed a report from Cleveland suggested that patients given no methotrexate compared favourably with a historic control group given that drug although other data support the use of GVHD prophylaxis. Attempts have been made to improve this rather dismal situation; Ramsey and colleagues in Minnesota reduced the incidence of GVHD to 21% by combining methotrexate with antithymocyte globulin and prednisolone. However, no survival difference was seen. Particular problems associated with the use of methotrexate are oral mucositis and delayed engraftment.

An immunosuppressive agent, cyclosporin A (CSA), has recently been widely used in BMT centres, particularly in Europe. This fungal metabolite has a selective action against post-thymic T-cells and has the advantage of lack of myelotoxicity. CSA prevents the synthesis of interleukin-2 by T-helper cells and in addition can reduce the responsiveness of cytotoxic T-lymphocyte precursors by inhibiting expression of interleukin-2 receptors. Several different administration schedules have been described. The protocol used at Seattle commences on day 1 with 1.5 mg/kg given i.v. every 12 hours until the patient has recovered from gastrointestinal toxicity related to conditioning, after which 6.25 mg/kg is given every 12 hours orally. The dose is slowly tapered after day 50 and discontinued after about 6 months of therapy. The major problem with cyclosporin usage is nephrotoxicity which is dose and plasma level-dependent. Accordingly levels should be measured at least twice weekly initially and radio-immunoassay kits and assays using high pressure liquid chromatography are available. The level of CSA can be affected by interaction with ketoconazole and phenytoin and its nephrotoxicity compounded by the use of nephrotoxic antimicrobials such as aminoglycosides. Levels taken 12 hours post-dose (trough) should be kept in the range agree with the laboratory and dependent on the assay used; adjustment must be made if the creatinine rise. Nephrotoxicity takes three main forms, the most common (80%) being an early reversible rise in urea and creatinine. Acute reversible renal failure has also been reported, as has the later occurrence of a micro-angiopathic haemolytic syndrome. Other side effects include hyperbilirubinaemia, abnormal hair and nail growth and neurological problems (tremor, myelopathy, cerebellar toxicity). In addition CSA is extremely expensive. The benefits for using CSA appear to be avoidance of the mucositis and myelotoxicity associated with methotrexate. The incidence of acute and chronic GVHD is not affected, although some data suggested the severity of the GVHD has been lessened. Faster engraftment is a very worthwhile benefit resulting in less use of blood product support, fewer febrile days and a reduction in hospital stay. The effect on engraftment is most clearly seen following BMT for aplastic anaemia. In previously transfused patients, Hows and her colleagues at the Hammersmith demonstrated engraftment in 21 out of 23 patients given CSA; in a historical control group given methotrexate, 26% failed to engraft and a similar number had late graft failure. The latter phenomenon has been seen when CSA is stopped in patients transplanted for aplastic anaemia and it is now recommended that CSA is continued for approximately 9 months in this situation. Recently a trial has been reported from Seattle comparing in a prospective randomised fashion CSA and CSA combined with methotrexate. A previous trial from that centre comparing CSA and methotrexate had failed to show a significant difference in GVHD or survival. However the combination of CSA and methotrexate did appear to significantly reduce the incidence of GVHD and influence survival. Only 3 of the 43 patients given CSA and methotrexate developed grade III GVHD, while none developed grade IV disease compared to 6 and 7 patients respectively out of the 50 patients given CSA alone. As might have been expected, there were more problems with mucositis and delay in recovery of granulocyte count with combined prophylaxis. A recent update of this study shows that the benefit appears to be confined to patients with chronic myeloid leukaemia; patients with acute myeloid leukaemia had a higher relapse rate. The combination of CSA and methotrexate also appears effective in reducing acute GVHD in patients transplanted for aplastic anaemia.

These data have to be compared with the results of the other recent approach to GVHD prevention, T-cell depletion. With the availability of monoclonal antibodies to T-cells it is possible to try and reduce GVHD by removing the cells which are felt to be important in its pathogenesis. The most popular approach has involved the in vitro treatment of the marrow prior to its infusion. This usually relies on the T-cell cytopathic effect of a monoclonal T-cell antibody, e.g. Campath I (or a cocktail of antibodies) and complement, although antibody linked to ricin and soya bean agglutinin has been used. T-cell depletion does appear to significantly reduce the incidence of GVHD and any that does occur is usually mild; furthermore a reduction in chronic GVHD is seen. However, a particular problem associated with this technique is graft failure, which occurs in approximately 10% of transplants involving fully matched donors, rising to over 50% in cases of HLA non-identity. The explanation for this may lie in the ability of donor T-cells to suppress the recipient's response to an infusion of marrow. Increasing the immunosuppression given pre-transplant (e.g. with total nodal irradiation) may result in less graft failure. A further difficulty which has recently been reported is an apparent increased incidence of leukaemic relapse in patients receiving T-cell-depleted marrows for chronic myeloid leukaemia and probably acute leukaemia. Thus, although T-cell depletion seems a powerful tool to prevent GVHD, its use is associated with considerable problems. Experience will define the best situations for its use – possibly patients who are at maximum risk for GVHD- and at present it would certainly seem wise to consider using alternative prophylaxis (e.g. CSA and methotrexate) in chronic myeloid leukaemia until more data are available.

A potential benefit of GVHD might be its association with a graft versus leukaemia effect. An increased incidence of leukaemic relapse has been reported in patients who do not develop acute or chronic GVHD. However, Seattle data on 204 patients with acute non-lymphoblastic leukaemia transplanted between 1976 and 1984 did not show a lower incidence of relapse in patients with severe acute GVHD. Patients with chronic graft versus host disease, on the other hand, do appear to have a lower incidence of relapse; a recent series from Italy demonstrated in addition a survival advantage, with 73% of patients with chronic GVHD being alive and disease-free at 2 years compared to a 36% survival in those without chronic GVHD. The most recent data from Seattle shows a reduced relapse rate and increased survival in patients with acute leukaemia transplanted in relapse and patients with chronic myeloid leukaemia transplanted post chronic phase who develop chronic GVHD. Patients with acute lymphoblastic leukaemia in first remission or chronic myeloid leukaemia in chronic phase who developed GVHD had a poorer survival.

Interstitial pneumonitis

This is a very serious complication of BMT occurring in up to 30% of cases transplanted for acute leukaemia, with a mortality rate of 80%. It tends to occur in the second and third month after transplant and is characterised pathologically by thickening of the alveolar wall with intra-alveolar haemorrhage oedema and hyaline membrane formation.

The causes are multifactorial; however, in most series 50–60% of cases are labelled idiopathic although chemoradiotherapy is felt to be involved. The remainder of cases are due to infections, cytomegalovirus accounting for the majority of these, with pneumocystis carinii, herpes simplex and varicella-zoster, and fungi also being documented. A recent large multicentre analysis by the International Bone Marrow Transplant Registry reviewing fully matched transplants for leukaemia sought to delineate risk factors. Patients transplanted relatively soon after diagnosis, who were prepared with total body irradiation at a slow dose rate (approximately 4 cGy per minute) and were given CSA to prevent GVHD had an 11% incidence. 36% of those transplanted later, who were given methotrexate and radiotherapy at a faster rate, developed interstitial pneumonitis. No protective effect was demonstrated in this series for fractionated irradiation but older patients and those with more severe GVHD were at increased risk.

The diagnosis should be confirmed by biopsy as discussed in Chapter 35. The management of idiopathic interstitial pneumonitis is wholly unsatisfactory, there being no definitive treatment, although benefit has been reported with steroid therapy. The management of the infectious cause of interstitial pneumonitis will be discussed in Chapter 35. Cytomegalovirus is the most common causative pathogen and the best treatment is prevention. A very low infection rate is found when a cytomegalovirus-negative patient and donor are involved and only cytomegalovirus-negative blood products are given to the recipient. In cytomegalovirus-positive recipients there may be a protective effect from receiving marrow from a cytomegalovirus-positive donor.

Failure of engraftment

This is thought to be due to residual recipient cytotoxic T-lymphocytes although a role for natural killer cells is also proposed. Generally the incidence is very low in fully matched recipients transplanted for acute leukaemia. However, the incidence rises in HLA-non-identical transplants, and in patients whose donor marrow has been depleted of T-cells.

In contradistinction to the above failure of engraftment and late rejection are very significant problems in patients transplanted for aplastic anaemia. Approximately half of previously transfused patients will experience these complications; avoidance of transfusion prior to transplantation can ensure engraftment. This is a difficult and potentially dangerous policy to institute and various regimens have been tried to ensure engraftment. Modified total body irradiation, total lymphoid irradiation and infusion of donor buffy coat cells have all been successful. The use of CSA has been shown to ensure engraftment but the occurrence of graft failure when the drug has been stopped has resulted in the recommendation that it be given for a longer period than when it is used in acute leukaemia.

Table 21.6 Manifestations (%) in patients with extensive chronic GVHD

Cutaneous	95–100	Contractures	40
Abnormal liver function tests	90	Oesophagitis	35
Dry mouth/mucositis	85	Serositis	20
Dry eyes	80	Enteritis	20
Bacterial infections	70	Myositis	10
Weight loss	50		

Chronic graft versus host disease (chronic GVHD)

Chronic GVHD occurs in 25–45% of patients who survive for more than 100 days following a BMT from a fully matched sibling. It is a multisystem disease, but can be found in localised forms involving only the skin or hepatic dysfunction. The incidences of the major manifestations in extensive chronic GVHD are shown in Table 21.6.

Older patients and those with a history of grade II–IV acute GVHD appear to be at increased risk for chronic GVHD. Changes affecting the skin are almost universal; the changes often commence with dryness and scaling of the skin which develops into areas of hyperpigmentation and/or hypopigmentation. If the process is not arrested, thickening of the skin ensues and contractures can result. Alopecia may occur, as may nail changes. Liver function test abnormalities include hyperbilirubinaemia as well as elevation of liver enzymes; hepatic failure is uncommon. Dryness of the eyes and mouth are other troublesome, common complaints. The diagnosis can be made most readily by skin biopsy. Treatment of patients with extensive chronic GVHD and normal platelet counts can be effective with prednisolone alone. The addition of azathioprine results in more infection and a poorer survival. Patients with chronic GVHD and platelets counts of less than $100 \times 10^9/l$ fare poorly on prednisolone alone and survival is increased by an alternating daily regimen of prednisolone and CSA. Infection prophylaxis with cotrimoxazole is important.

Outcome following BMT

A number of factors potentially affect the survival of patients following BMT. The disease status at the time of the procedure is most important, as is the age of the recipient. It is important to consider these when evaluating results from different centres where patients may have received differing conditioning and GVHD prevention regimens. Table 21.7 lists the 2–3 year survival figures for the disease at present treated commonly by allogeneic BMT. The figures represent the result of a

Table 21.7 Outcome of patients transplanted for the leukaemias or aplastic anaemia at 2–3 years

Disease	Status at BMT	Survival %	Relapse %
Acute non-lymphoblastic leukaemia	CR1	50	12–35
	CR2	30	
	CR2+	25	25
Acute lymphoblastic leukaemia	CR1	50	5
	CR2	35	34
	CR2+	20	73
Chronic myeloid leukaemia	CP	65	10
	Post-CP	20	60
Aplastic anaemia	Severe	60	

number of series from the major centres and collaborative groups. A trend towards poorer survival and a definitely increased relapse rate is seen when patients are transplanted following recurrent disease. Thus, although most patients with acute lymphoblastic leukaemia have been transplanted in second remission, the poorer results in adults have prompted several centres to transplant in first remission. As the numbers are small it has been difficult to demonstrate a benefit for the group as a whole. However, patients in high risk categories (e.g. high white count) probably do better, and of course patients may not necessarily obtain a second remission following relapse. More data are required but small studies of patients in first remission from acute lymphoblastic leukaemia have shown excellent survival results with a very low relapse rate. Results of BMT have to be assessed against the response that can be obtained with chemotherapy. Truly randomised trials are not possible, as all patients do not have a donor, but a large centre can use a group of patients treated with chemotherapy during the same period of study as controls. Four such studies have been reported from Los Angeles, Seattle, London and Houston. All agree that BMT offers the greater opportunity to avoid relapsed disease. For example, in the series reported from Champlin at UCLA there was a 40% relapse rate in the transplant group compared to a rate of 70% in the chemotherapy arm. Despite this no difference in survival was noted due to the morbidity of transplant-related complications. The group from the Marsden do feel their data show a survival advantage following BMT. A survival advantage can be demonstrated in the Seattle and Houston studies but the significance depends on the way the various groups of patients are analysed. The problem will be difficult to solve because of the innate inability to conduct a truly randomised

trial and the changing situation as regards improved results with chemotherapy and control of complications of BMT such as GVHD.

Patients treated with chemotherapy following relapse of acute lymphoblastic leukaemia, although often obtaining a remission, are seldom long-term survivors. BMT has been reported to offer the best chance of long-term survival in this situation, although a recent study from London showed no such benefit. The treatment of chronic myeloid leukaemia with chemotherapy has failed to alter the natural history of the disease with its inevitable progression to acute leukaemia. BMT can eradicate Philadelphia chromosome positive cells from the bone marrow and the results of transplantation in the chronic phase are very encouraging with a 69% three year actuarial survival.

Patients with severe aplastic anaemia treated only with supportive care have a 70% mortality; BMT dramatically reverses this figure. Encouraging results have been obtained recently with antithymocyte globulin, although only partial haematological responses are often obtained; this therapy is however very useful for older patients and those without a donor.

The future

Despite the world usage of allogeneic BMT many serious problems require to be solved. As patients are followed for longer periods an increased relapse rate has been found compared to the small earlier series. Superior conditioning schedules are being evaluated. The relative values and problems of the more recently described anti-GVHD prophylactic regimens – T-cell depletion and the combination of CSA and methotrexate – need to be defined and new approaches sought. New approaches to the treatment of cytomegalovirus pneumonitis and the use of colony-stimulating factors to shorten the cytopenic period may reduce the morbidity and mortality from infections. The problem of small family size in the Western world limits the availability of fully compatible sibling donors. Methods (e.g. using extended haplotyping) need to be developed to improve donor selection. Promising results have appeared in small studies involving transplantation in Hodgkin's disease, non-Hodgkin's lymphoma, myelodysplasia, storage and immunodeficiency disease; the list of disease in which BMT has been tried is increasing and the results require to be analysed critically.

AUTOLOGOUS BONE MARROW TRANSPLANTATION (auto BMT)

In the last 5 years tremendous interest has developed in the use of the patient's own marrow as rescue from the myelodestructive effects of high dose cytotoxic therapy. The concept has many appealing features: no donor is required, older patients can be treated and there should be no problem with graft rejection or GVHD. As with allogeneic BMT this technique will only be successful in patients with tumours that respond to chemotherapy/ radiotherapy. Thus this treatment has been used for the leukaemias, lymphomas and a number of other solid tumours. Marrow obviously has to be removed from the patient prior to the commencement of the cytotoxic treatment, which if given over several days necessitates freezing and storage of the marrow. This is technically feasible but requires considerable expertise. A major concern with auto BMT is that the patient's marrow may harbour residual disease.

Marrow harvest, manipulation and storage

The technique of bone marrow harvest and the general support of the patient is similar to that employed for allogeneic BMT except no GVHD prophylaxis is required. Decisions have to be made concerning the type of cytoreduction regimen to use which will determine the method of marrow storage. Various high dose cytoreductive schedules have been used (Table 21.3), some using chemotherapy alone, others the combination of chemotherapy and radiotherapy. Marrow stored at 4°C for 48–72 hours will reconstitute the marrow following reinfusion. The conditioning regimen has to be given during this short period of storage. Suitable protocols involve cyclophosphamide 60 mg/kg ×2 and radiotherapy or the use of high doses of an agent such as melphalan (140 mg/m^2) which has a short half-life. If any of the more complicated regimens are given, then the marrow will have to be stored frozen. The steps in this process are as follows: The marrow is concentrated to its buffy coat on a cell separator to which is added a freezing solution principally containing the cryopreservative agent DMSO. The marrow is cooled at a controlled rate of 1–3°C/minute; programmable apparatus for controlled-rate freezing is commercially available. The marrow is then stored in liquid nitrogen at −196°C until required. Prior to reinfusion the marrow should be thawed rapidly (40°C) and infused immediately to avoid toxicity from the DMSO. Progenitor cell studies should be carried out to monitor the kinetics of engraftment in auto BMT. A number of stem cell assays have been used but a dose of 10^3 CFU-GM/Kg appears to ensure efficient engraftment.

Most recently successful reports of engraftment have followed infusion of progenitor cells collected from peripheral blood by leukopheresis. It had long been appreciated that blood from patients with chronic myeloid leukaemia contains large numbers of stem cells and its infusion would result in marrow reconstitution. Successful engraftment following infusion of stem cells from the peripheral blood of patients with acute leukaemia, in remission recovering from the effects of chemotherapy, has recently been demonstrated. The theoretical possibility that fewer malignant stem cells may be present in a peripheral blood harvest remains to be proven by clinical studies.

If it were felt appropriate, purging of the marrow would be carried out on the buffy coat prior to its cryopreservation. The aim of purging in auto BMT is to remove the malignant cells whilst leaving normal stem cells intact. The two main methods employed are the use of monoclonal antibodies or pharmacological agents. The former depends on the presence of a tumour-specific protein; thus antibodies are available against lymphoblasts which are T or common ALL antigen positive. However, no specific antibody is available to selectively remove abnormal cells from the marrow of patients with acute or chronic myeloid leukaemia. A variety of methods are used to ensure cytotoxicity, including the addition of complement and the conjugation of the antibody to the toxin ricin. Apart from the non-availability of monoclonals for certain leukaemias, other disadvantages of this approach include the toxicity of complement to normal cells, the non-expression of the particular antigen by a variable proportion of the cells in the marrow, and antigenic modulation. Some of these problems can be at least partially overcome by using a combination of monoclonals. In view of the problems and lack of general applicability of the antibody approach, pharmacological purging has been evaluated. Most available data involve the use of 4-hydroperoxycyclophosphamide (4HC) which is an analogue of 4-hydroxycyclophosphamide, one of the cytotoxic metabolites of cyclophosphamide. 4HC can be reduced to hydroxycyclophosphamide inside cells but normal haemopoietic precursors may be less sensitive due to the presence of aldehyde dehydrogenase which inactivates hydroxycyclophosphamide. Animal experiments have demonstrated the efficacy of this compound although, as expected, the dosage of 4HC employed was critical: too low a dose and the animals died of leukaemia; too high a dose and marrow failure results. Interestingly, toxicity to CFU-C or CFU-GM does not appear to correlate with the ability of the treated marrow to subsequently engraft. The problems associated with marrow purging have led a number of groups to explore the use of auto BMT for acute leukaemia using unpurged marrow, fully realising that the latter may well contain residual leukaemia cells. Certainly the cytoreductive conditioning should decrease the leukaemic load and one could speculate that there might be a survival advantage for normal progenitors over the leukaemic clone when the marrow harvest is given to the patient. In an effort to maximise any such advantage, repetition of the whole procedure (after recovery) has been advocated. In practice, getting a patient through 'double' auto BMT has proved difficult, although the concept of in vivo purging of the second harvested marrow has appeal.

Clinical results of auto BMT acute leukaemia

In the case of acute myeloid leukaemia in first remission a number of small series have been reported. These have included a variety of cytoreductive regimes (chemotherapy alone or with TBI): patients were treated at varying time intervals from diagnosis and results have been reported using purged and unpurged marrow. Recently data collected from 18 European centres have been presented by the European Bone Marrow Transplantation Group (EBMTG). In acute non-lymphoblastic leukaemia 2-year relapse-free rates were superior for patients transplanted in first remission (67%) compared to those in second remission (41%). No effect was noted that was attributable to purging. However, promising results have been reported on small numbers of patients in second and third complete remission from acute non-lymphoblastic leukaemia treated in Baltimore with autologous marrow treated with 4HC.

In acute lymphoblastic leukaemia the actuarial relapse-free rate at 2–years was similar in the study from the EBMTG for patients transplanted in first (56%) and second remission (55%). Encouraging results have been reported using purging with anti-CALLA antibody, with one-third of patients continuing in remission mostly for over 1 year.

A study from Minnesota compared autologous and allogeneic transplantation in patients with high risk disease. Post-transplantation relapse was the major problem and an estimate of those likely to be 'cured' was not significantly different for either group (20 and 27%).

Generally auto BMT appears well tolerated with a procedure-related mortality of less than 10%. Recovery is delayed compared to allogeneic BMT, with an average time to a granulocyte count of $>0.5 \times 10^9/l$ of 21 days and a platelet count of $>50 \times 10^9/l$ of 27 days.

More data are still required, particularly in view of the heterogeneous nature of the patients treated in terms of risk factors, the types of conditioning regimens, and the influence or lack of effect of the different modalities of purging. Few, if any, of the trials to date have been controlled. The Medical Research Council has recently embarked on a study which randomises patients in first CR from acute myeloid leukaemia to an arm using auto BMT.

Autografting using cryopreserved cells from the peripheral blood of patients with chronic myeloid leukaemia in chronic phase has been used when patients entered blast cell transformation. Results from the Hammersmith group demonstrate that, although the patients were restored to chronic phase, relapse was the rule and the median duration of survival was only 26 weeks. The same group has autografted a small number of patients in chronic phase; the occasional patient achieved a negative Philadephia chromosome status.

Lymphomas

Many studies have now demonstrated the feasibility of auto BMT in non-Hodgkin's lymphomas (NHL). NHL is particularly heterogeneous as regards prognosis, which depends on a number of factors including histological grading, age, disease bulk, extranodal involvement and the presence of constitutional symptoms. Auto BMT has been tried at various stages of disease activity usually in intermediate or high-grade cases. The trials have used a variety of conditioning regimens and some have used purged marrow. Analysis of the available data has revealed a higher relapse rate in patients treated with more advanced, less chemotherapy-sensitive disease. A multicentre study had a zero 3-year survival in patients with disease refractory to primary conventional therapy, whereas those whose relapsed disease was still sensitive had a 36% actuarial three year survival. A study from the USA, which treated only patients with minimal disease after conventional therapy, indicated a 65% probability of disease-free survival for more than 11 months post-BMT.

Fewer patients with Hodgkin's disease have been treated with auto BMT. A variety of conditioning regimens have yielded a complete remission rate of around 50%. A relatively higher procedure mortality has been noted in some series compared to other auto BMT situations, probably reflecting that most patients have been heavily pretreated. Patient follow up is relatively short; the Bloomsbury Transplant Group report that 75% of their patients who achieved complete remission remain in treatment-free continuous remission with a median follow-up of 18 months. Better results should be obtained by improved patient selection and conditioning regimens as poor performance status and bulky disease have been identified as adverse risk factors. Marrow purging is usually less of an issue due to the low incidence of marrow involvement.

Future work will hopefully define the patient groups which will benefit from auto BMT and the optimal timing of the procedure, and will evaluate its efficacy compared to conventional chemotherapy and allogeneic BMT. Patients who have poor prognostic features may benefit from an auto BMT early in their disease. Large collaborative studies will be required to answer these questions. New in vitro techniques will be developed; an exciting recent finding has been ability of non-leukaemic clones to assume a survival advantage in long-term culture. Thus marrow infused following such culture may have been 'self purged', although it is possible that, as with an ex vivo procedure, the integrity of the stem cells has been altered and further work is obviously required to test the efficacy and toxicity of this approach. The use of growth factors to aid marrow reconstitution may be a significant advance in reducing morbidity and mortality from infections.

BIBLIOGRAPHY

Deeg H J, Storb R, Thomas E D 1984 Bone marrow transplantation: a review of delayed complications. British Journal of Haematology 57: 185–208

Forman S J, Blume K G 1984 Bone marrow transplantation for leukaemia. In: Goldman J, Priesler H D (Eds) Ch in haematology. 1: Leukaemias. Butterworth, p 322

Gale R P et al 1987 Risk factors for acute graft-versus-host disease. British Journal of Haematology 67: 397–406

Goldstone A H 1986 Autologous bone marrow transplantation. Clinics in Haematology 15 (1)

Gorin N C et al 1986 Autologous bone marrow transplantation for acute leukaemia in remission. British Journal of Haematology 64: 385–395

Kendra J et al 1981 Response of graft-versus-host disease to high doses of methylprednisolone. Clinical and Laboratory Haematology 3: 19–26

Petersen F B, Buckner C D 1987 Allogeneic and autologous bone marrow transplantation for acute leukaemia and malignant lymphoma: current status. Haematological Oncology 5(4): 233–245

Storb R et al 1986 Methotrexate and cyclosporine combined with cyclosporine alone for prophylaxis of acute graft-versus-host disease after marrow transplant for leukaemia. New England Journal of Medicine 314: 729–735

Sullivan K M, Witherspoon R P, Storb R et al 1988 Prednisone and azathioprine compared with prednisone and placebo for treatment of chronic graft-v-host disease: prognostic influence of prolonged thrombocytopenia after allogeneic marrow transplantation. Blood 72: 546–554

Weiner R S et al 1985 Risk factors associated with interstitial pneumonitis following allogeneic bone marrow transplantation for leukaemia. Transplantation Proceedings XVII: 470–474

22. Compromised host defence

K. S. Froebel   S. J. Urbaniak

The immune system is increasingly recognised to be a complex network of inter-reacting effector and controlling mechanisms. In this chapter we review the main immune defence mechanisms as they apply to clinical immunology. For simplicity we have subdivided the immune system into 1) the largely non-specific phagocytic system and 2) the specific humoral and the cell-mediated systems. A brief discussion of the complement system has been included in the section on humoral immunity. The reader will be aware, however, that there are multiple sites at which immune cells of one 'system' interact with cells or with soluble factors from another 'system'; thus the subdivisions are by no means independent of each other.

The present state of clinical immunology is such that, apart from the gross defects which, unless treated, are generally incompatible with survival beyond infancy, an immune deficiency is likely to be partial or secondary to another form of therapy and thus predispose an individual towards infections or neoplasms. Moreover, since immune deficiencies are comparatively rare, more sophisticated tests are not likely to be generally available but may be offered in the context of a research interest of a particular department. The tests may not be diagnostic but the results may augment a clinical impression and favour a particular approach to treatment. As even the basic immunological tests are time-consuming, samples usually need to be arranged in advance, and taken to fit in with the requirements of the laboratory.

It is our aim that after reading this chapter the clinician will have enough background understanding of the scope and limitations of clinical immune investigations to rationally and effectively use such services as are available.

THE PHAGOCYTIC SYSTEM

Phagocytosis is probably the most important but least apparent form of first-line immune defence in that phagocytic cells provide an ongoing surveillance system,

Table 22.1 Functions of the phagocytic cells

Function	Consequence
Neutrophils	
1. Phagocytosis	Removal of microorganisms and cellular debris
2. Migration	Rapid accumulation at a site of infection or trauma
3. Release of IL-1	Stimulation of inflammation, vasodilation, stimulation of cell-mediated immune system
4. Cytotoxicity	Killing of ingested microorganisms
Monocyte/Macrophages	
1. Phagocytosis	In situ for removal of microorganisms and cellular debris
2. Migration	Accumulate at site of infection in response to chemotactic factors released by neutrophils
3. Antigen presentation	Stimulates lymphocyte responses
4. Release of IL-1	Stimulates T-helper cell response
5. Cytotoxicity	Killing of ingested microorganisms Killing of tumour cells (dependent on lymphokine) Killing of antibody-coated target cells

scavenging invading organisms before they are able to colonise the host's body tissues (Table 22.1) Phagocytosis is mediated by two types of cell: the neutrophil, which is short-lived, spending in total about 10 hours in the bloodstream, and the monocyte/macrophage, which is long-lived and, apart from the blood monocyte, is located predominantly in the tissues in a variety of sessile and mobile forms. The ways in which the two cell types phagocytose organisms and cellular debris appear to be similar, although because of ease of access most in vitro investigations are carried out on blood-derived neutrophils.

Neutrophil functions important for effective phagocytosis

Migration to site of infection or inflammation

Neutrophils react to inflammation by responding to the

chemotactic properties of the complement components C3a and C5a and, with an extraordinary ability to contort themselves between cells, arrive rapidly and in vast numbers at a site of inflammation. The migratory properties of neutrophils are related to a group of membrane antigens associated with adhesion: CR3 (the receptor for the inactivated C3b), LFA-1 (lymphocyte-associated antigen) and a protein whose precise function is unknown, p 150.95. These antigens are heterodimers consisting of identical β subunits and distinct α subunits.

Binding of the organism to the neutrophil

This takes place via one of three surface receptors:

1. A non-specific receptor which can bind organisms directly
2. A receptor for the Fc-region of immunoglobulin which binds to the antibody part of an antibody-antigen complex
3. A receptor for the C3b component of complement (the CR1 receptor) which binds antigen-antibody-complement complexes.

The non-specific receptor is the least efficient of the three in terms of its binding avidity, but is arguably the most important since it can remove opportunistic organisms before they become clinically relevant. Binding via the CR1 receptor requires pre-activation of specific or cross-reacting antibody and is thus only a first line of defence if antibody is already present. Binding via the CR1 creceptor requires pre-activation of the complement cascade to generate C3b. The CR1 and Fc-receptors act synergistically, so enabling the binding of a target organism when the concentration of antibody is insufficient to effect binding alone.

Opsonising ability of plasma

The opsonising ability of antibody in the patient's serum varies considerably among individuals in a way that is poorly understood, but any investigation of phagocytic deficiency should be carried out in both the patient's and a control or standard reference serum. Phagocytosis takes place when pseudopods from the macrophage or neutrophil extend around the bound organism, fusing so as to engulf it in a discrete cellular vacuole known as a phagosome. The phagosome then fuses with the lysosomal granules present in the cytoplasm to form a phagolysosome.

Destruction of the ingested organism

Killing of an organism takes place within the phagolysosome by either an oxygen-independent or an oxygen-dependent mechanism. The oxygen-independent pathways are associated with broadly cytotoxic proteins present in neutrophil granules including collagenase, lysozyme and a group of low molecular weight proteins termed 'defensins'. Oxygen-dependent killing is associated with a respiratory burst, an oxidative pathway unique to neutrophils which involves the consumption of oxygen and glucose and the generation of highly reactive products: superoxide anions (O_2-) hydrogen peroxide (H_2O_2) and hydroxyl radicals $(.OH)$. The antimicrobial activity of H_2O_2 is probably due to the myeloperoxidase and chloride-dependent conversion to hypochlorous acid:

$$H_2O_2 + Cl^- + H^+ \rightarrow H_2O + HOCl$$

Other functions

Phagocytic cells have a number of important additional functions. Under certain conditions they have the ability to kill target cells by cytolytic mechanisms. Macrophages can be activated by a lymphokine released by activated T-cells to kill tumour cells. Peripheral blood monocytes can be cytotoxic in vitro in an antibody dependent reaction in which target cells coated with IgG antibody bind to the Fc-receptor of the monocyte. The importance of these mechanisms in host defence is unknown. Macrophages which have the HLA class II or DR antigen on their surface act as antigen-presenting cells, processing and displaying the antigen to the lymphoid immune system. When activated, they synthesise and release a group of molecules known collectively as interleukin-1 (IL-1), which in turn activates both the cell-mediated immune system via the T-helper cells, and the inflammatory system.

Investigation of the phagocytic system

The number of circulating neutrophils should be ascertained; this test should be repeated as an abnormality may be a consequence of disease and not the cause. A count of less than 0.5×10^9 neutrophils per litre of blood can lead to serious infections and a count of less than 0.2×10^9 per litre is likely to result in overwhelming life-threatening infection. In cyclic neutropenia, the number of neutrophils falls approximately every 21 d.

Most aspects of phagocytic function can be investigated (Table 22.2). Chemotaxis is measured in vitro by measuring the movement of neutrophils towards an agent such as C5a or in vivo by measuring their rate of accumulation at a site of abrasion – the 'skin window' test. The presence of membrane antigens associated with

Table 22.2   Investigation of neutrophils

Numbers and morphology

1. Count a) Raised
          b) Reduced

2. Morphology: presence/absence of large cytoplasmic granules
          a) Peroxidase stain: demonstrates azurophilic granules
          b) Wright's stain: demonstrates neutrophil-specific granules

3. Presence/absence of neutrophil-specific antigens

Function

1. Chemotaxis a) in vitro
              b) in vivo 'skin window'

2. Phagocytosis/killing in a) control serum
                          b) patient's serum

3. Reduction of NBT

4. Myeloperoxidase activity

5. Chemiluminescence

---

adhesiveness can be determined using monoclonal antibodies and fluorescence microscopy. Phagocytosis and killing should, if possible, be tested in relation to the organism against which the patient is particularly susceptible. This can be done microscopically by differential staining of live and dead organisms, either in a preparation in which the neutrophil can also be seen (to determine the amount of phagocytosis in relation to killing) or after removal of non-phagocytosed organisms. This latter approach is generally difficult because of the tendency for organisms to adhere to the surface of the neutrophil, but is useful for *Staphylococcus aureus*, as externally-bound bacteria can be removed by lysozyme. Phagocytosis should be determined in both a standard control serum and the patient's serum. Opsonisation and killing mechanisms can be investigated by measuring the production of superoxide to different stimuli, either in an automated assay, such as chemiluminescence, or in a simple slide test, by the reduction of yellow nitroblue tetazolium (NBT) to a blue formazan precipitate. Myeloperoxidase activity can be determined semiquantitavely using the 'Nadi' reagent on formalin fixed smears.

THE LYMPHOID SYSTEM

Lymphocytes are mediators of the adaptive or specific immune responses. A small pool of B$^-$ and/or T-lymphocytes is activated by an antigen; the pool expands by cell proliferation and differentiates to effect a response which is specific for the antigen. Suppressor T-cells eventually curtail the response, but a subpopulation of lymphocytes remains in the circulation as long-lived memory cells which, upon reactivation respond much more rapidly and more specifically to the same antigen.

The lymphoid system has two major compartments, the humoral, qr B-cell compartment, which responds to antigen by making specific antibody, and the cell-mediated compartment which covers all the immune responses mediated by T-lymphocytes.

Humoral immunity

The humoral, or antibody, response is the most important means of specific defence against bacteria. Pre B-cells go through a series of maturation steps before becoming mature B-cells capable of responding to antigen. Mature B-cells have on their surface membrane-bound immunoglobulin antibody molecules, the binding sites of which are specific for the antigen to which a particular cell is programmed to respond. When a B-cell meets and binds to its antigen, the cross-linking of the surface immunoglobulin molecules triggers the next stage of maturation. The B-cell replicates and differentiates into a clone of antibody-secreting plasma cells. In the primary response to antigen, antibody is predominantly of the IgM class. During activation rearrangement of the antibody-producing genes takes place resulting in a class switch to IgG. Any subsequent stimulation of memory B-cells (the final maturational stage) triggers the synthesis and release predominantly of IgG.

At its simplest, antibody acts by binding to the attachment sites of a microorganism and thus 'neutralising' it. Once bound, IgM antibody fixes complement and facilitates complement-mediated lysis of the organism (see below). IgG antibody is less efficient at fixing complement but facilitates the phagocytosis of microorganisms via the Fc-receptor on neutrophils and macrophages.

Complement

Complement is the name given to a group of proteins which, when activated, form part of a chain or cascade reaction, resulting in the lysis of target cells. The cascade is activated by one of two routes, the classical or the alternative pathway. Both lead to the cleavage and activation of the C3 component and eventually to the formation of a membrane-bound complex (C5–9) that lyses the cell to which it is bound.

Antibody and complement act very much in concert (hence the name). Antibody-antigen complexes, particularly of IgM but also IgGI and IgG3, activate the complement cascade and so promote destruction of the mircoorganism, either by direct lysis by the terminal complement complex C5–9, or by phagocytosis by binding of the complex to the CR1 receptor of the phagocyte. Neutrophils gather at the site of activation in response to the chemotactic properties of the C5a component of the complement cascade.

Investigation of humoral immunity

Investigation of humoral immunity should include both the B-cell/antibody system and the complement system (Table 22.3).

Table 22.3 Investigation of humoral immunity

1. Serum antibody and complement levels:
   Immunoglobulin classes
   IgG subclasses
   Isohaemagglutinins
   Complement components

2. In vivo antibody production:
   Specific immunisation with e.g. tetanus toxoid

3. Activation of complement cascade:
   CH50
   APH50

4. B-cells:
   Count SIg or CD19/20 positive cells
   In-vitro stimulation of immunoglobulin synthesis

The B-cell/antibody system

Measurement of isohaemagglutinins, the naturally occurring antibodies that cross-react with a range of environmental organisms, total serum immunoglobulins, particularly IgG, IgM and IgA and, if available, the IgG subclasses, will establish whether there is a total or a specific defect in antibody production. The relative importance of the IgG subclasses is not well understood, but IgG$_2$ may be particularly important in the defence against the polysaccharide capsular antigens on some bacteria. If a B-cell deficiency is suspected, the patient's ability to make new antibody in response to specific immunisation with, for instance, tetanus toxoid, may be determined.

Following these serological tests, the B-cells themselves may be investigated. B-cells normally represent 5–15% of circulating blood lymphocytes and can be identified using a specific antibody, either to their membrane surface immunoglobulin (SIg) or to one of the B-cell-specific antigens, followed by a fluorescein or enzyme conjugated second antibody. Using membrane immunoglobulin as the surface marker may give falsely high counts unless steps are taken to remove adsorbed

immunoglobulin, and to prevent non-specific binding of aggregates in the antibody. There are a number of B-cell-specific antigens, most of which are expressed at restricted stages of maturation (and are therefore useful for typing B-cell leukaemias) but two antigens, the CD19 and CD20 antigens (also known as B1 and B4) are weakly expressed at all stages of maturation.

The complement system

An investigation of possible complement deficiency should, if possible, distinguish between the two routes of activation. The CH5O and APH5O tests respectively measure the turnover of haemolytic complement activated by the classical and alternative pathways. A negative result in both indicates a deficiency in a component of the terminal lytic complex. Serum levels of several of the complement components may be measured, some of which are specific for one or other pathway: C2 and C4 are specific for the classical pathway, factor B is specific for the alternative pathway, while C3 is common to both. It is important that the tests are carried out serially, as reduced complement components or function may be secondary to inflammation or to immune complex formation and not due to a primary defect.

A summary of tests of humoral immunity is given in Table 22.3.

Cell-mediated immunity

The cell-mediated immune system is particularly important in the immune responses towards cell surface antigens such as viral or neoplastic antigens. T-cell responses are now known to be quite varied and essential for the proper functioning of the humoral and phagocytic systems. The main division of T-cells is into effector and controlling subtypes. The effector cells are the cytotoxic cell (Tc), which lyses tumour or virally infected cells after specific sensitisation, and the delayed type hypersensitivity cell (Td), which induces inflammation and is responsible for the 48-hour reaction after skin testing. The controlling functions of T-cells are mediated by the helper cell (Th), which responds to antigen presented by a macrophage and releases both effector T-cell and B-cell 'helper' factors, and the suppressor cell (Ts), which limits the overall response.

The T-helper factors are known generically as the interleukins (IL). To date six, IL-1 to IL-6, have been identified and sequenced. They are produced, and probably act, locally, and therefore to measure systemic blood levels may not be particularly informative.

The T-cell subpopulations can be partially distinguished by cell surface glycoproteins, known collectively as the CD-antigens. The most generally useful are the CD3, CD4 and CD8 antigens (also known as T3, T4 and T8) which are present respectively on all T-cells, on helper T-cells and on suppressor and cytotoxic T-cells. No antigen which is unique to the delayed hypersensitivity T-cell has been described. The CD antigens broadly describe the subsets in which the functional cells occur, but they themselves do not relate to the functional capability of the cell. Some CD antigens, however, function as receptors. The CD3 antigen forms part of the T-cell antigen receptor and the CD4 antigen is the receptor for human immunodeficiency virus (HIV), the causative agent of AIDS.

Measurement of cell-mediated immunity

Cell-mediated immune function can be tested in vivo or in vitro (Table 22.4), although the tests measure different subpopulations of T-cells. Skin tests measure antigen recognition and effector Td-cell function in vivo. The 48-hour cutaneous response to either a range of recall antigens such as purified protein derivative from tubercle bacillus (PPD), tetanus antigen, streptokinase-streptodornase and candida antigen, or to a new antigen such as dinitrochlorobenzene (DNCB) may be measured. The recall antigens (which can be applied as a battery using a Merieux applicator) test the memory T-cells' ability to respond to previously encountered antigens, while the DNCB tests the patient's ability to mount a delayed type hypersensitivity response to a new antigen.

T-cell function is tested in vitro by activating the cells with either a non-specific mitogen such as phytohaemagglutinin (PHA) or concanavalin A (Con A), or with a specific antigen such as PPD. In this case the responder cells are primarily Th-cells and the response can be measured in one of three ways: (1) most commonly, by measuring proliferation as the incorporation of ^{3}H-thymidine into DNA; (2) by assaying the supernatant for one of the lymphokines or interleukins produced by activated T-cells, such as interleukin-2 (IL-2) or macrophage migration inhibition factor (MIF); or (3) by observing the appearance on the T-cell membrane of activation markers such as receptors for IL-2 or for transferrin. As all of the functional responses of T-cells involve the interaction of more than one cell subpopulation, interpretation of abnormal results must be done with caution. For instance, successful stimulation with antigen presupposes that sufficient functional antigen-presenting cells are present in the cell culture vessel, and production of IL-2 depends on the cell being able to respond to IL-1.

T-cells and T-cell subsets can be enumerated using methods identical to B-cell enumeration. The CD antigens are expressed more strongly on T-cells than on B-cells and the subsets can be readily identified by incubating the cells with mouse monoclonal antibody to the CD antigen followed by a secondary fluorescein or enzyme conjugated anti-mouse antibody. The results should always be expressed as the absolute number of cells per litre of blood; thus a white cell differential count must be carried out on the same blood sample. Expressing helper and suppressor percentages as a ratio is much less informative, as the two cell subpopulations are not interdependent. HIV infection, for instance, causes a decrease in the number of Th-cells whereas CMV or EBV infection can result in a transitory increase of Ts-cells. In both cases the helper/suppressor ratio is reduced, but for different reasons.

T-cell-mediated cytotoxicity against virally infected target cells can be measured, although this is a complicated test and rarely available. Other cells which may be important in immune defence include the non-specific killer (NK) cell and the antibody-dependent cytotoxic (ADCC) cell which kills antibody-coated target cells following attachment through a receptor for the Fc-region of IgG. These cells can be tested in in-vitro functional assays against radiolabelled target cells; however their lineage is uncertain and it is likely that cells of different lineages have similar cytotoxic ability.

CLINICAL INFECTIONS IN THE COMPROMISED HOST

The immune compromised host is particularly vulnerable to infection. However, because of his immune

Table 22.4 Measurement of cell-mediated immunity

In vivo tests

1. 48-hour skin test response to recall antigens
2. Sensitisation with DNCB followed by 48-hour challenge

In vitro tests

1. Enumeration of T-cell subsets:
   Total T-cells
   T-helper
   T-suppressor/cytotoxic
   Activated T-cells

2. Proliferative response to:
   Mitogens
   Antigens

3. Lymphokine production:
   IL-2
   Migration inhibition factor

4. Cytotoxicity:
   T-cell cytotoxicity
   Natural killer cell activity (NK)
   Antibody-dependent cellular cytotoxicity (ADCC)

deficiency, the clinical presentation, the type of organism and the course of infection may all be very different from the normal individual. For instance in the absence of neutrophils the normal inflammatory response to infection, with accumulation of neutrophils and formation of pus, does not occur. The immune deficient patient is often infected with normally harmless commensals of the digestive tract such as *E. coli* or *Candida albicans* or with opportunistic environmental organisms such as *Pneumocystis carinii* or *Listeria monocytogenes*. A latent infection with CMV or EBV may be reactivated. The infections tend to be recurrent and are unusually virulent or persistent. It is therefore important that any underlying immune deficiency is identified as prompt antibiotic treatment may be vital in such patients.

Primary immune deficiency tends to manifest itself after 3 months of age when the protective effect of maternal IgG antibody transferred across the placenta diminishes. Infections tend to be of the skin in the form of eczema, or of the upper respiratory tract, often spreading to the lungs to cause pneumonia, to the meninges or the middle ear. Other symptoms may include diarrhoea and failure to thrive.

Since neutrophils, antibody and complement are the body's main resources for resisting bacterial infection, it is likely that recurrent bacterial infections are due to a defect in one of these systems.

Patients with neutrophil dysfunction are particularly prone to infections of the mucous membranes with, normally harmless enteric bacteria such as the *staphylococci*, faecal *streptococci* or *Pseudomonas aeruginosa*. A defect in neutrophil killing, such as in chronic granulomatous disease, predisposes particularly to infection with the catalase-producing bacteria such as the *Staphylococci*, *Klebsiella* and *Serratia*. Absent or deficient neutrophils also predispose an individual to invasive infection with the gastrointestinal yeasts *Aspergillus* and *Candida*.

Capsulated bacteria such as the *pneumococci* can resist phagocytosis unless they are opsonised with antibody or C3. Persistent or recurrent infections with these organisms may therefore suggest a defect in antibody production, antibody opsonisation or in C3. Antibody deficiency often presents in children as pneumonia or meningitis caused by pyogenic bacteria such as *Haemophilus influenzae*, pneumococci or streptococci. Adults may also present with persistent *Gardia intestinalis* or cryptosporidial infection, or with septic arthritis caused by *H. influenzae*. Recurrent upper respiratory tract infections may be due to an IgA deficiency. A lack of gut IgA may predispose to infection with enteroviruses such as hepatitis A, poliomyelitis or Echo virus.

Deficiency of the C3 component of the complement cascade also predisposes an individual to recurrent and sometimes life-threatening infections with pyogenic bacteria, presenting as septicaemia, pneumonia or meningitis. A deficiency in one of the late components, C5, C6, C7 or C8, tends to result in recurrent neisserial infections, particularly *N. gonorrhoeae* or *N. meningitidis*. In contrast, a deficiency in one of the early components, for instance C1, C4 or C2, may present as immune complex disease rather than as an infection. Symptoms include a lupus-like syndrome with a malar flush, arthralgia and fever, glomerulonephritis or chronic vasculitis. The most frequent complement component deficiency is of C1-inhibitor (C1-INH) which results in hereditary angio-oedema.

Cell-mediated immune mechanisms are important in the resistance against yeasts, fungi, cell-associated organisms such as viruses (which are presented to the T-cell on the surface of the infected cell) and mycobacteria. Deficient CMI may present in children as infection following immunisation with a live or attenuated virus. It can often result in systemic fungal infection with *Candida* or *Aspergillus*, or in particularly virulent infections with measles, *Herpes simplex* or cytomegalovirus. These last two may be due to reactivation of a latent infection. In AIDS the most common presenting infection in the USA and Europe is a particularly aggressive form of pneumonia caused by the opportunist parasite *Pneumocystis carinii*. Cerebral or lung lesions due to *Toxoplasma gondii* or *Cryptococcus neoformans* infection are also common.

CAUSES OF DECREASED HOST DEFENCE

Immune incompetence can be due to a variety of causes. It can be a primary congenital defect; it can by induced by chemotherapy, radiotherapy or surgery; it can be secondary to another disease, to malnutrition, to psychological stress, or to direct infection of lymphocytes by a lymphotropic virus such as human immunodeficiency virus (HIV).

Primary immune deficiencies

The primary immune deficiencies are categorised in Table 22.5. These occur rarely. Any which is severe enough to have clinical consequences will manifest itself in the first two years of life. Serious cell-mediated immune defects will become apparent soon after birth, while antibody deficiency may not be detected until the

Table 22.5 Summary of primary immune deficiencies

Syndrome	Laboratory abnormalities	Clinical consequences	Treatment
Global deficiencies			
1. Reticular dysgenesis	Failure of differentiation of haemopoietic stem cells Deficient T-cells, B-cells and phagocytes Autosomal recessive inheritance	Total inability to combat infection	Bone-marrow graft
Deficiencies of the phagocytic system			
1. Chronic granulomatous disease	Inability to produce free radicals Impaired intracellular killing X-linked recessive (rarely autosomal) inheritance	Repeated infections with catalase-producing bacteria Often skin sepsis	Symptomatic treatment of infections Granulocyte infusions
2. Myeloperoxidase deficiency	Autosomal recessive Increased oxidative metabolism Impaired killing	Susceptible particularly to *C. albicans* infection	Symptomatic
3. Deficiency of adhesion-associated antigens CR3 receptor deficiency	Poor chemotaxis, migration and phagocytosis Autosomal recessive	Recurrent pyogenic bacterial infections Delayed umbilical cord separation; gingivitis	Symptomatic
4. Chediak–Higashi syndrome	Large cytoplasmic inclusions Poor migration and killing Autosomal recessive inheritance	Recurrent pyogenic bacterial infections Partial albinism	Symptomatic Granulocyte infusions
5. Hyper IgE – recurrent infection (Job's syndrome)	High IgE; eosinophilia Abnormal chemotaxis	Susceptibility to bacterial and candida infections	Symptomatic
Deficiencies of the lymphoid system			
1. Severe combined immune deficiency	a) X-linked absence of T- and B-lymphocytes b) Can be autosomally inherited c) Adenosine deaminase deficiency	Partial or total absence of humoral and cell-mediated immunity. Life-threatening opportunistic infection Fatal within 6 months	Bone marrow transplant Red cell transfusions
2. Ataxia telangiectasia	CMI deficiency (60%) IgA, IgE deficiency (70–90%)	Presents at 1–4 yrs of age Lymphoproliferative malignancy common Prognosis variable	Symptomatic
Humoral immune deficiency			
1. Bruton's X-linked infantile agammaglobulinaemia	Failure of B-cell maturation	Recurrent sino-pulmonary infections	Human immunoglobulin
2. Common variable immune deficiency	X-linked or autosomal Reduced Ig production Reduced CMI responses	Presents at any age Recurrent pyogenic infections	Human immunoglobulin
3. Transient humoral insufficiency of the neonate	Insufficient passage of maternal IgG at birth	Increased risk of infection in first 6 months	Self correcting
4. IgA deficiency	Failure to secrete IgA Absence of serum IgA	Disorders of GI tract Chronic bronchitis Autoimmune disease Malignancies	Symptomatic

continues over

Table 22.5   *(cont'd)*

Syndrome	Laboratory abnormalities	Clinical consequences	Treatment
Cell-mediated immune deficiency			
1. Thymic hypoplasia/Di George Syndrome	Abnormal embryogenesis of 3rd and 4th pharyngeal pouches; absence of thymus and partial to total absence of CMI	Susceptible to viral infection and malignancy	Transplant of fetal thymus
2. Purine nucleoside phosphorylase (PNP) deficiency	Accumulation of guanosine which is toxic to T-lymphocytes Autosomal recessive	a) Variable susceptibility to infection b) Neurological abnormalities (25%)	Bone marrow transplant Red cell transfusions
3. Wiskott-Aldrich syndrome	X-linked platelet deficiency, reduced IgM, lack of monocyte IgG receptors	Thrombocytopenia B-cell lymphomas Eczema	Bone-marrow transplant
Complement component deficiencies			
C1q	Autosomal recessive	Glomerulonephritis; SLE syndrome; infections	⎫
C1r	Probable autosomal recessive	SLE syndrome	
C1s	?	SLE syndrome	
C4	Probable autosomal recessive	SLE syndrome, infections	
C2	Autosomal recessive	Recurrent bacterial infection, SLE, glomerulonephritis, juvenile rheumatoid arthritis	Component replacement
C3	Autosomal recessive	Recurrent pyogenic infections, glomerulonephritis, vasculitis	
C5 C6 C7 C8 C9	Autosomal recessive	Recurrent neisserial infections, SLE	
C1 Inhibitor	Autosomal dominant	Hereditary angiodema	⎭
Factor I	Autosomal recessive	Recurrent pyogenic infections	
Factor H	Autosomal recessive	Haemolytic-uremic syndrome	

maternal IgG has been absorbed at about 2–4 months of age. A primary immune deficiency can result from a failure at any stage of the differentiation pathway of haemopoietic stem cells through to immunocompetent myeloid and lymphoid cells (Table 22.5). Where the defect is in the white cell precursor pool, the resulting reticular dysgenesis means a blanket failure in the differentiation of lymphocytes, monocytes and neutrophils.

Primary deficiencies of all the known mechanisms of neutrophil function have been described. The best documented example is chronic granulomatous disease (CGD) (Table 22.5) which is usually inherited as an X-linked recessive disorder and which presents in the first two months of life, often as severe skin sepsis. The neutrophils ingest normally but are unable to produce the respiratory burst associated with bacterial killing. Many bacteria produce enough hydrogen peroxide themselves to induce self-destruction but CGD patients are particularly susceptible to infection with catalase-producing bacteria, since the catalase hydrolyses the bacterial hydrogen peroxide, thus enabling these bacteria to persist inside the neutrophils and produce the characteristic granulomas.

Primary defects of the lymphoid system

Severe combined immune deficiency. If the immune defect occurs at a stage of lymphoid differentiation which is before the division of the T-and B-cell path-ways, the effect is manifest in both the cellular and humoral systems as severe combined or Swiss-type immune deficiency (SCID). This deficiency occurs in approximately 1 in 40 000 births as a spectrum from total absence of T-and B-cells to the relative loss of (up to 50%) B-cells.

Congenital CMI deficiency. This can result from a failure either in the differentiation of the T-cell or in the thymic environment in which the T-cell matures. Primary deficiencies of CMI always manifest themselves in infants or children.

Congenital humoral immune deficiency. Also called Bruton's X-linked infantile agammaglobulinaemia, this is a defect in B-cell maturation resulting in either a complete absence of cells with B-surface markers or totally non-functional B-cells. Recurrent sino-pulmonary infections tend to begin in these patients at between 4 months and 2 years of age when the protection afforded by maternal IgG has been absorbed. The condition, which can also be autosomally inherited, is partially treatable with regular injections of human immuno-globulin.

Transient humoral insufficiency. This can occur in the neonate if there has been insufficient passage of maternal IgG at birth, or if there is a delay in the synthesis of endogenous immunoglobulin, possibly because of a premature birth. This condition usually corrects itself as the humoral system reaches maturity, but can be a source of diagnostic confusion.

Secondary immune deficiencies

With increasingly aggressive medical treatment for cancers, and with the increase in organ transplantation, medically induced secondary immune suppression is now relatively common and brings with it predictable *sequelae* in terms of immune deficiency. Secondary immune deficiency can also be a direct consequence of malignant disease, particularly in the case of lymphomas or leukaemias in which immunocompetent cells are swamped by non-functional lymphoid or myeloid cells. A deficiency can arise secondarily to infection with cytomegalovirus, or to protein malnutrition. While malnutrition is predominantly a problem in the Third World, it does have relevance in developed countries if there is an associated problem of malabsorption, such as in AIDS. Severe emotional stress such as bereavement or other significant loss is associated with an increased incidence of autoimmune disease and malignancy.

Drugs can become immunogenic, particularly if they attach to a protein molecule which acts as a 'carrier'. Antibody to the drug is generated which can lead to immune complex formation, activation of complement and inflammation, or to immune cytopenias such as autoimmune haemolytic anaemia. Neutrophil dysfunction can be secondary to a defect in another part of the immune system. Poor opsonising serum due to an antibody or C3 deficiency is often found to be the cause of reduced phagocytosis and slow accumulation at a site of infection may be the result of a C5 deficiency.

Impaired antibody synthesis can be secondary to aging, to malnutrition or to lymphoreticular malignancies. Malnourished patients have a reduced primary response to antigen although their immunoglobulin levels are normal. Multiple myeloma, chronic lymphatic leukaemia and, in its terminal stages, Hodgkin's lymphoma can all cause a secondary hypogammaglobulinaemia. Reduced immunoglobulin levels can also result from excessive loss of antibody due to a nephrotic syndrome or to burns.

The most common cause of secondary cellular immune deficiency is chemotherapy: either cytotoxic therapy given in the treatment of leukaemia or immunosuppressive therapy given in association with transplantation to reduce the risk of rejection of the graft. The patient becomes susceptible to bacterial, fungal and viral infections, with herpes viruses and cytomegalovirus being the major cause of mortality in the early (7–10 days) and intermediate (up to 12 days) post-transplant period. Immunosuppressive doses of corticosteroids may also be given for some intractable inflammatory conditions.

Acquired immune deficiency syndrome

Soon after the first reports of what is now termed the acquired immune deficiency syndrome (AIDS) appeared in 1981, it was apparent that there was an infectious agent which could be transmitted sexually, or by blood or blood products. The agent was identified in France and shortly after in the USA, with the first reports appearing in 1983. Since then several hundred isolates have shown human immunodeficiency virus (HIV) to be a family of RNA lentiviruses with a remarkably high degree of genomic heterogeneity. In 1986 a second, but closely related, family of AIDS-causing viruses was described. The two groups of viruses, termed HIV-1 and HIV-2 respectively, have some RNA sequence homology, but negligible antigenic cross-reactivity.

HIV-1 consists of approximately 10 000 bases of genomic RNA. Its primary target is the T-helper cell which it infects by binding to an epitope on the CD4 antigen. It has been shown that a subgroup of cells of the monocyte/macrophage lineage which have the CD4 antigen is also susceptible to HIV infection. More recently CD4 negative cells have been shown to be infected, including brain glial cells, fibroblasts and epithelial cells.

The hallmark of RNA retroviruses is their gene for reverse transcriptase, the enzyme which enables the virus to make complementary DNA copies of itself. In the HIV-infected cell, these copies either accumulate as free DNA or they integrate into the host's genomic DNA. In the integrated form activation of the virus is related to immune activation of the T-helper cell. For as long as the helper cell remains quiescent, the host is an 'asymptomatic carrier'. If activated, for instance by an unrelated infection, e.g. CMV, the T-helper cell is stimulated to divide and new HIV virions are formed which bud from the T-cell surface to infect further cells. HIV-infected T-helper cells, in which the viral genome also remains as unintegrated DNA, can form large, multinucleate cells which eventually die, liberating free infectious viral DNA. Viral replication is controlled at the translational stage by the products of two regulatory genes known respectively as 'tat' (transactivator of transcription) and 'art' (antirepressor activator). There is some evidence to show that similar regulatory proteins produced by other viruses can act on HIV. Thus activation and replication of HIV may be initiated indirectly by immunological stimulation of the host cell, or directly by interaction of viral regulatory proteins with the HIV genome.

The factors which govern whether viral DNA remains free or becomes integrated are not fully known, although in-vitro immune activation can lead to integration.

If the cellular immune system is still sufficiently intact, the expression of viral antigen on the helper T-cell surface can induce a cytotoxic-T-cell-mediated reaction against the infected helper T-cell. Thus the helper cell population can be gradually eliminated both by direct viral infection and by an autoimmune cytotoxic response.

The humoral immune system responds to HIV infection by making antibody, initially to viral envelope glycoprotein gp120, and subsequently to a major viral core protein, p24, and to the viral transmembrane protein, p41. Antibody may not appear in the plasma for up to 6 months after infection. Although the virus is immunologically 'silent' in the host, and the infection is undetectable by anti-HIV screening, the individual at this stage is still infectious.

Anti-HIV-1 antibodies appear to cross-react with all the isolates of HIV-1 which have been characterised. This is thought to be due to highly conserved regions within the envelope gene which determine the antigenic structure. Antibody from some individuals has been shown to neutralise the virus in vitro. It is not yet known, however, whether an anti-HIV positive individual can ever be said to have successfully overcome an HIV infection.

The proportion of individuals who are anti-HIV antibody positive who go on to develop full blown AIDS is still a matter of conjecture. Early estimates suggested a figure of 5–20%; however more recent estimates, which take into account the long incubation period of the virus in some patients, suggest that 85% or more of HIV-infected individuals will develop AIDS in the 15 years following exposure to the virus.

The immunological consequences of HIV infection are listed in Table 22.6. All the effects are a consequence of a debilitated helper T-cell population since they are dependent upon factors released by activated T-helper cells. Where the primary infection is in glial cells, very few immunological abnormalities may result.

Table 22.6 Immunological consequences of HIV infection

Effects on T-cells
1. Reduced number of circulating CD4 positive (T-helper) cells
2. Expression of activation markers on T-cells
3. Reduced proliferative response to mitogens, antigens and allogenic lymphocytes
4. Reduced suppressor cell activity
5. Reduced T-cell-mediated cytotoxicity
6. Reduced skin test responses

Effects on B-cells
1. Non-specific polyclonal B-cell activation
2. Reduced or absent antibody response to new antigens

Effects on neutrophils and monocytes
1. Reduced chemotaxis
2. Reduced cytotoxicity

Transmission of HIV

HIV is transmitted either as free virus or as a passenger within an infected cell. Free HIV-1 virions have been demonstrated in semen, blood, saliva, tears, breastmilk, cervical and vaginal secretions. Unequivocal transmission of infection has been associated only with blood, blood products, semen and, less frequently, from female to male via cervical/vaginal secretions. In blood and in the semen of infected men, HIV is also present in infected lymphocytes.

Sexual transmission occurs by rectal and vaginal intercourse. Infection may therefore be acquired by homosexual and heterosexual activity or following artificial insemination from an infected donor.

Blood-borne transmission occurs via parenteral introduction of infected blood or blood products. The main risk groups are haemophiliacs, recipients of a blood transfusion or organ transplant from an infected donor and recreational drug users who share needles, syringes or drug preparation equipment. The last group is particularly at risk if the syringe is 'flushed out' with blood before being passed on. Transmission of HIV by accidental 'needlestick' injury has occurred in health care and laboratory workers, although this is a rare event.

Maternal-fetal Intra-uterine and/or perinatal infection may occur in infants born to HIV-infected mothers, some of whom go on to develop AIDS. Transmission via breast milk may add to the viral inoculum received perinatally by the infant.

Factors influencing susceptibility to infection

Viral inoculum. Increased rates of infection are associated, in haemophiliacs, with the amount of commercial factor VIII concentrate received, and, in homosexuals, with the number of sexual partners and with being the recipient partner, indicating that a greater viral load is more likely to lead to infection.

Strain infectivity. The infectivity of different isolates of HIV-1 for lymphocytes and macrophages varies by several orders of magnitude, which suggests that different strains are more or less pathogenic.

Route of transmission. Infection among homosexuals is very much higher (88% of cases) than among heterosexuals (1% of cases). While some of this difference can be accounted for by promiscuity among homosexuals, it also suggests that anal intercourse, which with the associated tearing of the rectal mucosa provides HIV more direct access to the bloodstream, is more likely to result in infection than vaginal intercourse.

Health status of the recipient. Activated T-cells are more susceptible to infection by HIV than resting cells; thus an individual who is exposed to HIV is more likely to become infected if he/she has an intercurrent infection.

Epidemiology

Current figures show that the epidemiology of AIDS in the UK is broadly similar to the experience in North America. However, there is considerable regional variation in the proportions of patients and carriers in each risk category. In Scotland, for instance, 63% of sero-positive individuals are intravenous drug users and only 15% are homosexual or bisexual men, compared with 1.5% and 88% in the UK as a whole. In areas where a large amount of imported factor VIII is used, up to 75% of haemophiliacs are sero-positive, whereas in the west of Scotland, where all the factor VIII is prepared regionally, less than 15% are infected.

Transmission of HIV-1 by transfusion of blood or blood products has been virtually eliminated following the introduction of rigorous screening of donors (self-deferral), screening of donations for anti-HIV-1 and heat-treatment of factor VIII. A 'window' of several weeks remains however, if blood is donated by an infected individual who has not yet produced antibody.

Clinical immunology of AIDS

Diagnosis of AIDS is made on the basis of clinical symptoms and the evidence of HIV infection. The techniques used for direct identification of HIV in the hosts' tissues are not sufficiently sensitive to be diagnostic. However, antibody to HIV is virtually always present and therefore patients with repeatable anti-HIV antibody – confirmed using a test of different type to the initial test such as western blotting or immunofluorescence – are considered to be infected.

The clinical manifestations of AIDS have been classified by the Centre for Disease Control, Atlanta, Georgia, into four mutually exclusive groups (Table 22.7).

Table 22.7   CDC classification of HIV infection

Groups			Clinical symptoms
I			Acute infection
II			Asymptomatic infection
III			Persistent generalised lymphadenopathy
IV			Other disease
	A		Constitutional disease
	B		Neurological disease
	C		Secondary infectious disease
		C–1	Specified secondary infectious disease listed in CDC surveillance definition
		C–2	Other specified infectious diseases
	D		Secondary cancers
	E		Other conditions

A patient can be reclassified depending on the progression of his disease to a higher group number but can not be reclassified into a preceding group if his symptoms resolve.

Group I. Acute HIV infection is a mononucleosis-like disease associated with sero-conversion.

Group II. Asymptomatic HIV infection may or may not be associated with a deterioration of the immune system (see below).

Group III. Persistent generalised lymphadenopathy is defined as two or more palpable lymph nodes of 1 cm or larger at extra-inguinal sites, which persist for more than 3 months in the absence of a cause other than HIV infection.

Group IV. Those patients who have AIDS. These are divided into five subgroups, which may be further subdivided.

Subgroup A. Constitutional disease includes unexplained weight loss of more than 10% of base line, persistent fever or diarrhoea (without other cause) for more than 1 month.

Subgroup B. Neurological disease can present as unexplained dementia, myelopathy or peripheral neuropathy.

Subgroup C. Secondary infectious disease is defined as an infectious disease associated with HIV infection and/or an underlying defect in cell-mediated immunity. Patients are further subdivided according to specified infections: **Category C-1** includes: *Pneumocystis carinii* pneumonia, chronic cryptosporidiosis, toxoplasmosis, extra-intestinal strongyloidiasis, isosporiasis, oesophageal, bronchial or pulmonary candidiasis, cryptococcosis, histoplasmosis, mycobacterial infection with *Mycobacterium avium* complex or *M. kansasii*, cytomegalovirus, chronic mucocutaneous or disseminated *Herpes simplex* virus infection and progressive multifocal leuko-encephalopathy. **Category C-2** includes: oral hairy leukoplakia, multidermatomal *Herpes zoster*, recurrent *Salmonella* bacteraemia, nocardiosis, tuberculosis and oral candidiasis.

Subgroup D. Secondary cancers are defined as one or more of those known to be associated with HIV or defective cell-mediated immunity: Kaposi's sarcoma, non-Hodgkin's lymphoma (small, non-cleaved lymphoma or immunoblastic sarcoma) or primary lymphoma of the brain.

Subgroup E. Other conditions include patients with conditions not classified above that may be attributable to cell-mediated immune deficiency, including chronic lymphoid interstitial pneumonitis, or those that may be complicated by HIV infection.

Investigation of the immune system of anti-HIV positive patients with symptoms suggestive of AIDS is not diagnostic, but serves to add information as to the stage and progression of the disease. The single most important parameter is the number of T-helper cells in the circulation. An anti-HIV positive individual with less than 500×10^6 T-helper cells per litre of blood is more likely to develop full blown AIDS than if he had a normal helper cell count. The CD4 (helper cell) antigen is lost, while the patient may still have normal numbers of CD3-positive (Total-T) cells. As the disease progresses all the T-cell subsets are lost; in particular the CD4 subset may reach zero. Functional responses in vitro show a progressive reduction, followed by a progressive loss of skin-test responses.

The presence of antibody to the major core protein, p24, is associated with carrier status and loss of this antibody together with an increase in p24 antigen often predates the appearance of clinical symptoms.

Prevention and treatment

Attempts to produce a vaccine for AIDS are con-

founded by the heterogeneity of HIV. Added to this is the problem that, although antibody to gp120 is broadly cross-reactive, at least with HIV-1 isolates, it may not be protective, given that the virus has the capacity to remain immunologically 'hidden' inside a T-helper cell, a macrophage or a glial cell. Although gp120 appears to be the antigen recognised by both the humoral and the cell-mediated immune system, other antigens may also be of importance.

Attempts to treat AIDS by either immunostimulation (by IL-2 or interferon) or immunosuppression have failed since they either activate the cells containing the virus, or they aggravate the action of the virus by suppressing the immune system further. Similarly, irradiation of the lymphoid cells followed by a bone marrow graft has so far been unsuccessful since a reservoir of virus has always remained which has infected the grafted cells.

Present anti-viral agents such as acyclovir appear to be ineffective against HIV. A new generation of specific anti-retroviral agents needs to be developed. The first of these to be granted a licence, zidovudine (3'azido-3-deoxythymidine), acts by terminating the synthesis of viral complementary DNA, by competing with the natural DNA substrate, TTP (thymidine-5'-triphosphate). Thus, while this drug does not eliminate existing HIV, it inhibits the synthesis of new DNA copies and clinically retards the progression of the disease. Ultimately, the goal of therapy is not to retard but to prevent all expression of the virus, and to reconstitute the host's immune system.

Conclusion

The last 30 years has seen a vast accumulation of knowledge of how the various components of the immune system work. The more severe deficiencies can be treated by bone marrow, thymus or fetal liver transplant, and as techniques improve, including those of purging the transplant cells of unwanted subpopulations, this form of treatment may become more widespread.

Replacement therapy is possible for humoral deficiencies, and the introduction of intravenous preparations of immunoglobulin has greatly improved the tolerance of this treatment. The problem of histocompatibility severely restricts the use of replacement cellular therapy and there are still many unanswered questions in relation to antigen specificity, intracellular control and intercellular regulation. Genetic engineering is likely to play an increasing role in the future both in the understanding of immune deficiencies and in their treatment. The genetic repair of defective cells is probably still a long way off, but genetically engineered or modified antibodies and other immunological mediators are already available and are likely to be used increasingly in the more immediate future.

BIBLIOGRAPHY

Chapel H, Heaney M 1984 Essentials of Clinical Immunology. Blackwell Scientific Publications

Infections in Haematology 1984 In: Grant Prentice H (ed) Clinics in Haematology, vol. 13, no. 3. W B Saunders Co.

Laboratory Investigation of Immunological Disorders 1985 In: Thompson R A (ed) Clinics in Immunology and Allergy, vol. 5, no. 3. W B Saunders Co.

Tests of immune function 1986 In: Weir D M, Hertzenberg L A, Blackwell C, Hertzenberg L (eds) Handbook of Experimental Immunology, 4th edn. Blackwell Scientific Publications, pp 126.1–126.33

World Health Organization 1978 Immunodeficiency Report of a WHO Scientific Group. WHO, Geneva

23. Drugs used in the treatment of malignant haematological disorders

M. J. Mackie

The use of cytotoxic drugs has produced remarkable improvements in the prognosis of many haematological malignancies. However, they are associated with a variety of side effects which can affect most organs in the body (Table 23.1) and they should therefore be used only by physicians experienced in their administration.

Drugs are frequently used in combination, as single agents are generally unable to effect a cure. The aim of combination therapy is to achieve maximum cell kill within the range of tolerated toxicity; drugs are chosen that have some effect as single agents but whose toxicities ideally do not overlap. Such a broad approach should give a wide coverage of de novo resistant cells and prevent or slow the development of new resistance. Thus alternating schedules of non-cross-resistant drugs should be administered in optimal doses. The interval between schedules should be as close as possible but adequate recovery from myelosuppression must have occurred before the next cycle is given. For most agents the nadir of the white count is 10–14 days after administration of the drug(s). Recovery usually is under way by 21 days so that many regimens are given on a 28-day schedule. Infectious problems during the period of myelosuppression represent the greatest hazard to the patient and their management is discussed in Chapter 35. It is very important to explain to the patient and his general practitioner the possible side effects of therapy and the action that should be taken if these occur. Deterioration in a patient on cytotoxic therapy may be due to effects of treatment which are usually remediable if the appropriate action is taken quickly.

In addition to the short-term implications of chemotherapy, long-term sequelae such as infertility and second malignancies need to be considered. As regards the former, male patients should be offered the option of sperm banking if appropriate. All patients should be advised as to the risks of infertility, although these should be put in the context of the benefit of treatment. Sexual difficulties following chemotherapy can often be helped by frank discussion. Second malignancies,

Table 23.1 Organ toxicity of cytotoxic drugs

Organ	Toxicity	Drug
Lung	Disturbance of lung function Eventually fibrosis	Bleomycin Busulphan Cyclophosphamide Chlorambucil Nitrosoureas Methotrexate
Heart	Arrhythmias Cardiac failure	Doxorubicin Daunorubicin Mitoxantrone Cyclophosphamide
Nervous system	Peripheral neuropathy may include autonomic features and cranial nerve palsies	Vincristine Vindesine
	Encephalopathy Cerebellar signs	Methotrexate High dose Cytosine arabinoside
Skin	Pigmentation	Busulphan
Bladder	Haemorrhagic cystitis Bladder cancer	Cyclophosphamide Ifosfamide
Kidney	Failure	High dose Methotrexate
Pancreas	Pancreatitis	L-asparaginase
Bones	Osteoporosis Aseptic necrosis	Steroids
Marrow	Myelosuppression, leukaemia	Alkylating agents Antimetabolites
Liver	Fibrosis Veno-occlusive disease	Methotrexate Pre-marrow transplant conditioning, Azathioprine

usually acute non-lymphoblastic leukaemia or non-Hodgkin's lymphoma, occur in approximately 7% of patients. They are usually seen in patients who are apparently cured of the original disease, which was treated, on average, five years previously. Patients who have received treatment with both chemotherapy and radiotherapy are most at risk and the second neoplasm responds poorly to treatment.

Concern has been expressed over the years about the possible dangers of exposure of medical and nursing staff to these mutagenic and leukaemogenic drugs. Codes of practice for their safe reconstitution and administration have been devised and should be followed. Personnel involved in the giving of chemotherapy should be reassured that if they have been properly instructed in the administration of cytotoxic drugs any risk to them is very small and probably more theoretical than real. Individual cytotoxic drugs will be considered along with other members of their class (Table 23.2). The sites of action at the cellular level of the drugs are shown in Figure 23.1.

Table 23.2 summarises the main uses and toxicities of the principal members of each class of cytotoxic drug.

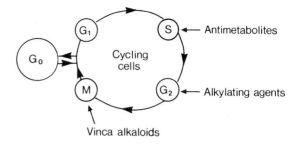

Fig. 23.1 Cell cycle and sites of action of various drugs. Resting cell (G_0); RNA and protein synthesis (G_1) prior to DNA synthesis (S) and preparation for mitosis (G_2); mitosis (M).

Schedules of administration are considered in the relevant chapters. However, it is essential that manufacturer's and appropriate literature are consulted before cytotoxic drugs are administered and that extreme care is taken in the calculation of the correct doses of the various agents.

Table 23.2 Alkylating agents. Indications, routes of administration and side effects.

Drugs	Indications	Route of administration	Side effects	Special precautions
All			Marrow suppression	Monitor FBC
Melphalan	Myeloma	p.o.		↓ dose if renal impairment
Mustine	Hodgkin's	i.v.	Vomiting Venotoxic	Fast-flowing drip
Chlorambucil	Chronic lymphatic leukaemia and lymphomas	p.o.	Pulmonary fibrosis, GI upset, rash, 'wasting syndrome'	
Busulphan	Chronic myeloid leukaemia and other myeloproliferative disorders	p.o.	Pigmentation, lung fibrosis, cellular atypia, cataracts, gynaecomastia, 'Addisonian state'	NB May cause prolonged severe myelosuppression
Cyclophosphamide	Lymphoma	p.o. i.v.	Vomiting, alopecia	
Ifosfamide	Lymphoma	i.v.	Bladder toxicity, bladder Ca, lung fibrosis, cardiotoxicity, inappropriate ADH secretion	Hydration, mesna additive with radiotherapy
Lomustine	Myeloma	p.o.	nausea, nephritis	NB Delayed thrombocytopenia
Carmustine	Hodgkin's	i.v.	Pulmonary fibrosis	
Amsacrine	Acute leukaemia	i.v.	GI upset Venotoxic	Infuse in dextrose via free-flowing drip. Use glass syringe to reconstitute drug
Procarbazine	Hodgkin's	p.o.	Reactions with alcohol	Care with alcohol

Alkylating agents (Table 23.2)

These form cross-links with DNA. An unsuitable im-onium ion is formed by activation of a chloroethyl side chain (most alkylating agents have two). This cross-links with DNA strands interfering with its function. Attempts are made to repair the lesion but cell death usually occurs, although mutations (leukaemogenic effect) can also take place.

It is certain members of this group which are particularly responsible for the most notorious side effects of chemotherapy as far as patients are concerned – vomiting and alopecia. Both these problems may have such an impact that the patient is unwilling to continue treatment. It is essential, therefore, to do everything possible to mitigate these side effects. Patients should be told that hair will regrow when treatment stops and be fitted for a wig (if desired) before there has been significant hair fall. Attempts at reducing hair loss by means of scalp cooling or a torniquet have been variably effective and are not thought appropriate for patients with leukaemia.

The management of vomiting is also difficult. There is a variance in the extent to which a regimen makes an individual patient vomit. A particular problem is so-called 'anticipatory vomiting'; in this very real phenomenom vomiting is precipitated by mere associations with chemotherapy (e.g. sight of the doctor!) occurring before the actual administration of the drug. This may be helped by drugs with an anxiolytic effect; a cannabis derivative, nabilone 1 mg, administered the night before chemotherapy and a further 1 mg 1 hour before the drugs are infused, helps some patients. Generally there is no panacea for cytotoxic-drug-induced vomiting; phenothiazines (e.g. chlorpromazine 10–25 mg i.v./i.m.) or metoclopramide (standard and high dose) help a proportion of patients. It is important not to rely on one dose of these drugs but to give repeated injections every 4–6 hours. The effects of these drugs may be augmented by concomitant administration of dexamethasone (10 mg intravenously before the chemotherapy and 10 mg intravenously or orally every 6 hours for four days after chemotherapy).

Mustine

This drug is used as part of the very successful MOPP regimen for treating Hodgkin's disease. It must be given intravenously as it is sclerosant to the veins and therefore it is imperative that a fast-flowing intravenous line is established before the drug is infused. It causes predictable myelosuppression and also severe vomiting.

Cyclophosphamide

This drug, which can be given orally or intravenously, is used for the treatment of lymphomas and leukaemias and also for conditioning prior to bone marrow transplantation. It requires activation by hepatic microsomes and metabolites with an alkylating action are excreted into the bladder. It has a number of side effects including myelosuppression, alopecia, haemorrhagic cystitis, bladder carcinoma, cardiac toxicity and inappropriate ADH syndrome. The likelihood of bladder toxicity can be minimised by ensuring that the patient has good renal function and is well hydrated. It can be used in conjunction with mesna, which combines with and inactivates the toxic derivative (acrolein) of cyclophosphamide. Bladder cancer tends to occur with prolonged usage and therefore this should be avoided. As regards cardiac toxicity, it should be appreciated that the effects of radiotherapy and anthracyclines are additive.

Ifosfamide

This is used for treatment of non-Hodgkin's lymphoma and is given either as a continuous intravenous infusion or daily as an intravenous fractionated dose. Side effects are vomiting, alopecia, myelosuppression and bladder toxicity. As regards the latter, the same measures can be employed that are successful in minimising cystitis from cyclophosphamide.

Nitrosoureas (lomustine, carmustine)

These drugs are used for the treatment of multiple myeloma and Hodgkin's disease. Lomustine (CCNU) is given orally and carmustine (BCNU) is given intravenously. A particular characteristic of these drugs is delayed myelosuppression in that the platelet count may not recover for 4 to 6 weeks. This drug is also leukaemogenic in animals and probably so in man.

Melphalan

This drug is used for the treatment of myeloma. It is usually given orally but has variable absorption by this route and can be given intravenously. The dose should be reduced in the presence of renal impairment and the main side effect is myelosuppression.

Chlorambucil

This medication, which is given orally, is used in chronic lymphatic leukaemia and Hodgkin's disease. Its

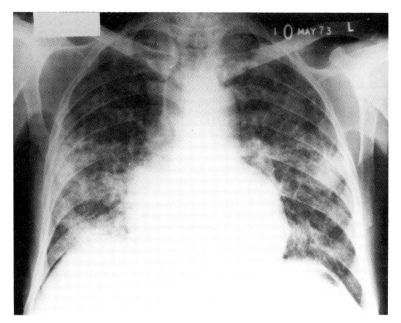

Fig. 23.2   Chest radiograph of busulphan-induced pulmonary fibrosis.

side effects include myelosuppression, pulmonary fibrosis, gastrointestinal upset, skin rash and rarely a 'wasting' syndrome.

Busulphan

This drug is used for the treatment of chronic myeloid leukaemia and other myeloproliferative disorders. It has also been advocated as conditioning prior to bone marrow transplant. It is given orally and may produce severe prolonged hypoplasia. Other side effects include pigmentation and an Addisonian-like state, pulmonary fibrosis (Fig. 23.2), cellular atypia, and cataract.

Anthracyclines/anthracenediones

These will be considered as a group. Doxorubicin (adriamycin) and daunorubicin are the most widely used cytoxic antibiotics. More recently mitoxantrone, a synthetic derivative (an anthracenedione), has been introduced. Several mechanisms of action may operate, including binding to DNA and cell membranes, conversion to free radicals, and chelation of metal ions. These effects lead to cell DNA and membrane damage. These agents are used to treat leukaemias and lymphomas. They must be given into a fast-flowing intravenous line but can be given as an infusion. The cytotoxicity of mitoxantrone is said to be enhanced in leukaemia if given 12 hours after the commencement of an infusion of cytosine arabinoside. The anthracyclines are metabolised by the liver and reduction of dosage is required if hepatic impairment is present. Side effects include myelosuppression, mucositis alopecia, extravasation necrosis (Plate 23) cardiotoxicity. There is some evidence that mitoxantrone causes less alopecia, cardiotoxicity and sclerosis of the veins. A radiation recall reaction has been observed with adriamycin in the skin, lungs and heart.

The cardiotoxicity may be acute with arrhythmias or pericarditis, or it may manifest later as chronic cardiac failure which is refractory to treatment. The injury causing the latter has a relationship to the dose of drug administered. The incidence of toxicity rises steeply once more than 550 mg/m^2 has been given. Different schedules of administration appear to have varying rates of toxicity. Additional risk factors are pre-existing heart disease, prior therapy with cyclophosphamide, and radiotherapy to the mediastinum. The best methods for monitoring possible cardiotoxicity are assessment of the ejection fraction and endocardial biopsy.

Antimetabolites (Table 23.3)

Methotrexate

This folate analogue inhibits dihydrofolate leading to a lack of tetrahydrofolic acid required for purine, nucleotide and thymidylate synthesis. It is used for treatment of non-Hodgkin's lymphoma and acute lymphoblastic leukaemia and can be given orally, intravenously or intrathecally as appropriate. The drug concentration and duration of exposure are important for the cytotoxic effect: 40–100% of the drug is excreted in the urine and during a constant plasma infusion 3% of the plasma level is achieved in the central nervous system. Methotrexate causes myelosuppresion and mucositis. Prolonged therapy may result in chronic liver disease and pneumonitis.

Central nervous toxicity occurs within intrathecal administration and may take the form of an acute arachnoiditis due to a chemical irritation or sub-acute paralysis, cranial nerve palsies, seizures or chronic demyelinating encephalopathy. The risk of central nervous system toxicity is increased if the patient has received cranial irradiation and intravenous methotrexate. Extreme care should be taken when checking the dose of intrathecal methotrexate to be administered. If an overdose is accidentally given intrathecally, cerebro-spinal fluid should be exchanged. High dose regimens of methotrexate require special care to avoid renal and severe gastrointestinal toxicity. The patient should have good renal function and be well hydrated. Depending on the exact dose to be administered, consideration should be given to alkylating the urine and monitoring blood levels to guide the duration of folinic acid rescue therapy. The dosage of the latter varies depending on the dosage of methotrexate: usually a dose of 10 mg/m^2 is given 4 times daily for 24–72 hours commencing at a set time (8–24 hrs) following the infusion of methotrexate at intermediate or high dose.

Cytosine arabinoside

This cytosine analogue has to be metabolised to its active form in ara-CTP which inhibits DNA synthesis. It is used in the treatment of acute leukaemia and can be given intravenously, subcutaneously or intrathecally. For systemic administration a number of low dose, conventional and high dose regimens are in use and the appropriate sections should be consulted. During infusion 40% of the plasma level is achieved in the central nervous system. Side effects of conventional doses are vomiting, myelosuppression, mucositis and hepatic dysfunction. With high dose regimens cerebellar toxicity may occur.

Azacytidine

This drug is a pyrimidene nucleoside and is used for the treatment of acute non-lymphoblastic leukaemia. It is given intravenously and side effects include myelosuppression, vomiting, hepatic toxicity and a neuromuscular syndrome.

Table 23.3 Antimetabolites: indications, routes of administration and side effects.

Drugs	Indications	Route of administration	Side effects	Special precautions
Cytosine arabinoside	Acute leukaemia	i.v. s.c. i.t.	Marrow suppression	Monitor FBC
	Non-Hodgkin's lymphoma		Vomiting, mucositis, hepatic, high dose–cerebellar	
Methotrexate	Acute lymphoblastic leukaemia	p.o. i.v.	Myelosuppression, mucositis, hepatic, renal, pneumonitis, central nervous system	Monitor FBC, renal function
	Non-Hodgkin's lymphoma			Avoid in renal failure, high dose-hydration, folinic acid rescue, alkaline urine, monitor levels
Thioguanine	Acute myeloid leukaemia	p.o.	Myelosuppression, hepatic, gastrointestinal	Monitor FBC
Mercaptopurine	Acute lymphoblastic leukaemia	p.o.	Myelosuppression, hepatic	Monitor FBC interaction with allopurinol
Hydroxyurea	Chronic myeloid leukaemia	p.o.	Myelosuppression, gastrointestinal	Monitor FBC
5-Azacytidine	Acute myeloid leukaemia	i.v.	Myelosuppression, gastrointestinal, hepatic	Monitor FBC

6-Mercaptopurine

This purine analogue requires conversion to an active metabolite which is incorporated into nucleic acids. It is given orally and used for the treatment of acute lymphoblastic leukaemia. Side effects include myelosuppression, nausea and hepatic toxicity. It is important to remember that allopurinol augments the action of mercaptopurine. A reduction of up to 75% of the dose of mercaptopurine should be made when both drugs are administered. The dose of mercaptopurine should also be reduced in the presence of renal impairment.

Thioguanine

This is a hydroxyl amine which inhibits ribonucleotide for the treatment of acute non-lymphoblastic leukaemia. It causes myelosuppression and the dose should be reduced in the presence of renal impairment.

Hydroxyurea

This a hydroxyl amine which inhibits ribonucleotide reductase. Its main use is in chronic myeloid leukaemia and other myeloproliferative disorders. It can cause myelosuppression and gastrointestinal upset. Patients receiving hydroxyurea develop a high mean corpuscular volume.

Miscellaneous drugs (Table 23.4)

Vinca alkaloids

These drugs are derived from the periwinkle plant and bind to tubulin, thus interfering with cell division. They are used for treatment of acute lymphoblastic leukaemia, lymphoid blast crises of chronic myeloid leukaemia, lymphomas and myeloma. These alkaloids are metabolised in the liver and excreted into the bile. They must be given intravenously and great care must be taken with the injection as any extravasation will result in tis-

Table 23.4   Other chemotherapeutic drugs. Indications, routes of administration and side effects of cytotoxic drugs.

Drug	Indications	Route of administration	Side effects	Precautions
Vinca alkaloids				
Vincristine	Acute lymphoblastic leukaemia		Sclerosant to veins	Ensure good venous access
Vinblastine	Lymphoma	i.v.	Neurotoxicity	Vinblastine, vindesine
Vindesine	Blast crisis of chronic myeloid leukaemia			less toxic than vincristine
	Myeloma		Myelotoxicity	Vinblastine, vindesine more toxic than vincristine
Anthracyclines, anthracenediones				
Adriamycin	Acute leukaemia		Marrow suppression, vomiting, sclerosant to veins, cardiotoxic	Monitor FBC
Daunorubicin	Lymphomas	i.v.		Ensure fast-flowing drip
Mitoxantrone				Monitor cumulative dose
Miscellaneous				
Etoposide	Acute myeloid leukaemia, lymphomas	p.o. i.v.	Marrow suppression, vomiting, alopecia	Monitor FBC
DTIC	Hodgkin's disease	i.v.	Marrow suppression, vomiting, sclerosant to veins	Monitor FBC
				Ensure good venous access
L-asparaginase	Acute lymphoblastic leukaemia	i.v.	Hypersensitivity, pancreatitis, hepatitis, decreased clotting factors	Can use another source of product
Bleomycin	Lymphomas	i.m. i.v.	Fever, pulmonary fibrosis, radiation recall, cutaneous	Watch cumulative dose. Monitor CXR, pulmonary function tests
Steroids	Acute lymphoblastic leukaemia	i.v. p.o.	Sodium and water retention, diabetes mellitus, mood disturbance, dyspepsia	Monitor blood pressure, urinalysis

sue necrosis. Vincristine is neurotoxic and this may be acute and painful; however, most commonly after repeated injections a degree of parasthesia is experienced and tendon reflexes are lost. More serious problems necessitating cessation of therapy are wrist or foot drop, cranial nerve palsies or paralytic ileus. It may also cause inappropriarily ADH secretion and alopecia but is not particularily myelosuppressive. Vinblastine is more myelosuppressive (especially as regards the white cells) but is less neurotoxic than vincristine. Vindesine is intermediate in terms of neurotoxicity and myelo-suppression.

Etoposide (VP16)

This is a semi-synthetic derivative of podophyllotoxin. Its exact mechanism of action is unclear but it is thought to inhibit DNA synthesis. It is used to treat lymphomas and acute non-lymphoblastic leukaemia. The drug can be administered intravenously or orally and causes alopecia, vomiting and myelosuppression. Peripheral neuropathy has also been recorded.

Dacarbazine (DTIC)

The mode of action of this drug is unknown. It is given intravenously and used to treat Hodgkin's disease. Its side effects are vomiting and myelsuppression and it is irritant to the skin and veins.

Steroids

These are non-myelosuppressive and derived from a cholesterol framework. The main endogenous steroid, cortisone, is not used for treatment of haematological malignancy, but useful analogues with increased glucocorticoid activity and reduced salt retention (pred-nisolone, dexamethasone) are employed therapeutically. The mechanism of cytoxicity is unclear but involves interaction with cytoplasmic receptor protein following which the steroid-receptor complex is modified and in-corporated into the nucleus. The number of receptors is variable and is thought to be an important factor governing responsiveness to steroids. It is used for the treatment of lymphoproliferative disorders. They are most often given orally when an enteric coated prepar-ation should be used, but they can also be given in-travenously. Side effects include salt and water retention, disturbances of glucose metabolism, im-munosuppression and dyspepsia. Longer-term problems include truncal obesity, osteoporosis, proximal muscle wasting and cataracts.

L-Asparaginase

This enzyme is purified from two bacterial sources — Escherichia coli and Eriwina carotova. L-asparaginase depletes cells of the essential amino acid L-asparagine. Tumour cells have a relative lack of L-asparagine syn-thetase and are thus more vulnerable than normal cells. Depletion of L-asparagine results in increased protein and DNA synthesis. It is used in the treatment of acute lymphoblastic leukaemia and can be given sub-cutaneously, intramuscularly or intravenously. Its main problem is sensitisation which can result in either localised reactions or anaphylaxis. These reactions have been reported particularly when repeated courses of high dose therapy are given and the intravenous route specifically is used. If reactions are obtained with one preparation, then the patient can be given the product from the other bacterial source. Other side effects include inhibition of protein synthesis which leads to a low albumin, fibrinogen (abnormal clotting studies), antithrombin III, insulin and lipoproteins. Acute pan-creatitis, abnormal liver function tests and cerebral dys-function have also been reported. Thrombosis has also been described following its use when combined with prednisone and vincristine. Fortunately the drug does not appear to be particularly myelotoxic.

Bleomycin

The mode of action of bleomycin is unclear. It is used for the treatment of lymphomas and can be given in-travenously, intramuscularly or into body cavities. It commonly causes a fever following its administration and may cause cutaneous problems and pulmonary fibrosis. It may also be responsible for irradiation recall reaction which can affect the skin, heart and lungs. As regards pulmonary toxicity the elderly, those patients who have received prior radiotherapy and patients given many courses (dose greater than 300 mg) are at risk of damage. Pulmonary function tests (especially the DLCO) should be monitored in addition to chest X-ray appearances. If pulmonary toxicity occurs, some cases respond to high dose steroids. Bleomycin is not myelotoxic.

Amsacrine (mAMSA)

This acradine derivative interferes with DNA function and is used for the treatment of acute leukaemias. It has to be given intravenously and must be drawn up in a glass syringe and infused in dextrose. It causes vomit-ing, alopecia and myelosuppression and is sclerosant to the veins. It can also cause abnormalities of the liver function tests and cardiotoxicity has been reported.

BIBLIOGRAPHY

Clendenium N J, Joliver J, Curt G A et al 1984 Cytotoxic drugs active in leukaemia. In: Goldman J M, Preisler H D (eds) Leukaemias, Butterworth, London, p 25

Coltman C A 1982 Treatment related leukaemia. In: Bloomfield C D (ed) Adult leukaemias. Martin Nijoff, The Hague, p 61

De Vita V T 1985 Principles of chemotherapy. In: De Vita V T, Hellman S, Rosenberg S A (eds) Cancer: principles and practice of oncology, 2nd edn. Lippincott, Philadelphia, p 257

Kearsley J H, Tattersall M H N 1986 Prevention or reduction of cytotoxic-induced nausea and vomiting. In: Williams C J, Whitehouse J M A (eds) Recent advances in clinical oncology 2. Churchill Livingstone, Edinburgh, p 221

Pindeo H M, Longo D L, Chabner B A 1987 Cancer chemotherapy and biological response modifiers, Annual 9. Elsevier Science Publishers

Disorders affecting all cell lines

24. Aplastic anaemia

M. Judge   J. A. Whittaker

Aplastic anaemia is bone marrow failure with consequent pancytopenia. It results from loss of haemopoietic stem cells and replacement by fatty tissue, and the term excludes cases of marrow failure secondary to malignant or other infiltrates and marrow fibrosis. Predictable marrow failure, induced by cytotoxic drugs and radiotherapy in the treatment of malignancy, is also excluded. Although there are many recognised aetiological factors, many patients have no identifiable precipitating event and must be termed idiopathic. Varying degrees of severity are defined and, although the definition of aplastic anaemia implies failure of all three haemopoietic cell lines (Fig. 24.1), some patients show reduction in only two of the formed elements. Another important feature is the varying degree of marrow cellularity which occurs in individual patients, which may lead to an unexpectedly cellular specimen in the face of severe pancytopenia. Except in the more severe cases, the term 'hypoplastic anaemia' is a more accurate label.

Classification and epidemiology

Three broad groups are recognised based on known aetiological factors or their absence (Table 24.1). Congenital aplastic anaemia is also called Fanconi's anaemia in recognition of the earliest description of this usually familial condition. Various congenital abnormalities and multiple chromosomal defects occur in some patients, but partial and non-familial types occur.

Acquired aplastic anaemia is subdivided into primary, or idiopathic where no definite cause is found, and secondary when a definite or likely agent can be identified. As more chemical toxins and drugs come under suspicion of causing aplasia and more exhaustive searches are carried out in new cases, the proportion of secondary cases increases. However, the long latency of aplasia often hinders accurate identification of the causative agent. The natural course and prognosis is similar for primary and secondary aplastic anaemia with the possible exception of post-hepatic aplasia.

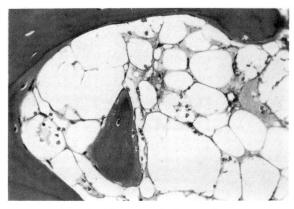

Fig. 24.1 Trephine biopsy in aplastic anaemia demonstrating almost complete absence of haemopoietic activity.

Table 24.1 Classification of aplastic anaemia

Congenital
e.g. Fanconi's anaemia

Acquired
  Primary (idiopathic)
  Secondary to
    Drugs
    Chemicals
    Radiation
    Viral – hepatitis
         – infectious mononucleosis
    Pancreatitis
    Autoimmune disease
    Pregnancy
    Paroxysmal nocturnal haemoglobinuria
    Eosinophilic fasciitis
    Graft versus host disease

The prevalence of aplastic anaemia shows marked variation between Western and Far Eastern countries. Surveys show an annual prevalence in the US and UK of 3–6 cases per million, 9 per million in Japan, and a rate of 13 per million in Sweden, while that of certain Chinese provinces is 20 per million. The sex ratio is approximately equal in Western countries, with a rising incidence in older patients, whereas four times as many men as women develop aplasia in the East and the incidence peaks between 20 and 40 years of age. Environmental differences are the likely cause of these variations, since Japanese people living in the US have an incidence similar to the US rate. Exposure to industrial toxins and the frequent use of chloramphenicol are both probable contributory factors. Reports of clusters of aplastic anaemia are surprisingly few, but detailed study of a group of four teenagers from the same school over a 7-year period showed only weak associations between the school and employment in the textile industry and agriculture.

Aetiology

Drug-induced

The most common cause of secondary aplastic anaemia is drug-induced marrow damage. The list of drugs implicated is long and ever-increasing, but a strong association exists for only a few, the major ones being chloramphenicol, phenylbutazones, anti-thyroid agents, gold, penicillamine and sulphas. Other less common agents are listed in Table 24.2.

Table 24.2 Drugs inducing marrow aplasia

Probable	Possible
Chloramphenicol	Phenobarbitone
Phenylbutazone	Indomethacin
Oxyphenylbutazone	NSAID
Gold	Amitryptiline
Penicillamine	Mianserin
Sulphonamides	Semisynthetic penicillins
Trimethoprim	Tetracyclines
Thiouracils	Griseofulvin
Phenothiazines	Ketoconazole
Chlorpropamide	Chloroquine
Quinacrine	Allopurinol
Hydantoins	Chlorpheniramine
Carbamazepine	Aspirin
Sodium valproate	
Thiazide diuretics	
Captopril	
Procainamide	
Levamisole	
Cimetidine	

Chloramphenicol. This is a definite cause of aplasia at an incidence of approximately 1 in 20 000 to 1 in 60 000 patients treated. The strong association was first noted within 5 years of its introduction in 1948, but it continued to be a popular widely used antibiotic until the 1960s, especially in Far Eastern countries. Reports from the American Medical Association in 1967 cited a strong link between it and aplasia in 44% of over 700 cases of aplastic anaemia.

A dose-dependent reversible marrow hypoplasia is probably due to inhibition of mitochondrial function and produces vacuolation and maturation arrest of precursor cells. This occurs at levels above 25 μg/ml of blood and resolves on withdrawal of the drug. This pharmacological effect primarily affects erythropoiesis and may be due to defective hepatic and renal clearance of the drug. An irreversible aplastic anaemia is a more rare effect unrelated to dose or duration of exposure to chloramphenicol and is presumed to be idiosyncratic. It often occurs weeks after exposure and the most likely mechanism is permanent damage to haemopoietic stem cells in genetically predisposed individuals. Chloramphenicol is a hydrocarbon containing a benzene ring which accounts for its considerable marrow toxicity. Topical use in eye drops and ointment has also caused marrow aplasia. Its systemic use is now restricted to the treatment of typhoid fever and severe ampicillin-resistant haemophilus influenzae infections, although it continues to be used topically, often inappropriately.

Phenylbutazone and oxyphenylbutazone. These are now among the most common culprits in drug-induced aplasia, with an incidence around 1 in 60 000 and a mortality rate of 50%. Elderly females are more at risk and pancytopenia usually occurs after many months of treatment with phenylbutazone. On the other hand, oxyphenylbutazone may induce aplasia at any time, independent of dose given.

The possible mechanisms of butazone-induced marrow damage include idiosyncratic reactions and stem cell membrane damage leading to immunological suppression of haematopoiesis.

Their use is now restricted, with oxyphenylbutazone being withdrawn altogether and phenylbutazone being licensed for the hospital treatment of ankylosing spondylitis only. Most of the non-steroidal anti-inflammatory drugs have been linked with cases of aplastic anaemia, but the relative risk is unknown.

Others. Amidopyrine, colchicine and penicillamine are all capable of inducing pancytopenia and gold induces a dose-dependent stem cell suppression in vivo and in vitro. Immune mechanisms may be more important in other patients, but a favourable response to chelation with dimercapral in some patients suggests a direct toxic effect from accumulated gold stores in macrophages.

Chemical toxins

Benzene and other organic aromatic hydrocarbons cause

dose-dependent marrow aplasia and, in spite of their known association with aplastic anaemia and leukaemia, many of these compounds continue to be used as solvents in industry and the home. Solvent, i.e. toluene, abuse in the form of glue sniffing has also become commonplace among teenagers. These substances are used as solvents for glue, cement, fat, nail varnish and paint and as diluents for paint and varnishes. The major industries involved are aircraft manufacture, petrol refining, glue making, dry cleaning and car repair, but the use of paint strippers and solvent fluids in the home may also be hazardous, particularly if ventilation is poor.

Long-term low dose exposure to benzene can induce a range of haematologic side effects from isolated anaemia, leukocytosis, lymphopenia, eosinophilia, leuko-erythroblastic anaemia and haemolysis to pancytopenia and acute leukaemia. Pancytopenia may be secondary to marrow hypoplasia or hyperplasia with myelodysplastic features. Some patients have moderate myelofibrosis.

Chronic exposure increases the risk of toxicity and the likely effect is to impair DNA synthesis at stem cell level and in differentiated cells, leading to maturation arrest in one or more haemopoietic lines. Characteristic chromosomal defects occur, including fragmentation and sister chromatid exchanges. Pancytopenia usually recovers when exposure ceases, but patients with myelodysplastic features have a worse prognosis since 15–20% can be expected to progress to acute leukaemia.

Some insecticides, particularly chlorinated hydrocarbons (DDT, lindane), organophosphates and carbonates, have been associated with hypoplastic marrow damage of varying severity, with leukaemic transformation in some. Children are more susceptible and these compounds are still used in popular household insecticides.

Viral infections

The association between viral infections and aplastic anaemia is difficult to test, but clues to a probable viral aetiology exist in some cases. Many viral infections cause transient leukopenia and mild pancytopenia in humans, and aplastic crises can be induced in mice by injecting Coxsackie virus and CMV. Intra-uterine rubella and CMV infections often lead to congenital hypoplasia of the marrow. The causative role of human parvovirus B19 infection in the aplastic crisis of hereditary spherocytosis and sickle cell disease is well established, but this virus does not seem to affect normal marrows, and does not cause persistent aplasia. Sera from patients with active infection showed marked inhibition of CFU-E growth, which was not evident when convalescent sera were used. Good epidemiological evidence and, recently, serological tests show a clear association between aplastic anaemia and non-A non-B hepatitis. Lack of detail on these agents has hampered investigation of their inhibitory effect on haematopoiesis, but clinically severe aplasia occurs with a bad prognosis in 80% or more of patients affected. Many of the reports of aplastic anaemia occurring with hepatitis A or B have lacked serological confirmation, but a definite association with hepatitis B has been shown. A number of cases of infectious mononucleosis with persisting pancytopenia have also occurred. Epidemiological links between HTLV1 infection and the high incidence of aplastic anaemia in the Orient have led some experts to postulate that a 'human retrovirus'-like agent may cause chronic aplastic anaemia.

Mechanisms of marrow damage by viruses include stem cell depletion, damage to stromal cells, membrane damage, which alters antigenicity, or direct inhibition of DNA replication. Marked chromosomal damage including total disruption is seen in post-hepatitic aplasia.

Radiation

Radiation induces predictable and dose-dependent marrow damage and haemopoietic tissue is second only to germinal epithelium in its radio-sensitivity. The severity and chronicity of the hypoplasia depends on the type of radiation (X rays and γ rays are more penetrating than α and β), the size and site of the irradiated field, the duration of exposure and whether or not prior cytotoxic therapy was used.

Whole body irradiation, such as that used for conditioning prior to marrow transplant or resulting from accidental exposure in reactor accidents, leads to permanent marrow aplasia at doses exceeding 700 rads. Fractionation as in TBI slightly reduces toxicity and allows therapeutic doses up to 1000 rads. Local irradiation of up to 4500 rads is used to treat breast cancers and results in permanent local marrow aplasia since microvascular damage prevents regeneration of vital stromal cells which could support migrating stem cells.

The more sensitive cells such as erythroblasts and lymphocytes show early mitotic arrest and chromosomal damage, but anaemia is a late occurrence because of the prolonged erythrocyte life span. Leukopenia and later thrombocytopenia are the earliest changes occurring within the first week, and stromal marrow cells are relatively radio-resistant. After 3–6 weeks of aplasia, surviving progenitor cells may repopulate the marrow and, although some patients have chronic hypoplasia, many recover normal function with some persisting chromosomal damage. Recovery is more likely if the exposure is less than 400 rads.

Rarely, aplastic anaemia has occurred after long-term low dose exposure in physicians, or in patients given spinal irradiation (for ankylosing spondylitis) or thorotrast dye.

Other causes

PNH (paroxysmal nocturnal haemoglobinuria) is an acquired haemolytic process due to membrane lysis by activated complement which coats blood cells. Marrow hypoplasia may occur at the onset of PNH or predate it by some years and transformation to acute leukaemia may follow.

A rare recently described condition known as diffuse or eosinophilic fasciitis shows a striking association with haematological disorders ranging from eosinophilia to aplasia and acute leukaemia. It is a connective tissue disease, manifested by cutaneous and fascial plaques and fibrosis, which occurs in late middle age and responds to steroid therapy.

Pathogenesis

Advances in the treatment of severe aplastic anaemia over the past 15 years have shed some light on the probable mechanisms of marrow failure. The observation that pre-transplant immunosuppression and anti-lymphocyte globulin can alone restore marrow function suggests an autoimmune basis, but the mechanisms are unknown. These treatments are not effective in all patients and produce a transient response in others, and other factors must be involved. A unifying theory suggests that an initial foreign substance may act as a hapten on the haemopoietic cell membrane stimulating auto-immune destruction or activation of suppressor T-lymphocytes. These T-cells release colony-inhibiting activity (CIA) which suppresses haemopoietic stem cell maturation. Transient or persistent exposure would explain the variable outcomes and the failure to detect such a reaction.

Surprisingly, natural killer lymphocyte activity (NKa) is depressed in severely aplastic patients, even before transfusion. These are the large granular lymphocytes (LGL) with T-cell features which react with the LEU 11 monoclonal antibody and after successful treatment their function returns to normal.

The explanation would seem to be that the subset of LGL which survives in aplastic anaemia is an immature NK cell sensitive to lymphokines and interferon, both of which are raised in aplastic anaemia. The more mature LGL with spontaneous NKa is lacking and whether this is a primary or secondary event is not known. A specific condition of suppressor T-cell lymphocytosis (T γ lymphocytosis) with associated leukopenia and anaemia has been described recently. In vitro culture studies in aplastic anaemia indicate low colony-stimulating and burst-promoting activities (CSA, BPA) and these patients' serum shows increased 'releaser activity' as a secondary response to the maturation block. Erythropoietin is also raised.

Other factors with inhibitory effects on CFU-GEMM growth and stimulatory effects on marrow macrophage activity exist in patients' serum and these appear to be produced by peripheral blood monocytes and B-cells. This complex network of interacting factors will take some time to disentangle. A favourable response to immunosuppression in some aplastic patients infers that their stem cells can react to the high levels of CSA and BPA once inhibitory factors have been removed. A poor response to immunosuppressive therapy might indicate that stromal cells in the marrow micro-environment may be damaged in the aplastic process. Their inability to produce growth factors for the haemopoietic stem cells in spite of high CSA/BPA would explain a failure to respond to steroids or ALG.

Clinical features

Complications of pancytopenia are the usual presenting features in patients with aplastic anaemia. The main complaints are of increasing tiredness and pallor, fever secondary to respiratory or other infections, and bruising and bleeding due to low platelets. In retrospect, a gradual decline in well-being is evident and investigations may have been delayed. A history of drug ingestion, exposure to toxic chemicals or of likely viral infection in the preceding months may be forthcoming and should be vigorously sought. A detailed family history, especially of haematologic, skeletal or congenital defects must also be taken.

Physical examination usually reveals pallor, petechiae, bruises and possibly oral or retinal haemorrhages in addition to signs of specific infection which may arise in the mouth, skin, chest or perianal areas. Rectal examination is contraindicated. The presence of jaundice suggests either concurrent viral or drug-induced hepatitis and hepatomegaly may occur. However, post-hepatitic aplasia may follow mild hepatitis and occur many weeks later, so that its significance is missed. Splenomegaly is unusual in aplasia at diagnosis and if present should lead to a search for PNH or chronic haemolytic process (e.g. hereditary spherocytosis with aplastic crises). Skin and subcutaneous nodules suggest a diffuse fasciitis, but this is a very rare condition. Skin pigmentation, mental retardation and thumb hypoplasia in a child suggest Fanconi's anaemia.

Laboratory investigations

Pancytopenia is the hallmark of aplastic anaemia, though some patients may have depression of only two cell lines at diagnosis. A normochromic anaemia always occurs and non-specific red cell changes with some macrocytes may be seen on the blood film. A low reticulocyte count in absolute numbers is typical, though occasionally the percentage value may be misleadingly high. Thrombocytopenia is invariable with a count below $80 \times 10^9/l$ in most cases. Bleeding complications do not usually occur when the platelet count exceeds $20 \times 10^9/l$, unless infection is also present.

Neutropenia occurs in all patients, but lymphocyte numbers may not be affected and the overall white cell count may thus be normal. Monocytopenia is common. Eosinophilia is very rare and suggests eosinophilic fasciitis, especially if the immunoglobulins are also raised.

Criteria for the categories of severe and moderate aplastic anaemia are given in Table 24.3.

Table 24.3 Criteria in aplastic anaemia

| | Two of the following values | |
	Severe	Moderate
Haemoglobin and reticulocytes	<10 g/dl	≤10 g/dl
	$<20 \times 10^9/l$	$<60 \times 10^9/l$
Granulocytes	$<0.5 \times 10^9/l$	$<1 \times 10^9/l$
Platelets	$<20 \times 10^9/l$	$<50 \times 10^9/l$
	+ a hypocellular (<25%) or acellular marrow biopsy	

An important feature is the increase in serum iron and transferrin saturation, which may be a useful early finding in drug-induced aplasia. Ferrokinetic studies show characteristic delayed clearance of labelled injected iron and increased uptake in the liver. Chromium-labelled red cells have a normal life span in the early untreated aplastic patient, but later in the course of continuing hypoplasia the red cell life span may be reduced to one-third of normal through a combination of haemorrhage, haemolysis and transfusion. Marrow aspiration usually yields a dilute bloody sample with scant marrow granules. These show variable but increased fat content, conspicuous macrophages and reticulin cells, often with phagocytosed material, lymphocytes and plasma cells. However, even in severe aplastic anaemia, early myeloid and erythroid cells may be present in unexpected numbers, but maturation is not evident and

dyserythropoiesis is common. Iron stores are increased and non-ringed sideroblasts may be seen. Focal hypercellularity may lead to sampling errors and further aspirates at different sites are useful. Trephine biopsy (Fig. 24.1) of the marrow is the most reliable indicator of marrow cellularity and this too should be obtained from more than one site. As well as providing reliable detail of marrow cellularity, biopsy will also reveal malignant infiltrates or abnormal fibrosis which may be the underlying cause of the aplasia in a given patient. Nests of residual myelo- and erythroblasts may resemble erythroleukaemia or refractory anaemia with excess blasts, and an aplastic presentation of acute lymphoblastic leukaemia is well recognised. Repeat sampling, ferrokinetic studies and a consistent blood picture will usually clarify the diagnosis.

There is a compensatory elevation of erythropoietin levels in plasma and urine in aplastic patients. Part of this rise is thought to be due to increased oxygen affinity of haemoglobin secondary to a deficiency of red cell 2,3-diphosphoglycerate. Serum B_{12} and folate levels are normal and a sucrose haemolysis test should be performed on all new cases.

Treatment

Severe aplastic anaemia carries a grave prognosis and, since the pathophysiology is still poorly understood, various therapies, mostly directed towards immunosuppression, have had limited success.

The natural course of the disease itself is unpredictable with spontaneous remissions occurring in some patients. Yet, even when a cause is identified and removed, patients may follow an inexorable downhill course.

All of these factors make evaluation of treatments difficult, but guidelines to the most appropriate treatment for a given patient, depending on severity, age and available resources, exist in most centres. Comparative results are now being published on long-term survival in specific treatment groups, comparing antilymphocyte globulin (ALG) to marrow transplantation (BMT).

At diagnosis, a detailed historical search for a possible cause is rarely of therapeutic interest, but removal of a suspected drug, chemical toxin or radiation source may be followed by recovery.

During the investigative phase, various supportive measures are started, plans for definitive treatment made and any spontaneous improvement can be observed.

Supportive treatment

Prevention and control of bleeding may be the prime consideration and simple measures to reduce the risk include careful oral hygiene, using a soft toothbrush, pre-scribing of laxatives and hormonal suppression of men-struation. Aspirin and intramuscular injections are for-bidden. The occurrence of major bleeding or the appearance of retinal haemorrhages necessitate the infu-sion of random or single HLA-matched donor platelets, the latter to reduce the risk of sensitisation. If BMT is being planned, irradiated blood products should be used, but avoidance of all transfusions prior to transplant is desirable. Serious bleeding is uncommon when the platelet count exceeds $20 \times 10^9/l$ in a well patient, and platelet prophylaxis should not be needed. Both infec-tion and severe anaemia increase the risk of bleeding when the platelet count might otherwise be considered safe and it then warrants prompt correction. Symptoma-tic anaemia is corrected with packed cell transfusion and haemoglobin maintained at the lower end of the normal range. Patients with mild hypoplastic anaemia or partial recovery may not need regular transfusion, lessening the risks of viral hepatitis and haemosiderosis. In those with a high transfusion requirement, intravenous or con-tinual subcutaneous desferrioxamine reduces iron over-load.

Infection is common in severely neutropenic patients and is a major cause of death in chronic aplastic anaemia. It tends to arise at unusual sites such as the mouth, skin, groin and perianal regions and often in-volves organisms of low pathogenicity such as *Staphylococcus epidermidis*, bacteroides and fungal or-ganisms, e.g. *Candida albicans*.

Pathogenic organisms such as *Klebsiella*, *Pseudomonas proteus* and *E. coli* can cause fulminant, rapidly fatal sep-sis with early cardiovascular collapse. They may not induce local inflammatory changes, so that physical signs are few (due to absence of neutrophils), and fever may be a relatively late development. Quite apart from prompt and aggressive antibiotic treatment, prophylactic antibiotics may be used to reduce the risk of serious in-fection (Ch. 35).

Resistant infection may respond to granulocyte in-fusions from partially HLA-matched donors (i.e. family members) obtained by leukopheresis. This is a tem-porary measure only and carries a potential risk of CMV infection if the donor is positive for CMV antibodies.

The intensive supportive care and subsequent specific therapy of patients with severe aplastic anaemia neces-sitates the insertion of an indwelling central venous catheter, e.g. Hickman catheter.

Steroid therapy

Anabolic steroids, androgens and corticosteroids have all been used in treating aplastic anaemia. A favourable response to testosterone was recognised in the late 1950s, but after many attempts to assess the role of androgens in aplasia, it is accepted now that they have limited activity and have not proven effective in controll-ed trials. Oxymethalone is occasionally useful in mild to moderate aplastic patients who are not suitable for BMT and have failed to respond to ALG. A gradual improvement in blood counts over some months may persist when it is stopped. Continued treatment causes significant toxicity in the form of virilisation, severe acne, fluid retention, hyperlipidaemia and hepatic damage. Hepatic toxicity includes cholestatic jaundice, peliosis, hepatitis and hepatocellular carcinoma. These drugs probably exert their effect on stem cells by induc-ing differentiation.

Corticosteroids were used in the past for two reasons. It was known that excess endogenous and exogenous steroid induced a leukocytosis, but this effect was the result of a shift from the marrow pool to the peripheral blood and not due to haemopoietic stimulation. In high doses they are immunosuppressive and might be ex-pected to reverse immunologic suppression of haemopoiesis. One trial yielded a response rate of 40% after 1 year's treatment, but many other controlled studies do not show long-term benefit and some reveal increased mortality at 6 and 10 months of treatment. Steroids may reduce the rate of complications of pancy-topenia by improving vascular stability and prolonging of red cell life span, but these effects may not balance the long-term toxicity.

There have been anecdotal reports of a good response to acyclovir in steroid-refractory patients when other op-tions were not available, but it has not been the subject of a controlled trial.

Antilymphocyte globulin

Antilymphocyte or antithymocyte globulin (ALG, ATG) was first produced and used as immunosuppressive pre-transplant conditioning in aplastic anaemia patients. It was noted that some patients recovered autologous mar-row function after failure of engraftment and further randomised studies confirmed a significant remission rate in patients treated with ALG alone. Most studies show a consistent 50% rate of sustained improvement within 3 months and a dramatic increase in long-term survival of 60% or more of patients treated.

Although these results suggest an autoimmune basis for severe aplasia, the mechanism of action of ALG and ATG is unknown. Among other suggested modes of ac-tion are a direct stimulatory effect on stem cell proliferation or activation of accessory marrow cells with release of specific growth factors. Many responders show only partial recovery, while some relapse and may respond to a second course of treatment.

ALG is usually given with high dose prednisolone or androgens, both of which are claimed to improve response and survival rates. However, recent reports fail to show any enhancement of ALG effect. Prednisolone is nevertheless justified to prevent allergic reactions and serum sickness after ALG. Transient drops in the platelet count on starting ALG also necessitate the use of daily prophylactic platelets during therapy and ALG must be given through a central catheter.

In-vitro colony growth following T-cell depletion has not proven a reliable predictor of response to ALG, but other pre-treatment factors which influence outcome have been identified. Good prognostic indicators were ALG treatment within 16 weeks of diagnosis, a higher pre-treatment marrow cellularity and better CFU-GM growth in vitro. Surprisingly, in those treated within the first 16 weeks of diagnosis, older patients (mean age 75 years) fared better than younger ones (mean 25 years). It would seem that ALG is effective only in those patients with a reserve of progenitor cells and the overall dose or duration of ALG therapy is irrelevant.

It is notable that even with good and sustained responses to ALG, haematologic recovery is always incomplete. Platelet and granulocyte counts remain lower than normal, macrocytosis and marrow hypocellularity with increased mast cells also persist, and in-vitro CFU-GM and BFU-E growth is suboptimal.

There is a suspicion that late sequelae such as the development of PNH and acute leukaemia are more likely in ALG treated patients.

Bone marrow transplantation (See Ch. 21)

The only truly curative treatment for severe aplastic anaemia is replacement of haemopoietic tissue by allogeneic or syngeneic marrow transplantation.

The earliest marrow transplants were performed in Seattle in the early 1960s from identical twin donors. Each of the six aplastic patients was transplanted without any immunosuppressive preconditioning and all were successful, with engraftment and recovery of marrow function. An intrinsic defect in haemopoietic stem cells seemed to have been corrected. However, it was reported in the 1970s that some syngeneic BMTs failed, but were successful on second syngeneic transplantation after high dose cyclophosphamide immunosuppression.

Progress in the understanding of the major histocompatibility antigens on lymphocytes led to allogeneic BMT from HLA-identical siblings using cyclophosphamide preconditioning. Initially used in patients who had failed to respond to ALG and other treatments, this resulted in a 45% cure rate. Failures were due to graft rejection, acute graft versus host disease or the advanced stage of the illness.

Marrow rejection occurred in 36% and most of these patients died. Mixed lymphocyte reactivity (between donor and recipient lymphocytes) in vitro and low cell counts in the infused marrow were identified as the major factors in rejection. However, as more patients were referred and transplanted prior to transfusions, it became clear that graft rejection never occurred in the untransfused patients and consequently survival extended to 90%. Rejection therefore is due mainly to sensitisation of the patient to minor histocompatibility antigens after blood transfusion. Preconditioning in multi-transfused patients now includes total body irradiation and the practice of post-BMT buffy coat infusions (from donor) has been dropped in most centres. The problems of graft rejection have now been largely solved, but acute and chronic graft versus host disease (GVHD) are still major problems.

The advent of cyclosporin A, a T-lymphocyte suppressor initially used to prevent renal transplant rejection, has reduced the incidence and severity of GVHD as well as preventing graft rejection post-BMT. It is used in the immediate pre-BMT phase and for 6 months post-BMT in most centres and seems to obviate the need for total body irradiation in preconditioning in aplastic patients. Some transplant centres routinely use intermittent methotrexate for the 3 months post-BMT as GVHD prophylaxis.

Acute GVHD is treated with high dose methylprednisolone, reducing the doses rapidly over 2 weeks. Further relapses are usually controlled with additional immunosuppression by ALG, methotrexate or azathioprine with continuing low dose steroids. Acute GVHD is more common in multi-transfused patients. Chronic GVHD continues to affect up to 40% of aplastic patients after allogeneic BMT and shows a similar frequency in non-transfused and transfused patients. It is treatable in all patients and most lead a full, active life.

Late graft rejection after withdrawal of cyclosporin occurs in some patients and it seems prudent to continue cyclosporin for 12 months. Most respond to its reintroduction. Purging of marrow with a T-cell monoclonal antibody (CAMPATH I) reduces the incidence of GVHD, but is associated with a higher graft failure rate. Figures from Seattle show a 74% long-term survival in patients who engraft and the Hammersmith experience is of 76% long-term survival in cyclosporin-primed patients.

Prospective studies comparing ALG and allogeneic BMT in severe aplastic anaemia have shown fairly similar response rates and, allowing for the drawbacks of each mode of therapy, the follow-up guidelines have been suggested by Thomas and the Seattle team:

1. Any patient with a normal identical twin should be transplanted immediately and, if engraftment does not occur, a second syngeneic BMT with cyclophosphamide preparation should be done.
2. Patients under 40 with an HLA-matched sibling should have an allogeneic BMT and transfusions should be avoided if possible.
3. In the absence of an HLA-matched sibling, ALG should be given and, failing that, a second course may induce a response while an extended family search or search for an unrelated HLA match is carried out. Over the age of 50, ALG should be the treatment of choice, since BMT complications are more frequent in this group. Between the ages of 40 and 50, a clear-cut advantage for either ALG or BMT is not evident.

Haplo-identical BMT is very rarely used in aplastic anaemia, but has been combined with ALG and androgen therapy in some studies.

A few reports of marrow recovery in aplastic patients after infusion of fetal liver cells suggest successful engraftment of fetal stem cells which are immuno-competent, but this has not been followed up.

Congenital hypoplastic anaemia

The combination of inherited or familial aplastic or hypoplastic anaemia, certain visceral and skeletal defects, pigmentation and physical or mental retardation is called Fanconi's anaemia. All features may not be present, but multiple chromosomal breaks, duplications and chromatid exchanges are invariable. The anaemia is diagnosed in children under 10 years and renal hypoplasia with absent or hypoplastic thumbs are characteristic features. The cytogenetic abnormalities render these children very sensitive to myelotoxic agents and transformation to acute leukaemia is not uncommon

in their second decade. Spontaneous recovery of marrow function may occur, but the management of marrow failure in these patients should be the same as for idiopathic aplastic anaemia. Irradiation should be avoided.

Pure red cell aplasia

Failure of erythropoiesis with normal white cell and platelet production is a rare condition. Like aplastic anaemia, it may result from drug or chemical exposure and may be idiopathic or congenital. An association with a thymoma occurs in 50% of cases and rarely myasthenia gravis or SLE may occur also.

In-vitro studies show normal BFU-E growth, but failure of differentiation with absent CFU-E colonies. Surface marker studies reveal an increase in large granular T-lymphocytes and low levels of natural killer (NK) activity. Remission, if it occurs, leads to normalisation of lymphocyte subsets, and it seems pure red cell aplasia is immunologically mediated, possibly via a clonal excess of LGL. It has also complicated both B- and T-cell CLL and a history of autoimmune disorders may occur. It usually runs a chronic course with severe transfusion-dependent anaemia. Immunosuppression with prednisolone, azathioprine or cyclophosphamide is often beneficial and ALG has been used successfully. Removal of a thymoma produces remission in 50% of thymoma-related red cell aplasias, but relapse is not uncommon. Splenectomy has been recommended – the response is partial and slow, although subsequent immunosuppression may be more effective than before.

Congenital pure red cell aplasia is termed Diamond-Blackfan anaemia and it is usually diagnosed in the first few months of life. It can be sporadic or familial and, in contrast to the acquired forms, culture studies show deficient BFU-E growth.

Life-long red cell transfusion is usually required and iron overload is a serious complication. Spontaneous remission is said to occur in 25% of cases, but many are steroid-responsive. Allogeneic BMT may be indicated if no improvement occurs by the mid-teens.

BIBLIOGRAPHY

1986 Aplastic anaemia in the Orient. British Journal of Haematology 62: 1–6
Cametta et al 1982 Aplastic anaemia. New England Journal of Medicine 306: 645
Conall Thomas E 1984 Acquired severe aplastic anaemia: progress and perplexity. Blood 64 (2), 325–328
Geary G C 19 Aplastic anaemia. Balliere Tindall, London
Heimpel H, Gordon Smith E, Heit W, Kubanek B 19 Aplastic anaemia: pathophysiology and approaches to therapy. Springer Verlag, London

Linet M et al 1985 An apparent cluster of aplastic anaemia. Archives of Internal Medicine 145: 635–639
Speck B et al 1986 Treatment of severe aplastic anaemia. Experimental Haematology 14: 126–132
Williams, Beutler, Erslev, Lichtman 19 Haematology, 3rd edn. McGraw Hill, New York
Young, Levine, Humphries (eds) 19 Progress in clinical and biological research, vol. 148. Aplastic anaemia. Alan R Liss, New York

25. Myelodysplastic syndromes

J. A. Whittaker   M. Judge

Myelodysplastic syndromes (MDS) have been described under a variety of names since the beginning of this century. Perhaps most attention has been devoted to the preleukaemias, a group of disorders characterised by the subsequent development of acute myeloid leukaemia (AML) and often presenting with multiple cytopenias in the presence of a hypercellular marrow. Increasingly it has become clear that there is a group of disorders with similar characteristics to the preleukaemias which do not necessarily transform to AML. To facilitate description and comparison, the FAB group have classified these disorders as MDS (Table 25.1). Thus, as a general term, MDS is preferable to preleukaemia, as by no means all patients will develop leukaemia, but it must be remembered that similar morphological appearances may be seen after cytotoxic or immunological damage to bone marrow.

Unfortunately, the older terms varied in their usage, making exact comparison difficult. For example, in the RA group, some older studies have excluded patients with hypocellular bone marrow.

Classification

In the FAB classification, refractory anaemia (RA) and refractory anaemia with sideroblasts (RAS) are similar groupings with much the same predisposition to transform to AML and this is particularly so for patients with defects in the granulocyte and megakaryocyte cell lines. Those defects more closely related to leukaemia were previously described under a variety of names including 'atypical' leukaemia, oligoblastic, smouldering or subacute leukaemia, sub-acute or chronic myelomonocytic leukaemia, chronic erythraemic myelosis and refractory anaemia with excess of blasts. The great majority of, or possibly all, patients previously falling into these categories are now covered by the FAB classification as refractory anaemia with excess blasts (RAEB), RAEB in transformation (RAEB-T) and chronic myelomonocytic leukaemia (CMML).

Table 25.1 Classification of the myelodysplastic syndromes

FAB	Previously used names
Refractory anaemia (RA)	Aregenerative anaemia
Refractory anaemia with sideroblasts (RAS)	Idiopathic refractory sideroblastic anaemia Sideroachrestic anaemia
Refractory anaemia with excess blasts (RAEB)	Refractory anaemia with excess of myeloblasts
RAEB in transformation (RAEB-T)	'Atypical' leukaemia Smouldering leukaemia
Chronic myelomonocytic leukaemia (CMML)	Oligoblastic leukaemia Chronic erythraemic myelosis Sub-acute myeloid leukaemia

Incidence

The incidence of these disorders is difficult to estimate reliably and considerable variation is apparent even in recently published series. This is because most authors have simply collected a series of patients without regard for the incidence of the disorder. The Leukaemia Research Fund's Data Collection Study, at present in progress, indicates a provisional incidence similar to that of AML. Table 25.2 gives comparative figures for the five subdivisions of FAB collected from previously published reports.

While RAEB-T represents only a small proportion

Table 25.2 The comparative occurrence of the subtypes of the myelodysplastic syndromes

	(%)
Refractory anaemia (RA)	30–45
Refractory anaemia with sideroblasts (RAS)	15–20
Refractory anaemia with excess blasts (RAEB)	10–20
RAEB in transformation (RAEB- T)	5–10
Chronic myelomonocytic leukaemia (CMML)	10–20

(<5%) of all AML, there is a suggestion that AML in patients over 50 years is preceded by preleukaemia and one estimate that 30% of acute myelomonocytic leukaemia (FAB M4) has an initial preleukaemic phase. As the populations of developed countries live longer, more MDS is certain to be seen and already in elderly populations MDS is as common as CLL, with an approximate incidence of 1:1000 in those over 65 years.

When preleukaemia occasionally occurs in children and young adults, it is associated more often with chromosomal changes (see below).

Pathogenesis

Most MDS show dyspoiesis in two or even three cell lines, suggesting a defect in the multipotent haemopoietic stem cell. This is supported by colony growth patterns and karyotype studies, but the exact nature of the production of this defect is unknown and similarly there is no real evidence to explain why the various subtypes of MDS develop from this stem cell defect.

CMML is almost always a dyspoiesis of one cell line, although erythroid and megakaryocytic defects have been reported, and has a low (or ? absent) tendency to transform to AML. Although it is now included in the MDS, on these and other grounds one can make a case for its classification as a myeloproliferative disorder.

Leukaemogenesis

Carcinogenesis has long been considered to be a two-step process including initiation and promotion steps, and both may result from contact with chemicals, radiation or oncogenic viruses. Many agents are both initiators and promoters, causing irreversible changes in the cell and rendering the cell susceptible to a tumour-promoting agent. Promotion appears reversible, but if a threshold exposure is exceeded, recognisable malignant change results. This change may be multifocal or of a single focus which may show multiple clones of aberrant cells with different genetic and phenotypic characters. Oncogenes, probably involved in growth regulation in normal circumstances, may become aberrantly expressed if transported to a new site on the genome by chromosomal translocation (cellular oncogenes), by virus (viral oncogenes) or by mutation or amplification. Thus, the detection of non-random chromosomal abnormalities is important in any malignancy, as it may indicate associations with known oncogenes.

Cytogenetic abnormalities

Non-random abnormalities similar to those seen in

AML occur in at least 40% of MDS patients, but none are unique and the most common occur in AML with about the same frequency, except perhaps for the 5q-defect which is much more commonly found in MDS. However, the translocations seen in AML (for example 8:21 and 15:17) and the Philadelphia chromosome have not been seen in MDS. The presence of karyotype abnormalities in MDS appears to have prognostic value, but disappearance of abnormal clones is reported and not all patients show a rapid development of leukaemia.

Monosomy 7 (−7) is the most frequent specific defect described for 15–18% of patients with the preleukaemic syndrome in the older literature and one of the commonest now seen in MDS. It also occurs in AML, but with a slightly lower frequency. In childhood, it is associated with a specific myeloproliferative disorder characterised by a hypoproliferative bone marrow, pancytopenia associated with defective neutrophil chemotaxis and recurrent infection followed by a progressive evolution to AML. Leukaemic transformation in Fanconi's anaemia also may be associated with the development of a clone of cells lacking a number 7 chromosome.

Chromosome 7 seems to have particular haematological importance and the 7q− abnormality is also relatively frequent, occurring in about 5% of MDS and AML patients. Chromosome 7 is the site of the cellular homologue of the erb-B oncogene, which may code for the epidermal growth factor receptor.

5q− is the third most common defect in MDS and when it occurs in isolation is usually associated with a refractory anaemia with a slight excess of blasts. Patients, who are more commonly women, also usually have a macrocytic anaemia, bone marrow erythroid hyperplasia and thrombocytosis, sometimes with poorly-lobed megakaryocytes. Granulocyte and macrophage production appears normal. Patients usually have a chronic course with a low incidence of leukaemic change.

Trisomy 8 is a frequent defect occurring in about 20% of MDS and AML patients. It is of interest to note that two cellular oncogenes are situated on the long arm of chromosome 8, the c-myc and c-mos oncogenes.

20q− has been reported relatively frequently (6.5%) in patients with the preleukaemic syndrome; it also occurs in AML and may be a frequent accompaniment of polycythaemia rubra vera.

Haemopoietic Progenitors

Cell culture in vitro is useful in the diagnosis and assessment of prognosis of MDS, but variation in the technique used makes comparison difficult. Abnormalities of colony growth in vitro are compatible with a gradual replacement of normal haemopoietic cells by an abnormal clone which occurs via an intrinsic stem cell defect, giving the new clone a growth advantage, either by insensitivity to normal feedback regulation or by inhibiting normal haemopoiesis.(For a detailed review see Francis & Hoffbrand, 1985.)

Granulocyte-macrophage colonies (CFU-GM)

Bone marrow cultures from patients with RA, RAEB and CMML show a reduction in colony and cluster growth and attempts have been made to use these findings to classify MDS into prognostic groups. It is possible to separate patients into leukaemic and non-leukaemic groups, but it is debatable whether this gives better prognostic information than simply separating patients according to the percentage of blast cells in blood and bone marrow.

In the preleukaemic syndrome, about two-thirds of patients have reduced or absent colonies with normal or reduced cluster growth, a pattern similar to that seen in aplastic anaemia or to the 'low growth' or 'no growth' patterns described in AML. The remaining one-third of patients show the characteristic 'leukaemic' growth pattern of absent colonies associated with a great increase in clusters.

RAS is associated with an essentially normal growth pattern, while RAEB and CMML can be separated on the basis of culture findings. In CMML, there is generally a very large increase in the number of colonies and clusters with an excess of solitary cells, while RAEB patients show growth patterns similar to those seen in the preleukaemic syndrome.

Culture pattern does not correlate well with transformation rate, although high colony-stimulating activity has been associated with a high risk of early leukaemic transformation.

Erythroid colonies (BFU$_E$ and CFU$_E$).

Erythroid colonies are generally decreased in blood and marrow cultures from MDS patients, but as yet this information has not given help with prognosis.

Clinical Features

Patients with MDS are generally over 50 years of age and mostly over 60. One clear exception is MDS in childhood associated with monosomy 7, an atypical form of MDS with a high risk of leukaemic transformation. MDS is most often diagnosed by chance on routine blood examination, but may present with infection, especially mouth ulcers, or with haemorrhage. There are usually no physical signs, although 20% of patients have a modest splenomegaly and some patients present with the signs of haemorrhage and/or infection reflecting partial bone marrow failure. Specific clinical signs of

leukaemia are rare, except for the occasional occurrence of skin rashes and deposits in CMML.

Haematological and morphological findings

Blood

Changes in both blood and bone marrow are essentially non-diagnostic (Table 25.3). All three cell lines are usually involved, except in CMML (see below), and the red cells show hypochromasia with appreciable numbers of ovalocytes and macrocytes and sometimes poikilocytosis with or without tear drop forms. There is occasional red-cell stippling and punctate basophilia. Often, a few nucleated red blood cells are seen and occasionally circulating normoblasts can be identified. Anaemia is usual, but 5–10% of patients have a normal haematocrit and in most patients the reticulocyte count is unexpectedly low for the haemoglobin concentration. A number of red cell enzymes are reduced, especially pyruvate kinase, and fetal haemoglobin may be increased. There is also an alteration in the expression of red cell membrane antigens, especially a reduction in the amount of A1, and rarely there is a positive acidified lysis test.

Table 25.3 Haematological findings and MDS subtypes

	RA	RAS	RAEB	RAEB-T	CMML
Blood					
Haemoglobin	R	R	R	R	N/R
Neutrophils	N/R	N/R	R	R	I
Blasts (%)	<1	<1	<5	>5	<5
Platelets	N/R	N/R	R	R	N/R
Marrow					
Dyserythro-poiesis	Moderate	Marked	Marked	Marked	None to Minor
Sideroblasts (%)	<15	>15	<15	<15	<15
Granulo-poiesis	N*	N*	I	I	Greatly increased
Blasts (%)	<5	<5	5–20	20–30	5–20
Megakaryo-cytes	N*	N*	I	I	I

N = Normal; R = Reduced; I = Increased; * Usually

Neutrophils

Neutropenia is most commonly seen, but occasionally there is a monocytosis or neutrophil leukocytosis. Neutrophils often show nuclear and cytoplasmic anomalies, occasionally the Pelger Huet defect and rarely hypersegmentation. Defective granulation is frequent, usually in the form of loss of primary granules, paralleled by a loss of peroxidase activity. In CMML, 'intermediate' or 'paramyeloid' cells with features of monocytes and myelocytes may be seen in the blood and marrow.

A variety of neutrophil functional defects are seen, especially associated with the monosomy 7 defect where reduced bacteriocidal and phagocytic function is common and disordered chemotaxis is also encountered.

Lymphocytes

Lymphocytes in MDS are not morphologically abnormal, but functional defects include impairment of T-cell function.

Platelets

More than half of MDS patients are thrombocytopenic, although very occasionally thrombocytosis is seen. When examined with the electron microscope, platelets show vacuolation, defective or absent microtubules, dilated canalicular systems and giant platelet granules which do not participate in the normal release reaction during aggregation. Platelet function may be abnormal with a prolonged bleeding time in the presence of an adequate platelet count.

Bone Marrow

In MDS, the marrow is of normal or increased cellularity and only occasionally is cellularity reduced. Granulopoiesis is often left-shifted, making it difficult to count the percentage of blasts accurately. Erythropoiesis may show megaloblastosis and dyserythropoiesis with multinucleate forms, cytoplasmic vacuolation, nuclear budding, karyorrhexis and, rarely, internuclear bridging in erythroblasts. Abnormal sideroblasts are seen in RAS and less commonly in other types. A predominance of non-ring or intermediate sideroblasts may be important, as there are claims that under these circumstances transformation to acute leukaemia may be more frequent.

When blasts are present, they are often agranular and frequently accompanied by abnormal promyelocytes with blue-grey cytoplasm, in which fine nuclear chromatin and pale nucleoli are often seen.

Giant megakaryocytes are frequent with a reduced number of lobules and fragmented nuclei. Often micromegakaryocytes as small as 800 μ are present which may be mistaken for primitive granulocytes. Some have suggested that when more than 10% of megakaryocytes are mono- or binucleated, there is a high risk of transformation to acute leukaemia.

Marrow histology. Marrow histology is useful, especially for a more accurate assessment of marrow cellularity. Fibrosis is sometimes present and provides a useful differentiation from aplastic anaemia in hypocellular marrows. Some authors have claimed that small foci of blasts and promyelocytes can be identified more easily, especially when the blast count is low.

Special Haematological Features

There is considerable overlap between the various subtypes of MDS, but there are a number of discriminatory features.

Refractory anaemia (RA)

RA is heterogeneous, although only a minority of patients have abnormalities of granulocytes and megakaryocytes. Before making the diagnosis of RA, it is important to exclude alcoholism, as many alcoholics show macrocytosis and thrombocytopenia.

In RA, the blood shows the changes described above, but in particular reticulocyte counts may be low. Blast cells are usually absent or present at counts of less than 1%. The marrow is hypercellular or normocellular with or without non-ring sideroblasts and ring sideroblasts up to 15%. It also shows erythroid hyperplasia, variable dyserythropoiesis and occasionally dysgranulopoiesis. The marrow contains less than 5% of blasts in which Auer rods are not seen. The rate of leukaemic transformation is uncertain, but probably around 30%, although in one series it was 56%. Leukaemic change occurs especially in those patients with minor changes in the granulocytic and megakaryocyte lines, although it may occur even in patients who only show macrocytosis without anaemia. In addition, red cell aplasia, not normally classed with MDS, is a preleukaemic syndrome, especially in the elderly, but rates are lower than for RA at about 10–15%.

Refractory anaemia with ring sideroblasts (RAS)

This group of disorders was previously classified as primary or idiopathic acquired sideroblastic anaemia, but it remains uncertain whether all the disorders covered by these terms should be included as RAS, although both the acquired and the genetic defect show similar abnormalities in DNA synthesis and in haemsynthesis. In addition, the RAS group now includes a few patients with abnormalities of the granulocyte and megakaryocyte cell lines.

RAS patients show a dimorphic anaemia with an increased or normal MCV. Morphological changes are mainly in the red cell series, where ring sideroblasts represent more than 15% of the nucleated red blood cells. Megaloblastosis occurs in more than 50% of patients.

Refractory anaemia with excess of blasts (RAEB)

The RAEB subgroup includes some patients with what was previously called sub-acute, oligoblastic or smouldering leukaemia.

Blood and marrow changes in RAEB are similar to those in RA, but the blood is more typically pancytopenic with less than 5% of blasts which lack Auer rods. The marrow shows erythroid hyperplasia with a variable sideroblastosis, usually of non-ring forms and 5–20% of myeloblasts. The marrow may resemble M6 AML, causing diagnostic difficulty. The FAB group have proposed that if marrow erythroblasts are 50% or more with greater than 30% myeloblasts, then the condition should be classified as M6 AML.

Patients with large spleens and palpable livers are said to have a poorer prognosis with progression to RAEB-T or AML.

Refractory anaemia with excess blasts in transformation (RAEB-T)

The FAB definition includes patients with more than 5% of blasts in the blood and 20–30% of marrow blasts, and the group includes some patients with conditions previously called sub-acute, oligoblastic or smouldering leukaemia.

Chronic myelomonocytic leukaemia (CMML)

CMML is a difficult disorder to categorise, as it shows features both of myelodysplasia and of atypical myeloproliferative disease.

Characteristically, the blood shows a monocytosis greater than $1 \times 10^9/l$ and usually between 5 and $10 \times 10^9/l$. There is a marrow proliferation of immature myeloid cells, but with far fewer blasts (5–25%) than in M4 AML patients, and the spleen is usually moderately enlarged. Monocytes show nuclear abnormalities including convolutions and hypersegmentation. Paramyeloid cells are frequent and some patients have immature granulocytes in the blood. Skin deposits and gum hypertrophy occur very infrequently and rarely there is an associated nephropathy. There is a high incidence of polyclonal hyperimmunoglobulinaemia and occasionally monoclonal proteins are seen. Serum uric acid and Vitamin B_{12} levels are often high. In addition, the serum and urinary lysozyme are raised.

There is an overlap with RAEB, RAEB-T and M4 AML, although all of these conditions show a greater blast cell proliferation than that seen in CMML. In addition, some cases of Ph negative CML may cause diagnostic difficulty, although here the blood and marrow monocytosis is usually much less pronounced.

CMML usually has an indolent course with modest anaemia which may require blood transfusion. Some patients transform to frank M4 AML, but the risk of this transformation is difficult to assess, although patients who transform are said to have high levels of immature blood granulocytes and bone marrow blasts of 20% or more at diagnosis. However, under such circumstances these patients may not be clearly distinguishable from those with RAEB-T.

Aplasia-leukaemia syndrome

There are various associations between marrow hypoplasia and leukaemia. (For a full review of this and other variant MDS, see Geary, 1986.)

1. Rarely, typical idiopathic aplastic anaemia may terminate as acute leukaemia, although this is more common in constitutional Fanconi aplasia and aplasia secondary to benzene. In the context of aplastic anaemia, paroxysmal nocturnal dyspnoea is regarded by some as a stage in the process of leukaemic transformation.
2. Acute leukaemia may present in a hypoplastic phase making exact diagnosis difficult, although leukaemia patients usually show more than 30% of blasts in trephine biopsy of bone marrow. Most patients are elderly and represent about 5% of all AML.
3. MDS may present with a hypoplastic bone marrow and there is some limited evidence that the risk of acute leukaemia is higher in pancytopenic patients' hypercellular marrows than in those with hypoplasia. However, if only patients with trilineage MDS are included, the difference is less.

Secondary myelodysplasia

There is an increasing incidence of AML following the use of cytotoxic drugs, especially alkylating agents and procarbazine. AML occurs in about 10% of patients treated for Hodgkin's disease and in more than 15% receiving myeloma treatments with the combination of alkylating agents and radiotherapy appearing to be particularly leukaemogenic. About three-quarters of the patients have a myelodysplastic phase.

There are some differences between this secondary MDS and the primary disorder. Macrocytosis and dyserythropoiesis are especially common in secondary MDS. The marrow is more likely to be hypocellular and to show reticulin and even collagen fibrosis, a feature which is associated with a shorter transition time to AML. Karyotypic anomalies are often multiple and are more common than in primary MDS.

Prognosis

Generally, prognosis for MDS patients is poor and this relates chiefly to their advanced age, increasing anaemia and the problems presented by granulocytopenia and thrombocytopenia. Other poor prognostic features are an increasing number of blasts in blood and bone marrow, significant enlargement of the liver or spleen and the presence of complex karyotype anomalies. Most studies of MDS report a median survival of less than 30 months, a figure which is only slightly better than current survival prospects for adult patients with AML. However, fewer than 10% of MDS patients survive for more than 10 years, compared with a projected figure of about 30% for AML patients treated with modern chemotherapy regimens. Most MDS patients are elderly and die from marrow failure or its indirect effects of infection and/or haemorrhage. The percentage of patients transforming to AML varies with MDS subtype and it is uncertain whether the number of patients transforming would be greater if patients survived longer. The five FAB subtypes (Table 25.3) separate into two distinct prognostic groups, with RA and RAS patients showing a much better survival than those with RAEB or RAEB-T, where survival is often less than 6 months. The majority of transformations are to M2, M4 or M6 AML, with transformations to ALL extremely unusual.

CMML presents a much wider prognostic spectrum, with many patients surviving in satisfactory health for a number of years, but a few transforming early to frank M4 AML(see above).

Treatment

Before treatment is even considered for an MDS patient, the physician would do well to consider what is likely to be achieved, and patient assessment will centre mainly on age, general condition and the subtypes of MDS. Most MDS patients are elderly and many myelodysplastic syndromes are not life-threatening even for patients with a degree of thrombocytopenia and neutropenia. Consequently, most patients are best managed with supportive care only, with specific treatment reserved for those with RAEB-T or frank AML transformation.

However, the clear exception is patients of less than 50 years of age where an 86% complete remission rate has been reported with daunorubicin and cytosine arabinoside used intensively before progression to frank AML has occurred. In addition, patients under 50 years should be considered for early bone marrow transplant if a suitable donor is available.

Otherwise there is a long experience of disappointing treatment results, especially for transformed disease. Remission rates are low and generally below what would be expected for age-matched patients with de novo AML.

Low dose cytosine arabinoside

In MDS, an abnormal clone appears to be in a state of arrested differentiation along a normal maturation pathway and consequently differentiation inducers may help to overcome the defect, although the alternative hypothesis that the abnormal clone arises from a misprogrammed stem cell makes differentiation induction less rational. The presence of inappropriate surface markers on granulocytes and monocytes in MDS suggests that differentiation is abnormal rather than arrested normal.

Some reports have suggested that Ara C at very low dosage acts as a differentiation inducer in vitro but others have questioned whether its action in vivo is anything other than a cumulative myelosuppression. The result for most patients is severe pancytopenia before any marginal benefit is obtained and the use of cytosine arabinoside should be confined to patients with RAEB-T or transformation to AML, where several authors have reported remission rates of 30% following 14 to 21 days' treatment at 10 mg/m^2.

Retinoids

Retinoic acid is known to prevent chemically-induced skin cancers in mice and hundreds of retinoid analogues have been tested for their ability to cause regression of skin papillomas. Retinoids are known to inhibit the proliferation of many cell types and in some cells to allow differentiation of morphologically and functionally mature cells with granulocyte and monocyte characters. Retinoids have been effective in producing differentiation both in vitro and in vivo in a few patients with M3 AML. These findings lead to their use in MDS, where there is some evidence of improvement, with a reduction in blast cell number and an increase in haemoglobin concentration, leukocytes and platelets. However, these improvements seem only to occur at high dosage which is associated with hepatotoxicity, hyperkeratosis and hyperostosis when used for prolonged periods.

Some observers have suggested using combinations of true inducers such as retinoic acid with cytotoxic agents which slow the rate of replication of the stem cell, thus rendering it susceptible to the action of inducers. At present, there is no evidence that this is practical.

Vitamin D₃

1:25 dehydroxy vitamin D_3 has been used clinically, but without real evidence of improvement. Vitamin D_3 suppresses the proliferation of murine and human AML cells and allows the differentiation of some leukaemia cell lines in vivo with predominantly monocyte differentiation.

Biological differentiation inducers

A number of proteins, mostly produced by macrophages, T-lymphocytes and various cultured cell lines, produce differentiation factors for normal myelopoiesis. Most have not been tried therapeutically, although endotoxin, which may be an inducer of granulocyte CSF, is currently being studied.

Supportive treatment

Many patients will require transfusion, but care is needed and automatic transfusion should be avoided in view of the risks of a high iron load in recurrently transfused patients. Platelet infusion should be reserved for the treatment of clinical bleeding and should not be given simply because MDS patients have low platelet counts.

Infection, which can threaten life in elderly patients with marrow failure, requires scrupulous treatment (Ch.35).

BIBLIOGRAPHY

Bennett J M, Catovsky D et al 1982 Proposals for the classification of the myelodysplastic syndromes. British Journal of Haematology 51: 189–199

Francis G E, Hoffbrand A V 1985 The myelodysplastic syndromes and preleukaemia. In: Recent advances in Haematology, vol 4. Churchill Livingstone, Edinburgh, pp 239–267

Galton D A G 1984 The myelodysplastic syndromes. Clin. Lab. Haematol. 6: 99–112

Geary C G 1987 Myelodysplasia. Morphology, clinical presentation and treatment. In: Whittaker J A, Delamore I W (Eds) Leukaemia. Blackwell, Oxford

Jacobs A 1985 Myelodysplastic syndromes: pathogenesis, functional abnormalities and clinical implications. Journal of Clinical Pathology 38: 1201

Jacobs A 1987 Myelodysplasia and preleukaemia – pathogenesis and functional aspects. In: Whittaker J A, Delamore I W (Eds) Leukaemia. Blackwell, Oxford

Nowell P C 1982 Cytogenetics of preleukaemia. Cancer Genetics and Cytogenetics 5: 265–278

Ruutu T 1986 The myelodysplastic syndromes. Scandinavian Journal of Hematology, Supplement 45, vol.36

26. Polycythaemia

R. J. G. Cuthbert   C. A. Ludlam

The term 'polycythaemia' embraces a group of disorders characterised by elevation of the packed cell volume, haemoglobin and red cell count. Polycythaemia can be subdivided into the true polycythaemias, in which there is an absolute increase in the red cell mass (RCM), and the relative polycythaemias, in which the red cell mass is normal and the rise in packed cell volume (PCV) is secondary to reduced plasma volume (PV). Table 26.1 gives a full classification of the polycythaemias. The most significant feature common to all the polycythaemias is the considerable risk of vascular occlusive events including stroke, myocardial infarction, peripheral vascular disease and venous thrombo-embolism.

Pathogenesis of vascular occlusive lesions in the polycythaemias

The vascular lesions occurring in polycythaemia include occlusion of major arteries or veins and in some cases obstruction of the microvasculature. The frequency of these occlusive events increases exponentially as the PCV rises (Fig. 26.1) This relationship is strongest for primary proliferative polycythaemia (PPP, otherwise known as polycythaemia rubra vera) but can also be demonstrated in patients with idiopathic erythrocytosis, secondary polycythaemia and relative polycythaemias. Indeed, data from the Framingham epidemiological studies show that even in individuals who are not diagnosed as having polycythaemia the risk of stroke is greater in those with high-normal PCV than those with low-normal PCV. The reason for this is not completely clear but relates at least in part to the change in whole blood viscosity associated with elevation of the PCV.

Whole blood viscosity

The major determinant of the whole blood viscosity (WBV) is the PCV, which reflects the red cell concentration. The white blood cells, platelets and plasma proteins contribute negligible effects unless they are grossly elevated. The influence of the PCV on the WBV is further accentuated by a fall in the shear rate of the blood (Fig. 26.2). The shear rate is lowest in venous blood where the rate of blood flow is lowest. Thus as the rate of blood flow falls the WBV rises.

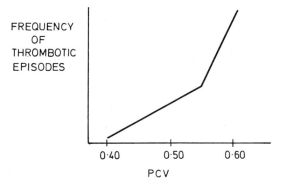

Fig. 26.1 Relationship between frequency of thrombotic episodes and packed cell volume in primary proliferative polycythaemia. (Reproduced by permission of Dr T. C. Pearson)

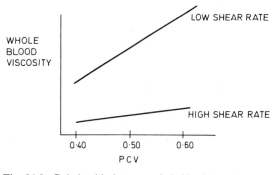

Fig. 26.2 Relationship between whole blood viscosity and packed cell volume at different shear rates. The shear rate can be shown to be significantly higher at high rates of blood flow. (Reproduced by permission of Dr T. C. Pearson)

Table 26.1 Classification of the polycythaemias

True

1. Primary proliferative polycythaemia

2. Secondary

(a) Hypoxaemia:	Altitude
	Chronic lung disease
	Cyanotic congenital heart disease
	Heavy smoking
	Congenital methaemoglobinaemia
	High affinity haemoglobinopathies
	Red cell enzyme defects
	Cobalt poisoning

(b) Inappropriate rise in erythropoietin:		
Renal	Renal parenchymal cysts
	Polycystic kidneys
	Hydronephrosis
	Renal cell carcinoma
	Post renal transplant
	Chronic glomerulonephritis
	Barrter's syndrome
Liver	Hamartoma
	Hepatocellular carcinoma
	Alcoholic liver cirrhosis
Others	Cerebellar haemangioblastoma
	Uterine fibromyoma
	Ovarian carcinomas
	Phaeochromocytoma
	Bronchial carcinoma

| (c) Hypertransfusion: | Overestimation of blood loss |
| | Neonatal – twin-twin – placenta-fetus |

3. Idiopathic erythrocytosis

Apparent

Overt fluid loss
Relative polycythaemias
High-normal red cell mass
Physiological variant

Cerebral circulation

The rate of blood flow in the cerebral circulation is abnormally low in polycythaemias compared with the rate of blood flow in other vascular trees. At increased haemoglobin levels the arterial oxygen-carrying capacity is increased. Consequently the rate of blood flow falls by physiological vasoconstrictor mechanisms, resulting in a normal degree of cerebral oxygen delivery. A further rise in PCV in this situation may lead directly to the increased risk of thrombotic events by producing a dangerous rise in whole blood viscosity.

Circulation to limbs

The rate of blood flow in the limbs rises as the PCV falls when polycythaemia is treated. However, there may be no significant change in oxygen transport to the limb tissues, because the benefit of reducing the WBV is offset by the reduction in oxygen-carrying capacity as the PCV falls. Despite these physiological observations a significant minority of patients with intermittent claudication derive benefit from treatment to reduce their PCV. Therefore elective arterial surgery should be considered only after the PCV is brought down to normal.

Platelet vessel wall interaction

In PPP (unlike other causes of polycythaemia) abnormal platelet function may contribute to the pathogenesis of vascular occlusive lesions. Microvascular lesions such as erythromelalgia, gangrene and ulceration of the toes, livedo reticularis and transient ischaemic attacks are not uncommon in PPP (and essential thrombocythaemia). Many of these symptoms are significantly improved by anti-platelet drugs such as aspirin, and by reducing the platelet count to normal.

Occasionally platelet emboli can be observed migrating along vessels of the retina during episodes of transient visual disturbance. This suggests that platelet sludging is involved in the pathogenesis of these microvascular lesions. Platelet aggregation studies have shown that patients with PPP often have reduced responses to ADP and serotonin, increased frequency of spontaneous platelet aggregation in vitro and reduced inhibition of platelet aggregation by prostaglandin-D_2. Abnormalities of plasma and platelet B-thromboglobulin, which are reversible by aspirin therapy, have also been observed. Thus abnormal platelet function may play a role in the pathogenesis of large vessel as well as microvasculature occlusion in PPP. Other factors such as hypertension and atherosclerosis, which also occur at increased frequency with increasing age, may also contribute to vascular occlusive events in the polycythaemias.

Measurement and interpretation of packed cell volume, red cell mass and plasma volume in the polycythaemias

Packed cell volume

Accurate estimation of the PCV can be done by the microhaematocrit method in which the relative proportion of red cells to buffy coat and plasma are measured in a standard centrifuged capillary column of blood. Estimations of PCV on automated electronic blood counters are usually calculated from the MCV or other cell-size measurements and are adequate for most clinical purposes.

The PCV is taken as a guide to the presence and degree of polycythaemia. However, when the red cell mass is grossly elevated the PCV becomes less reliable an indicator of the severity of true polycythaemia, since the PCV does not correlate directly with the RCM. Occasionally patients may present with a normal or even reduced PCV. This may be due to gross splenomegaly causing an increase in total PV and splenic red cell pooling, or because of a recent bleeding episode. In the presence of iron deficiency (a relatively commonly recognised phenomenon at presentation) there is a microcytic hypochromic blood picture and the red cell count will be more markedly elevated than the haemoglobin or PCV.

Samples must be taken for PCV measurements without venous occlusion. Application of a tourniquet causes a rise in venous pressure leading to leakage of crystalloid from plasma. Consequently the PV is reduced and overestimation of the PCV may result.

Red cell mass and plasma volume

Once the presence of an elevated PCV is confirmed, it is necessary to estimate the RCM and PV to establish what type of polycythaemia is present. The RCM is estimated by measuring the degree of dilution of a suitably labelled, known volume of concentrated red cells. [51]Chromium or [99]technetium are the most suitable radio-isotopes for labelling red cells. The PV is estimated by a similar dilution technique using [125]iodine-labelled albumin. Both estimations can be carried out simultaneously.

Interpretation of results

Interpretation of RCM and PV for each individual depends on comparing the observed values with the values expected for that individual in health. Commonly RCM and PV are expressed in terms of body weight,

i.e. l/kg. In obese patients the linear relationship between weight and blood volume is lost because adipose tissue is relatively less vascular than other tissues, so that the estimate of blood volume tends to be low in relation to body weight.

Blood volume correlates more closely with lean body mass than body weight, but estimation of lean body mass is a cumbersome procedure which is not practicable as part of routine procedure. However reference values for lean body mass based on age, height and sex are available (Geigey Scientific Tables). Expression of blood volumes in terms of estimated lean body mass is useful to ensure that true polycythaemia is not underdiagnosed in obese individuals.

The reference values for RCM, PV and calculated whole blood volume for adult males and females are given in Table 26.2. These values apply only to subjects living at sea level.

Table 26.2 Reference ranges for blood volume estimations in normal adults

	Male	Female
Red cell mass	0.025–0.035 l/kg	0.020–0.030 l/kg
Plasma volume	0.040–0.050 l/kg	0.040–0.050 l/kg
Total blood volume	0.060–0.080 l/kg	0.060–0.080 l/kg

PRIMARY PROLIFERATIVE POLYCYTHAEMIA

Primary proliferative polycythaemia (PPP) is a neoplastic condition in which there is excessive production of erythropoietic cells causing an absolute rise in the red cell mass. There is very often associated increased production of granulocytes and platelets. One of the myeloproliferative disorders, this condition is now recognised to be due to a clonal stem cell defect.

Aetiology and pathogenesis

The underlying cellular defect causing malignant proliferation in PPP is unknown. There is an overlap with other myeloproliferative disorders. Many patients with idiopathic erythrocytosis will progress to PPP. Genetic factors may operate in some cases: the prevalence in Jews of Eastern European origin is much higher than in those from other regions; occasional familial occurrence has been observed in other populations. PPP is predominantly a disease of middle age and later life. Less than 5% of cases present below the age of 40 years. There is a slightly greater incidence in males. No causal association between environmental factors, such as ionising radiation, toxins or infectious agents, has been identified.

Two lines of investigation have been useful in proving the clonal nature of PPP. Studies of females with PPP who are heterozygous for two iso-enzymes of glucose-6-phosphate dehydrogenase demonstrate that one iso-enzyme is present in >90% of haemopoietic cells, whereas equal distribution of both iso-enzymes is present in non-haemopoietic tissues. This suggests that the abnormal proliferative stem cell clone giving rise to PPP predominates in the marrow at the expense of normal stem cell activity.

Bone marrow culture studies have demonstrated the presence of two populations of red cell progenitor cells: normal CFU-E activity requiring erythropoietin for in vitro erythropoietic growth, and a second population which, although responsive to erythropoietin, will form colonies in its absence – autonomous mutant clones.

Clinical features

PPP may present as an incidental finding when a full blood count is done for an unrelated condition, or splenomegaly is identified unexpectedly. Alternatively it may present with the insidious onset of non-specific symptoms. In some cases it is first recognised after a major vascular occlusive event. Table 26.3 lists the commonest presenting features of PPP.

The salient features on clinical examination are facial plethora and splenomegaly–present in 70% of patients at presentation. The spleen slowly increases in size as the disease progresses. Other recognised findings are

Table 26.3 Common presenting features of primary proliferative polycythaemia

	Pathogenesis
Headache Dizziness Lethargy Blurred vision Loss of concentration Mental impairment	Increased cerebral blood viscosity
Weight loss Night sweats Hyperuricaemia and gout	Hypermetabolic state
Epistaxis	Abnormal platelet function
Pruritus	? Increased histamine
Splenic pain	Splenomegaly
Cebrovascular disease Peripheral vascular disease Acute myocardial infarction Venous thrombo-embolism	Increased whole blood viscosity/abnormal platelet function

acne rosacea, urticaria, leg ulcers, conjunctival infection, and retinal vein engorgement with or without retinal haemorrhages. The liver is enlarged in about 50% of patients at presentation. Hypertension is found in up to 30% of patients.

Vascular occlusive lesions

About a third of patients present with some form of vascular occlusive phenomenon. These represent the most serious complications of PPP. The frequency of arterial and venous occlusive events is roughly equal.

Cerebrovascular complications range from transient ischaemic attacks to complete stroke or sudden death. The cerebral circulation is four times more commonly affected than the coronary circulation. However, myocardial infarction is a well-recognised cause of severe morbidity and mortality. Peripheral vascular lesions range from digital ischaemia to severe lower limb arterial insufficiency, thrombosis and gangrene. Painful, burning sensation (erythromelalgia) of the soles, and less commonly the palms, may occur. It is often associated with thrombocytosis resulting in local microcirculatory embarrassment.

Venous occlusion resulting in deep venous thrombosis in the limbs, as well as visceral venous thrombosis (e.g. mesenteric vein, splenic vein, hepatic vein or portal vein) may occur. In the retina tortuous distended veins may be observed due to the effects of hyperviscosity. Occasionally even papilloedema may be observed. Retinal vein thrombosis may result in serious impairment of vision.

Hyperviscosity causing reduced cerebral blood flow may lead to other cerebral symptoms. These include headache, dizziness, feeling of fullness in the head, loss of concentration and overt intellectual impairment. These symptoms are usually alleviated by reduction of viscosity.

Bleeding

Abnormal bleeding is a less frequent complication of PPP compared with other myeloproliferative disorders, particularly essential thrombocythaemia. Spontaneous haemorrhage is rare, and most abnormal bleeding episodes follow trauma or surgery. These may occur due to abnormal platelet function or less commonly, due to coagulation defects (see below).

Pruritus

This is a well-recognised complication of PPP, affecting about 15% of patients at presentation. It is usually generalised but may be localised to the trunk or limbs. Characteristically it is provoked or exacerbated by warmth, such as entering a hot room, or following a hot bath. However, occasionally it may also be provoked by cold ambient temperature such as contact with water.

The pathogenesis of pruritus in PPP is not entirely clear. Histamine levels are elevated in over 90% of PPP patients with itch, and increased basophil and histamine turnover has been reported. However, similar findings have been recorded in chronic myeloid leukaemia and acute leukaemias which are not associated with pruritus. The itch rarely responds satisfactorily to antihistamine therapy. Thus other factors are almost certainly involved in its pathogenesis.

Gout

The increased cell turnover in PPP often leads to excessive accumulation of uric acid. Hyperuricaemia is observed in about 75% of patients and about 10% have symptomatic gout. Acute classical gout is the most common complication. Tophaceous gout, ureteric calculus and chronic renal impairment have occasionally been observed.

Peptic ulceration

Several studies have reported an increased incidence of peptic ulceration. Histamine has been suggested as a possible pathogenic factor. However, in a recent report the incidence of peptic ulceration was found to be no different than in a comparable non-PPP control population.

Hypertension

Hypertension is usually considered to be an incidental finding in PPP. Hypertensive patients who develop PPP are more easily controlled following definitive treatment of the polycythaemia.

Laboratory investigations

Red cell changes

A haemoglobin (Hb) level above about 18 g/dl with a packed cell volume (PCV) in the range of 0.50–0.60 and a total red cell count (RCC) of 5.5–6.5 × 10^{12}/l indicates the presence of erythrocytosis. The definitive diagnosis of polycythaemia, however, requires estimation of the red cell mass (RCM) and plasma volume (PV). The red cell lifespan is normal in PPP. This confirms that the elevated RCM is due to increased red cell production rather than excess accumulation. As the disease progresses, however, the red cell lifespan tends to shorten. This is due to increased rate of splenic destruction and ·a reduction in survival advantage of the abnormal erythroid clones.

White cell changes

The total white cell count is usually moderately elevated in the range 15–25 × 10^9/l. This is due to elevation of granulocytes, mainly neutrophils. Relatively few immature granulocytes are detectable in the peripheral blood. The presence of basophilia suggests development of a transitional myeloproliferative disorder (see below). Characteristically the leukocyte alkaline phosphatase activity is increased to about 100–400 and is >100 in 50% of patients. This is in contrast to chronic myeloid leukaemia in which the LAP is usually markedly depressed.

Platelet changes

The platelet count is characteristically elevated to 500–2000 × 10^9/l; 66% of patients have a platelet count of more than 400 × 10^9/l. Platelet morphology is often abnormal, with variation in platelet shape and size, including the presence of large, bizarre forms. Platelet function may be abnormal and this is reflected in abnormalities of in-vitro tests. These functional changes may give rise to abnormal bleeding or microvascular occlusive lesions such as gangrene of toes or erythromelalgia.

Bone marrow

Characteristically there is gross erythroid hyperplasia with normoblastic erythropoiesis. Micronormoblastic changes due to iron deficiency may be recognised, especially after venesection or chronic bleeding. The amount of stainable iron and the number of sideroblasts in the marrow are greatly reduced (often to nil) since all the marrow iron stores tend to be used up by the rapidly proliferating clone. There is often accompanying increased myeloid and megakaryocyte activity which correlates with the peripheral granulocyte and platelet counts.

Trephine marrow biopsy shows dramatic increased cellularity with >90% of the marrow space occupied by haemopoietic cells and concomitant reduction in fat spaces. Stains for reticulin show an overall increase in reticulin fibril density but retention of the normal pattern of distribution. Occasionally minor increases in coarse reticulin may be seen.

Other features

No specific chromosomal abnormalities have been recognised in several cytogenetic studies of untreated patients with PPP. However, following ^{32}P therapy minor chromosomal defects such as partial deletions, aneuploid lines, and C-group anomalies may be recognised. None of these has been shown to have diagnostic or prognostic value.

The serum B_{12} level is often increased. This is due to elevation of B_{12}-binding capacity due to increased transcobalamin III which is synthesised by granulocytes. The increase in transcobalamin III reflects the size of the granulocyte mass and tends to rise further as the disease progresses.

Occasionally folic acid deficiency (due to the high rate of marrow turnover) occurs if dietary folate is limited. Multiple minor abnormalities of coagulation function may be detected in PPP. These are rarely of clinical significance, although occasionally they may contribute to abnormal bleeding.

Diagnosis

In all instances it is essential to make a positive diagnosis of PPP and to exclude, so far as possible, all other causes of erythrocytosis. Increased PCV, splenomegaly, granulocytosis and thrombocytosis strongly support a diagnosis of PPP. All patients should have a RCM and plasma volume estimation to establish true polycythaemia (Table 26.4). In addition further investigation to exclude secondary polycythaemia is necessary before the diagnosis can be confidently established. If all the diagnostic criteria cannot be met and secondary polycythaemia is excluded, a diagnosis of idiopathic erythrocytosis should be made.

Table 26.4 Diagnostic criteria for primary proliferative polycythaemia

1. Normal pO_2
    + Elevated red cell mass
    + Splenomegaly

or

2. Normal pO_2
    + Elevated red cell mass
    + Any two of the following: Platelet count $>400 \times 10^9/l$
    White cell count $>12 \times 10^9/l$
    Leukocyte alkaline phosphatase >100
    B_{12} >900 ng/l
    B_{12}-binding capacity >2200 ng/l

These diagnostic criteria are based on the Polycythaemia Vera Study Group protocols of management of PPP.

Using these criteria the false positive rate is $<0.5\%$. However, since these criteria are used for clinical trials, they do not cater for the false negative rate and so some patients just outside the criteria may actually have the disease. This must be borne in mind when each individual patient's clinical management is being planned.

Course and prognosis

PPP can generally be followed through distinct phases, each merging into the next. Initially there is a proliferative phase in which elevated PCV, granulocytosis and thrombocytosis occur. A minority of patients then enter a stable phase in which the peripheral blood remains relatively stable with little or no treatment. During this phase haemopoietic marrow is gradually being replaced by fibrotic tissue. Eventually the spent phase is reached in which there is extensive marrow fibrosis and consequent pancytopenia and hepatosplenomegaly due to compensatory myeloid metaplasia. The change from the proliferative or stable phases to the spent phase may be marked by development of a transitional myeloproliferative disorder. During the late proliferative, transitional and spent phases, transformation to acute leukaemia may occur.

In the absence of treatment the prognosis for PPP is poor, with median survival of 18 months. The major cause of morbidity and mortality in untreated or inadequately treated patients is vascular occlusion. Effective reduction of the PCV results in improvement in the median survival to 10–15 years by reduction of the early mortality from vascular complications. Up to 60% of patients, however, will eventually die from cerebral or coronary events. It is not clear whether by effective treatment life is extended into the age group where the risk of mortality from these diseases is high or whether the polycythaemia itself is an influencing factor.

Between 10 and 25% of patients will eventually experience transformation of PPP to myelofibrosis. This is often manifested by progressive splenomegaly, the development of anaemia or pancytopenia, and increasing proportions of immature cells in the peripheral blood, producing a leuko-erythroblastic blood picture. There is no correlation between the mode of treatment and development of myelofibrosis.

The concept of a stable transitional myeloproliferative disorder is also recognised in which there are features of both PPP and myelofibrosis. In this situation there is elevation of the red cell mass, splenomegaly, a leuko-erythroblastic blood picture and a hypercellular marrow. Transition to overt myelofibrosis eventually occurs.

Acute myeloid leukaemia (AML) is a well-recognised late complication of PPP. It is manifested by rapidly progressive anaemia, thrombocytopenia and the appearance of blasts in the peripheral blood. 1–2% of patients treated by venesection alone will develop an acute leukaemic transformation. In contrast, it is reported from the Polycythaemia Vera Study Group that treatment with radiophosphorus or chlorambucil is associated with a significantly higher risk of acute leukaemic transformation. The majority of transformations are M1 or M2 (FAB classification), whereas M6 transformation is surprisingly rare. Acute lymphoblastic leukaemia has been reported. The risk of AML is greater in patients progressing to myelofibrosis. The response to treatment of AML developing secondary to PPP is much poorer than to that of AML arising de novo. The precise influence of radiophosphorus or chlorambucil in the induction of leukaemic transformation is not fully evaluated. However, patients with PPP are known to develop abnormal clones detectable by cytogenetic studies. Their rate of formation is accentuated by 'leukaemogenic' treatment. One of these abnormal clones may relate to the development of leukaemia.

Treatment

The aims of treatment are:

1. Reduction and maintenance of PCV at a level that will substantially reduce the risks of vascular occlusive events. There is a significant risk of vascular complications even if the PCV is modestly increased and therefore it should be maintained at less than 0.45 or a haemoglobin of less than 13 g/dl.
2. Control of thrombocytosis.
3. Reduction of the mortality from acute leukaemic transformation by avoiding chlorambucil, and judicious use of radiophosphorus.

Venesection

The advantages of venesection are prompt symptomatic relief and reduction of the risk of vascular occlusive episodes associated with a grossly elevated PCV. It is probably the treatment of choice in patients less than 50 years of age who have relatively normal white cell and platelet counts. In otherwise healthy patients, 400–450 ml of blood are removed at 5–7 day intervals until the PCV is less than 0.40. More rapid reduction of the PCV can be achieved by daily or even twice-daily venesection, with plasma volume replacement with colloid and crystalloid. In the elderly there is an increased risk of major thrombotic events if aggressive venesection

is conducted. However, more conservative venesection of 150–200 ml with plasma volume replacement, conducted at 5–7 day intervals, has been demonstrated to be relatively safe. The PCV can then be maintained in the region 0.35–0.44 by less frequent, regular venesection. The interval between venesections required for maintenance therapy is usually 2–4 months. Iron deficiency is an inevitable consequence of venesection, and the haemoglobin should not be allowed to fall below 12 g/dl.

The main disadvantage of venesection is a potentially greater risk of thrombotic events, as demonstrated in the early Polycythaemia Vera Study Group reports. This may have been due to inadequate maintenance of the PCV below 0.45 in the venesection arm of the treatment protocols. The other main disadvantage is the frequency of attendance required by patients to achieve adequate, safe treatment.

Radiophosphorus

A single dose of ^{32}P of 112 MBq/m^2 is an effective, convenient method of bringing the PCV under control. In addition it provides a method of controlling thrombocytosis. Occasionally, for complete control of the PCV, a second, smaller dose is required after about 3 months. The effect is relatively prolonged compared with venesection alone. However, repeat doses may be required at 12–18-month intervals.

The major disadvantage of radiophosphorus is that its use is associated with a six to ten fold increased risk of development of AML compared with treatment by venesection alone. This increased risk begins 4–5 years after the first dose of radiophosphorus and thus may potentially be responsible for premature death in a substantial proportion of patients in their 60s and 70s, even if its use is confined to the treatment of PPP in the 'elderly'. However, half of the radiophosphorus-associated cases of AML occur more than 11 years after the start of treatment. Thus radiophosphorus is still considered to have a useful role in the treatment of elderly patients.

Chemotherapy

The early Polycythaemia Vera Study Group reports of the use of chlorambucil in the treatment of PPP showed a very high risk (10–15-fold greater than venesection alone) of leukaemic transformation. Thus chlorambucil is now considered to be absolutely contra-indicated in PPP. However, this excess of acute leukaemias has not been demonstrated by the use of busulphan which is also an alkylating agent. An initial evaluation of hydroxyurea has shown no excess of malignancies compared with venesection alone after a minimum of 5 years follow-up and this may, therefore, be an alternative form of chemotherapy.

The main indication for chemotherapy is control of thrombocytosis, in conjunction with venesection for control of the PCV. It may also be used alone in situations in which venesection is contra-indicated, such as severe cardiac disease, or when venous access is difficult.

General approach to treatment

Figure 26.3 outlines possible therapeutic strategies for patients with PPP. Venesection should be considered as first-line treatment of PPP. However, if this form of treatment is used, it is essential that the PCV is consistently maintained below 0.45. Occasionally some patients have such a rapid rise in PCV after venesection that it is impossible to provide adequate treatment by venesection alone. In this situation the addition of chemotherapy or radiophosphorus is recommended to reduce the venesection requirements. In the UK a Medical Research Council-sponsored multicentre trial of treatment of PPP has so far shown no differences in mortality between treatment by venesection, radiophosphorus or busulphan. However, this trial is in its infancy compared with the Polycythaemia Vera Study Group trials. Most physicians would agree that, in view

of the reported leukaemogenic effects of chlorambucil and radiophosphorus, use of myelosuppressive agents in PPP requires caution. In the elderly radiophosphorus remains first choice treatment, despite the increased risk of AML, because treatment by venesection alone is associated with a higher mortality from thrombosis.

Treatment of other aspects of PPP

Hyperuricaemia and gout. The risk of renal complications of hyperuricaemia are greatest following chemotherapy or radiophosphorus therapy. Thus allopurinol should be administered before myelosuppressive therapy and in all patients with hyperuricaemia. The uric acid level should be monitored regularly in all patients.

Pruritus. Pruritus often improves as the peripheral blood counts return to normal after definitive treatment; particularly after chemotherapy or radiophosphorus. Occasionally antihistamines provide some relief. Other forms of treatment attempted with limited success include H_2 blockers (cimetidine and ranitidine), cholestyramine, simple analgesics, aspirin and nocturnal sedatives. Avoidance of precipitating and exacerbating factors such as heat or cold damp atmospheres may obviously be of benefit.

Peripheral vascular disease. Erythromelalgia often responds promptly to definitive treatment to reduce the PCV. Control of thrombocytosis and antiplatelet therapy

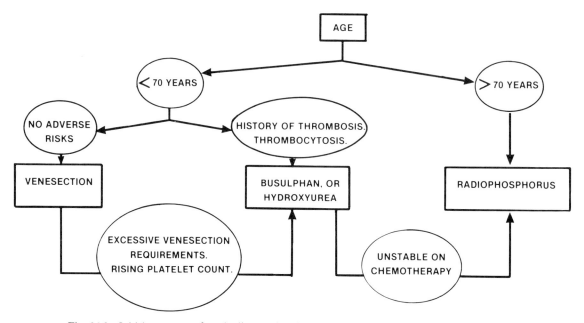

Fig. 26.3 Initial treatment of newly diagnosed patients with primary proliferative polycythaemia.

with aspirin and/or dipyridamole often produce dramatic improvement in symptoms due to sludging in small vessels in individuals with thrombocytosis. Surgical treatment of peripheral vascular disease should be postponed until full assessment of the response to reduction of the PCV is possible. If peripheral vascular problems persist when the PPP is under control, they must then be treated on their own merits.

Surgery in PPP. Untreated patients have a 75% increased risk of major haemorrhage or thrombosis following surgery. This is associated with up to 30% mortality. In contrast, patients whose PPP is completely controlled do not have an increased risk of bleeding or thrombosis. Elective surgery, therefore, should be postponed until PPP has been under control for 2–3 months. When emergency surgery is required, rapid haemodilution by venesection and plasma volume replacement with crystalloid and albumin solution is appropriate prior to operation.

IDIOPATHIC ERYTHROCYTOSIS

Patients who are found to have a raised PCV and RCM but do not have the parameters necessary to make a diagnosis of PPP or secondary polycythaemia are diagnosed as having idiopathic erythrocytosis.

On follow-up, up to 40% progress to PPP between 6 months and several years after presentation. Thus it is likely that a significant proportion have PPP, in an earlier phase, when first diagnosed. The pathogenesis is not clear in the subgroup who do not progress to PPP.

Clinical features

The condition predominantly affects males. 20% or more are asymptomatic and diagnosed when a raised PCV is recognised during the investigation of an unrelated problem. The clinical complications are dominated by vascular occlusive events, particularly peripheral vascular disease and venous thromboembolism. Abnormal bleeding, thrombocytosis and splenomegaly do not occur. The incidence of vascular complications correlates with the PCV.

Management

Reduction of the PCV to below 0.45 is as vital for patients with idiopathic erythrocytosis as those with PPP. Control of the PCV is by venesection alone. If overt PPP develops it is treated as outlined above.

SECONDARY POLYCYTHAEMIA

Secondary polycythaemia is diagnosed when elevation of

PCV and RCM is a consequence of some identifiable condition (Table 26.1). Broadly the causes can be subdivided into those with an appropriate increase in erythropoietin, e.g. secondary to hypoxaemia, and those in which there is an inappropriately elevated erythropoietin, e.g. secondary to renal disease.

Appropriately increased erythropoietin production

Chronic hypoxic lung disease

The majority of patients with chronic hypoxic lung disease demonstrate an inverse relationship between arterial pO_2 and the PCV. In most cases the clinical features are dominated by the primary disease. However, it is incorrect to assume that the rise in Hb, RCM and PCV is an appropriate response to chronic hypoxia for which no treatment is required. When the PCV rises above about 0.75, optimal compensation for hypoxia is exceeded and patients become exposed to the risks of increased whole blood viscosity. The median survival of polycythaemic patients with hypoxic lung disease is 18–30 months. Treatment of individuals to reduce a very high PCV leads to reduced blood viscosity, right heart work and pulmonary arterial pressure, along with improved exercise tolerance and alleviation of symptoms of hyperviscosity such as lethargy, headache and impaired concentration.

The best treatment to reduce the PCV is probably domiciliary oxygen administered for at least 15 hours per day. Alternatively, cautious venesection results in significant improvement in cardiorespiratory function once the PCV enters the range 0.55–0.52. Further venesection down to a PCV of 0.44 will not provide any further benefit. Therefore venesection is recommended only when the PCV is above 0.55, and treatment is aimed at maintaining the PCV between 0.52 and 0.55. Occasionally symptoms of hyperviscosity persist at PCV values below 0.55, in which case further cautious venesection should be performed until symptoms are controlled. Although venesection considerably improves symptoms, there is no evidence that it improves long-term survival.

Cyanotic congenital heart disease

In some patients with cyanotic congenital heart disease, the haemoglobin, RCM and PCV may be grossly elevated; occasionally the PCV may reach 0.80. Thrombotic lesions, involving particularly the cerebral and pulmonary circulations, are commonly identified in post-mortem studies of such patients. Cautious venesection with plasma volume replacement results in reduced peripheral vascular resistance (by reducing blood viscosity) leading to increased cardiac output and improved systemic blood flow. This may be particularly important before cardiac surgery. Thus, as in chronic hypoxic lung disease, the rise in PCV in cyanotic congenital heart disease can be considered to be overcompensation for the reduced arterial pO_2, so that the increased oxygen-carrying capacity is offset by the haemodynamic disadvantages of the increased whole blood viscosity. The optimal level at which the PCV should be maintained has not been established in patients with cyanotic congenital heart disease and is probably different in different shunt disorders and for different individuals.

Smoking

Very heavy smokers have elevated PCV which returns to normal if they stop smoking. The rise in PCV is due mainly to elevation of the RCM. This is due to chronic accumulation of carboxyhaemoglobin which reduces the blood's oxygen-carrying capacity, resulting in stimulation of erythropoiesis. In addition these individuals may develop hypoxia (even in the absence of overt lung disease) due to nocturnal pulmonary hypoventilation. Abrupt changes in smoking habits may lead to rapid changes in PCV. Heavy smoking initially causes a fall in plasma volume by an unknown mechanism. This tends to return to normal as the smoking habit remains constant. As the PCV may rise to 0.55 or higher, smokers are at risk of vascular occlusive events due to the increased blood viscosity as well as the adverse effects on the vessel wall.

Altitude

The changes in PCV occurring at altitude are variable and depend on several factors including the rate of ascent, altitude attained and the duration of stay. Initially the PCV falls due to fluid retention and fluid shift from the extravascular to the intravascular compartment. Subsequently diuresis occurs and the PCV returns to normal, or a state of relative polycythaemia due to haemoconcentration is established. This may last 10–15 days. Eventually the chronic hypoxic drive leads to the development of true polycythaemia. Polycythaemia developing in visitors to high altitude carries considerable risk of vascular occlusive episodes, the frequency of which correlates with the PCV. However, indigenous populations living at high altitude do not have this increased risk of thrombotic disease. Interestingly, Peruvians who ascend to high altitude develop a shift in their oxygen dissociation curve to the right, true polycythaemia often associated with pulmonary hypertension, and experience chronic mountain sickness. In contrast, Sherpas who ascend to high altitude maintain a normal PCV by developing a shift in their oxygen dissociation curve to the left. The reasons for these differences in physiological response to the hypoxia of high altitude are not fully understood.

High affinity haemoglobinopathies

More than 30 high affinity hemoglobinopathies have now been identified. The increased oxygen affinity leads to reduction in the amount of oxygen released from haemoglobin in the tissues causing chronic tissue hypoxia. This stimulates erythropoiesis and results in a rise in PCV. In chronic methaemoglobinaemia relative tissue hypoxia results, with a consequent rise in PCV.

Diagnosis depends on laboratory identification of the abnormal Hb and demonstrating left shift of the oxygen dissociation curve. A family history of polycythaemia should alert the physician to consider this group of disorders. Patients with high affinity haemoglobinopathies tend to have a high output cardiac state with increased cerebral blood flow. Thus it is rare for the increased PCV and RCM to cause significant hyperviscosity or vascular occlusive episodes. No specific treatment is available for these disorders.

Red cell enzyme defects

Very rare causes of secondary polycythaemia include 2,3-DPG deficiency. In one family this was due to a defect in 2,3-DPG mutase. The consequence of 2,3-DPG deficiency is a shift of the oxygen dissociation curve to the left leading to relative tissue hypoxia which stimulates erythropoiesis. No specific treatment is available.

Congenital deficiency of the red cell enzyme Met Hb reductase is a rare cause of polycythaemia in which the Met Hb level rises to 20–50%. Severely affected individuals have symptoms of chronic hypoxia, associated with a rise in PCV, and a consequent increased risk of vascular occlusive events. The diagnosis is confirmed by identifying deficiency of red cell Met Hb reductase. Treatment with ascorbic acid 500 mg daily, which acts as a reducing agent, leads to clearing of Met Hb and resolution of the cyanosis and polycythaemia.

Inappropriate erythropoietin production

This group contains several rare causes of secondary polycythaemia. Some patients present with the clinical features of the primary condition, but many present with polycythaemia and are later found to have a primary condition during routine investigation of the polycythaemia. Treatment of the primary condition leads to rapid resolution of the polycythaemia. Although these conditions are rare causes of polycythaemia, they must be confidently excluded when the cause of polycythaemia is not obvious.

Renal causes of polycythaemia

Investigation of the renal tract is an essential part of the assessment of unexplained polycythaemia. The main lesions which stimulate erythropoietin production resulting in a rise in PCV are listed in Table 26.1. The commonest causes in this group are renal cell carcinoma, in which erythropoietin or erythropoietin-like substances are secreted by the tumour, and renal parenchymal cysts, in which anatomical distortion of renal tissue may cause local tissue hypoxia leading to stimulation of erythropoietin production. Post renal transplant the PCV may transiently rise to about 0.65. This is secondary to excessive erythropoietin production by the graft, which usually adjusts to normal within a few weeks. The importance of the rise in PCV post-transplant is that the consequent rise in blood viscosity leads to a considerable risk of thrombotic events including jeopardy to the graft.

Liver causes of polycythaemia

Hepatocellular carcinoma is a very rare cause of polycythaemia in the UK. However, in Hong Kong, where hepatoma is relatively more common, about 12% of patients have a raised PCV. In contrast, in Africa, where hepatoma is also relatively common, a raised PCV is rare. This may be because of the high prevalence of anaemia from unrelated causes in African populations at risk for hepatoma. In patients who have liver cirrhosis, the sudden development of polycythaemia is highly suggestive of the development of hepatoma. However, even uncomplicated liver cirrhosis may occasionally cause polycythaemia, due to increased erythropoietin production by damaged hepatocytes. If a patient with liver cirrhosis has splenomegaly due to portal hypertension, a mistaken diagnosis of PPP may be made. Portosystemic anastomosis may occasionally cause a rise in PCV by shunting blood into the systemic circulation.

Hypertransfusion

Over-estimation of the volume of a blood transfusion will obviously cause a rise in PCV. This is dangerous because the sudden rise in blood viscosity in a system which has had no time to compensate produces considerable risk of vascular occlusive episodes. In addition the overloading of the vascular system may provoke acute pulmonary oedema.

Hypertransfusion of neonates occasionally occurs at the time of delivery by imbalance in twin-twin interaction with the placenta, or excessive placental transfusion directly into the delivered infant.

RELATIVE POLYCYTHAEMIAS

Relative polycythaemia can be defined as a rise in PCV due to contraction of the PV associated with normal RCM. This may occur acutely or develop slowly, depending on the aetiology. A classification of the relative polycythaemias is given in Table 26.5.

Table 26.5 Classification of the relative polycythaemias

Primary plasma volume contraction	
Dehydration	
Capillary leak	– Septicaemia
	Anaphlyaxis
	Snake venom poisoning
Loss of albumin	– Nephrotic syndrome
	Liver disease
	Protein-losing enteropathy
Others	– Oedema
	Effusions
	Ascites
Primary contraction of the vascular compartment	
Hypoxaemia	– Heavy smoking
	Sudden ascent to altitude
	CO poisoning
	CN poisoning
Idiopathic stress polycythaemia (Gaisböck's syndrome)	
Others	– Hypertension
	Phaeochromocytoma
	Pre-eclampsia
	Head injury
	Stroke

Pathogenesis

Primary contraction of the plasma volume

In most cases the cause is obvious loss of fluid from the intravascular space. The body compensates by cardiovascular mechanisms such as increased cardiac output and vasoconstriction to maintain the circulation. The majority of cases are acute.

Primary contraction of the vascular compartment

Constriction of the venous capacitance vessels leads to central hypervolaemia. The body compensates by bringing about a reduction in plasma volume resulting in a rise in the PCV. Acute hypoxaemic stimuli, such as ascent to altitude, carbon monoxide poisoning or heavy cigarette smoking, stimulate sympathatic/adrenal activity which raises cardiac output and causes venoconstriction, with centralisation of blood volume, and consequently haemoconcentration by a fall in PV.

Stress polycythaemia

In idiopathic stress polycythaemia (Gaisböck's syndrome) similar mechanisms to those outlined above operate. Psychological stress may be an important factor in many cases, but it is difficult to assess objectively and therefore difficult to prove.

Clinical features

Idiopathic stress polycythaemia commonly affects middle-aged males who have very active, stressful lifestyles. Obesity, diabetes, excessive alcohol consumption, smoking, hypertension, and hyperuricaemia and gout are common associated findings. Specific treatment of hypertension may cause a fall in PCV. Similarly, removal of other 'stresses', particularly smoking and alcohol, may also bring about improvement in the PCV.

Patients with idiopathic stress polycythaemia are at increased risk of serious vascular occlusive episodes and have a six-fold higher mortality rate than age-matched controls. It is difficult to establish how much increased blood viscosity due to elevated PCV contributes to this, since many of the associated features are known risk factors for stroke and acute myocardial infarction. However, there is some evidence that controlling the PCV reduces the risk of vascular occlusive events.

Investigations

The diagnosis depends on estimation of RCM and PV.

The RCM is usually within the normal range, although often at the upper range of normal. The PV is consistently reduced. Exclusion or correction of causes of primary PV contraction should be conducted before RCM and PV studies are initiated.

Assessment of the associated features such as hypertension, diabetes and hyperuricaemia should be performed. Granulocyte and platelet counts and leukocyte alkaline phosphatase activity are normal, and splenomegaly is absent.

Treatment

Treatment is aimed at correcting the associated features and reducing the 'stressful' stimuli such as smoking, alcohol, hypertension and psychological stress.

However, control of the PCV often requires venesection. Usually the patient feels better after venesection, although at least part of this may be placebo effect. Once the PCV is reduced to 0.45 or less, maintenance venesection is often only required at 3–4 month intervals. In the future effective long-acting venodilators may be useful in bringing about more 'physiological' control of the condition.

Although many patients feel better and improved cerebral blood flow can be demonstrated after venesection, there are no reported data to indicate whether control of the PCV improves long-term prognosis. No reported studies indicate which is the best approach to management, although a Royal College of Physicians-sponsored multicentre study is in progress to address this question.

BIBLIOGRAPHY

Berk P D, Goldberg J D, Donovan P B et al 1986 Therapeutic recommendations in polycythaemia vera based on Polycythaemia Vera Study Group protocols. Seminars in Haematology 23: 132–143

Harrison B D W, Stokes T C 1982 Secondary polycythaemia: its causes, effects and treatment. British Journal of Diseases of the Chest 76: 313–340

Ibister J P 1987 The contracted plasma volume syndromes (relative polycthaemias) and their haemorheological significance. Clinical Haematology 1: 665–693

International Committee for Standardisation in Haematology 1980 Recommended methods for measurement of red cell and plasma volume. Journal of Nuclear Medicine 21: 793–800

Kaplan M E, Mack K, Goldberg J D et al 1986 Long term management of polycythaemia vera with hydroxyurea: a progress report. Seminars in Haematology 23: 167–171

Landaw S A 1986 Acute leukaemia in polycythaemia vera. Seminars in Haematology 23: 156–165

Pearson T C 1987 Rheology of the absolute polycythaemias. Clinical Haematology 1: 637–664

Pearson T C, Guthrie D L 1984 The interpretation of measured red cell mass and plasma volume in patients with elevated PCV values. Clinical and Laboratory Haematology 6: 207–217

Pearson T C, Messinezy M 1987 Polycythaemia and thrombocythaemia in the elderly. Clinical Haematology 1: 355–387

Weatherly-Mein G, Pearson T C, Burney P G J, Morris R W 1987 The Royal College of Physicians Research Unit, polycythaemia study. I. Objective, background and design. Journal of the Royal College of Physicians of London 21: 7–16

27. Myelofibrosis

C. A. Ludlam

Myelofibrosis is a disorder characterised by increased fibrosis within the marrow, splenomegaly and extra-medullary haemopoiesis. It is usually considered to be one of the myeloproliferative disorders, although in many ways it should not be included in this group of conditions. There is substantial evidence that the other myeloproliferative disorders,chronic myeloid leukaemia, polycythaemia rubra vera and essential throm-bocythaemia are due to malignant clonal proliferation of one or more of the pluripotent cells, giving rise to erythropoiesis, myelopoiesis or megakaryocytes. These disorders may transform to myelofibrosis. Until recently it was considered that in primary myelofibrosis there is malignant clonal expansion of fibroblasts and that other myeloproliferative disorders transformed to myelofibrosis because the malignant pluripotent clonal cell line dedifferentiates to include the fibroblast line. Recent evidence now supports the view that in myelofibrosis the fibrosis is reactive or secondary to other events in the bone marrow rather than being a primary malignant process.

Extra-medullary haemopoiesis is characteristic of myelofibrosis and can always be demonstrated in the spleen and usually the liver, but it may also be observed in lymph nodes and occasionally at other sites, e.g. kidney. The mechanism causing this is unknown.

Pathogenesis

The aetiology of this enigmatic condition is obscure. Recent studies have suggested that the primary abnormality in myelofibrosis may be an autonomous proliferation of abnormal megakaryocytes. In the early or cellular stage of myelofibrosis the bone marrow reveals a marked increase in megakaryocytes which often have bizarre features. The cells are often larger than normal with well-defined multilobed nuclei. In normal developing megakaryocytes various proteins, e.g. fibrinogen, Btg, and platelet-derived growth factor (PDGF),are synthesised and then stored

in alpha granules(Ch.30). Recent evidence suggests that in myelofibrosis this packaging mechanism may be defective and that these proteins may diffuse out of the megakaryocyte. The resultant local increase in concentration of PDGF would be a potent stimulus to marrow fibroblast proliferation. Further evidence that this may be the operative mechanism is derived from the grey platelet syndrome. In this very rare congenital platelet disorder alpha granules are absent, presumably due to a defective packaging mechanism in the megakaryocyte. Excessive marrow fibrosis is also a feature of this condition, possibly by a mechanism similar to that operative in myelofibrosis.

Circulating immune complexes and paraproteins are occasionally observed in patients with myelofibrosis. This has led to the speculation that the fibrosis is secondary to an underlying lymphoproliferative disorder. As the clinical manifestations and rate of progression of myelofibrosis are very variable, it may well be a heterogeneous group of conditions characterised by fibroblastic proliferation in the marrow.

History

The clinical presentation of patients is very variable. Some will be asymptomatic and diagnosis will be made following a full blood count for some unrelated condition. Most individuals, however, present with weight loss along with increasing abdominal distension. This often develops slowly, sometimes over many years, and the increasing abdominal girth is due principally to splenomegaly and to a lesser extent the accompanying hepatomegaly. In the later stages of the condition ascites may accumulate. Post-prandial fullness and reflux oesophagitis are common symptoms. Patients may present with splenic infarction or have this as a complication at some time following diagnosis. Mucocutaneous bleeding is sometimes observed due to thrombocytopenia. Arterial or venous thrombosis may be presenting features either due to a high platelet count or because these cells are hyperactive. A huge increase in splenic venous blood flow predisposes to portal hypertension and resultant ascites and oesophageal varices; these are often late manifestations. Some patients merely present with the symptoms of anaemia, others with gout due to hyperuricaemia, and others may be intolerant of heat because of their hypermetabolic state.

Examination

The typical patient has a distended abdomen which contrasts markedly with the emaciated spindly arms and legs. Usually the spleen is grossly enlarged, sometimes extending to fill almost the whole abdomen, although in some patients it may be only marginally enlarged. The liver is usually increased in size and firm in character. In those individuals who have undergone splenectomy the liver may rapidly increase in size almost to the pelvic brim. Ascites is only rarely observed at diagnosis but when present it is secondary to portal hypertension; this may occasionally be massively exacerbated by a splenic vein thrombosis. Lymphadenopathy is found in a few individuals. Cardiac failure may be present partially due to the shunting of a large proportion of the cardiac output through the spleen. Thrombocytopenic purpura and echymoses may be observed.

Investigation

The haemoglobin may be normal or markedly reduced. Several different mechanisms contribute to the anaemia. Production of red cells may be reduced despite some additional cells being produced in the spleen. An element of increased red cell destruction may result from intrinsic red cell abnormalities which slow passage of erythrocytes through the enlarged spleen where a significant proportion of red cells will be pooled. The anaemia will be exacerbated by the dilutional effect of a marked increase in the plasma volume observed in individuals with grossly enlarged spleens. Folate deficiency may aggravate the degree of anaemia. Bleeding, particularly into the gastrointestinal tract as a result of varices or thrombocytopenia, may worsen the anaemia. The total white count may be normal, reduced as a result of splenomegaly, or increased as a part of the myeloproliferative disorder. As nucleated red cells are present in the circulating blood the total leukocyte count estimated by automatic blood counters will need to be corrected, as normoblasts may be counted as leukocytes. Thrombocytopenia may result from decreased production, abnormal fragmentation of the megakaryocytes or folate deficiency. Up to 90% of the

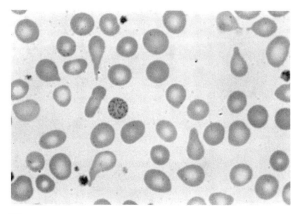

Fig. 27.1 Blood film changes in myelofibrosis; note tear drop, rod cells and basophilic stippling.

circulating platelets may be pooled within a grossly enlarged spleen.

The peripheral blood film exhibits characteristics that are almost diagnostic of myelofibrosis. The film is leuko-erythroblastic and the presence of many tear drop cells along with some anisopoikilocytosis is strongly suggestive of the diagnosis (Fig. 27.1). The number of nucleated red cells is very variable and they may exhibit a small degree of dyserythropoiesis. The majority of leukocytes will be of myeloid origin and most will be mature forms, although some myelocytes and metamyelocytes will be observed and up to 5–10% blasts may be present. Platelets may exhibit bizarre morphological features, with many being much larger than normal with vacuoles. Patients will be predisposed to bleeding not only from thrombocytopenia but also because such platelets may be functionally impaired. Leukocyte alkaline phosphatase is increased and this may be of value in distinguishing the condition from chronic myeloid leukaemia where it is characteristically very low.

Bone marrow aspirate is often unsuccessful, being a 'dry' tap due to the fibrotic change in the marrow. A trephine biopsy will reveal a marrow of usually increased cellularity with some degree of fibrosis (Plates 24–26). The histological features are very variable. At one end of the spectrum hyperplasia of all three cell lines will be observed, with virtually no fat spaces, and abnormal megakaryocytes are often greatly increased in number. In this cellular phase of the disorder the degree of fibrosis may not be prominent. At the other end of the spectrum the marrow is densely fibrotic with very few normal marrow elements being visible.

A fibrotic reaction may also be observed in other myeloproliferative disorders as well as a reaction to carcinomatous infiltration (Plates 27, 28) particularly from breast and prostate. Radiotherapy may also induce fibrosis. Disseminated tuberculosis may be found in association with increased marrow fibrosis and splenomegaly. Occasionally it may be unclear as to whether or not the patient also has underlined myelofibrosis. In these circumstances the patient should be treated with antituberculous chemotherapy and if the fibrosis and splenomegaly progress, this will confirm the diagnosis of myelofibrosis.

Radiological examination may reveal an increase in bone density, particularly noticeable in the vertebrae. Increased trabeculation may be observed in the proximal shafts of both femur and humerus.

Iron kinetic assessment can be attempted using ^{59}Fe but interpretation of the results is often difficult. With the use of surface counters uptake of iron into the sacrum (bone marrow) will be negligible, whereas that into the spleen will be markedly increased initially, due to the extramedullary haemopoiesis followed by a decline due to the liberation of red cells into the circulation. In patients presenting with atypical features of myelofibrosis, iron kinetic studies may provide additional evidence to support the diagnosis. Such studies are not helpful in prognosticating as to whether splenectomy will be helpful or not. The degree of red cell pooling in the spleen can be assessed using ^{51}Cr-labelled red cells and plasma volume increase measured with ^{125}I albumin.

An increase in serum B_{12} concentration may be observed due to an increase in transcobalamin III which is synthesised by leukocytes. Immune complexes may be detected in some individuals and in an occasional patient a paraprotein will be found.

The diagnosis of myelofibrosis is straightforward if the patient presents with splenomegaly, peripheral blood demonstrating the characteristic leuko-erythroblastic change along with many tear drop cells and extensive fibrosis in the marrow. Some patients may have features of other myeloproliferative disorders, particularly primary proliferative polycythaemia and essential thrombocythaemia. In these instances it may be difficult to pigeonhole the patient into one of these diagnostic groups and the individual is said to have a transitional disorder. As patients with other myeloproliferative disorders may transform to myelofibrosis and if they present during this transformation, features of both conditions may be present. A period of observation will demonstrate whether the condition is transforming into myelofibrosis or whether it is a true transitional disorder. Other diagnoses to be considered, particularly in a patient without splenomegaly, are carcinomatous infiltration of the bone marrow, previous radiotherapy and tuberculosis.

Management

Most patients with myelofibrosis will have had the condition for a long time prior to diagnosis. Some will initially have been diagnosed as having another myeloproliferative disorder that progresses to myelofibrosis but in the majority of patients no history suggestive of a prior disorder is ellicited. In the majority of instances the myelofibrosis will be only slowly progressive and immediate chemotherapy or splenectomy is not indicated.

At presentation folate deficiency should be corrected and patients started on allopurinol. Symptomatic anaemia should be corrected by red cell transfusion and acute bleeding due to thrombocytopenia will respond to platelet therapy, although large numbers may need to be given because of the splenomegaly.

Chemotherapy may occasionally be helpful in patients with the cellular type of myelofibrosis, especially those with a marked leukocytosis. A small dose of alkylating agent, e.g. busulphan 2 mg daily, may halt progression, although thrombocytopenia may be a troublesome side effect of this drug. Chemotherapy is sometimes indicated following splenectomy when both the platelet and white counts may rise dramatically predisposing the patient to thrombosis.

Splenectomy can have a very beneficial result for the patient but deciding the best time to have the surgery is often difficult. Removal of the spleen will reduce the pooling of blood cells, decrease red cell haemolysis and reduce the dilutional effect of the increased plasma volume. Splenectomy should be considered for any patient with progressive splenomegaly, particularly if this is associated with marked abdominal discomfort or splenic infarction. Thrombocytopenia can usually be alleviated by splenectomy, which should be considered in any patient in whom this is sufficient to cause bleeding. Occasionally recurrent infections are observed due to a leukopenia and splenectomy may be beneficial in this circumstance.

Although anaemia will respond to red cell transfusions, a time may be reached, possibly exacerbated by the development of allo-antibodies, when the patient requires transfusions every few weeks. Splenectomy often results in a dramatic fall in the requirement for transfusions.

The timing of splenectomy is often difficult. The incidence of complication is proportional to the size of the spleen. There is always reluctance to advise splenectomy early in the disorder when the spleen is small, because the patient is unlikely to be suffering any ill effects. At the other extreme the removal of a spleen which fills most of the abdomen, particularly if there have been previous infarcts, will be hazardous. There may also be other debilitating features such as poor general health and cardiac failure. With modern anaesthetic techniques and a surgeon experienced in splenectomies, most patients can undergo this procedure provided they are carefully prepared prior to operation and closely monitored afterwards.

It is often worth assessing platelet function with a bleeding time and aggregation studies prior to operation, because if this is markedly reduced there may be major haemorrhage at or after surgery. If platelet function is demonstrably deranged, platelet transfusion immediately prior to operation or after the splenic pedicle has been tied will be of benefit. Abnormal platelet function may also predispose to post-operative venous thrombosis and therefore, if the platelet count rises towards $1000 \times 10^9/l$ use of aspirin and or heparin should be considered.

Splenic size can also be reduced by local radiotherapy. This is usually of only temporary benefit, as the organ increases in size again, but it may be of value to tide the patient over a difficult period or occasionally prior to splenectomy.

Prognosis

The outlook for an individual with myelofibrosis is very variable and ranges, on average, between 3 and 6 years. Some patients have very static disease and with splenec-

tomy may survive for more than 10 years. Others have a much more rapidly progressive condition, carrying a poor prognosis, with the spleen perceptibly enlarging over a period of a few months. A transformation to acute myeloid leukaemia is sometimes observed but this responds poorly to intensive chemotherapy. Death usually results from progressive marrow failure, with anaemia that cannot be effectively treated with red cell transfusions, thrombocytopenia and resultant bleeding or leukopenia and overwhelming infection.

ACUTE MYELOFIBROSIS

This is an uncommon disorder in which the patient presents with an acute illness associated with fever, anaemia and often thrombocytopenic purpura. The spleen may be impalpable or only slightly enlarged. Bone marrow aspiration results in a 'dry' tap, whilst a trephine biopsy reveals a marrow containing a predominance of immature blast-like cells and increased deposition of fibrin. These primitive cells may be immature megakaryocytes and can be shown by chromosome studies to be a clonal proliferation.

Initial therapy should be directed to treating infection and correcting anaemia and symptomatic thrombocytopenia. The condition carries a poor prognosis but therapy as for acute myeloid leukaemia may be appropriate.

BIBLIOGRAPHY

Barosi G 1987 Chronic myelofibrosis and myeloid metaplasia. The spectrum of clinical syndromes. Haematologica (Pavia) 72: 553–562

Ellis J T, Peterson P, Geller S A, Rappaport H 1986 Studies of the bone marrow in polycythaemia vera and the evolution of myelofibrosis and second haematological malignancies. Seminars in Haematology 23: 144–155

Kelsey P R, Geary C G 1987 Management of idiopathic myelofibrosis. Clinical and Laboratory Haematology 9: 1–12

Lewis S M 1985 Myelofibrosis: pathophysiology and clinical management. Dekker, New York

28. Erythrocyte and leukocyte abnormalities in the neonate

E. A. Letsky

Throughout gestation and in the first few weeks of life there are dynamic changes occurring in the composition of the circulating blood of the human fetus and neonate. By approximately 6 months of age a relatively stable population of so-called adult red cells is established. During childhood, adolescence and into old age, the responses to haematological stimuli are in essence similar. It is only the changing susceptibility to various disease processes at different times of life which creates broad separations between the clinical practice of paediatric and adult haematology. In contrast, the blood of the neonate has unique characteristics. It is changing from day to day and these changes differ in magnitude and quality depending on the gestation and birth. There are marked physical, metabolic and antigenic differences between the fetal red cell and the adult red cell. In addition, interactions between fetal and maternal circulations have to be considered in the differential diagnosis of any haematological abnormality.

DEVELOPMENTAL HAEMATOPOIESIS

ERYTHROPOIESIS

Erythropoiesis in the human embryo can be detected 2–3 weeks after conception. Blood islands form in the yolk sac, the peripheral cells of which differentiate to form the first blood vessels, the central cells becoming the primitive haemocytoblasts. Prior to this, the embryo obtains oxygen by diffusion until its volume makes this process inadequate and a circulatory system is essential to maintain in-utero respiration.

All blood cells are derived from the mesenchyme, and haematopoiesis in intra-uterine life is conventionally divided into three periods: mesoblastic, hepatic and myeloid (Fig. 28.1).

The earliest blood cells have megaloblastic features. They are nucleated and contain haemoglobins which are virtually confined to the mesoblastic period – the embryonic haemoglobins – and unlike the later

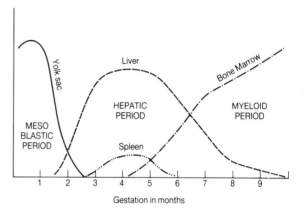

Fig. 28.1 Stages of haematopoiesis in the developing embryo and fetus.

erythropoietic cells do not appear to be under the influence of erythropoietin.

Normoblastic red cell production begins in the liver by about the fifth week of gestation, taking over from the yolk sac. The liver appears to be the major site of erythropoiesis in human fetal life, but blood production in the liver starts to fall off at about 24 weeks' gestation and very little haemopoietic activity is detectable in the liver at birth.

Erythropoiesis in the bone marrow can be detected as early as 9–11 weeks' gestation and by about 28 weeks' gestation this is the major blood-producing organ. Haemopoietic tissue in the bone marrow continues to increase until term, and even after birth, when increase in haematopoietic tissue produces marrow expansion which can easily be seen in the bone of the skull.

During the second trimester particularly, secondary sites of haematopoietic tissue are found in various connective tissues, the thymus, kidney and spleen (Fig. 28.1). The total contribution from these secondary sites is probably quite small, and certainly negligible at birth.

Control of erythropoiesis in the fetus is only partially

influenced by maternal factors and appears to be mainly under the influence of fetally produced erythropoietin, at least in the hepatic and myeloid phases. It is thought that the fetal liver may be the source of erythropoietin throughout most of intra-uterine life.

DEVELOPMENTAL CHANGES IN HAEMOGLOBINS

With the establishment of erythropoiesis there is production of a series of different haemoglobins. These are embryonic, fetal and adult haemoglobins. There are three embryonic haemoglobins – Hb.Gower 1 and 2 and Hb.Portland. They disappear by 12 weeks' gestation and it is thought that they are restricted to the primitive red cells produced in the yolk sac (Table 28.1). Fetal haemoglobin Hb.F ($\alpha_2 \gamma_2$) can be detected in the blood from embryos of 6–12 weeks' gestation.

Table 28.1 Globin chain composition of human haemoglobins

Haemoglobin	Globin composition	Site of production	Stage of development
Gower 1	$\varsigma_2\varepsilon_2$		Embryo
Gower 2	$\alpha_2\varepsilon_2$	Yolk Sac	Embryo
Portland	$\varsigma_2\gamma_2$		Embryo
Fetal	$\alpha_2\gamma_2$		Embryo
Fetal	$\alpha_2\gamma_2$		Fetus
Adult	$\alpha_2\beta_2$	Liver	Fetus
Hb.A$_2$	$\alpha_2\delta_2$	Bone Marrow	Fetus
Fetal	$\alpha_2\gamma_2$		Adult
Adult	$\alpha_2\beta_2$	Bone Marrow	Adult
Hb.A$_2$	$\alpha_2\delta_2$		Adult

From the time when hepatic erythropoiesis is established Hb.F ($\alpha_2 \gamma_2$) forms the major respiratory pigment throughout intra-uterine life, but from as early as 8–10 weeks' gestation it is possible to detect about 5–10% of adult haemoglobin – Hb.A ($\alpha_2 \beta_2$).

Between 32 and 36 weeks' gestation the production of Hb.A increases co-incident with a sharp decline in Hb.F production (Fig. 28.2). The decrease in Hb.F results in a level of Hb.F of less than 10% at 3 months of age and the adult level of Hb.F of less than 1% by 6 months to 1 year in the vast majority of infants.

The decline of fetal haemoglobin in the newborn period appears to be strictly regulated. The switch from Hb.F to Hb.A synthesis occurs around 32 weeks' gestation and it is important to realise that this is not related to birth but is based on post-conception age. It follows then that the relative concentration of Hb.F and Hb.A in cord blood will depend on gestation. Babies

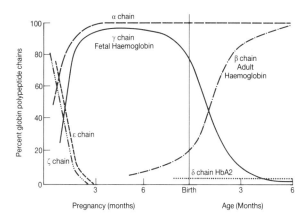

Fig. 28.2 Developmental changes in human haemoglobins.

born at 32–34 weeks have a mean of 90% Hb.F, while those born at term will have 70–80% Hb.F.

The molecular basis of this changeover from fetal to adult haemoglobin is at the centre of current investigation and has excited much interest in recent years. In spite of this, studies have failed to produce a clear picture of events at the cellular level during the haemoglobin 'switch'.

Hb.A$_2$, the minor adult haemoglobin, is detectable in utero in the third trimester in small amounts, and reaches its adult level of about 2.5% by 6 months of age. The intracellular distribution of the haemoglobins produced during the hepatic period has not been studied in detail, but Hb.A is present in most, probably all, of the red cells, although the amount varies from cell to cell.

Hb.A is detectable in very small quantities at 6–8 weeks' gestation, but a slight increase in beta chain production at 12–20 weeks results in a level of approximately 10% Hb.A which persists until 32 weeks' gestation – the time of the Hb.F → Hb.A switch. The fact that measurable amounts of Hb.A are present at around 18 weeks' gestation and that fetal blood-sampling carries acceptable risks to the continuance of the pregnancy is the basis of the late prenatal diagnosis of the clinically important beta globin chain defects, homozygous beta thalassaemia and sickle cell disease.

The efficiency of oxygen delivery to the tissues is directly related to the interactions of haemoglobin with 2,3 diphosphoglycerate (2,3-DPG). High concentrations of 2,3-DPG push the oxygen dissociation curve to the right and facilitate oxygen delivery to the tissues. The reduction in the oxygen affinity of Hb.F by interaction with 2,3-DPG is only a fraction of that produced by the same concentration of 2,3-DPG with Hb.A. The effect of this reduced reaction of Hb.F with 2,3-DPG ensures that the oxygen affinity of fetal blood does not drop below that of its mother. This facilitates binding of oxygen from the maternal circulation in the placenta villi. More than half of the oxygen bound in the placenta by the fetal blood can be released to fetal tissue because the tissue oxygen levels in the fetus are much lower than those in the maternal tissues.

In the first few weeks of extra-uterine life there is a progressive increase in the delivery of oxygen to the tissues. This is brought about by the interactions of several factors. There is a gradual replacement of Hb.F by Hb.A, an increase in 2,3-DPG levels which shifts the oxygen dissociation curve to the right, and, of course, increased availability of oxygen. The net result of these changes is that although the haemoglobin level in the term infant falls from 17 g/dl to 11 g/dl in the first 12 weeks of life, the oxygen delivery to the tissues at 3 months is greater than that in the newborn infant.

Changes in red cell metabolism during development

Studies of metabolism of cord blood red cells of term and premature infants show many differences from adult blood. However, the red cell is a dying cell from the moment it enters the circulation and the activity of most enzymes decreases with age so that the increased metabolic rate of fetal red cells may just be a reflection of the younger cells in the cord blood. No specific isozymes have been identified on electrophoresis of fetal red blood cell enzymes.

Glycolysis

Although there is increased activity of many of the glycolytic enzymes in the cord blood, allowing for the younger mean red cell age, the rate of glucose consumption appears to be decreased compared with adult cells. This appears to be related to the reduced activity of phosphofructokinase. Galactose utilisation, on the other hand, is increased in the neonate with considerable increase of galactokinase activity.

The levels of 2,3-DPG are similar in cord and adult blood, but newborn and adult red cells differ in the metabolism of this compound. 2,3-DPG plays an important part in regulating the oxygen affinity of Hb.A but has little effect on the affinity of oxygen for Hb.F (see above).

Pentose phosphate pathway

The response of the hexose monophosphate shunt in cord blood of term and premature infants appears to be normal and is stimulated by oxidants, but the red cells of the newborn are particularly susceptible to oxidant-induced injury. Increased peroxide formation leads to glutathione instability and the development of methaemoglobin and Heinz body formation.

Although the levels of glutathione peroxidase are inappropriately low for the young cells present in cord blood, no direct relationship between this deficiency and the peroxide sensitivity of fetal red cells has been proved.

It is probable that it is the cumulative effect of several factors which is responsible for the newborn cells' susceptibility to oxidant damage. This would include reduced levels of methaemoglobin reductase and catalase, reduced levels of membrane SH groups and decreased levels of membrane antioxidants such as Vitamin E (see below).

MORPHOLOGY OF CELLS IN THE NEWBORN

The normal appearance of the red cells in a stained blood film of cord blood is very different to that of the young child or adult. There are striking variations in size and shape and there are some very large cells by normal adult standards. It is quite usual to see occasional nucleated red cells, moderate numbers of spherocytes, target cells, crenated cells, burr cells and fragments. These appearances are thought to be due to immaturity of splenic circulation resulting in a 'post-splenectomy' picture. Examination of the cells by interference/contrast microscopy reveals an increased number of cells with pits and craters on the surface, probably due to cytoplasmic vacuoles. By approximately 8 to 9 weeks of life the red cells of the newborn are indistinguishable from those of the adult.

Red cells

In the premature infant there are increased numbers of nucleated red cells at the time of birth. These nucleated red cells persist in the circulation longer in the premature compared to the term infant. It must not be forgotten that increased numbers of nucleated red cells above these expected levels are seen in haemolytic disease, with hypoxia and after haemorrhage.

White cells

The total white cell count at birth ranges from 9–36 × 10^9/l, with a mean of 15–20 × 10^9/l. There is usually a rise in the total white cell count in the first few hours and than a gradual fall to a mean of 12 × 10^9/l per cu mm by the end of the first week of life (Table 28.2).

Table 28.2 Normal leukocyte counts in the first month of life

Age	Total leukocytes Mean	(Range)	Neutrophils Mean	(Range)	%	Lymphocytes Mean	(Range)	%	Monocytes Mean	%	Eosinophils Mean	%
Birth	18.1	(9.0– 30.0)	11.1	(6.0–26.0)	61	5.5	(2.0–11.0)	31	1.1	6	0.4	2
12 hours	22.8	(13.0–38.0)	15.5	(6.0–28.0)	68	5.5	(2.0–11.0)	24	1.2	5	0.5	2
24 hours	18.9	(9.4–34.0)	11.5	(5.0–21.0)	61	5.8	(2.0–11.5)	31	1.1	6	0.5	2
1 week	12.2	(5.0–21.0)	5.5	(1.5–10.0)	45	5.0	(2.0–17.0)	41	1.1	9	0.5	4
2 weeks	11.4	(5.0–20.0)	4.5	(1.0–9.5)	40	5.5	(2.0–17.0)	48	1.0	9	0.4	3
1 month	10.8	(5.0–19.5)	3.8	(1.0–9.0)	35	6.0	(2.5–16.5)	56	0.7	7	0.3	3

Numbers of leukocytes $\times 10^9/l$

neutrophils include band forms and a small number of metamyelocytes and myelocytes in the first few days of life.

Granulopoiesis

Significant granulopoiesis does not take place until the myeloid period of haematopoiesis. There are very few circulating granulocytes in the first 20 weeks of gestation. During the last trimester the numbers increase rapidly and at term the total count is greater than in adults (Table 28.2).

In the first 24 hours of life the absolute numbers of neutrophils in the blood rise in both term and premature infants. The count remains relatively stable during the first few days but then starts to fall by the end of the first week. During these first days of life the differential count shows a predominance of polymorphonuclear neutrophils. Sometime between the fourth and seventh day in the term infant the lymphocyte becomes the predominant cell and remains so throughout early childhood. In the first few days of life the granulocytes total approximately 60% of the total white cells and it is not unusual to see a fair proportion of 'young' forms circulating. Band-forms and myelocytes are commonly seen, but occasional promyelocytes and even blast cells have been observed in healthy term infants, although these immature forms are more frequently observed in the premature neonate. Blast cells may also be seen in the infected neonate. These normal alterations in the neutrophil count in the first few days of life limit its value in the diagnosis of neonatal infection.

Factors other than bacterial infection which significantly alter the neutrophil response during the first week of life include maternal hypertension, maternal fever prior to delivery, haemolytic disease, intraventricular haemorrhage and birth asphyxia. The usual response to bacterial infection in the neonate is profound neutropenia but there is much overlap between physiological changes and the various disorders which may alter the total or differential white cell counts in the first few days of life.

Eosinophils

In the term infant the mean absolute eosinophil count is $0.267 \times 10^9/l$ (2.2%) during the first 12 hours of life. This rises gradually and reaches a mean of $0.483 \times 10^9/l$ by the end of the first month of life. Premature infants have very low levels indeed at birth. A progressive increase takes place after the first few days of life, reaching $0.900–1.650 \times 10^9/l$ at the end of the first month. Premature babies who fail to progress have a marked eosinopenia.

Lymphopoiesis

In contrast to granulocytes, circulating lymphocytes can be identified from the third fetal month and by 20 weeks' gestation the numbers reach a maximum of $10 \times 10^9/l$. Thereafter there is a decrease in the numbers to reach approximately $3 \times 10^9/l$ at term.

The proportion of T- and B-lymphocytes in cord blood is similar to that found in adult blood, but the total number of B-, T- and null cells is higher than in adults because of the greater absolute total white cell count in neonates.

Neonatal lymphocytes undergo a greater degree of spontaneous transformation into blasts and up to 3 months of age incorporate larger amounts of thymidine than adult lymphocytes. The lymphocytes of the newborn may be less active in effector functions than adult lymphocytes, for reasons related to the immaturity of the immune system in the neonate.

Platelets

Megakaryocytes, from which the platelets are derived, can be seen in the yolk sac as early as 5 weeks' gestation; they can be seen in the liver until term and in the bone marrow from 12 weeks' gestation in increasing numbers. The platelet count from the thirtieth week of gestation is similar to that in the adult and should be within the normal adult range (150–450 × 10⁹/l) in the term neonate. The premature infant should also have a normal platelet count in the absence of any complication, although there is some conflicting data on this matter.

Disseminated intravascular coagulation (DIC) is a common result of the complications of prematurity and could give rise to low platelet counts which are not due to the premature state per se.

PHYSIOLOGICAL ANAEMIA OF INFANCY

After birth the haemoglobin level falls over the first weeks of life. The decrease in haemoglobin is more rapid and profound in premature infants than in those born at term and has been termed the physiological anaemia of prematurity.

Before the differential diagnosis and management of true neonatal anaemia can be discussed, some knowledge of the factors influencing the physiological values is required.

TERM INFANTS

The site and timing of sampling, and the treatment of the cord and placenta will all affect the haemoglobin values in the newborn infant.

The umbilical arteries constrict shortly after birth, preventing blood flow from the infant to the mother, but the umbilical vein remains open allowing blood flow in the direction of gravity. If the infant is held below the level of the placenta and clamping of the cord is delayed, then maximum blood gain possible will be achieved, but if the infant is held above the placenta, then transfusion of blood from the placenta to the infant may be prevented or will be very small in volume indeed.

In the first few hours after birth an increase in haemoglobin is observed, even if the cord clamping is not delayed, but the magnitude of the increase depends directly on the amount of placental transfusion.

With so many factors exerting a measurable effect it is not surprising that cord blood haemoglobin concentrations show wide variations in apparently normal term infants. Most values fall within the range of 14–20 g/dl with a mean of 16.8 g/dl (Table 28.3). After the initial increase in haemoglobin during the first 24 hours of life the level returns to the cord blood haemoglobin value by 1 week of age (Table 28.3). At birth the reticulocyte count is around 5% with a range of 2–7%. The proportion is usually less than 1% at the end of the first week, showing an abrupt fall after the first 3 days. Nucleated red cells are present in the blood for the first 4 days of life in relatively small numbers, about 1 per 10 000 erythrocytes. The common practice of expressing the erythroblasts as a percentage of the white cells is very inaccurate because of the variability of the white cell count; however, the term infant has an average of 7.3 nucleated red cells per 100 leukocytes at birth (range 0–24). More nucleated red cells are seen in the blood of premature infants. After the first week of life the haemoglobin falls progressively in the next 1–3 months of life. By 8 to 12 weeks the haemoglobin will fall as low as 11.4± 0.9 g/dl in infants born at term. The fall in haemoglobin is due for the most part to the decrease in red cell mass. This is a combination of the effect of the reduced red cell life span in the newborn and a striking decrease in marrow erythroid activity.

The reticulocyte count falls rapidly from birth and remains at less than 1% from the end of the first week until around 6 weeks post-natally. Erythropoietin is not detectable during this period. Erythroblasts in the bone-marrow decline sharply during the first week. The sharp fall in erythropoietin activity after birth is considered to be a physiological reaction to the greater availability of oxygen. Together with the shortened red cell life span and increasing haemodilution accompanying growth, the

Table 28.3 Normal red cell values during the first week of life in the term infant.

	Cord blood	Day 1	Day 3	Day 7
Haemoglobin (g/dl)	16.8	18.4	17.8	17.0
Packed cell volume (PCV)	0.53	0.58	0.55	0.54
Red cell count (× 10¹²/l)	5.25	5.8	5.6	5.2
Mean corpuscular volume (MCV fl)	107	108	99.0	98.0
Mean corpuscular haemoglobin concentration (MCHC g/dl)	31.7	32	33	33
Mean corpuscular haemoglobin (MCH pg)	34	35	33	32.5
Reticulocytes per cent of red cells	4.7	3.7	1.3	0.1
Nucleated red cell count (per cu mm)	500 (7.3/100 WBC)	200	0.5	0

fall in haemoglobin concentration is easily accounted for. The neonate is still capable of responding to increased demand during the first few weeks of life. Hypoxic and anaemic infants do not show the decrease in erythroid activity observed in the healthy newborn and continue to produce erythropoietin. The initial cord blood haemoglobin concentration has no effect on the level to which the haemoglobin falls. Recovery begins when a level of about 10–11 g/dl is reached.

The erythroid activity in the bone marrow starts to increase after 3–4 weeks, but there is a delay in recovery of the haemoglobin level because the rate of red cell destruction still exceeds production and continued rapid growth results in expansion of the blood volume and haemodilution. Erythropoietin becomes detectable in the serum by 8–12 weeks after birth, the erythropoietin activity in the bone marrow is comparable to the adult level of activity and the haemoglobin level begins to rise. By 6 months of age a mean level of about 12.5 g/dl is achieved in normal infants in whom there is no evidence of iron deficiency. This level is maintained until 2 years of age, after which there is a gradual increase up to puberty.

Racial differences must be borne in mind in determining normal haemoglobin values during childhood. It has been shown that Negro children show mean haemoglobin levels of 0.5–1.0 g/dl lower than Oriental and Caucasian children throughout childhood; these levels do not depend on social or nutritional factors.

PREMATURE INFANTS

The newborn premature infant experiences a fall in haemoglobin which by 4–8 weeks of age greatly exceeds that of healthy term infants. It is not known to be associated with any abnormalities in the infant and therefore has been termed the 'physiological anaemia of prematurity'. This early anaemia of prematurity has been distinguished from the late anaemia which is generally accepted to be the result of nutritional deficiencies, particularly iron deficiency, and does not manifest itself until 3–5 months of age, well clear of the neonatal period. This late anaemia will not be discussed except in terms of possible prevention.

The early physiological anaemia of prematurity remains poorly understood in spite of active investigations by many workers in the past and current research in the area of oxygen delivery in the immature infant. Oxygen availability in the premature infant appears to be the key question in deciding whether or not therapy with transfusion is necessary.

After the first 24 hours of life, when it is not unusual to observe a rise in haemoglobin of 1–2 g/dl, as a result of placental transfusion and poor oral fluid intake, the haemoglobin remains relatively constant for several days and then falls gradually, reaching its lowest level between 4 and 10 weeks post-natally. The rapidity and magnitude of the fall in haemoglobin varies directly with the degree of immaturity of the infant. In infants with birth weights 1200–2350 g the haemoglobin will fall to 9.6 ± 1.4 g/dl, while in those with birth weights less than 1200 g the haemoglobin falls to 7.8 ± 1.4 g/dl.

It would appear that the newborn infant is capable of regulating its own rate of erythropoiesis in response to needs. We know that in utero the fetus produces its own erythropoietin independent of maternal influence. Infants born anaemic do have a reticulocytosis much above the normal range for gestation. Small-for-dates infants who have suffered intra-uterine hypoxia demonstrate increased erythropoiesis. In addition, infants with respiratory insufficiency or with cyanotic congenital heart disease rarely develop the physiological anaemia associated with prematurity. Although the cord haemoglobin will affect the levels in the weeks after birth, the minimum haemoglobins reached are largely similar, indicating that the signal for marrow activity to return is grossly the same for all premature infants. Those with lower haemoglobin levels at birth will reach their nadir more rapidly than those born with higher haemoglobins. How does the premature infant tolerate such large falls in haemoglobin without compromising supplies of oxygen to the tissues? The adaptive changes which could be brought into play include a higher cardiac output, improved oxygen-unloading capacity, redistribution of blood flow and a greater oxygen extraction.

After the first week cardiac output does not change significantly during the first 3 months of life. In contrast to the falling haemoglobin, the oxygen delivery to the tissues is constantly increasing from the moment of birth. This increased oxygen release results from a right shift of the oxygen dissociation curve as the fetal haemoglobin falls and red cell 2,3-DPG rises. The magnitude of this shift is of profound physiological significance for both term and preterm infants. For example, a healthy premature baby of birth weight around 1500 g, with a cord haemoglobin of approximately 15.0 g/dl, can actually have doubled its oxygen delivery to the tissues by 10 weeks of age in spite of a fall in the haemoglobin to 8.0 g/dl.

In summary, between 4 and 12 weeks of age the oxygen conveying capacity of the blood is decreased because of the rapid fall in haemoglobin but this is offset by the increasing capacity of the haemoglobin to release oxygen to the tissues. The low haemoglobin concentration in most premature infants between 1 and 3 months of age should be considered normal and the term anaemia is inappropriate.

The premature infant is more prone to develop nutritional deficiencies than the term infant because of rapid growth and diminished reserves. Factors that can accentuate the anaemia of prematurity are iron, folate, Vitamin B_{12} and Vitamin E deficiency. Another factor of increasing importance in modern Special Care Baby Units is frequent blood sampling for laboratory studies.

Iron in the premature infant

The role of iron in the pathogenesis of the anaemia of prematurity has excited interest for almost 50 years. As a result of innumerable investigations a clearer picture has emerged from the initial confusion. Iron deficiency is not likely to play a part in the early anaemia of prematurity unless there has been perinatal blood loss or repeated blood sampling has been performed for laboratory investigations. It follows then that the administration of medicinal iron will not prevent the initial fall in haemoglobin. However, unless the premature infant is given iron supplements sometime in the first 2–4 months of life, an anaemia – the so-called late anaemia of prematurity – will inevitably develop due to iron deficiency. The time of the anaemia will depend on the initial haemoglobin level and the rate of growth. In general, infants with normal haemoglobin levels at birth will have depleted their iron stores and will therefore have a limited rate of haemoglobin synthesis by the time they have doubled their birth weight. Approximately 75% of the infant's total body iron is contained in the haemoglobin of the circulating and developing red cells. Infants who are anaemic at birth and have a decreased red cell mass will have reduced iron reserves.

There is now a consensus of opinion that all premature infants, and particularly those weighing less than 1500 g at birth, require supplemental iron to prevent the development of late anaemia due to iron deficiency. Cord blood haemoglobin level, birth weight and bloodletting in the first weeks of life will determine the timing of the development of iron deficiency.

Iron supplements in low-birth-weight infants should be given as follows, starting on the 15th day of life:

– 2 mg/kg per day for infants 1500–2500 g birth weight

– 3 mg/kg per day for infants 1000–1500 g birth weight

– 4 mg/kg per day for those less than 1000 g birth weight

and these supplements should be continued for at least 12–15 months after birth. If the infant is receiving adequate Vitamin E in relation to polyunsaturated fat in the diet, then the early introduction of supplemental iron will cause no adverse effects (see below).

Copper

More than 90% of the copper normally present in plasma is bound to ceruloplasmin. Ceruloplasmin also facilitates the absorption of iron and the release of iron from body stores. Copper is also necessary for iron metabolism within erythroid precursors. Copper deficiency mimics iron deficiency with the production of a hypochromic microcytic anaemia but it also produces neutropenia. The term infant has abundant hepatic copper stores, sufficient to maintain him through the first 6 months of life. These stores are accumulated in the last 12 weeks of fetal life. The premature infant is born with marginal copper stores, and severe symptomatic copper deficiency may develop by 2–3 months in those infants fed cow's milk products with inadequate copper content. It is recommended that the infant receive 80 μg of copper per kg per day and most infant formulas have been supplemented appropriately.

The diagnosis of copper deficiency anaemia is made by the demonstration of low serum copper (less than 40 μg/dl) or low ceruloplasmin values (less than 15 mg/dl), together with megaloblastoid bone marrow changes, vacuolated erythroid precursors and maturation arrest in the granulocyte series. Anaemia and neutropenia due to nutritional copper deficiency will respond promptly to the administration of 400–600 μg of copper per day in a 1% copper sulphate solution.

Vitamin E

Alpha tocopherol (vitamin E) is a fat-soluble dietary factor first shown to be required for successful reproduction in rats and now known to be an essential nutrient for all animals, including humans. Vitamin E has been the subject of extensive investigations over the past 40 years or so and in animals the signs and symptoms of vitamin E deficiency, including effects on the reproductive system, have been the subject of many reviews. Effects of deficiency of vitamin E do not readily occur in the adult human being, presumably because tissues do not easily become depleted and there is a wide distribution of alpha tocopherol in foodstuffs. Vitamin E deficiency syndromes have been described in neonates and particularly in premature neonates. The reason for this is that all newborn infants are in a state of relative tocopherol deficiency and the smaller the infant at birth the greater the lack of vitamin E.

A mother at term has a vitamin E level, on average, of around 9 mg/l, whereas her newborn's value is considerably lower at 2 mg/l. Term infants with a birth weight of 3500 g have vitamin E body stores of 20 mg, while babies with a birth weight of 1000 g will have stores of vitamin E amounting only to 3 mg. There is a direct relationship between the maternal level of vitamin E and that of her infant but a newborn baby never has a value in excess of 6 mg/l, which is considered to be the lowest limit of normal for older children and adults.

Vitamin E is a potent antiperoxidant at the cellular level. Deficiency of this vitamin results in an increased rate of cell membrane lipid peroxidation which, in the case of the red cell, can lead to a shortening of the red cell life span and a haemolytic anaemia.

It has been shown that the dietary requirement for vitamin E increases when the intake of polyunsaturated fatty acids (PUFA) increases. Although the breast-fed infant will quickly attain normal adult levels of vitamin E, there is considerable variability in achieving normal vitamin E status in the artificially-fed infant. This results in part from the PUFA content of the artificial formulas. Most infant formulas contain quantities of linoleic acid, an 18-carbon fatty acid with two unsaturated double bonds, far in excess of the quantities found in breast milk.

The first reports of the association of vitamin E deficiency with haemolytic anaemia in the premature neonate came from the USA in the late 1960s. These infants were aged 6–10 weeks and had been fed proprietary formulas with a high PUFA content. The administration of vitamin E to affected infants resulted in a prompt increase in the haemoglobin level and a fall in the reticulocyte count.

It was clear that the severity of the haemolysis in the premature infant was related to the level of vitamin E and the PUFA content of the diet (E:PUFA ratio). The lack of reports from the United Kingdom is probably a reflection of the lower PUFA content of our proprietary formulas at that time and hence a higher E:PUFA ratio.

It became evident through the passage of time that it was not just the high PUFA and low vitamin E content of the diet which were predisposing factors to haemolysis in the premature infant. It has become common practice to supplement infant feeding with iron to prevent the development of late anaemia (see above). Iron acts as a catalyst in the non-enzymatic auto-oxidation of unsaturated fatty acids and can result in the peroxidation of red cell membrane lipids. It has been shown that iron-fortified formulas can trigger a haemolytic anaemia in the infant who receives large

quantities of PUFA with inadequate amounts of vitamin E.

There are, therefore, three important variables in the diet which affect the development of haemolytic anaemia associated with lack of vitamin E in the premature infant:

1. Polyunsaturated fatty acid composition
2. Presence of added iron
3. Vitamin E content.

The interactions of these equally important factors may help to explain the marked variability in the incidence of vitamin E deficiency haemolytic anaemia from nursery to nursery and the virtual lack of a problem in the United Kingdom. It should be appreciated that vitamin E deficiency may contribute to the magnitude of the physiological anaemia in all non-supplemented premature infants. The commercial formulas have for the most part corrected the potential problem by reducing the content of linoleic acid and increasing the concentration of vitamin E. Breast milk has a very low content of linoleic acid.

The problem of the triad of factors (iron, PUFA and vitamin E levels) contributing to anaemia in premature infants is now well recognised and haemolysis can be prevented in one or more of three ways:

1. Introduction of iron can be delayed
2. A water soluble form of vitamin E can be administered to overcome the malabsorption of the natural vitamins
3. Formulas with a low PUFA content or human milk can be fed to small premature infants.

The removal or correction of just one of the contributing triad will prevent any significant haemolysis or anaemia in the premature neonate.

It has been suggested that vitamin E supplements may also reduce the incidence of two serious complications of oxygen administration in the premature infant, namely retrolental fibroplasia (RLF) and bronchopulmonary dysplasia (BPD). These suggestions are based on a large number of animal experiments that have demonstrated that vitamin E-deficient animals suffer more oxygen-induced damage to their lungs and CNS, as well as the red cells, than animals fed on a controlled vitamin E-supplemented diet.

Reports of a reduction in incidence, severity and duration of RLF in the human neonate associated with vitamin E-supplementation have appeared in recent years. Preliminary studies suggesting that the intramuscular administration of a water-dispersible preparation of DL alpha tocopherol during the acute phase of therapy for respiratory distress syndrome prevented the development and modified the severity of BPD, await confirmation from large combined studies.

Intraventricular haemorrhage and vitamin E

About 40% of newborn babies under 32 weeks' gestation develop ultrasound evidence of periventricular haemorrhage within the first 3 days of life. This bleeding may be confined to the sub-epidural region where it originates or it may rupture into the ventricles or brain parenchyma. It has been suggested that parentral vitamin E may prevent the progression to intraventricular haemorrhage in the pre-term infant.

Folic acid

Serum and red cell folate levels are higher in the newborn than in the normal adult regardless of birth weight or gestation, but fall quickly to levels which are often below normal adult ones within several weeks of birth. This fall occurs more rapidly in the premature than in the term infant, since subnormal levels are reached within the first few weeks of life, whereas low levels do not develop in the term infant until after 6 months of age. Controlled studies, however, have failed to demonstrate any alteration in the early anaemia of prematurity by giving routine folate supplementation. The normal premature infant absorbs folic acid easily and although there is no general recommendation for the prophylactic use of folic acid in newborn, a dietary provision of 20–50 μg per day would ensure sufficiency. Half a litre of almost any infant formula daily would provide this amount of folic acid.

Megaloblastic anaemia associated with folic acid deficiency has been observed in infants with chronic diarrhoea, chronic infection, infants and children receiving goat's milk and in infants receiving anticonvulsants.

In those infants whose dietary intake would be predictably poor, such as the very immature or those with chronic diarrhoea or recurrent infections, it would appear wise to give parenteral folic acid at periodic intervals.

Vitamin B_{12}

Serum B_{12} levels in all neonates are generally higher than in maternal serum. This is the result of active transfer of vitamin B_{12} across the placenta to the fetus at the expense of maintaining maternal vitamin B_{12} serum levels. This makes little impact on the mother's own reserves because adult stores are of the order of 3000 μg or more and vitamin B_{12} stores in the newborn infant are about 50 μg.

Because of these low storage reserves and because of poor dietary intake of vitamin B_{12} during the period of rapid growth most premature infants will end up with lower than normal adult levels by the fourth or fifth month of life. There is probably no significant relationship between deficiency of vitamin B_{12} and the early anaemia of prematurity (cf. folic acid and iron deficiency).

The haemoglobin, red cell counts and haematocrit are similar in deficient and replete premature infants. Any supplements of these essential nutrients that are given to premature infants in the first few weeks of life are to prevent the late anaemia due to deficiencies, which would inevitably develop by the fourth or fifth months of life.

PATHOLOGICAL ANAEMIA IN THE NEONATE

True anaemia in the neonate can result from haemorrhage, haemolysis or failure of red cell production. Significant anaemia at birth is usually due to severe immune haemolysis or haemorrhage. Anaemia that becomes apparent after 24 hours is most often due to internal or external haemorrhage or non-immune haemolytic disorders. Infants with impaired red cell production do not usually develop anaemia until after 3 weeks. Reference red cell values in the first week of life, for healthy term infants, are given in Table 28.3. The rise in haemoglobin in the first 24 hours is due to shift of fluid from the intravascular to extravascular space (see above). An infant with a capillary haemoglobin below 14.5 g/dl in the first post-natal week should be regarded as anaemic.

ANAEMIA RESULTING FROM HAEMORRHAGE

The causes of anaemia due to blood loss in the early neonatal period can be divided broadly into three categories: haemorrhage due to obstetric accidents, occult blood loss and internal bleeding (Table 28.4).

Obstetric accidents

Umbilical vessels

Rupture of a normal umbilical cord may occur in an unattended precipitous delivery. Anaemia in the infant can result from haemorrhage from the cord and from internal bleeding due to the fall. The cord can also rupture in a normal delivery if there are vascular abnormalities such as an aneurysm, or if the cord is abnormally short or entangled around the fetus. Traction with forceps can result in rupture of the normal cord.

Table 28.4 Conditions associated with anaemia in the newborn due to blood loss.

Obstetric accidents	Rupture of normal umbilical cord
	Haematoma of cord or placenta
	Incision of placenta during Caesarean section
	Placenta praevia
	Abruptio placentae
Malformations of placenta and cord	Rupture of anomalous vessels
	Rupture of abnormal umbilical cord
	Velamentous insertion
	Vaso praevia
Occult Haemorrhage	Before birth or during delivery
	Feto–maternal Spontaneous
	Traumatic
	amniocentesis
	External cephalic version
	Feto–placental
	Twin-to-twin
Internal haemorrhage	Intracranial
	Cephalhaematoma
	Retroperitoneal
	Ruptured liver
	Ruptured spleen
	Pulmonary
Iatrogenic blood loss	

Haematomas of the cord, although rare, may contain large volumes of blood and a fetal mortality of over 45% has been reported associated with such blood loss.

Velamentous insertion of the umbilical cord has been reported to occur in 1% of all pregnancies. The umbilical vessels are unprotected and insert into the edge of the placenta; the vessels may rupture spontaneously or during labour, but most velamentous insertions of the cord do not rupture. The condition is more common in twin than in singleton pregnancy and where there is a low-lying placenta.

The perinatal mortality rate, if the abnormal vessels do rupture, is high, many of such infants being still-born.

Placenta

Massive fetal haemorrhage can be associated with accidental incision of the placenta at Caesarean section, placenta praevia or abruptio placentae.

Lower segment Caesarean section with anterior placaentae can result in direct placental injury. The placenta and membranes should always be examined from the fetal side, following Caesarean section, for damage. Should such evidence be found the haemoglobin of the infant should be estimated at birth and again 12 to 24 hours later, because the initial haemoglobin may be normal. These estimates should also be carried out on all neonates born to mothers with unusual vaginal bleeding, placenta praevia or abruptio placentae. Placenta praevia is associated with anaemia in approximately 10% of the offspring and although abruptio placenta often results in intra-uterine death, anaemia may well be present in surviving infants. Multilobed placentae may be associated with anomalous vessels crossing the internal os termed vaso praevia. The infant is in double jeopardy with vaso praevia for the vessels may well be compressed as well as lacerated during the second stage of labour. The perinatal death rate ranges from 58 to 80% in these cases, the majority of infants being stillborn. In the minority born alive, death often occurs during the first 24 hours because of unrecognised severe anaemia.

Occult haemorrhage before and during delivery

Feto-maternal haemorrhage

Small numbers of fetal erythrocytes commonly enter the maternal circulation at some time during pregnancy. Occasionally these losses are of such magnitude as to cause anaemia, shock and, rarely, stillbirth. This mode of occult blood loss is probably the commonest cause of anaemia in the newborn.

Kleihauer test

The acid elution technique of Kleihauer and Betke is the simplest and most commonly used method for demonstration of fetal cells in maternal blood. It depends on the fact that fetal haemoglobin at low pH resists acid elution, whereas adult cells lose their haemoglobin leaving, after appropriate staining, some deeply pigmented fetal cells in a sea of maternal ghost cells. In adults only 1% of the total haemoglobin is HbF. This small amount is restricted to approximately 8% of the total red cells. These cells are termed F cells. They contain very small amounts of HbF for the most part. A very occasional maternal cell may contain up to 30% fetal haemoglobin, but even a rare cell such as this is unlikely to cause confusion with a fetal cell which will contain 60–80% of fetal haemoglobin at term and stain deeply in a Kleihauer preparation. A rough quantitation of the volume of fetal blood lost, if small, can be made by comparing the number of fetal cells counted over a fixed period of time, with standard films made of known volumes of fetal blood mixed with adult blood. If the loss is large enough to figure as a percentage of the maternal cells, then a rough quantitation of the volume can be made using the fact that a fetal red cell count of 1% in the maternal circulation is indicative of a haemorrhage from the fetus in the range of 50 ml. The identification of fetal cells by the acid elution method is limited in some situations. Where there is ABO blood group incompatibility between maternal and fetal red cells, the fetal cells may be rapidly removed from the maternal circulation by maternal antibody. Genetic conditions which result in raised levels of fetal haemoglobin in the mother, such as hereditary persistence of fetal haemoglobin, sickle cell disease and heterozygous beta thalassaemia, may give rise to difficulty in interpreting the results of the acid elution technique, and methods based on differential agglutination should be used.

The physiological increase in maternal fetal haemoglobin of from 1.5 to 5.7% during pregnancy gives rise to a faint positive stain in maternal red cells which is not easily confused with fetal cells which contain 60–80% fetal haemoglobin and stain intensely. Fetal haemoglobin is relatively stable and as well as resisting acid elution, the basis of the Kleihauer technique, also resists alkali denaturation. The alkali denaturation technique, however, is not as sensitive as the acid elution technique and cannot be used in the same way to quantitate fetomaternal bleeds, because this would involve estimation of the total alkali-resistant haemoglobin in the maternal circulation. A bleed of 50 ml would raise the total fetal haemoglobin in the maternal circulation by only 1%. On the other hand, this technique, unlike the Kleihauer, is a rapid valuable bedside method for identifying the source of vaginal blood losses. Strong alkali is added to a sample of the blood and the time it takes to denature to methaemoglobin (brown) is compared with the time taken by a similarly treated sample of normal adult blood. Although spontaneous feto-maternal bleeding usually occurs in the last trimester and there is an increased incidence during labour and delivery, transplacental fetal blood losses have been identified as early as 4 to 8 weeks' gestation and there may be chronic small blood losses throughout pregnancy as well as acute losses at or near parturition.

The mechanism of passage of fetal cells into the maternal circulation is not fully understood. Erosions in the placental villi through which the cells could pass and a correlation between occult placental haemorrhages and fetal red cells in the circulation have been demonstrated. Occult fetal haemorrhages are associated with trauma incurred at amniocentesis, prenatal diagnostic fetal blood sampling, intra-uterine transfusion and external version of the fetus.

Feto-maternal transfusion may sensitise the mother during pregnancy where there are differences between fetal and maternal red cell antigens. In the case of possible Rhesus D incompatibility, the mother should be given an appropriate dose of Rhesus anti-D immune globulin to prevent such sensitisation. Usually such invasion of her circulation has no immediate adverse effect on the mother, but maternal transfusion reactions to the fetal blood have been described.

Feto-placental haemorrhage

In some instances the blood lost from the fetus may not pass into the maternal circulation but may accumulate in the substance of the placenta or retroplacentally.

Approximately 20% of the infant's blood volume may be lost into the placenta when there is a tight nuchal cord. Holding the infant above the placenta before clamping the cord at delivery will result in continual loss of blood into the placenta. Decreased blood volume in infants delivered by Caesarean section compared with those delivered vaginally has been shown, presumably due to holding the infant above the placenta.

Twin-to-twin transfusion

In multiple pregnancy with dichorionic placentae vascular anastamosis is uncommon. With monozygotic twins a monochorial placenta is present in 70% of cases and twin-to-twin anastamosis occurs in almost every instance. It has been estimated that significant twin-to-twin transfusion occurs in 15% or more of all monochorial twins. The twin transfusion syndrome results in anaemia in the donor and polycythaemia in the recipient. There is significant morbidity and mortality in both the donor and the recipient. The condition should be suspected in any pair of identical twins in whom the haemoglobin difference is greater than 5 g/dl at birth. In dizygotic twins the haemoglobin difference is no greater than 3.3 g/dl. The donor twin's haemoglobin may range from 3.7 to 18 g/dl, while haemoglobin values as high as 20 to 30 g/dl have been recorded in the recipient twin. If there has been chronic haemorrhage from one twin to the other there will be marked difference in birth weight and organ size as well as haemoglobin levels. There may be hydramnios in the polycythaemic twin's sac and oligohydramnios in the other. Disseminated intravascular coagulation has been described in the liveborn of sets of twins with a macerated stillborn sibling. The anaemic twin may develop congestive cardiac failure whereas the plethoric twin may suffer from hyperviscosity and hyperbilirubinaemia, and kernicterus has been described (see p. 282).

Internal haemorrhage

Damage to organs during traumatic delivery is the usual cause of internal bleeding in the neonate. The common sites of major haemorrhage are the subaponeurotic and subperiosteal spaces of the cranium, the cerebral ventricles and subarachnoid space, liver, spleen, kidney and lungs.

Typical clinical signs of internal bleeding occur 24 to 72 hours after birth, although problems can occur immediately after delivery.

Blood loss into the subaponeurotic space can be much greater than into the subperiosteum because it is not confined by periosteal attachments and can spread over the whole calvarium, but both forms of bleeding into the scalp can result in severe anaemia. Neonatal exsanguination has been described. On recovery from these enclosed haemorrhages, jaundice usually develops and may be severe enough to warrant exchange transfusion.

Life-threatening complications result from bleeding into the ventricles and subarachnoid space, particularly in the premature infant, and the outcome in terms of permanent damage in the surviving infant is unpredictable. The clinical manifestations of an intracranial haemorrhage include changes in vital signs, seizures, hypothermia, apnoea, a bulging fontanelle and anaemia. The quantity of blood lost into the spinal fluid may amount to as much as 15% of the infant's blood volume. The diagnosis of subarachnoid haemorrhage in premature infants is difficult because of the frequency of traumatic taps. Rupture of the liver probably occurs more often than is clinically appreciated after traumatic delivery. If the haemorrhage remains confined within the capsule of the liver, although there may be abdominal swelling, decreased blood volume and anaemia, the haematoma may subside and the babe recover without complications. Should the capsule rupture, usually 24–48 hours, but occasionally up to 4 days, postdelivery, the infant goes into shock coincident with the escape of blood into the peritoneal cavity. On examination, upper abdominal distension and shifting dullness will be found and straight X-rays of the abdomen may reveal free fluid. The prognosis is poor but some infants have survived with prompt surgical repair and blood transfusion.

Splenic rupture is unusual in the newborn infant, but can occur after a difficult delivery, or during exchange transfusion, most commonly in association with an enlarged spleen due to erythroblastosis fetalis. Rarely the condition has been described in large, healthy infants after an apparently normal delivery.

Traumatic, particularly breech, deliveries are also associated with haemorrhages into the kidneys, adrenals and retroperitoneal space. Adrenal haemorrhage, like splenic rupture, has also been described following the normal delivery of a large infant. Such haemorrhage will be accompanied by signs of renal insufficiency. Bluish discoloration of the skin of the flank overlying a palpable mass will suggest retroperitoneal haemorrhage, and should be differentiated from a solid tumour such as neuroblastoma. Bleeding into the retroperitoneal space can also be caused by perforation or rupture of an umbilical artery by catheterisation.

Premature infants on ventilation support may haemorrhage into the lungs and develop profound anaemia–often accompanied by DIC. Respiratory distress increases with impairment of perfusion and ventilation. Prognosis is poor and mortality is high.

MANAGEMENT OF ACUTE AND CHRONIC BLOOD LOSS

The main differential diagnoses of pallor in the newborn and their clinical signs are listed in Table 28.4. It is essential to have a planned programme of management on delivery of a pale, distressed infant, as follows:

1. Maintain the airway and administer oxygen if necessary.
2. Insert an umbilical catheter and take blood for haemoglobin estimation, grouping, bilirubin, DAT and cross-matching.
3. Administer a plasma expander, 20 ml/kg, promptly to maintain blood volume (normal saline will do, if plasma or blood are not easily available).
4. If the arterial and venous pressure have not returned to normal, repeat the procedure with whole blood of the appropriate group, correcting acidosis as required.
5. Search for the cause of haemorrhage:

Table 28.4 Pallor in the newborn – differential diagnosis.

Acute blood loss	Asphyxia	Haemolytic disease
Blood pressure ↓	Response to oxygen and IPPV	Hepatosplenamegaly
Tachycardia	Bradycardia	
Rapid shallow respiration	Recession	
Acyanotic	Cyanosis	Jaundice
	Moribund appearance	Positive Coombs' test
Drop in haemoglobin	Stable haemoglobin	Anaemia

– careful examination of infant
– examination of placenta and cord
– maternal blood Kleihauer.

Infants who have suffered chronic blood loss in utero vary in their clinical state at delivery from a hydropic infant with severe anaemia, requiring immediate resuscitation, to an asymptomatic, mildly anaemic, thriving neonate who will require oral iron supplements only to raise the haemoglobin and replenish iron stores.

If replacement transfusion is required, the amount of blood needed can be calculated from this simple formula:

Volume of whole blood required (ml) = wt (kg) × desired rise in Hb × 6

Acute, severe blood loss during delivery results in a pale, shocked, hypovolaemic infant at birth with a normal haemoglobin initially, falling rapidly within 6–8 hours. Jaundice and cyanosis are absent and the babe will respond to plasma volume expanders.

Special care and precautions should be taken when events known to be associated with, or to cause, fetal bleeding during pregnancy have occurred. For example, an unexpected maternal history suggestive of a transfusion reaction indicates loss of incompatible fetal cells into her circulation. Other conditions associated with fetal blood loss include twin pregnancies, abruptio placentae, vaso praevia, placenta praevia and amniocentesis.

The newborn infant who suffers internal hemorrhage following traumatic delivery rapidly deteriorates in to hypovolaemic shock 24–72 hours following delivery.

ANAEMIA DUE TO HAEMOLYSIS IN THE NEONATE

The essential feature of a haemolytic process is a shortening of the normal adult red cell life span of 100–120 days. By this definition virtually all term (RBC life-span 80–100 days) and all premature (RBC life-span 60–80 days) infants suffer from haemolysis.

In the adult the classical triad of anaemia, reticulocytosis and hyperbilirubinaemia are the usual basic laboratory findings in any haemolytic process. In the newborn, however, features of haemolysis are more variable and in particular anaemia is usually not the presenting feature. Usually a haemolytic process is first detected in the investigation of jaundice occurring during the first week of life. To make the situation even more confusing, so-called physiological jaundice regularly occurs in the newborn period because of the transient impaired hepatic bilirubin conjugation and increased bilirubin production. In the absence of haemolysis, bilirubin levels of 205 μmol/l are seen in term neonates with a peak at 4 days and levels of 255

μmol/l peak at 7 days in premature infants. These levels are exceeded and clinical jaundice usually appears before 36 hours of age in the presence of haemolysis. Jaundice due to haemolysis in the newborn period can occur despite minimal changes in the haemoglobin level and without reticulocytosis so that occasionally hyperbilirubinaemia is the only manifestation of neonatal haemolytic disease. Haemolysis is common in the newborn period and has multiple aetiologies which can be grouped broadly into three large categories: isoimmunisation, congenital defects of the red cell and acquired defects. In most parts of the world the most important cause of haemolytic disease in the newborn is the production of maternal red cell antibodies against incompatible red cell antigens of her fetus.

CONGENITAL HAEMOLYTIC DISEASE

Hereditary red cell morphology (membrane) disorders

Hereditary spherocytosis

For an account of this condition see Chapter 11. A few points only will be made, which have special relevance for the newborn period.

Approximately 50% of cases of hereditary spherocytosis will develop significant jaundice due to haemolysis in the first week of life, but the anaemia is mild and values of less than 10.0 g/dl are unusual. The diagnosis is confirmed by laboratory evidence of haemolysis together with increased incubated red cell osmotic fragility plus family studies. The finding of spherocytes in the blood film does not mean that the owner of that blood suffers from hereditary spherocytosis. There is a long list of conditions which can injure the erythrocyte membrane, producing variable numbers of spherocytes. These include: immunohaemolytic anaemia and haemolytic transfusion reactions with a positive Coomb's test; *Clostridium welchii* septicaemia and other infections such as CMV; severe burns; and spider, bee and snake venoms, etc. In the newborn period, however, there is only one common condition which might be confused with hereditary spherocytosis and this is haemolytic disease of the newborn due to ABO incompatibility.

The finding of the typical ABO blood group combination (O mother with A or B infant) plus an immune anti-A or Anti-B antibody in the maternal serum, together with a lack of family history, should help the paediatrician to arrive at the correct diagnosis. Other conditions such as cytomegalovirus infections are not likely to be confusing because of the special characteristics and diagnostic features. It would be misleading, however, to suggest that the diagnosis is always easy.

The main stumbling block is the variable severity of the condition in close family members.

Prevention of kernicterus in the neonatal period is the most important aspect of therapy as with any haemolytic anaemia, whatever the cause. Splenectomy should be delayed, if possible, until 5 years of age when the maximum risk of overwhelming pneumococcal or *H influenzal* infections has passed. Once the diagnosis is made, the babe should be maintained on daily oral supplements of folic acid to meet the requirements of the increased marrow turnover until the spleen is removed.

Hereditary elliptocytosis

Elliptical cells are present in the circulation of normal individuals and may number up to 15%. Those who have more than 25% and up to 75% are described as having the disorder hereditary elliptocytosis.

Elliptocytosis probably results from several genetic determinants, one of which is linked to the Rh blood group locus. Homozygous hereditary elliptocytosis is associated with severe haemolytic anaemia in the neonatal period. Heterozygotes show much greater variation in clinical expression of the condition, ranging from no anaemia or evidence of haemolysis to relatively severe haemolysis with splenomegaly and jaundice. This clinical variability probably reflects underlying genetic heterogeneity. The condition is clearly heterogeneous from a clinical, genetic and biochemical point of view (See Ch. 11).

Generally elliptocytosis is an incidental finding in the unrelated investigations of a haematologically healthy child. Occasionally the condition may present as neonatal jaundice with or without anaemia. The blood film in these cases usually contains a high proportion of poikilocytes and pyknocytes instead of a high proportion of elliptocytes. Morphologic diagnosis may not be revealed until the cells from an exchange transfusion have been cleared. Many of the cases with more severe haemolysis also have significant numbers of circulating spherocytes.

The most important aspect of management again is the prevention of kernicterus by phototherapy and exchange transfusion. If there is significant haemolysis, folic acid supplements should be given. The severe forms of hereditary elliptocytosis behave clinically in the same way as hereditary spherocytosis. The anaemia will respond to splenectomy, which should be delayed until 5 years of age.

Hereditary stomatocytosis

This is a condition in which there is relative failure of the Na^+ K^+ pump because of passive permeability to the cations resulting in the influx of Na^+ exceeding the loss of K^+, so that the cells swell due to the progressive gain of cations and water. The defect is probably located in the membrane and something to do with the skeleton but it has not been defined. The condition is characterised by variable numbers of stomatocytes in the circulating blood, but they are not unique to this disorder. There is a spectrum of clinical severity similar to that seen in hereditary elliptocytosis. It may present in the neonatal period with severe jaundice requiring treatment.

Red cell enzyme abnormalities

Haemolytic anaemia and haemolysis of neonatal red cells resulting in jaundice without anaemia has been described in association with many inherited enzyme defects but only two of these are of clinical significance – glucose-6-phosphate dehydrogenase (G6PD) deficiency and pyruvate kinase (PK) deficiency.

Glucose-6-phosphate dehydrogenase deficiency

This condition is the most frequent inherited enzyme defect and affects millions of people worldwide (Ch. 11).

Further discussion of this fascinating and common deficiency in general terms is inappropriate here, but it does have an important role as a cause of haemolysis, jaundice and anaemia in the newborn period in special care nurseries all over the world.

G6PD deficiency and neonatal haemolysis

G6PD is the key enzyme on the pentose phosphate shunt which provides reducing substances that protect the red cell membrane, its haemoglobin and metabolic systems from the deleterious effects of oxidation. The hexose monophosphate pathway in cord blood appears to be sound and is stimulated by oxidants. Nevertheless the red cells of the normal newborn are particularly susceptible to oxidant injury. It is not surprising, then, that neonatal jaundice is so often apparently associated with G6PD deficiency. The problem is further exacerbated by the newborn's temporary inability to cope with the breakdown of haem and conversion to conjugated bilirubin. G6PD deficiency per se does not necessarily always result in neonatal jaundice. The usual causal factors are infection (common) and drugs (less common) but recently there have been more and more frequent reports of haemolysis associated with G6PD deficiency where no known oxidant stress can be found. For instance, it was once thought that Black term infants with G6PD deficiency (Gd^{A-}) did not show any increased incidence of haemolysis or neonatal hyper-bilirubinaemia, without a known stimulus such as administration of vitamin K or painting the umbilical stump with brilliant green or methyl violet antiseptic, but a report from Nigeria shows a clear association between G6PD deficiency and the incidence of neonatal jaundice. The authors of this report conclude that because of the undoubted difference in incidence of neonatal jaundice between Afro-American and West African newborns associated with the Gd^{A-} variant, there must be some, as yet, unidentified environmental factor responsible. Similar unexplained differences in incidence have been described from different areas in Greece associated with Gd^{Mediterranean} variants. The fact that G6PD deficiency is found in association with neonatal jaundice does not exonerate the paediatrician from looking for the oxidant stimulus. One unique mechanism which may cause haemolysis in a G6PD infant in the neonatal period is the effect of maternal ingestion of haemolysis-inducing drugs which may have little or no effect on her own blood. Fatal hydrops fetalis has been reported in one case of G6PD deficiency in a Chinese infant whose mother ate fava beans and ascorbic acid. The investigation of G6PD deficiency in the neonatal period should always involve enzyme assay of maternal as well as neonatal blood, because an established reticulocyte population in the babe's blood may well give near normal levels of G6PD activity, especially in the A− variety. Special stains of the peripheral blood using methyl violet may reveal Heinz bodies – the product of oxidative degradation of globin – and typical fragmented cells, but these factors are of limited value in diagnosis in neonatal blood. The important feature of management in the neonatal period is prevention of kernicterus and the problem in the vast majority of cases is a temporary one. Parents of an affected babe should be given a list of the potentially dangerous oxidant drugs and toxins, some of which can be bought over the counter, such as aspirin and moth balls (naphthalene). Because many of the parents have limited understanding of written English (Greek, Turkish, Semitic and Oriental origins), steps should be taken to make sure that they understand what is written down. There is no need for folic acid maintenance in these cases as the chronic haemolysis is insignificant.

The rare type of G6PD deficiency resulting in chronic severe haemolysis presents early in the neonatal period and requires exchange transfusion in the first hours of life. There is a continued requirement for folic acid and usual maintenance therapy and care throughout life.

Pyruvate kinase deficiency

This is an autosomal recessive disorder that occurs in all ethnic groups, although documented cases have come mainly from persons of north European stock.

The block of glycolysis at the lower end of the Embden-Myerhof pathway results in an accummulation of 2,3-DPG, a shift of the oxygen dissociation curve to the right and a reduction in oxygen affinity, which means that oxygen delivery to the tissues in the presence of PK deficiency may be normal or near normal even with levels of haemoglobin between 6 and 8 g/dl. Clinically child may thrive and only require the occasional transfusion.

Many cases of PK deficiency go undiagnosed for months or even years until the blood is examined for one reason or another but PK-deficient newborns often develop haemolytic jaundice and require phototherapy and exchange transfusion to prevent kernicterus. The diagnosis at this stage is made by finding a low enzyme concentration and intermediate levels in the parents, who are not anaemic and have no evidence of haemolysis. The neonatal blood film has no special characteristics to suggest PK deficiency, except for an exaggeration of the normal neonatal morphology in the presence of increased marrow activity. A child requiring regular transfusion to thrive normally may improve dramatically in terms of transfusion requirements with the small rise in haemoglobin achieved post-splenectomy.

Haemolysis due to haemoglobin disorders

Haemoglobinopathies are divided into two broad groups: the haemoglobin variants and the thalassaemia syndromes (See Ch. 12). Both are defects of globin. The variants result from either single or multiple amino acid substitutions in one or other of the globin chains of normal human haemoglobins. The thalassaemia syndromes are conditions where there is defective synthesis of structurally normal globin chains.

The two most important haemoglobinopathies clinically and numerically are sickle cell disease HbS/S and homozygous beta thalassaemia – thalassaemia major. Both are beta chain defects and therefore do not usually cause problems until between 3 and 6 months of age when the beta chain of adult haemoglobin (HbA($\alpha_2\beta_2$) normally becomes predominant (See Fig. 28.2).

Haemoglobin variants

Since the description of the structural defect in sickle haemoglobin hundreds of variants of haemoglobin have been described. Most of them do not affect function significantly. The most common after HbS are HbC, D Punjab and E. They are all beta chain defects which are not usually detectable before 3 to 6 months of age and do not cause problems in the newborn period. However, there is an increased incidence of hyperbilirubinaemia in babes with HbS/S sickle cell disease, probably as a result of the small amount of sickle cells present at birth. Massive sickling with severe jaundice has also been described, occasionally with a fatal outcome. These episodes are triggered by anoxia and severe infection. Diagnosis in the newborn period is made by haemoglobin electrophoresis on agar gel pH 6.2. This separates HbF and A, which run together on conventional cellulose acetate Hb electrophoresis at pH 8.2. On agar gel electrophoresis only two bands of HbF and HbS are seen in sickle cell disease HbS/S, whereas three distinct bands of HbA, F and S are seen in the case of sickle cell trait. Once the diagnosis of HbS/S is made, daily folic acid supplements should be prescribed and the parents warned of the signs of sickling infarcts and the conditions which precipitate them in the young infant, so that they can seek prompt medical treatment and advice early in any potential sickling crisis.

Thalassaemia syndromes

This group of disorders constitutes the most common inherited single gene defect in the world. They are caused by a quantitative defect in synthesis of one or other of the various chains of normal human haemoglobins and result in the production of small red cells with an inadequate haemoglobin content (Ch. 12).

Alpha thalassaemia

The alpha chain is common to all three circulating human haemoglobins, $HbA(\alpha_2 \quad \beta_2)$, $HbA_2(\alpha_2\delta_2)$ and $HbF(\alpha_2\gamma_2)$. Alpha thalassaemia can therefore present at birth. Alpha chain production is under the control of four genes – two on each of homologous chromosomes. Alpha thalassaemia results usually from deletion of one or more of these genes. The condition is very common in Oriental and Negro populations. The clinical severity of the various forms of alpha thalassaemia depends on how many of these genes are deleted. Alpha thalassaemia trait results from deletion of one or two genes. The condition with one gene deleted (α^+ trait) results in no clinical manifestation and no obvious abnormality on initial screening of the blood. The diagnosis can only be made by globin chain synthesis and gene mapping. Alpha^0 thalassaemia (two genes missing) will produce typical thalassaemic indices and mild anaemia, especially under haematologic stress such as pregnancy, infection, etc.

HbH disease is the chronic haemolytic anaemia resulting from deletion of three of the four alpha genes. Sufferers are not usually transfusion-dependent. Folic acid supplements and timely splenectomy, in more severe cases, will help to maintain a reasonable haemoglobin level. The condition can present at birth and the usual precautions to prevent kernicterus should be taken. It is not widely appreciated that these individuals are susceptible to increased haemolysis induced by the same oxidant drugs which provoke haemolysis in G6PD-deficient individuals. Parents of a child with HbH disease should be given the same list of drugs and toxins to avoid. Diagnosis is made usually by finding a typical fast band of HbH (β_4) on haemoglobin electrophoresis in the adult and a similar band of HbBarts (γ_4) in the newborn. Typical Hb inclusions are seen in a film of an incubated reticulocyte preparation. The diagnosis is confirmed by DNA analysis and gene mapping.

Alpha thalassaemia major is the condition in which all four alpha genes are deleted and no alpha chains are made at all. This condition is incompatible with extra-uterine life and pregnancy ends in a hydrops which may be stillborn or lives a maximum of a few hours. The condition was first defined in a Chinese baby born at St. Bartholomews Hospital. The haemoglobin was found to be made up entirely of tetramers of the γ chain of fetal haemoglobin, no alpha chains being made. This haemoglobin – γ_4 – has accordingly been called HbBarts and the condition described as HbBarts hydrops.

The chromosome on which both alpha genes have been deleted is found only rarely in Negroes. For this reason HbH disease and HbBarts hydrops almost never occurs in Black populations. It occurs quite frequently in eastern Mediterranean populations and reaches a maximum incidence in Thailand. Parents at risk should be identified early in pregnancy. They will have either alpha thalassaemia trait with typical indices or Hb.H disease. Women carrying an alpha thalassaemia hydrops have a high incidence of life-threatening hypertension and difficult vaginal deliveries. The condition can be diagnosed by amniotic fibroblast or trophoblast DNA analysis and termination of the non-viable child carried out before these complications become a problem.

Gamma thalassaemia

In the same way that gamma chain variants may cause transient haemolysis in the first weeks of life, gamma thalassaemia can have a similar effect, producing a mild to moderate anaemia at birth with reduced levels of (HbF) fetal haemoglobin which may require transfusion therapy.

ACQUIRED HAEMOLYTIC DISEASE

Anaemia associated with infection

Both intra-uterine and post-natal acquired infections are associated with anaemia and other haematological abnormalities in the neonatal period. Although these changes are sometimes produced by marrow suppression, severe neonatal infection is usually accompanied by haemolysis. Sometimes, particularly in acquired bacterial sepsis, the haemolytic process develops because of infection-induced small vessel damage and resulting disseminated intravascular coagulation (DIC). This is a common complication of neonatal infection. DIC is always secondary to some other pathological process and in the newborn is commonly associated with asphyxia, respiratory distress syndrome, hypovolaemia and hypothermia, as well as with infection. Infants with DIC are very sick. Anaemia is only one of the many haematological and other problems arising from and associated with this process. The mainstay of management is to treat the underlying cause. Intra-uterine infections commonly associated with haemolytic anaemia include toxoplasmosis, cytomegalovirus, congenital syphilis and rubella. The haemolytic process here is thought to arise from reticulo-endothelial hyperplasia or direct injury to the red cell membrane. Occasionally an antibody produced against the infecting organism cross-reacts with an antigen on the surface of the red cell, an apparent auto-antibody, which may give a positive direct Coomb's test.

The clinical and haematological picture in congenital infection may resemble that seen with HDN due to blood group incompatibility. Hepatosplenomegaly, anaemia with reticulocytosis and large numbers of circulating erythroblasts plus jaundice and hyperbilirubinaemia are common features. The laboratory distinction can usually be made by finding increased IgM, a negative direct Coomb's test and antibody titres against specific infecting microorganisms, and direct harvesting of the infective agent from urine or blood. Clinically there are distinctive features of congenital infection, such as chorioretinitis and cerebral calcification.

Severe infection in the neonate can produce some very bizarre changes in the blood which accompany anaemia, whether the anaemia be due to haemolysis or suppression of erythropoiesis. There may be thrombocytopenia and bruising in the absence of DIC together with leukocytosis and an increase of circulating immature white cells and even frank blasts.

Congenital malaria

All three species of the human malaria parasite are known to cause congenital infections. In endemic areas up to 9% of newborn infants may be affected. Severe fetal infection is incompatible with life and parasites can be found in the brain, liver and spleen as well as in the red cells of the still-born infant. The transfer of parasitised maternal red cells often presumably takes place at delivery, so that the babe is apparently normal at birth and sometimes does not present until weeks or even months post-natally with the maternally acquired infection, unless a careful search for the offending parasite is made. Malaria in the pregnant woman, because it is so unusual, causes great concern in the United Kingdom, but the possible transfer of infection to the fetus is not widely appreciated. Treatment should be instituted immediately if there is any suggestion that there has been transfer of maternal parasites. In any case there should be careful supervision of the infant for at least 2 months post-delivery.

Haemolytic anaemia due to maternal autoimmune disease

The rare combination of autoimmune haemolytic anaemia (AIHA) and pregnancy carries great risks to both the woman herself and the fetus. The degree of haemolysis in the fetus depends mainly on the amount and avidity of the transferred antibody for the fetal red cells. Although pregnancy may result in exacerbation of disseminated lupus erythematosus, up to 50% of women with this condition are reported to improve during pregnancy, especially in the third trimester. Haemolytic anaemia, leukopenia and thrombocytopenia have all been observed in infants of women with active disease, presumably due to IgG antibody involved in the disease process crossing the placenta. Administration of prednisolone 2 mg/kg/day to the mother with active AIHA prenatally may both reduce maternal haemolysis and reduce neonatal morbidity. Management of the newborn as in other cases of neonatal haemolysis is directed primarily to anticipating and treating hyperbilirubinaemia to prevent kernicterus.

ANAEMIA IN THE NEONATE DUE TO IMPAIRED PRODUCTION OF RED CELLS

Congenital red cell aplasia (Diamond-Blackfan syndrome)

There have been well over 200 reports of this condition in the literature since it was first described in 1936. The disorder has been called chronic congenital regenerative anaemia, pure red cell aplasia, erythrogenesis imperfecta, congenital hypoplastic anaemia and chronic idiopathic erythroblastopenia. Evidence suggests that the disorder is secondary to either a lack of erythroid stem cells or immune suppression of stem cell differentiation. Inheritance appears to follow an autosomal recessive pattern in most of the cases so far reported. It is not a common cause of anaemia in the neonatal period, but 25% of reported cases present with pallor of the newborn, although diagnosis has not been made until up to 6 years of age. Anaemia is manifest in 90% of cases by the end of the first year of life. The diagnosis should be suspected in any newborn with anaemia and reticulocytopenia (0–2%), together with normal platelets and leukocytes. Confirmation of the diagnosis is obtained by examination of a bone marrow aspirate which reveals virtual absence of erythroid precursors. One-third of patients have physical abnormalities and the paediatrician may be alerted to the possibility of this diagnosis by finding triphalangeal thumbs, characteristics of Turner's syndrome or other musculo-skeletal anomalies. Once the diagnosis is established, treatment with steroids should be started as soon as possible. The chances of remission on this therapy are increased the earlier it is commenced. Management in the neonatal period is not a problem but long-term support with blood-transfusion and inevitable iron-loading should be avoided if at all possible by early institution of Prednisolone as soon as the diagnosis is made.

CONGENITAL LEUKAEMIA

Infiltration of the bone marrow with proliferating white cells prevents adequate erythroid production in this rare condition which may present with anaemia in the neonatal period. It has been the custom to designate leukaemia diagnosed within a few days of birth as congenital and that detected during the first 4–6 weeks as neonatal. However, cell kinetics in leukaemia suggest that leukaemia presenting at 4 weeks must have originated in utero; therefore the term 'congenital leukaemia' should be applied overall to leukaemia in the neonatal period. The incidence is unknown but there are more than 100 reported cases. Congenital leukaemia is usually myeloid or myelomonocytic in sharp contrast to the high incidence of lymphoblastic leukaemia in the older child. There is an increased incidence in association with Down's syndrome (as with other chromosome abnormalities in older children) but there is in addition an unexplained transient myeloproliferative disorder in association with Down's syndrome. There is no relationship between radiologic examination during pregnancy and neonatal leukaemia. There has not been any reported case of congenital leukaemia in an infant born to a mother suffering from leukaemia.

The newborn bone marrow response to anoxia, infection or severe haemolysis often results in a leuko-erythroblastic blood film with increased numbers of immature cells of all cell series in the circulating blood. This picture may be confused initially with congenital leukaemia. With true congenital leukaemia skin manifestations are the most frequent clinical finding at birth. More than 50% of cases have leukaemic skin nodules, varying in size from 0.2 to 3.0 cm and slate blue in colour, in addition to petechiae and purpura. Hepatosplenomegaly is common. Examination of the blood reveals anaemia, thrombocytopenia and a total leukocyte count often above 150 000 per cu m with many circulating myelocytes. The bone marrow aspirate shows sheets of undifferentiated myeloblasts. I disagree with many investigators who suggest the posterior iliac crest as the aspiration site of choice, although it is possible to obtain a good sample in some cases from that site. A representative sample is best obtained from the tibia of a newborn babe in the first week of life, especially if the babe is premature.

Myeloblasts in the blood are uncommon and granulocyte maturation is complete in leukaemoid reactions secondary to infection, inflammatory disease and severe HDN. Neuroblastoma may also present as anaemia in the neonate, secondary to bone marrow infiltration. Examination of bone marrow which will show clumps of metastatic tumour cells and estimation of catecholamines will establish the diagnosis.

The prognosis is poor in true cases of congenital leukaemia with or without therapy. Most infants die within a few days to months of diagnosis. Death is commonly due to respiratory failure.

The only condition which will cause genuine problems in differential diagnosis after examination of blood and bone marrow and after exclusion of infection, inflammatory disease and severe haemolysis is the transient myeloproliferative syndrome usually associated with Down's syndrome. This condition will recover spontaneously.

HAEMOLYTIC DISEASE OF THE NEWBORN

Haemolytic disease of the newborn (HDN) is a condition in which the life span of the infant's red cells is shortened by the action of specific antibodies derived from the mother. The immune antibodies in the maternal plasma are immunoglobulins of the IgG subclass and therefore – unlike the naturally occurring antibodies of the ABO blood group systems (IgM) – are able to cross the placenta.

Although HDN can theoretically occur in any situation where the mother lacks a paternally derived antigen which her baby carries on its red cells, there is no doubt that prior to the introduction of the specific immunoglobulin for the prevention of RhD haemolytic disease, RhD HDN was by far the most important form of HDN in terms of clinical severity and frequency in Caucasian populations. Since introduction of prophylaxis the numbers of babes affected by severe HDN have plummeted and the proportion of HDN due to antibodies other than Anti-D have risen, but the most severe cases with very rare exceptions are still caused by Anti-D antibodies. Other Rh antibodies which can cause HDN are anti-c and rarely Anti-E, in which case the mother is usually Rh(D) positive.

THE RHESUS BLOOD GROUP SYSTEM

This is the most complex of the blood group systems. It is characterised by more than 30 known antigens and a much larger number of complex alleles. The Rh antigens are most probably lipoproteins and they are confined to the red cell membrane. The system was first described by Landsteiner and Wiener in 1940.

The Wiener system proposed that the Rh phenotype is determined by a single genetic locus with many alleles. The Fisher-Race system, on the other hand, assumes that the inheritance of the Rh antigens is determined by three pairs of allelic genes, C-c, D-d, E-e, acting on three closely linked loci. Despite expansion over the years, the Fisher-Race system does not cover all the reactions which have been observed within the Rh system, but because the CDE/cde nomenclature is easy to use and enables practical visualisation of how a given sample of cells will react with available antisera, the World Health Organization has recommended that the Fisher-Race system be adopted.

A number of variants exist for each of the common Rh antigens, e.g. D^u, C^w, C^x, E^w. The D^u antigen is of particular importance and is common in Black populations. In most individuals the D^u antigen differs from the normal D only in that there are fewer antigenic sites per red blood cell, and the D^u antigen will react weakly and variably with the various anti-D antisera. There are, however, some D^u variants which have both a qualitative and quantitative defect. Such individuals can make anti-D antibodies and should be identified. If a structural D variant is excluded, then it is not necessary to treat the D^u individual as Rhesus D negative for transfusion purposes. Similarly D^u individuals with a straightforward weakly expressed normal D antigen are not considered candidates for either antenatal or postnatal prophylaxis with passively administered anti-D immunoglobulin. If, however, there are no facilities for excluding structural D^u variant, then it is safer to treat all D^u individuals as Rh (D) negative.

Basically, therefore, there are considered to be six antigens and the main combination of genes at the three loci are:

$$\left.\begin{array}{l} \text{CDe or } R_1 \\ \text{cDE or } R_2 \\ \text{CDE or } R_z \\ \text{cDe or } R_o \end{array}\right\} \text{Rh(D) Positive}$$

$$\left.\begin{array}{l} \text{cde or r} \\ \text{Cde or r}' \\ \text{cdE or r}'' \\ \text{CdE or } r_y \end{array}\right\} \text{Rh (D) negative}$$

This classification follows the convention that possession of a D gene and antigen is termed Rh positive whereas absence of a D gene and antigen is termed Rh negative.

$$\left.\begin{array}{l} \text{DD homozygous} \\ \text{Dd heterozygous} \end{array}\right\} \text{Rh Positive}$$

dd   Rh negative

It follows that any Rh positive offspring of an Rh negative mother has to be heterozygous Dd, Rh positive having received a D antigen from the father but a d antigen from the mother. It also follows that if the father is homozygous Rh(D) positive then he can only have Rhesus positive children; whereas if he is heterozygous (Dd) Rh positive there is a 50:50 chance of him fathering a Rh negative babe which will not be affected by maternal anti-D.

Approximately 15% of the Caucasian population of the United Kingdom are Rh (D) negative, and the remaining 85% are Rh (D) positive.

Difficulties in determining the zygosity of an Rh positive individual arise from the fact that there is no antiserum which will identify the d antigen. Probabilities of genotype are worked out from reactions with the five available antisera which react with C-D-E and c and e antigens and frequencies of combinations of these antigens derived from population studies. This is why the report on paternal blood for Rhesus genotyping will always be preceded by the word 'probable'.

RHESUS HAEMOLYTIC DISEASE OF THE NEWBORN

The disease begins in intra-uterine life and may result in death in utero. In live-born infants the haemolytic process is maximal at the time of birth and thereafter diminishes as the concentration of maternal antibody in the infant's circulation declines. During pregnancy the fetal and maternal circulations are separate. Red cells are not thought to cross the placental barrier in sufficient numbers in normal circumstances. Oxygen, nutrient and waste exchange takes place by diffusion across the intervillous space. IgG antibodies cross the placenta freely carrying protection in the form of passive immunity for the fetus against infective agents to which the mother has had a healthy immune response. Following delivery of the neonate, rupture of the placental villi and connective tissue at separation allows escape of fetal blood cells into the maternal circulation prior to constriction of open-end maternal vessels. This is when sensitisation takes place in the majority of cases unless prevented.

Prevention of Rh D HDN

The stimulus for primary induction of antibody formation has been shown to be Rh (D) positive fetal cells entering the maternal circulation. If Rhesus anti-D immune globulin is injected into the mother, the antibody coats the fetal Rh (D) positive antigen sites and the coated cells are rapidly removed from the maternal circulation by cells of the reticulo-endothelial system. Maternal immune system cells are prevented from producing antibody against the fetal Rh (D) positive cells in the presence of adequate antibody.

Fetal cells in the maternal circulation can be identified and quantitated crudely using the Kleihauer technique.

Prophylaxis against rhesus haemolytic disease (UK recommendations)

Anti-D immunoglobulin should be administered to any non-sensitised Rh (D) negative woman as follows:

1. Post-delivery, if she gives birth to an Rh(D) positive infant.
2. Post-therapeutic abortion or identified spontaneous abortion.
3. Ante-natally at 28 and 34 weeks' gestation if she has no living children.
4. To cover antenatal procedures such as amniocentesis.
5. If she threatens to abort or miscarry.

Post-partum anti-D. All Rh (D) negative women who give birth to an Rh (D) positive babe and who have produced no identifiable antibodies should receive a standard dose of 500 iu anti-D within 72 hours of delivery; this is an arbitrary time. If a woman is sent home without receiving anti-D it is well worth giving the anti-D if she is identified as being at risk – certainly within the first week of delivery and probably up to 3 to 6 weeks post-partum. The half-life of fetal cells in the maternal circulation is approximately 40 days.

A Kleihauer examination of fetal cells within the maternal circulation should be carried out to make sure that the estimated bleed is no more than 4 ml, which will be covered by the standard dose of 500 iu. If a larger loss of fetal cells into the mother's circulation has occurred, a proportionally larger dose of anti-D immunoglobulin should be administered. In the vast majority of cases fetal losses into the maternal circulation are less than 1.0 ml.

Post-abortion anti-D. The D antigen has been shown to be present on fetal red blood cells as early as 38 days post-conception. It has been reported that transplacental haemorrhage occurs in 20% of cases undergoing therapeutic abortion, 4% of which are associated with a bleed of more than 0.2 ml into the maternal circulation. The volume of fetal blood crossing into the maternal circulation following spontaneous abortion is usually less than 0.1 ml. Many women in the past developed antibodies following early terminations or spontaneous abortions. Therefore, all women who have a therapeutic or identified spontaneous abortion should receive a standard dose of 250 iu anti-D regardless of possible group of fetus or Kleihauer estimation.

Antenatal anti-D. It is estimated that approximately 1% of Rh (D) negative women may be sensitised during the antenatal period due to transplacental passage of fetal red cells in apparently non-eventful pregnancy without any invasive procedures. Ideally all non-sensitised Rh (D) negative women should receive antenatal prophylaxis in every pregnancy. In the United States and Canada, where supplies of anti-D are abundant, Rh (D) negative women receive 1500 iu of anti-D at 28 and 34 weeks' gestation in all pregnancies. In the United Kingdom, where supplies are limited, antenatal prophylaxis is confined to those women who have no living children and the dose they receive is less, namely 500 iu at 28 weeks' and 34 weeks' gestation. It is important to repeat therapy, once instituted, at 6-week intervals because it has been shown that very low levels of passively administered anti-D may enhance antibody formation in the presence of an antigenic stimulus. If an Rh (D) positive fetus is delivered at term, it is obvious that anti-D should be administered in the usual way, even if antenatal prophylaxis has been given.

Prophylaxis of antenatal procedures. Invasive procedures such as amniocentesis fetal blood sampling, which may encourage transplacental fetal red cell invasion of the maternal circulation, should be covered by passively administered anti-D. The dose to be given is 250 iu up to 22 weeks' gestation and 500 iu thereafter. External versions of breech presentations are very rarely performed nowadays, but these should be similarly covered with administration of anti-D.

Threatened abortion. A standard dose of anti-D should be given, the amount depending on gestation, and theoretically this prophylaxis should be repeated at 6-week intervals throughout the pregnancy.

Reasons for failure of prophylaxis

Injection not given. The non-identification of the woman at risk and failure to administer prophylaxis appropriately remains the most potent cause of failure of prophylaxis.

Inadequate dosage of anti-D. There are still some centres which do not perform a routine Kleihauer to identify those women who require more than the standard 500 iu. Mistakes can be made and rigid quality control must be applied to all laboratories who attempt to quantitate fetal cells in the maternal circulation.

Prior sensitisation. There are a number of women who have been antenatally sensitised but who do not have any identifiable antibody at the time of delivery, even if enzyme-treated Rh D positive cells are used in the test system. In this case any passively administered anti-D will be ineffective once the maternal immune system has been primed.

Injection badly given. Unless the injection is given deeply intramuscularly it will not be absorbed appropriately and will fail to have the desired effect.

MANAGEMENT OF HAEMOLYTIC DISEASE OF THE NEWBORN

ASSESSMENT OF THE RH NEGATIVE PREGNANT WOMAN

All Rh (D) negative women should be screened as a minimum at booking, at 28 weeks, 34 weeks and at delivery, and if no active anti-D antibody production is detected, the woman receives prophylaxis as described above.

If a woman has antibodies at booking or if antibody is detected on subsequent testing, the pregnancy becomes high-risk. Since the number of sensitised pregnancies has fallen dramatically, most peripheral centres will only see one or two women at risk per year and while this is fortunate in general and an advance in terms of public health, it means that very few groups now have expertise in monitoring progress, instituting therapy, prime-timing of delivery and in the skilled procedures of intra-uterine fetal transfusion.

It is essential that any woman at risk, once identified, should at least have her case drawn to the attention of one of the expert referral centres, so that collective experience may be applied to her case.

Disasters occur when a woman is referred for urgent treatment late in a sensitised pregnancy with a frank or incipient hydrops in utero, which may well have been prevented by earlier intervention. Not only are most centres untutored in the techniques of intra-uterine transfusion and other fetal therapy, they are unfamiliar with interpreting the significance of a maternal antibody concentration, amniotic fluid bilirubin and other methods of monitoring severity of disease in the fetus.

MONITORING SEVERITY OF DISEASE IN THE FETUS

Maternal antibody quantitation

The detection of anti-D antibodies in the maternal circulation alerts the clinician to a possible problem. It does not reveal the group of the fetus and whether it is of risk of severe HDN. Of more significance is whether the antibody concentration is rising. In addition, the zygosity of the father and previous history are important prognostic factors. There has been much interest recently in the method of antibody quantitation following the introduction of a standard preparation of anti-D. Large numbers of sera can be examined by an automated procedure. This does away with observer error in interpreting IAT and also with manual dilution errors, but is not really vastly superior in other ways. It is very important, however, for the units who see only relatively few cases. It has been shown that if the antibody is quantitated at less than 4 iu/ml then there is no indication for further investigation or intervention.

Because techniques of antibody determination vary from laboratory to laboratory it is essential that those concerned with managing the case are familiar with the methodology and reliability of the method used in their local laboratory. In the end, the antibody is only an indication of a potential problem and indicates the necessity or otherwise of further invasive procedures. It should be remembered that every amniocentesis carries the risk of stimulating increasing antibody concentration by releasing further fetal cells into the maternal circulation.

Amniotic fluid bilirubin

Principle and biochemical basis

In a normal pregnancy unconjugated bilirubin is present in the amniotic fluid, the concentration decreasing towards term. This is presumed to be due to some leakage of the normal breakdown products of fetal haemoglobin in their transplacental passage to the maternal liver, which converts fetal bilirubin to the non-toxic water-soluble form. The amniotic fluid is, to a large extent, a fetal product, with the infant swallowing it and excreting into it. In a pregnancy complicated by fetal haemolytic disease, the bilirubin concentration in amniotic fluid rises above the known normal level for gestation. This raised concentration of bilirubin is directly related to the severity of haemolysis. By measuring total bile pigment and the spectroscopic curve with quantitation of $\triangle 450$ nm value it is possible to assess the severity of fetal haemolytic disease.

A more accurate picture of the progress of the disease can be obtained if serial measurements are performed.

Unfortunately, normal ranges and abnormal amniotic △450 nm bilirubin values are not widely available or reliably interpretable before 22–24 weeks' gestation. After 34–35 weeks' gestation the amniotic fluid becomes increasingly cloudy and it is not possible to obtain reliable spectrophotometric measurements of bile pigment.

Amniocenteses for bilirubin content are usually carried out at 2-week intervals between 22 and 34 weeks' gestation. By plotting the △450 nm values on a specially prepared graph, relating Liley's zones of severity to gestation, it is possible to predict the outcome of the pregnancy and to take the appropriate measures when needed, e.g. intra-uterine transfusion or premature delivery of the fetus.

The △450 nm is plotted on a graph against gestational age. The graph is divided into three zones, following Liley's concept.

1. Rh (D) Negative or mildly affected fetus

2. Indeterminate – usually moderately severe disease

3. Severe disease impending fetal death.

Special problems

Contamination of the amniotic fluid with fresh or altered blood diminishes the value of the prognosis. This may be seen directly by the eye but sometimes only from the spectral curve. For this reason the amniotic fluid should be scanned in a spectrophotometer from 320 to 700 nm to detect pigments other than bilirubin, e.g. methaemoglobin or oxyhaemoglobin. Altered blood classically gives a peak at 405 nm and fresh blood (oxyhaemoglobin) at 413 nm. Later in gestation meconium may interfere with spectrophotometric amniotic fluid examination, but after 34 weeks the bile pigment estimations tend to be unreliable anyway because of increasing turbidity in the amniotic fluid. One of the main sources of error in assessing severity of haemolytic disease, in addition to contamination by pigments other than bile products, is incorrect gestational age. It is therefore very important to have the gestational age checked by ultrasound in the early weeks following conception in these high-risk pregnancies.

Fetal cord blood sampling

If other parameters (rapidly rising maternal antibody concentration, or previous intra-uterine fetal death) indicate that severe fetal haemolytic disease before 22 weeks' gestation is to be expected, earlier action may have to be taken. This would involve umbilical cord blood sampling at 18 weeks' gestation, when the blood group, haemoglobin, PCV, DAT, etc can be estimated directly and intravascular transfusion administered if indicated. Normal haematological values have been established for cord blood samples obtained at 18–24 weeks' gestation.

However, until skills of safe fetal cord sampling have spread to many more obstetric centres, estimation of amniotic fluid bilirubin will continue to play an important part in management of haemolytic disease of the fetus.

Ultrasound examination

The introduction of ultrasound techniques has facilitated to an enormous extent the investigation and management of the fetus at risk of serious HDN. The use of X-rays and their potential hazards can now be abandoned.

With real time ultrasound scanning the growth of the fetus can be monitored. In particular the abdominal circumference can be plotted on a normal growth chart to detect the first signs of abnormal abdominal swelling due to underlying hepatosplenomegaly. Early ascites and scalp oedema can also be visualised on the scanning screen. Detailed examination of the heart will detect early signs of stress and incipient failure.

All the foregoing investigations give indirect information of the seriousness of the problem. In some cases with a history of previous intra-uterine death early in gestation, or evidence of rapidly progressive disease, a direct sample of fetal blood can be taken to confirm the blood group, check the haemoglobin, DAT, etc.

TREATMENT OF ESTABLISHED HAEMOLYTIC DISEASE OF THE NEWBORN

The aim is to prevent hydrops in utero and to time delivery so that the infant has a maximal chance of survival. Over the past 10 years there have been dramatic improvements in the care of the preterm infant and so the old adage 'better in than out' is no longer true in many situations. Many babes delivered at 28 weeks' gestation survive, with no long-term handicap, and it is unusual for those of 32 weeks' gestation or more to present any more than routine problems for the average Special Care Baby Unit.

Measures to suppress haemolytic disease in utero

Plasma exchange to reduce maternal antibody titre

Regular plasmapheresis two to three times weekly, from

as early as 10 weeks' gestation, has been reported to reduce the severity of fetal haemolytic disease. Although the anti-D levels may be reduced initially, the levels rise very rapidly when the plasma exchanges are discontinued. There are many practical problems. Results from various centres are conflicting. The reports from groups who believe plasmapheresis to be beneficial are not convincing because the outcomes are not compared with any suitable control group. Indeed overall the survival rate of infants is no better than from those centres who do not use plasmapheresis.

Intra-uterine transfusion

Death of the fetus from severe anaemia may be prevented by the introduction of compatible adult donor cells into the fetal circulation by various methods. The factors which are important in determining the need for and timing of intra-uterine transfusion are:

1. The level and trend of bilirubin content of amniotic fluid
2. The gestation
3. The past obstetric history.

Intra-peritoneal transfusions (IPT)

Since the first description of successful intra-uterine transfusion by Liley in the early 1960s techniques have improved considerably.

It is possible to administer the first intraperitoneal transfusion from as early as 22–23 weeks' gestation, but the outlook for fetuses developing hydropic changes at an early gestational age remains extremely poor, possibly because fetal ascites prevents adequate absorption of transfused red cells through the lymphatics.

Intravascular tranfusion (IVT)

In 1981 Rodeck and colleagues in London described a technique for direct intravascular transfusion which can be performed as early as 18 weeks' gestation, under either direct fetoscopic vision or ultrasound guidance. The umbilical cord is entered and a pure fetal blood sample obtained for haematological and biochemical analysis (see above). Group O Rh (D) negative packed red cells are introduced into the lumen of the vessel at a rate of 1–3 ml per minute. The quantity of blood transfused is determined by the estimated fetal blood volume, the pretransfusion fetal haematocrit and the concentration of donor cells.

The transfusions are started as early as 18 weeks' gestation, if indicated, and repeated at 1–3-week intervals

until 32 weeks. Delivery is planned in collaboration with expert neonatal and haematological advice.

A survival rate of 84%, in a series of 50 fetuses referred before 25 weeks' gestation, has been reported from a centre using these measures.

Combination of IPT and IVT

It is now the practice at Queen Charlotte's Maternity Hospital to combine the two techniques of intra-uterine transfusions from 22 weeks' gestation onwards. The advantage is that the interval between transfusions can be prolonged. Immediate correction of anaemia is achieved by the intravascular transfusions and the haemoglobin level can be maintained by the slower absorption of intraperitoneally introduced packed red cells.

MANAGEMENT OF THE BABY AFTER BIRTH

Cord blood should be taken at delivery for:

1. ABO Rh (D) grouping
2. Direct antiglobulin test (Coomb's test)
3. Serum bilirubin
4. Haemoglobin.

Babies born after a series of intra-uterine transfusions often have a normal haemoglobin at delivery, negative direct antiglobulin test and group as Rh (D) negative because of successful replacement of fetal red cells by transfused donor blood combined with suppression of fetal marrow. They often only require phototherapy to control jaundice of prematurity and maybe a top-up transfusion to correct anaemia several weeks after delivery. The main problems are not haematological but those arising from immaturity.

On the other hand, those infants who have not received intra-uterine treatment may be born severely anaemic – even hydropic – and will rapidly accumulate dangerous concentrations of bilirubin if prompt measures are not taken to prevent this. The main risk to the neonate is that of kernicterus, arising from hyperbilirubinaemia. The liver of the neonate does not produce glucuronyl transferase and cannot convert bilirubin to an excretable form. Consequently bilirubin accumulates and if not removed (by exchange transfusion) will collect in the tissues, causing jaundice and brain tissue damage. Deeply jaundiced infants often exhibit signs of damage to the central nervous system. These signs develop usually after the age of 36 hours. At any time after this the infant which has previously behaved normally becomes increasingly lethargic and reluctant to feed and may exhibit opisthotonos and develop a high pitched cry. At this stage in 70% of cases, respiration becomes irregular, the infant grows cold and dies. Those who recover have permanent brain damage characterised by variable deafness, visual impairment, spasticity and mental retardation.

Management and prevention of hyperbilirubinaemia

Exchange transfusion

In addition to controlling existing hyperbilirubinaemia exchange transfusion corrects anaemia and blood volume abnormalities. The first exchange transfusion also washes out about one-third of the anti-D antibody in the neonatal circulation. A two-volume exchange (1700 ml per Kg) will remove 85–90% of the infant's circulating Rh (D) positive cells which would otherwise contribute to the bilirubin pool. However, a two-volume exchange transfusion removes only 25% of the infant's total bilirubin due in the main to the fact that a large part of the total bilirubin is in the extravascular compartment. Maximum reduction of the bilirubin is achieved by a two-volume exchange for a single procedure. There is no point in increasing the volume but after the exchange transfusion serum levels rapidly rebound to 70–80% of the pre-exchange values.

Criteria for exchange transfusion

Clinical evidence at delivery of severe disease such as pallor, petechiae and hypersplenomegaly are indications for immediate exchange transfusion without waiting for cord blood results. If the cord haemoglobin is less than 8.0 g/dl or the bilirubin more than 100 μmol/l the exchange transfusion should be instituted within 1 hour of birth.

The baby who does not require immediate exchange should be monitored haematologically at regular 3–4 hour intervals with particular reference to the bilirubin. A rapidly rising bilirubin is an indication for exchange. There are charts available at all SCBU to indicate the levels of bilirubin at which exchange should be undertaken related to the birth weight and gestation, so that kernicterus will be prevented.

Other measures to reduce hyperbilirubinaemia

Phototherapy

Phototherapy is effective in reducing the serum unconjugated bilirubin concentration in newborn infants. When exposed to blue light bilirubin is readily converted into less lipophilic, smaller water-soluble compounds. Used alone in the mildly affected baby or

following exchange transfusion in the more severely affected, it will reduce peak bilirubin levels and the need for further exchange transfusion. This is a major advance in the treatment of all types of indirect hyperbilirubinaemia in the infant.

Despite initial concerns to the contrary the procedure seems to carry no major side effects. Because there is a risk of retinal damage all babes should have their eyes protected. Phototherapy increases evaporative water loss therefore extra fluid should be administered. Loose green stools are an indication of the excretion of the photobilirubin isomer. These should cause no concern unless there is bowel stasis. Under these circumstances the unstable isomer is converted back to the stable toxic unconjugated isomer and is reabsorbed.

Albumin administration

The binding of bilirubin to albumin is of importance in the prevention of bilirubin encephalopathy. There are no controlled trials which show that the administration of albumin reduces the number of exchange transfusions required, or the incidence of kernicterus, but administration of albumin before or during exchange transfusion significantly increases the amount of bilirubin removed and increases the albumin-binding capacity of the infant's plasma after the exchange transfusion.

Albumin should not be added to blood used to exchange a severely anaemic or hydropic baby, because the resulting increase in plasma colloid pressure may precipitate or augment heart failure.

Other causes of feto-maternal allo-immunisation

In theory, any fetal red-cell antigen may cause allo-immunisation if the mother lacks that antigen. Thus any red-cell antigen which the father possesses and the mother lacks, if inherited by the fetus, can cause maternal allo-immunisation. Ideally, all pregnant women should have their blood tested in the 12th, 28th and 34th weeks of pregnancy for antibodies to red-cell antigens. These examinations not only alert the obstetrician to possible cases of haemolytic disease of the newborn (HDN), but also identify the mother for whom there may be difficulty in providing compatible blood quickly in an obstetric emergency.

Rhesus blood group c and E

Within the Rhesus blood group system the most immunogenic antigens after D are c and E. These antibodies are found most usually in women who are

Rh (D) positive and lack the c and E antigens, e.g. those women who have the genotype CDe/CDe (R₁R₁). The management of HDN due to allo-immunisation by antigens other than anti-D is the same as that for RhD HDN and there is no way as yet of preventing these conditions. Some cases of HDN due to anti-c are as severe as anti-D HDN and may end in hydrops if intra-uterine transfusions are not given. Anti-E antibodies, in my experience, never cause severe HDN, but may cause considerable difficulty in cross-matching if not identified.

Theoretically, prevention of allo-immunisation to other red-cell antigens by transfusion or pregnancy could be prevented in a similar manner to that with anti-D. In practice it would be very time-consuming and costly to Rh phenotype all women in pregnancy and to produce sufficient quantities of anti-c and anti-E from male 'volunteers' by injections of incompatible blood to produce the appropriate immunoglobulin.

Kell blood group

The Kell red-cell blood group is a good example of a system which occasionally causes problems. 95% of the British population are Kell negative (kk); the remaining 5% are Kell positive and the majority are heterozygous Kk. Only 1 in 500 individuals is found to be homozygous KK positive. The antibody anti-K is usually found in patients who have had multiple transfusions, either as a large number of donations to cover a single traumatic incident or as recurrent supportive therapy over a long period. When anti-K is found in antenatal sera, the majority of patients have a history of transfusion but the husband's blood should be tested to determine his Kell status; usually he is Kell negative which indicates transfusion allo-immunisation, providing that extramarital pregnancy can be excluded. Occasionally, the husband is Kell positive but statistically he is likely to be heterozygous Kk. If he is one of the rare 1 in 500 KK homozygous Kell positive, then all the children he fathers will be Kell positive and at risk of HDN from maternal anti-K. There is no difficulty in finding blood for intra-uterine or exchange transfusion as 90% of the population are kk Kell negative.

Kell haemolytic disease can be very severe and rapidly fatal in utero at relatively early gestation.

It would appear that amniotic fluid bilirubin levels are unhelpful in assessing severity of disease and the disease process is one of erythroid hypoplasia rather than haemolytic anaemia.

Fetal cord blood sampling is recommended in all cases thought to be at risk so that Kell grouping can be established and haematocrit can be directly measured at a time when appropriate management can be planned.

ABO blood group

Even before the striking reduction in RhD HDN due to prophylaxis the most frequent cause of HDN was the haemolysis due to ABO incompatibility. Although the incidence in Great Britain and the USA has been found to be approximately 2% of all births, in only 1 in 3000 births does severe ABO HDN occur. Mild cases not requiring exchange transfusion are identified in 1 in 150 births. Less than 5% of affected newborns require phototherapy, and in only the very rare case is exchange transfusion required. There is a 1 in 3 chance in marriage that the husband's red cells will be ABO incompatible with the wife's serum. However, the husband may be heterozygous in respect of the allele for the incompatible antigen, for example AO rather than AA (homozygous), so that the chance of ABO incompatibility between fetal red cells and maternal serum is 1 in 5.

It is therefore surprising that ABO HDN is relatively uncommon. There are several factors which explain this. A and B-like substances are widespread in vegetable and animal life. The agglutinins, anti-A and B, are often called natural antibodies, which is strictly a misnomer because they develop during the first few months of life, probably as a result of exposure to A- and B-like substances elaborated by gram-negative bacteria which colonise the gut. Naturally occurring anti-A and anti-B are usually IgM immunoglobulins which will not cross the placenta. The maternal antibody can only cause HDN if it is of the IgG type.

Group O women who have had ABO-incompatible pregnancies may have anti-A or B which is IgG (immune antibody). Also group O individuals who have been vaccinated or immunised with preparations derived from hog stomach or pneumococcal vaccine which contain an A substance may develop immune lytic IgG anti-A antibody which can persist for some years (hog pepsin is used in the preparation of TAB and diphtheria toxoid). But even if the group O mother has a high titre of lytic IgG anti-A or anti-B antibody, it is unlikely to cause problems for the ABO-incompatible fetus in utero because the A and B antigens, unlike Rh antigens, are present not only on the fetal red cells but on cells of all other tissue and body fluids. Neutralisation of maternal antibody by soluble fetal antigens and by antigens carried on cells other than the red cells will help to protect the incompatible fetal red cells.

Another factor which may help to protect the fetal red cells is that the A and B antigens, although detectable in the 5 week embryo, do not have the antigenic strength of adult red cells in the neonate and therefore will not react fully with antibody which crosses the placenta.

The vast majority of cases of HDN due to ABO incompatibility occur in group O mothers with A or B infants, because group O individuals make more avid antibody and are more likely to produce immune antibody; unlike Rh disease, 40–50% of cases occur in firstborn infants and the disease does not become more severe with each subsequent pregnancy.

Antenatal screening

Serological evaluation of the mother should be carried out at approximately 16 weeks. All Rh negative women should be screened again at 28 and 34 weeks. Ideally, all women should be screened again at these times in order to identify those who have IgG antibodies which might lead to other forms of HDN, e.g. Kell, c and E. Although determinations of lytic IgG and anti-A and anti-B titres do not give a good indication of the severity of the likely outcome of ABO maternal/fetal incompatibility, routine serological evaluation will detect some cases of lytic anti-A and anti-B in maternal serum and if potent antibodies are found this will alert the obstetrician to examine cord blood to enable HDN to be diagnosed as soon as possible after birth.

The serological investigations which should be carried out are routine grouping and an indirect Coomb's test to detect IgG antibodies in maternal serum. When these are found, they should be characterised in terms of specificity and titre by standard serological techniques.

Neonatal screening

It is very important to anticipate, identify and treat HDN, because if haemolysis and subsequent jaundice are managed effectively the prognosis is excellent. The direct antiglobulin test (Coomb's test) should be carried out routinely on all cord bloods of babies born to mothers who have an IgG blood-group antibody identified in antenatal screening. The specificity of the antibody will usually have been identified in the maternal blood by testing the serum with a mixed panel of red cells which bear a variety of antigens. Affected infants should have cord blood haemoglobin and bilirubin levels estimated and exchange transfusion should be initiated where appropriate.

Apart from the occasional case with a history of other previously affected infants and/or lytic IgG in the maternal serum, screening of cord blood for ABO incompatibility is not usually performed. The diagnosis of ABO HDN is usually made in the work-up of a ma-

ture infant who develops jaundice in the first 24 hours of life. In fact, the diagnosis may be quite difficult to make because the DAT test is not usually positive and there may be a very mild degree of anaemia, although such infants can develop a marked reticulocyte response and occasionally go on to develop jaundice of a severity which may lead to kernicterus. The confirmation of the diagnosis is made by finding IgG lytic antibody of the appropriate blood-group specificity in the maternal serum. The blood film characteristically has large numbers of spherocytes.

If exchange transfusion is undertaken in ABO HDN, then fresh group O donor blood of the same Rh type as the infant should be used: the plasma containing anti-A and anti-B may be removed and replaced with fresh platelet-rich group AB plasma. Alternatively group O cells of the appropriate Rh type recovered from a bank of frozen cells may be used, the cells being suspended in plasma protein fraction (PPF) or albumin to which bilirubin will bind.

Because HDN may occasionally arise unexpectedly, either because IgG antibodies were not detected in the maternal serum even late in pregnancy, or because screening was not carried out at all, and due to the difficulties in the diagnosis of some cases of HDN due to ABO sensitisation, it might seem that the ideal approach to screening for HDN would be to carry out an Hb, DAT, and estimation of serum bilirubin on all newborn infants. However, this is impractical and it would certainly not be cost-effective. Hence, neonatal screening is reserved for those infants who are born of mothers known to have IgG antibodies, those with a previous history of HDN for any reason, and as part of the work-up for those who become jaundiced in the neonatal period.

POLYCYTHAEMIA IN THE NEWBORN INFANT

Polycythaemia in the neonatal period has been recognised as a relatively common occurrence over the last 10 to 15 years. Laboratory testing of the blood as a screening procedure at birth or in the first day of life reveals many cases, only a fraction of which develop overt clinical signs attributed to hyperviscosity.

Controversies centre around the need, or not, for screening all neonates within hours of birth for indications of this potential problem and whether or not prophylaxis of those symptomless babes considered to be at risk has any effect on the incidence of late manifestation such as cerebral defects affecting motor co-ordination and perhaps intellectual performance.

There is confusion among clinicians about which infants are likely to suffer effects in the neonatal period and which infants, symptomatic or not, will have sequelae.

Definition

Polycythaemia and hyperviscosity are not synonymous terms (see Ch. 2). Three factors – the deformability of the red cells, the plasma viscosity and the haematocrit – determine the viscosity of the blood. Of these factors the most important dependent variable affecting whole blood viscosity in the neonate is the haematocrit. There is an almost linear relationship between viscosity and haematocrit below a haematrocrit of 60–65%, but the relationship becomes exponential at higher haematocrits. The blood of all infants with a central venous haematocrit of 65% or more will, on in-vitro testing, prove to be hyperviscous; in contrast hyperviscosity is never demonstrated in vitro using blood of neonates with haematocrits below 60%. Blood with haematocrit values between 60 and 64% proved to be hyperviscous on in-vitro examination in up to 23% of cases in one series, presumably because of the other variables which affect hyperviscosity. The red blood cells of the healthy neonate are less filterable than those of normal adults. At low pH or in conditions of reduced oxygen tension the newborn red cells become even less filterable. Some babies have been shown to have hyperviscous blood on the basis of marked reduction in red cell filterability. In contrast, plasma viscosity in normal newborns and adults has been found to be virtually identical. Increases in osmolality and lipid concentrations will result in increased whole blood viscosity.

Incidence

The reported incidence of neonatal 'thick blood syndrome' varies considerably depending on the criteria used for diagnosing the condition. A venous haematocrit of 65% or more is the generally accepted screening test today, but the peripheral venous haematocrit is significantly higher than the umbilical venous haematocrit; the viscosity of umbilical venous blood is considerably elevated only when the haematocrit is over 65%, and therefore if a *peripheral* venous haematocrit of over 65% is used as a diagnostic screening test of hyperviscosity, the condition will be overdiagnosed. This may account for the fact that the majority of infants reported to have high venous haematocrits remain asymptomatic. The overall incidence of hyperviscosity is not well established and reported incidences vary from 4.0% down to 2.34%. More recently a study of healthy, appropriate-for-gestational-age newborns, found only 0.45% to have venous haematocrits above 65%. These reported differing incidences probably depend on sampling sites, patient population and cord clamping practices.

Aetiology

The aetiology of hyperviscosity syndrome in the neonatal period is multifactorial but the causes can be divided into two main groups – active and passive (Table 28.5).

Table 28.5 Neonatal polycythaemia

Active (Increased intra-uterine erythropoiesis)	Passive (Erythrocyte transfusion)
Placental insufficiency	Maternal – fetal
Maternal diabetes	Twin-to-twin
Neonatal thyrotoxicosis	Delayed cord clamping
Congenital adrenal hyperplasia	Unattended delivery
Chromosome abnormalities	

The active form occurs in those circumstances where the fetus, in response to intra-uterine hypoxia and other stimuli, produces an increased number of red cells. The passive forms of neonatal polycythaemia refer to those circumstances in which the fetus receives a red cell transfusion. This may be either maternal in origin, twin-to-twin or result from delayed clamping of the cord.

Impaired placental function with resultant intra-uterine hypoxia appears to be a major factor in many of the conditions associated with active neonatal polycythaemia, which include small-for-gestational-age and post-mature infants, pre-eclampsia, severe maternal heart disease and maternal smoking. Maternal drugs such as propranolol have been incriminated, but polycythaemia in the infant is probably due to the condition for which the mother is being treated. Hyperinsulinaemia in the fetus is associated with increased levels of erythropoietin. Polycythaemia occurs frequently in the infants of mothers with both overt and gestational diabetes. Down's syndrome, trisomy 13 and trisomy 18 have all been associated with neonatal polycythaemia, thought to be due to increased fetal erythropoietin activity. In Down's syndrome marked elevation of erythropoietin concentration has been reported.

In normal term infants the most frequent cause of polycythaemia is delayed clamping of the cord. Morbidity and mortality in the polycythaemic recipient twin in fetus-fetus transfusion is at least as high as in the anaemic donor twin. Infants with polycythaemia range in gestational age from 33 to 43 weeks. The condition is characteristically associated with the more mature infant, since the haematocrit rises with gestation. There is a higher incidence among the term small-for-gestational-age infants and in post-mature infants compared with appropriate-for-gestational-age term infants.

Clinical findings

The standard evaluation of newborn infants in most centres would not detect the majority of those who have polycythaemia and they may therefore be at risk for hyperviscosity syndrome. When quiet these infants may not appear plethoric and it is only when roused and active that they become very flushed or cyanosed. The signs usually become evident within the first 24 hours as the haematocrit rises due to a physiological decrease in plasma volume. The most consistent findings in newborns with established hyperviscosity are lethargy and hypotonia within 6 hours of birth, poor suck and vomiting, difficulty in arousal, irritability when aroused, poor response to light, tremulousness and ease of being startled. Some of these central nervous system signs and symptoms may be a result of the metabolic abnormalities – hypoglycaemia and hypocalcaemia – commonly associated with polycythaemia rather than the direct result of hyperviscosity itself. Observed complications include hyperbilirubinaemia with kernicterus and heart failure, as well as the other problems due to vascular occlusion (Fig. 28.3). Respiratory distress and cyanosis together with congestive cardiac failure may be severe enough to simulate cyanotic congenital heart disease.

Hyperbilirubinaemia is attributed to an increased red cell mass leading to increased bilirubin production. Thrombocytopenia is often observed but it is not associated with laboratory evidence of DIC and is thought to be due to local aggregation of platelets in the sluggish peripheral circulation. In the full-blown hyperviscosity syndrome sludging and formation of thrombi in the peripheral circulation lead to characteristic clinical manifestations due to tissue anoxia, depending where the circulation is compromised. Seizures may occur, and priapism and testicular infarction, renal vein thrombosis, renal failure, gangrene, distal bowel obstruction and necrotising enterocolitis have all been described.

Late neurological sequelae described have included running and laughing fits, fine motor and speech abnormalities, spastic diplegia and significant neurodevelopmental abnormalities.

However, most publications agree that in untreated neonatal polycythaemia with minor or no symptoms, significant late neurological manifestations are very rare.

Management

It is clear from the available literature that all

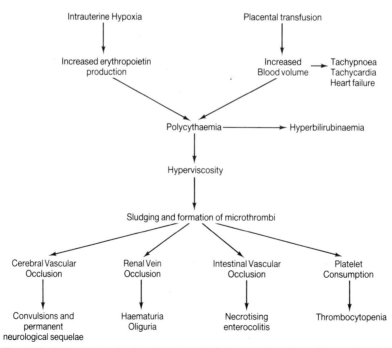

Fig. 28.3 Pathogenesis of polycythaemia and clinical manifestations of hyperviscosity in the newborn infant.

symptomatic infants with hyperviscosity require treatment in order to relieve the immediate clinical symptoms and to avoid late neurological sequelae. Dramatic improvement has been observed in patients with respiratory disturbance, cardiac failure, gastrointestinal and CNS signs and symptoms. The aim is to lower the haematocrit and thereby the viscosity. Partial exchange transfusion is performed removing whole blood and replacing it with equal volumes of fresh frozen plasma to achieve a haematocrit of 55%, which is considered to be a 'safe' level.

The formula used to calculate the volume to be exchanged (ml) is

$$\text{Total blood volume} \atop \text{(ml)} \times \frac{\text{(Observed Hct − desired Hct)}}{\text{Observed Hct}}$$

The problem of management arises in those neonates who have been identified as having significant polycythaemia with or without hyperviscosity, who are symptom-free. These infants may be at risk particularly of late neurological sequelae. Do these patients receive 'prophylactic' exchange transfusion? Some paediatricians are in favour of universal screening and prompt treatment of any neonate with polycythaemia. Others have been unable to demonstrate any significant benefit in babies with hyperviscosity but with no symptoms who have undergone partial exchange transfusion, compared with a control untreated group. An increased incidence of necrotising enterocolitis following exchange transfusion has been reported by several groups but never confirmed. It is felt by some that this fact should be taken into consideration before plasma exchange becomes an accepted treatment for all patients with hyperviscosity.

Until further experience is available the benefits of prophylactic exchange transfusion must remain speculative. The additional information available to date serves to make the problem more, not less, complex and speculation continues.

Screening

There is no doubt that all neonates at special risk of developing hyperviscosity should be screened within the first hours of life. Because of the changing haematocrit in the first few hours it has been suggested that blood sampling should be delayed until 8 hours post-delivery. Symptoms are not usually present at birth, but develop during the first 24 hours when the concentration of red cells rises secondary to absorption of excess plasma. It is very unusual for symptoms to develop after the first 48 hours of life. The infants to be screened include small- and large-for-gestational-age infants, infants of

diabetic mothers, of mothers with pre-eclampsia and other placental insufficiency syndromes, and twins. The haematocrit is the preferred screening method for hyperviscosity. A capillary haematocrit of more than 65–70% is taken to indicate the need for venous haematocrit. All those infants with a venous haematocrit of more than 65% will have hyperviscous blood, as well as a small proportion of those with venous haematocrits between 60 and 65%. In laboratories with the facility, viscosity of the blood should be measured in these infants. The infants should be carefully examined for symptoms and signs of hyperviscosity. In addition the blood sugar, calcium and bilirubin should be estimated. In this respect infants of 3–4 days gestation may develop hyperbilirubinaemia because of transient polycythaemia, but will not be polycythaemic any longer at the time of identification.

Ideally all infants should be screened for polycythaemia in the first few hours of life, but it is not the practice in most units to perform a capillary or venous haematocrit on all healthy, appropriate-for-gestational-age term infants. Where this has been performed, a variable incidence of polycythaemia in these otherwise healthy infants of between 0.45 and 4.00% has been reported.

Suggested practical approach

Healthy term infants appear to be at little risk of polycythaemia and hyperviscosity and need not be routinely screened. In units where only the babes known to be at risk of significant polycythaemia are screened the paediatrician must remain constantly alert to early clinical signs of the condition. In those identified polycythaemic babes with mild or no symptoms of hyperviscosity, keeping the babe warm and well hydrated is probably all that is required to prevent sludging in the peripheral circulation. All infants with significant symptoms should undergo partial exchange with fresh frozen plasma in order to bring the haematocrit down to a safe level of 55%.

BIBLIOGRAPHY

Chauhan P M, Kondlapoodi P, Natta C L 1983 Pathology of sickle cell disorders. Pathology Annual 18: 253–276

Freedman M H 1984 Congenital failure of haematopoiesis in the newborn infant. Clinics in Perinatology 11: 417–431

Glader B E 1987 Diagnosis and management of red cell aplasia in children. Haematology and Oncology Clinics of North America 1: 431–447

Pearson H A 1987 Sickle cell diseases: diagnosis and management in infancy and childhood. Pediatric Review 9: 121–130

29. Haematological changes in systemic disease

R. J.G. Cuthbert   C. A. Ludlam

The haemostatic and haemopoietic systems play an essential role in the maintenance of the body's physical integrity. This requires the ability to respond to a wide variety of external influences, and the precise regulation of production of mature blood cells and clotting factors in health is quite remarkable. It is not surprising that, since these systems are so intimately involved in normal homeostasis, haematological changes accompany other physical disturbances caused by many systemic diseases. This chapter discusses haematological changes occurring in systemic disorders, with particular emphasis on changes which may present to the haematologist.

ANAEMIA OF CHRONIC DISORDERS

The anaemia of chronic disorders (ACD) is associated with chronic infections, chronic inflammatory diseases and malignancy. There are characteristic haematological and ferrokinetic changes common to the anaemia of all these conditions, suggesting that the underlying pathogenetic mechanisms may be the same or similar in each. However, anaemia associated with renal, liver and endocrine disorders does not have the characteristic changes in iron metabolism seen in ACD and discussion of these conditions is dealt with separately.

Haematological changes (Table 29.1)

Mild-moderate normochromic normocytic anaemia becomes apparent over the first few weeks of the illness. The haemoglobin rarely falls below 8–9 g/dl in uncomplicated cases. Occasionally hypochromic red cells are seen on the blood film, but microcytic cells are rarely seen. The degree of fall in the haemoglobin reflects the degree of activity of the underlying condition and it returns to normal on resolution of the primary condition. There are no characteristic changes in leukocytes or platelets, although these may also be affected independently by the primary condition. Plasma iron is reduced and this is accompanied by reduction in the

Table 29.1 Characteristic laboratory findings in anaemia of chronic disorders

Normochromic (or hypochromic) normocytic anaemia
Decreased plasma iron
Decreased total iron-binding capacity (TIBC)
Decreased percentage saturation of TIBC
Increased plasma ferritin
Increased bone marrow iron – increased macrophage iron
      reduced proportion of
      sideroblasts
Decreased iron absorption from the gut
Increased free erythrocyte protoporphyrin
Increased plasma copper
Increased plasma caeruloplasmin

total iron-binding capacity (TIBC) and in percentage saturation of TIBC. Plasma ferritin is elevated. Bone marrow iron stores are elevated with increased iron in macrophages, but reduced proportions of sideroblasts. Morphologically erythropoiesis is normoblastic.

Pathogenesis

The pathogenesis of ACD is very complex. Several experimental observations have been made and these are described as follows:

Iron metabolism and ferrokinetic studies

Plasma iron turnover is increased with greater utilisation of transferrin iron. Consequently transferrin saturation is reduced and the supply of iron from plasma to bone marrow for haemoglobin synthesis is impaired. Thus the proportion of sideroblasts is reduced, free erythrocyte protoporphyrin is increased, and a population of poorly haemoglobinised hypochromic red cells is produced. The main reason for reduction in plasma iron may be impairment of iron flow from the tissues to plasma transferrin, possibly as a result of defective release of iron from macrophages. This is further reflected in reduced intestinal absorption of iron due to defective transfer from intestinal mucosal cells to transferrin.

The molecular basis for these changes in iron handling in ACD has not been fully worked out but two main schools of thought exist:

Lactoferrin. Lactoferrin is an iron-binding protein present in neutrophil granules, amongst other tissues. It is present at high concentration at inflammatory sites containing large numbers of neutrophils. Lactoferrin competes with transferrin for free iron, and because of its higher iron affinity removes iron directly from transferrin. Lactoferrin-bound iron is then transferred to macrophages, leading to reduction in the iron pool available for haemoglobin synthesis. Interleukin-1 stimulates release of lactoferrin from the specific granules of neutrophils. Thus as a consequence of the inflammatory response lactoferrin-mediated sequestration of iron may occur.

Ferritin. Another component of the inflammatory response is increased synthesis of apoferritin. This results in increased iron uptake, reflected in elevation of plasma ferritin. Consequently less plasma iron is made available for transferrin saturation and subsequent transfer to developing red cells. The main physiological control of apoferritin synthesis is the plasma concentration of ionic iron. But this is overridden during the inflammatory response. This is probably also mediated by interleukin-1.

Red cell survival

The red cell lifespan (assessed by ^{51}Cr-labelled red cell studies) in ACD is moderately reduced to about 80 days. Cross-transfusion studies have shown that normal red cells transfused into a patient with ACD have a reduced lifespan, whereas patient red cells transfused into a healthy volunteer survive normally. This suggests that a factor or factors extrinsic to the red cell are responsible for reduced red cell survival in ACD. This may be due to general increased activity within the macrophage-monocyte phagocytic system (reticulo-endothelial system), which can be observed in many inflammatory, infectious and neoplastic conditions. Macrophages normally clear effete red cells, which are recognised by an unknown mechanism. This system of red cell clearance is probably exaggerated in ACD so that the augmented macrophage activity leads to clearance of minimally affected red cells. The role of interleukin-1 in stimulating augmented macrophage activity may be important.

Erythropoiesis

The modest reduction in red cell lifespan observed in patients with ACD could easily be compensated for by increased erythropoiesis in normal marrow. Thus some impairment of erythropoiesis must be involved in the pathogenesis of ACD. One factor limiting erythropoiesis has already been discussed, i.e. limitation of iron for haemoglobin synthesis. However, the rate of iron turnover in ACD is normal and the degree of ineffective iron turnover is much lower than expected for the degree of anaemia, suggesting that other factors are involved. Most studies in which erythropoietin has been measured have shown that plasma erythropoietin levels are reduced in ACD. However, interestingly, erythropoietin levels rise in response to hypoxic stimuli in patients with ACD. It has been suggested that the set level of erythropoietin secretion is down regulated in ACD and that this may be mediated by interleukin-1.

Clinical significance

The main importance of ACD is its recognition. In addition it is important to recognise that other factors may account for anaemia in patients with infections, inflammatory or neoplastic conditions. ACD rarely requires treatment in itself since the anaemia is usually asymptomatic and the clinical features are dominated by the primary condition. No specific treatment is available, although recombinant erythropoietin is being evaluated. Thus at present for those few patients with symptomatic anaemia red cell concentrate transfusion is the only possible treatment.

MALIGNANCY

Haematological changes commonly occur in malignant diseases and in fact nearly all malignancies will produce changes in the blood at some stage of the illness (Table 29.2). It is not uncommon for the haematological complications to be the presenting feature of malignancy, and they may be present for a considerable time before the malignant condition becomes clinically apparent. In addition the haematological changes of malignant disorders may mimic almost any primary haematological disorder.

Anaemia

Anaemia is present in at least 50% of patients with solid tumours at presentation. A variety of types of anaemia may be seen:

Anaemia of chronic disorders. This is the most common form of anaemia in patients with malignant disease. It may occur in both localised and disseminated tumours. The degree of anaemia correlates roughly with the total extent of the tumour.

Table 29.2 Haematological changes in malignant diseases

Red cells	Anaemia of chronic disorders
	Iron deficiency anaemia
	Megaloblastic anaemia
	Leuko-erythroblastic anaemia
	Micro-angiopathic haemolytic anaemia
	Autoimmune haemolytic anaemia
	Sideroblastic anaemia
	Secondary myelofibrosis
	Polycythaemia
Leukocytes	Neutrophilia
	Leukaemoid reaction
	Eosinophilia
	Monocytosis
	Lymphopenia
Platelets	Thrombocytosis
	Thrombocytopenia
Coagulation	Disseminated intravascular coagulation
	Primary fibrinolysis
	Deficiency of liver-derived coagulation factors
	Thrombosis
	Thrombophlebitis migrans

Leuko-erythroblastic anaemia. This is associated with metastatic disease of the bone marrow. It may occur in any solid tumour but is most characteristic of carcinomas of breast, prostate or stomach, and oat cell carcinoma of the lung. Occasionally the malignancy is occult at presentation, leading to difficulty in distinguishing it from a myeloproliferative disorder. Bone marrow trephine biopsy often leads to the correct diagnosis.

Iron-deficiency anaemia. Chronic blood loss, often combined with poor nutrition, leads to iron-deficiency anaemia in a large proportion of patients with malignant diseases. Carcinomas within the gastrointestinal tract are the most common cause, but chronic haematuria due to renal tract malignancies or bleeding due to thrombocytopenia may also be responsible.

Megaloblastic anaemia. Folate deficiency due to poor nutrition, impaired absorption or increased utilisation by a rapidly dividing tumour may occur. Gastric carcinoma secondary to achlorhydria may be associated with vitamin B_{12} deficiency.

Micro-angiopathic anaemia. Intravascular haemolysis with red cell fragmentation commonly occurs in association with disseminated intravascular coagulation (DIC) in patients with a variety of malignant diseases. Mucin-secreting tumours, such as carcinoma of the stomach, ovary, gall bladder or bronchus, commonly produce this picture. The haemolytic-uraemic syndrome is a rare complication of disseminated malignancies.

Autoimmune haemolytic anaemia. Although this is a well-recognised complication of lymphoproliferative dis-

orders, it may occasionally be associated with solid tumours. Ovarian carcinoma is the most common cause but it has also been described in gastrointestinal, renal, lung and breast carcinomas. Warm or cold antibodies may occur but the specificity is rarely characterised. Eradication of the tumour leads to remission of the haemolytic process.

Polycythaemia

Although anaemia is a more common complication of malignant diseases, erythrocytosis may occasionally occur. However, malignancy is a very rare cause of polycythaemia. This has been described in Chapter 26.

Leukocyte changes

Neutrophil leukocytosis is the commonest white cell change in malignant diseases. Occasionally this may be grossly exaggerated with outpouring of granulocyte precursors into the peripheral blood; this is known as a leukaemoid reaction. Distinguishing a leukaemoid reaction from chronic granulocytic leukaemia is possible by demonstration of elevated neutrophil alkaline phosphatase activity and absence of the Philadelphia chromosome. Tumour products may directly or indirectly (via interleukin-1) stimulate granulopoiesis and outpouring of neutrophils from the bone marrow pool. Eosinophilia is a characteristic finding in Hodgkin's disease, and less commonly is recognised in patients with solid tumours such as ovarian carcinoma or various disseminated malignancies. Monocytosis may occur in patients with solid tumours. Lymphocytosis rarely occurs in malignant diseases apart from lymphoproliferative disorders.

Platelet changes

Thrombocytosis. Elevated platelet counts occur in up to 66% of patients with malignant disease. Platelet production is increased about twofold. This may be due to a generally reactive marrow state, or it may occur secondary to chronic blood loss leading to iron deficiency. Thrombocytosis may be identified before a malignancy becomes clinically obvious (Ch. 30).

Thrombocytopenia. This is usually a manifestation of disseminated intravascular coagulation in malignancy or a consequence of bone marrow metastatic invasion or secondary myelofibrosis.

Haemostatic disturbances

Bleeding. Disseminated intravascular coagulation is the common reason for haemostatic failure in patients with malignant diseases. Prostatic carcinoma is the most common malignancy associated with DIC. In particular, surgical intervention causing release of thromboplastins from the tumour may provoke abnormal bleeding. Other malignancies including stomach, colon, lung, ovary, breast and gallbladder carcinomas may cause DIC.

Chronic DIC. This represents the compensated state, and clinical bleeding usually does not occur. Fibrinogen/fibrin degradation products are elevated, the platelet count is usually moderately depressed, and fibrinogen is normal or only modestly reduced. The prothrombin time and partial thromboplastin time are similarly normal or only moderately prolonged. Clinical bleeding may occur if this fine balance is disturbed, e.g. surgery, infection, mucosal ulceration, trauma, etc. Treatment of the primary condition leads to resolution of the haemostatic defects.

Acute DIC. Catastrophic bleeding with hypo-fibrinogenaemia and thrombocytopenia is most characteristic of acute promyelocytic leukaemia. Less commonly solid tumours may provoke these changes. This is usually due to further provocation factors such as sepsis or major tumour lysis.

Other factors

Extensive liver disease due to metastatic infiltration may lead to impaired synthesis of coagulation factors. Vitamin K deficiency may result from broad spectrum antibiotic therapy causing depopulation of vitamin K-producing bacteria in the bowel. Rarely tumours secrete abnormal proteins with anticoagulant properties. Primary fibrinolysis may be provoked by chemotherapeutic agents such as doxorubicin, daunorubicin, etc. Large or rapidly progressive tumours may erode blood vessels causing catastrophic, often terminal, bleeding. Highly vascular tumours may themselves bleed.

Thrombosis and hypercoagulability

The incidence of venous thrombo-embolism is increased in patients with malignant disease. Up to 40% of such patients experience post-operative deep venous thrombosis (compared with up to 25% of patients with non-malignant conditions). Malignancy may be discovered in patients who survive pulmonary embolism; this may not become apparent until several months after the thrombotic episode.

The pathogenesis of thrombosis in malignancy is complex. Activation of coagulation with low grade DIC and secondary fibrinolysis probably occurs most frequently. Increased platelet aggregability may also contribute. The tumour itself probably triggers the clotting process by production of procoagulant products, e.g. mucin contains sialic acid residues which may trigger the intrinsic activation pathway, trypsin from pancreatic tumours may enzymatically activate clotting factors, thromboplastins released from prostatic tumours may activate the extrinsic pathway.

Treatment of thrombosis and hypercoagulability is difficult. Removal of the tumour will result in resolution. Anticoagulation with warfarin and/or heparin requires caution as the incidence of bleeding complications is higher than for non-malignant conditions. Antiplatelet therapy with aspirin and/or dipyridamole has been advocated by some, but again there is a significant risk of complications, particularly gastrointestinal bleeding.

RHEUMATOID DISEASE:

Haematological changes are common in rheumatoid disease, either as a direct complication of the disease itself or as a complication of treatment (Table 29.3).

Table 29.3 Haematological complications of rheumatoid disease

Anaemia	Anaemia of chronic disorders
	Iron deficiency anaemia
	Folate deficiency
	Autoimmune haemolytic anaemia
Leukocytes	Neutrophilia
	Neutropenia – especially in Felty's syndrome
	Impaired neutrophil function
Platelets	Thrombocytosis
	Immune thrombocytopenia
	Impaired platelet function
All cell lines	Felty's syndrome
	Drug-induced pancytopenias
	e.g. gold
	penicillamine
	phenylbutazone
	indomethacin

Anaemia

A variety of mechanisms may contribute to anaemia in rheumatoid disease. Anaemia of chronic disease is particularly common and is usually present during phases of acute active disease. Not uncommonly it is further complicated by iron deficiency due to chronic blood loss associated with non-steroidal anti-inflammatory drug therapy. Poor nutrition may cause impaired iron and/or folate intake and thus contribute to the anaemia. Bone marrow suppression by gold or penicillamine results in pancytopenia. Felty's syndrome (discussed below) may also complicate the anaemia.

Leukocytes

There are no characteristic changes in leukocytes in patients with rheumatoid disease, although neutrophilia often occurs during acute disease activity. Impairment of chemotaxis of neutrophils has occasionally been recognised.

Platelets

Thrombocytosis is commonly observed in patients with rheumatoid disease. The rise in platelet count tends to parallel the degree of disease activity. The pathogenesis is unknown. Thrombocytopenia is a relatively rare complication in the absence of complications such as drug-induced bone marrow suppression or Felty's syndrome.

Felty's syndrome

Felty's syndrome is a complication of chronic seropositive rheumatoid disease. It is characterised by long-standing polyarthritis, splenomegaly, leukopenia due to hypersplenism, lymphadenopathy and weight loss. There is usually severe, destructive, active arthritis associated with rheumatoid nodules and vasculitic lesions, particularly vasculitic leg ulceration. Felty's syndrome is also associated with clinical evidence of impaired immunity, with increased incidence of recurrent serious bacterial infections such as cellulitis, septic arthritis, pneumonia and septicaemia.

Histologically the spleen has a mononuclear infiltration and hypertrophied germinal centres. Diffuse lymphocytic infiltration of the portal tracts of the liver may also occur.

Anaemia is due mainly to ACD but is often accompanied by splenic red cell sequestration. Characteristically there is severe leukopenia with neutrophil counts of less than $1.0 \times 10^9/l$ and accompanying lymphopenia. The pathogenesis of the neutropenia is complex and includes splenic sequestration, impaired bone marrow production, shift to the marginating pool and also autoimmune destruction. Mild-moderate thrombocytopenia due to hypersplenism usually also occurs. The bone marrow shows marked left shift of granulopoiesis with impaired maturation to segmented neutrophils. The marrow tends to be hypercellular due to myeloid hyperplasia. No characteristic changes in erythroid activity or megakaryocytes are seen.

Treatment of Felty's syndrome is difficult. Splenec-

tomy usually results in improvement in the peripheral blood counts, but this may not improve the frequency of infectious episodes. Splenectomy is possibly most beneficial in patients with detectable neutrophil-bound IgG. Other forms of treatment, such as gold, penicillamine, plasmapheresis, corticosteroids, androgens or splenic irradiation, have produced variable, usually disappointing results.

SYSTEMIC LUPUS ERYTHEMATOSUS

Systemic lupus erythematosus (SLE) is a multi-system autoimmune disorder associated with a variety of haematological complications.

Anaemia

Anaemia of chronic disease, although recognised in patients with SLE, is usually very mild in the uncomplicated situation. In patients with lupus nephritis the anaemia of chronic renal failure may be present. Autoimmune haemolytic anaemia occurs in some patients with SLE, and may occasionally precede other manifestations of the disease by months or years. The Coomb's test is usually positive for both complement and anti-IgG. Rarely patients with very florid acute SLE may develop severe hypoplastic anaemia.

Leukocytes

Leukopenia is frequently present in patients with SLE. Neutropenia and accompanying impairment of neutrophil function may occur. An immunological basis for the neutropenia has been reported in some series. Mild-moderate lymphopenia can frequently be explained by an autoimmune process with the presence of cytotoxic anti-lymphocyte antibodies. Leukocytosis in response to infection or other insult is often impaired in SLE. Mild eosinophilia associated with dermatological complications is occasionally seen.

Platelets

Up to 40% of patients with SLE have mild-moderate thrombocytopenia with platelet counts of less than $100 \times 10^9/l$. Severe thrombocytopenia is present in up to 10% of patients, but serious haemorrhagic complications of thrombocytopenia are quite rare. Increased platelet-bound IgG is commonly found in thrombocytopenic patients, suggesting similar autoimmune mechanisms to ITP. Rarely, specific antibodies to megakaryocyte membrane proteins have been recognised. There is a strong correlation between thrombocytopenia and the presence of anticardiolipin antibodies in SLE. It is possible that these antibodies which react with phospholipid are directly attacking platelet membrane. Treatment of thrombocytopenia is along the same lines as treatment of isolated ITP, although immunosuppression with agents such as azothiapine or cyclophosphamide may be required more frequently.

The lupus anticoagulant

The lupus anticoagulant phenomenon is due to the presence of auto-antibodies against phosphodiester groups present in several body systems. Phospholipid is required for binding of calcium ions to vitamin K-dependent clotting factors. The lupus anticoagulant, by binding to such phospholipid, can interfere with in vitro coagulation tests. The lupus anticoagulant is detectable in up to 25% of patients with SLE. It may also occur in isolation or in association with other conditions (Table 29.4).

Table 29.4 Conditions associated with the lupus anticoagulant

Autoimmune disorders	SLE Rheumatoid disease Behçet's disease
Infections	
Lymphoproliferative disorders	
Drugs	Chlorpromazine Procainamide
Individuals without underlying diseases	

Despite causing prolongation of in vitro coagulation tests the lupus anticoagulant is associated clinically with an increased incidence of thrombosis. This may be venous thrombo-embolic disease or arterial thrombosis. Clinical complications include cerebral thrombosis, myocardial infarction, mesenteric artery thrombosis, peripheral vascular thrombosis, deep venous thrombosis and pulmonary embolism, renal vein thrombosis, mesenteric vein thrombosis and hepatic vein thrombosis. There is also an association with recurrent first or mid-trimester abortion due to multiple placental infarcts.

Investigations

The presence of the lupus anticoagulant is often first recognised in the laboratory by identifying prolongation of the partial thromboplastin (PTT) time, which is not corrected by addition of an equal volume of normal plasma. The prothrombin time (PT) is very often normal, but using serial dilutions of thromboplastin there is progressive prolongation of the patient's PT to a much greater degree than in control plasma, because the lupus anticoagulant becomes relatively more potent as the concentration of thromboplastin is reduced. A platelet neutralisation test may also be used to identify the lupus anticoagulant. When normal platelet phospholipid is added to the PTT test system, prolongation of the PTT by the lupus anticoagulant is corrected. The anticardiolipin antibody test is often performed in patients with SLE, and there is a strong association with the presence of the lupus anticoagulant.

Treatment

The optimal prevention and treatment of complications associated with the lupus anticoagulant are not known. Long-term anticoagulation with warfarin is recommended for patients who have had a thrombotic episode, since there is a high risk of further thrombosis. Successful pregnancies in patients who have had recurrent abortions have been managed by administration of antiplatelet drugs such as aspirin to reduce the occurrence of placental infarcts, and corticosteroids to attempt to suppress the titre of antiphosphodiester group antibodies. Long-term antiplatelet and/or immunosuppressive therapy, and plasmapheresis, have also been advocated.

OTHER CONNECTIVE TISSUE DISORDERS

Haematological changes are commonly found in many of the collagen-vascular or connective tissue diseases. Anaemia of chronic disorders is common to virtually all of them. Table 29.5 lists the haematological changes seen in these disorders. Occasionally these conditions present to the haematologist because of changes in the blood, or because there is clinical mimicry of a primary haematological disorder.

RENAL DISEASE

A variety of haematological complications accompany renal disorders. In addition generalised systemic disorders may involve both the blood and the kidney, such as occurs in several micro-angiopathic disorders: haemolytic-uraemic syndrome, malignant hypertension, severe pre-eclampsia, etc.

Anaemia of chronic renal failure

In chronic renal failure anaemia develops gradually and

Table 29.5 Haematological complications of some connective tissue disorders

Ankylosing spondylitis	Anaemia of chronic disease (ACD) Bone marrow hypoplasia secondary to spinal irradiation (now obsolete treatment of ankylosing spondylitis) AML
Polyarteritis nodosa	ACD Micro-angiopathic haemolytic anaemia Bleeding from mucosal surfaces Eosinophilia
Scleroderma	ACD Bleeding from telangiectases – iron deficiency anaemia B_{12} or folate deficiency due to small intestinal involvement Haemolytic anaemia – rare Thrombocytopenia
Polymyalgia rheumatica/Temporal arteritis	Constitutional symptoms, weight loss, sweats, anorexia ACD may occur with minimal muscle symptoms – steroid responsive Grossly elevated ESR
Reiter's disease	ACD Neutrophilia
Wegener's granulomatosis	Recurrent severe epistaxis – normal platelet count ACD Neutrophilia
Dermatomyositis	ACD Leukocytosis
Sjörgren's syndrome	Strong association with lymphoma

the degree of anaemia correlates to a large extent with the degree of uraemia. However, other factors may complicate the anaemia of chronic renal failure causing it to increase in severity.

Haematological changes

The haemoglobin varies within the range 5–12 g/dl depending on the severity of uraemia and the presence or absence of complicating factors. It is normochromic normocytic in character, but in addition burr cells and marked poikilocytosis are seen on the blood film. Burr cells are a characteristic finding in renal failure and arise as a consequence of some undetermined influence by uraemic plasma in red cell membrane phospholipid arrangement. The presence of significant numbers of spherocytes and schistocytes may point to a pathogenic factor, such as micro-angiopathy, or reflect a complic-

ation of the renal failure such as DIC. Hypersegmentation of neutrophils, even in the absence of vitamin B_{12} and folate deficiency, is an occasional observation in renal failure. There are no characteristic morphological or numerical changes in platelets. The bone marrow appears remarkably normal and the striking feature is the virtual absence of erythroid hyperplasia in patients with severe anaemia.

Clinical features

The clinical picture is dominated by the complications of uraemia. The incidence of symptomatic anaemia is variable and many patients appear to tolerate severe anaemia reasonably well due to the compensatory effects of increased 2,3-DPG production by the red cells. Splenomegaly is recognised in a significant percentage of patients on long-term dialysis.

Pathogenesis

The pathogenesis of anaemia in chronic renal failure is complex (Table 29.6). Different factors may be more important in some conditions than others. By far the most important factor, however, is impairment of the production of erythropoietin by the kidneys. Plasma erythropoietin activity is inappropriately low, and the anaemia virtually always improves in patients given exogenous erythropoietin. The cause of impaired erythropoietin production is not completely understood but probably relates to destruction of the erythropoietin-secreting cells of the renal tubules.

Table 29.6 Factors contributing to anaemia in chronic renal failure

Major factors	Impairment of erythropoietin production Inhibitors of erythropoiesis Haemolysis
Other factors	Iron deficiency Folate deficiency Chronic blood loss Osteitis fibrosa Recurrent infection – ACD Aluminium toxicity Expanded plasma volume

Other factors which may contribute to anaemia in chronic renal failure are as follows:

Inhibition of erythropoiesis

Uraemic plasma factors may cause inhibition of erythropoiesis within the bone marrow. The nature of these inhibitory factors is not known. Some improvement in anaemia may follow the initiation of dialysis in the earlier stages of chronic renal failure, implying that these inhibitory factors are dialysable. Erythroid progenitors from patients with renal failure have a normal in vitro growth response in the absence of the uraemic plasma, providing further evidence for the existence of these inhibitory factors. However, the clinical significance of such inhibitors of erythropoiesis is cast in doubt since nearly all patients with chronic renal failure have a favourable response to administration of recombinant erythropoietin.

Haemolysis

The red cell lifespan is shortened in virtually all patients with chronic renal failure, even in the absence of a micro-angiopathic aetiology. The red cell lifespan is correlated with the degree of uraemia, and may be shortened to half normal. Cross-transfusion studies of the type described above in the ACD section have demonstrated that an extra corpuscular defect is responsible for the shortening of the red cell lifespan. A number of defects of red cell metabolism, which are reversible by removal of the red cells from the uraemic plasma, can be demonstrated. Decreased Na^+-K^+ ATPase activity leads to leakage of K^+ ions out of and Na^+ ions into the red cell. Consequently increased auto-haemolysis and increased osmotic fragility occur. Impairment of intracellular glycolysis, glutathione metabolism and the pentose-phosphate pathway may occur. Reduction in glutathione concentration and reduced NADPH generation lead to increased susceptibility to oxidative stress. Consequently Heinz body formation and acute intravascular haemolysis may occasionally be induced by oxidative drugs such as sulphonamides or, previously, the oxidant chloramine in tap water. The majority of these metabolic changes probably relate to the presence of acidosis in chronic renal failure.

Hypersplenism is a not infrequent problem in patients with chronic renal failure. Obviously consequent red cell sequestration may further exacerbate the shortening of red cell survival.

Iron deficiency

Chronic gastrointestinal blood loss is common in patients with chronic renal failure. It is usually due to recurrent gastric erosions and not uncommonly to overt peptic ulceration. The presence of a haemostatic defect may augment the problem. Nutritional iron deficiency is also relatively common, at least at presentation. Blood loss during haemodialysis is a major problem and may contribute significantly to the anaemia of chronic renal failure in patients treated in this way.

Other factors

Folic acid is dialysable and it is important to supplement the diet with oral folic acid tablets. Folate deficiency may be exacerbated by impaired dietary intake, especially in patients requiring a protein-restricted diet. Hyperparathyroidism causing osteitis fibrosa may lead to impaired bone marrow function. Parathyroidectomy and/or 1,25 dihydroxy vitamin D therapy may result in some improvement. Aluminium toxicity is a former problem of dialysis because of the use of tap water as a source of the diasylate. Anaemia was often the first indication of aluminium toxicity and was of microcytic hypochromic character. Aluminium probably interferes with haem synthesis and/or transport of transferrin-bound iron to the developing red cell. Aluminium toxicity is reversible if recognised at an early stage, by desferrioxamine chelation therapy. Recurrent infection is a frequent problem in patients with chronic renal failure, and thus ACD may further complicate the anaemia of chronic renal failure.

Treatment

Renal transplantation, as well as reversing the uraemia, results in increased erythropoietin production and reversal of the anaemia. Dialysis may lead to some improvement in the anaemia, at least in the early stages. Peritoneal dialysis is more effective in this respect, since it avoids the problem of chronic blood loss.

Supplementation of iron and folate as appropriate may produce some improvement. Removal and avoidance of oxidative stresses may reduce the degree of haemolysis. Blood transfusion will be required for symptomatic anaemia but it has a limited role; since its benefits are short-lived, multiple transfusions will be required and iron overload may ensue. Splenectomy is occasionally considered for patients with hypersplenism associated with excessive transfusion requirements but the significant surgical risk limits the potential for this form of treatment.

Androgenic steroids stimulate erythropoiesis by a direct effect on the bone marrow. They may also augment residual renal and extrarenal erythropoietin production. However, they have a limited therapeutic role due to excessive toxicity. Although cobalt salts stimulate erythropoiesis, they have no therapeutic role in treatment of the anaemia of chronic renal failure due to excessive toxicity.

The most important advance in the management of anaemia of chronic renal failure has been the production of recombinant erythropoietin. Production in quantities large enough for therapeutic use is now possible. Administration of recombinant erythropoietin leads to rapid improvement in the anaemia irrespective of the cause of renal failure. Some patients attain normal haemoglobin levels and all patients become transfusion-independent. Iron and/or folate supplementation may be required to cater for the sudden increased rate of erythropoiesis. Toxic effects are limited but hypertension has been observed in some patients. There is a theoretical risk of an increased incidence of vascular occlusive events due to the sudden rise in packed cell volume.

Haemostatic defects in chronic renal failure

A bleeding tendency is commonly observed in chronic renal failure. This is due mainly to impaired platelet function, although thrombocytopenia and coagulation defects may also occur (Table 29.7). Prolongation of the bleeding time is accompanied by defective in vitro platelet aggregation, defective clot retraction and defective platelet release reactions. These abnormalities are reversed or at least improved by dialysis, suggesting that toxic substances in uraemic plasma are affecting platelets adversely. A further observation is loss of balance of the prostaglandin I_2/thromboxane A_2 balance due to reduced prostaglandin synthesis within the platelet and increased PGI_2 synthesis in the endothelium. The functional effect is similar to the influence of aspirin on platelet function.

DDAVP maybe of value in treating haemorrhage; its mode of action is unknown but it causes a shortening of the bleeding time. The effect of DDAVP is to stimulate the release of large multimers of von Willebrand factor from endothelial cells. The high concentration of these may then overcome the platelet defects involved in platelet-vWf-vessel wall interaction, with consequent stimulation of in vivo platelet aggregation.

A variety of defects of coagulation may be observed

Table 29.7 Haemostatic dysfunction in chronic renal failure

Platelet defects	Prolonged bleeding time Impaired platelet aggregation in vitro Thrombocytopenia
Coagulation defects	Increased VIIIC, vWF, VII, X, fibrinogen Decreased XII, XI, prothrombin, XIII Decreased fibrinolytic activity Decreased antithrombin III, protein C Dysfibrinogenaemia

in renal failure. Prolongation of the thrombin time due to FDPs or dysfibrinogenaemia may occur. Prolongation of the PT and PTT occasionally occur. Increased concentrations of factor VIIIC, vWF, factor VII and factor X have been observed. Fibrinogen may be elevated and fibrinolytic activity depressed before dialysis, with return to normal after initiation of dialysis. Depression of antithrombin III and protein C activity have also been observed. The net effect of these coagulation defects is a predisposition to thrombosis which may exist at the same time as the predisposition to bleeding associated with impaired platelet function. Haemodialysis with heparin anticoagulation may further predispose to bleeding.

Administration of antiplatelet agents such as aspirin may reduce the risk of thrombosis in patients with chronic renal failure, but the risks of bleeding may then outweigh any therapeutic benefit. Dialysis with lower doses of heparin reduces the haemorrhagic complications of heparin administration and may also decrease the thrombotic tendency due to excessive platelet activation.

Thrombocytopenia occurs in a variable number of patients with chronic renal failure due mainly to complications such as sepsis, DIC, hypersplenism or drug toxicity. Occasionally thrombocytopenia is recognised in the absence of an obvious cause and is attributed to the uraemic state itself.

Leukocyte abnormalities in chronic renal failure

Neutrophilia associated with myeloid hyperplasia of the bone marrow is relatively common and elevated levels of colony-stimulating factors can be demonstrated. Hypersegmentation without megaloblastic marrow changes may occur, the mechanism being unknown. Impairment of neutrophil function due mainly to depressed chemotactic activity secondary to toxic factors in uraemic plasma has been recognised. Occasionally sudden sequestration of neutrophils within the lungs occurs at the onset of haemodialysis. This may provoke adult respiratory distress syndrome. It may be brought about by activation of complement during dialysis, leading to generation of large quantities of C5a which causes granulocyte aggregation and adherence to pulmonary vascular endothelium.

Lymphopenia due to selective depletion of B-lymphocytes may occur in uraemic patients. It is usually corrected by dialysis. There is no apparent impairment of immunoglobin production, and the specific response to neo-antigens is retained. However, depression of helper T-lymphocyte activity and cutaneous anergy are demonstrable.

Table 29.8 Abnormalities of haemostatic function in nephrotic syndrome

Increased fibrinogen
Increased levels of factors V, VII, VIIIC, X
Decreased levels of factors XI, XII
Decreased plasminogen
Decreased α_1 antitrypsin
Increased α_2 macroglobulin
Increased α_2 antiplasmin
Decreased antithrombin III
Thrombocytosis
Increased platelet aggregation in response to ADP, collagen

Nephrotic syndrome

A number of defects of haemostatic function may occur in patients with nephrotic syndrome (Table 29.8). Clinically a considerably increased risk of venous thrombo-embolic disease is recognised. There is also a high risk of renal vein thrombosis. Predisposition to arterial thrombosis may also occur. The increased level of some coagulation factor, as outlined in Table 29.8, is a result of the general increase in liver protein synthesis. Anti-thrombin III is lost in the urine due to the glomerular leak. Hyperlipidaemia, which commonly occurs in nephrotic syndrome, may lead to the increased tendency for platelet aggregation.

LIVER DISEASE:

Liver disease causes a variety of changes in the blood. Viral hepatitis is discussed in the section on viruses (p. 316). The haematological changes occurring in chronic liver disease are variable and complex. They may be further complicated by the presence of portal hypertension, drugs, alcohol, infection and hypersplenism.

Anaemia in chronic liver disease

Moderate anaemia is a common manifestation of chronic liver disease. It is usually normochromic and macrocytic. The haemoglobin rarely falls below 10 g/dl in the uncomplicated case. The MCV usually lies within the range 100–115 fl. The macrocytes are poorly filled with haemoglobin, being described as 'thin'. They appear as circular discs on the blood film and show less anisopoikilocytosis than the macrocytes of megaloblastic anaemia. There is a variable number of target cells and polychromatic cells present in the blood film. The degree of anaemia, macrocytosis and concentration of target cells roughly correlates with the severity of liver

dysfunction. The bone marrow is hypercellular due to macronormoblastic erythroid hyperplasia. There are no characteristic changes in granulopoietic or megakaryocytic activity.

The pathogenesis of the anaemia of chronic liver disease is not completely clear. There is no aetiological association with deficiency of vitamin B_{12} or folic acid. Moderate shortening of the red cell lifespan has been reported in some studies. No immunological mechanism for this has been demonstrated. Despite erythroid hyperplasia of the bone marrow erythropoiesis is inadequate to some extent. The reason for this remains unknown. Anaemia may be further exacerbated by hypersplenism and increased plasma volume associated with portal hypertension.

Changes in haematinic factors in chronic liver disease

Serum vitamin B_{12} is usually normal but may be elevated due to release from damaged hepatocytes. Vitamin B_{12} absorption is normal and there is no evidence of impaired utilisation by the bone marrow. Folic acid deficiency is not uncommon due to impaired dietary intake, particularly in patients with alcoholic liver disease. Thus folate deficiency may complicate, but does not cause, the anaemia of chronic liver disease. Iron absorption is increased in patients with chronic liver disease. Siderosis can be demonstrated in a proportion of patients but it rarely reaches a degree severe enough to adversely affect the myocardium, pancreas or other tissues. Iron deficiency due to chronic blood loss, usually secondary to peptic ulceration, is more commonly seen, and may also complicate the anaemia of chronic liver disease.

Zieve's syndrome

A syndrome of acute haemolytic anaemia associated with jaundice, hyperlipidaemia and hypercholesterolaemia may occur after excessive alcohol consumption in patients with alcoholic fatty liver or cirrhosis. The red cell membrane content increases during these attacks and this is associated with increased red cell membrane instability leading to haemolysis. The plasma cholesterol and lipid concentrations fall when alcohol consumption stops and this leads to reversal of the red cell membrane defect.

Leukocyte changes in chronic liver disease

Leukopenia is commonly seen in patients with chronic liver disease. This is mainly due to neutropenia, although mild lymphopenia may also occur. The cause of depression of neutrophil and lymphocyte counts is not known. However, in some patients it can be explained by the presence of hypersplenism.

Platelet changes

Thrombocytopenia is a common manifestation of chronic liver disease. The platelet count is often within the range $60-100 \times 10^9/l$, but severe thrombocytopenia may also occur. The cause is unknown, although it may be further exacerbated by hypersplenism. Defects of platelet function may also occur. Spontaneous bleeding is rarely directly due solely to the thrombocytopenia or platelet dysfunction.

Coagulation defects in chronic liver disease

A variety of changes in the coagulation system occur in liver disease (Table 29.9) and these have a complex relationship to one another. The liver is the major site of synthesis of the clotting factors and impaired synthesis leading to deficiency of these proteins may occur in chronic liver disease. Malabsorption of vitamin K may result from prolonged cholestasis. Fibrinogen synthesis may be depressed and dysfibrinogenaemia may also occur. A state of low grade DIC is commonly recognised in chronic liver disease. Impaired clearance of activated clotting factors may underly this. In addition impaired clearance of activators of fibrinolysis may lead to increased fibrinolytic activity.

Table 29.9 Haemostatic dysfunction in chronic liver disease

Thrombocytopenia
Impaired platelet function
Impaired synthesis of coagulation factors
Dysfibrinogenaemia
Impaired clearance of activators of fibrinolysis
Impaired synthesis of antithrombin III, protein C
Low grade DIC

Despite these complex changes spontaneous bleeding is uncommon in patients with chronic liver disease, and its occurrence is a poor prognostic sign. Treatment of acute bleeding episodes is based on replacement therapy with fresh frozen plasma and/or cryoprecipitate, and platelet concentrates. Intravenous vitamin K should also be administered, although it will not influence the immediate clinical state. Prothrombin complex solutions have also been used but these contain activated clotting factors which may provoke thrombosis and/or DIC. They may also carry a high risk of transmission of hepatitis viruses, with potentially serious implications for patients who already have serious liver dysfunction.

MALABSORPTION

The main haematological changes occurring in patients with malabsorption are due to deficiency of iron, folic acid, vitamin B_{12} or vitamin K.

Coeliac disease (Table 29.10)

Folic acid deficiency is the most common haematological complication of coeliac disease and occurs in 60–90% of patients at presentation. It is accounted for principally by impaired absorption directly due to villous atrophy. However, brush border enzymes are required to deconjugate polyglutamated folate and these are deficient in coeliac disease. The enterohepatic recirculation loop is broken in coeliac disease and this may lead to further depletion of folate stores.

Co-existent iron deficiency is not uncommon and may lead to a dimorphic blood picture with a combination of oval macrocytes and hypochromic microcytes. Vitamin B_{12} deficiency is much less common, but may occur in severe, extensive coeliac disease which involves the terminal ileum.

Hyposplenism is frequently recognised in coeliac disease and occasionally is the presenting feature when Howell-Jolly bodies, target cells, microspherocytes, nucleated red cells and Pappenheimer bodies are recognised on the peripheral blood film. The cause of splenic atrophy remains unknown.

Vitamin K deficiency, leading to prolongation of the prothrombin time, is recognised in 30–70% of patients at presentation. Spontaneous bleeding, however, rarely occurs.

Patients with coeliac disease have a considerable risk of developing a T-cell lymphoma of the small intestine in middle or later life. Unfortunately this risk is not reduced by a gluten-free diet and reversal of the villous atrophy. The response to treatment is poor even with aggressive combination chemotherapy. An increased risk of small intestinal carcinoma is also recognised.

Bacterial overgrowth syndromes

Bacterial overgrowth in the small intestine may occur due to functional or anatomical small intestinal stasis. A syndrome of diarrhoea, weight loss, crampy abdominal

Table 29.10 Haematological complications of coeliac disease

Folate deficiency
Iron deficiency
Hyposplenism
Vitamin K deficiency
Vitamin E deficiency
Gastrointestinal lymphoma
Vitamin B_{12} deficiency

pain and malnutrition may then occur. The increased population of bacteria, particularly anaerobes, causes deconjugation of bile salts leading to fat malabsorption, direct damage to the intestinal mucosa causing malabsorption of all nutrients, and chronic intestinal blood loss resulting in iron deficiency. Anaerobic bacteria also utilise vitamin B_{12} leading to megaloblastic anaemia. Interruption of the enterohepatic recirculation loop may cause further depletion of vitamin B_{12} stores. Folic acid deficiency characteristically does not occur because of increased production by bacteria. Similarly vitamin K deficiency is not a feature of bacterial overgrowth.

The diagnosis is confirmed by small intestinal aspiration and culture. Rapid clinical improvement follows administration of broad spectrum antibiotics. Surgical correction of the blind loop may subsequently be required. If this is not possible, intermittent 1–2 week courses of antibiotics prevents relapse of the condition in the majority of cases.

Pancreatic insufficiency

The pancreas facilitates absorption of vitamin B_{12} by the action of its proteolytic enzymes in hydrolysing salivary R-factor from vitamin B_{12}. This makes more vitamin B_{12} available to bind to intrinsic factor. The alkaline pH of the duodenum, which is maintained by pancreatic bicarbonate secretion, promotes further intrinsic factor B_{12} binding. Over 50% of patients with pancreatic insufficiency have decreased serum vitamin B_{12} levels. However, overt megaloblastic anaemia is uncommon.

ENDOCRINE DISORDERS

Thyroid diseases

Thyroid dysfunction does not usually cause haematological changes and thus major haematological abnormalities should rarely be attributed solely to thyroid disease. The relationship between thyroid hormones and erythropoiesis is well recognised. By stimulating an increase in basal metabolic rate, thyroid hormone leads to increased tissue oxygen requirements. A rise in red cell mass is recognised in hyperthyroidism and a fall in red cell mass occurs in hypothyroidism. In addition thyroid hormones directly stimulate an increase in the rate of erythropoiesis, which is associated with a detectable rise in plasma erythropoietin concentration. In vitro erythroid colony growth is augmented by addition of thyroid hormone but only in the presence of erythropoietin.

Hypothyroidism

About one-third of patients with hypothyroidism are anaemic at presentation. The anaemia is mild-moderate, the haemoglobin rarely falling below 10 g/dl. A significant proportion of patients have mild-moderate macrocytosis with an MCV in the range of 95–105 fl. The anaemia improves following thyroxine replacement therapy. It is probably related to reduced erythropoiesis consequent on thyroxine deficiency. In females it may be complicated by iron deficiency due to menorrhagia. There are no characteristic changes in leukocytes in hypothyroid patients. Impaired platelet function and mild reduction in factor VIII concentration may occur, leading to a von Willebrand-like syndrome with bruising, menorrhagia and prolonged post-operative bleeding. This is reversed by thyroxine replacement therapy, but platelet and cryoprecipitate transfusions may be required for the very rare acute bleeding episode.

Hyperthyroidism

A slight rise in packed cell volume may occur in patients with hyperthyroidism but overt polycythaemia does not occur. A proportion of patients have iron deficiency anaemia. Impaired iron utilisation by erythroid precursors may occur in severe, prolonged hyperthyroidism, and this is reversed by treatment of the primary condition.

Moderate neutropenia may occur in untreated hyperthyroidism. Agranulocytosis is a well-recognised complication of anti-thyroid drugs such as carbimazole, methimazole and thiouracil. It is associated with the presence of anti-neutrophil antibodies, and is reversible on withdrawal of the offending drug. Rarely, more serious prolonged aplastic anaemia may occur. There are no characteristic changes in platelets or haemostatic function in hyperthyroidism.

Pituitary disease

Mild to moderate normochromic normocytic anaemia may occur in hypopituitarism. The patient may present for investigation of anaemia due to the characteristic pallor of hypopituitarism. The anaemia is reversed by adequate replacement therapy with thyroxine, corticosteroids and sex hormones.

Adrenal disease

Normochromic normocytic anaemia is a common complication of Addison's disease. However, it is frequently masked at presentation by the patient's dehydrated state, leading to haemoconcentration. Neutropenia and relative lymphocytosis may also occur. These changes are reversed by adequate replacement therapy. Cushing's disease is associated with neutrophil leukocytosis, lymphopenia, and eosinopenia in many patients. The neutrophilia is a consequence of increased outpouring from the bone marrow and shift from the marginating to the circulating pool stimulated by the corticosteroids. There is an increased incidence of infective episodes in Cushingoid patients, suggesting an immunosuppressive effect of the excessive corticosteroids. No associated increase in incidence of malignancies, however, is seen. Impaired platelet function occasionally occurs and this may exacerbate the purpura associated with skin atrophy. Paradoxically there is an increased incidence of venous thrombo-embolism and post-operative thrombosis. Increased levels of factors II, V, IX, XII, and VIIIc may occur, and this may be involved in the pathogenesis of the thrombotic tendency.

Diabetes mellitus (Table 29.11)

Red cell changes

Hyperglycaemia results in a rise in intracellular glucose causing alteration in intracellular carbohydrate metabolism and consequent alterations in red cell function. There is progressive non-enzymatic glycolysation of Hb A at the N-terminus of the beta-globin chains. Such glycolysated haemoglobin, termed Hb A1c, has an increased oxygen affinity due to left shift of the oxygen dissociation curve. This may result in mild impairment of tissue oxygen delivery if the Hb A1c level rises to about 6–8%. This may be particularly important in diabetic keto-acidosis when the availability of 2,3-DPG is reduced due to the acidosis and deficiency of inorganic phosphate. Hyperlipidaemia also causes reduced availability of 2,3-DPG by an unknown mechanism.

The rise in intracellular red cell glucose concentration adversely affects the red cell enzyme pathways, leading to accumulation of other sugars, particularly sorbitol and fructose. These sugars cause reduced red cell deformability and increase the tendency for red cell

Table 29.11 Haematological dysfunction in diabetes mellitus

Increased haemoglobin A$_1$C
Shift to left in oxygen dissociation curve for haemoglobin
Increased tendency to red cell aggregation
Increased whole blood viscosity
Depression of erythropoiesis
Impairment of neutrophil function
Impairment of cell-mediated immunity
Disseminated intravascular coagulation
Platelet hyper-reactivity
Increased fibrinogen

aggregation, causing a net increase in whole blood viscosity. This, along with the accelerated rate of atheroma formation, may contribute to the increased incidence of vascular occlusive events in diabetic patients.

Anaemia is not uncommon in patients with diabetes. Erythropoietic activity is depressed during the hyperglycaemic state, and improves with strict glycaemic control. Chronic blood loss from the gastrointestinal tract, renal failure due to diabetic nephropathy or pernicious anaemia may contribute to the anaemia.

Leukocyte changes

Impairment of neutrophil function has been reported in some studies. Chemotaxis, phagocytosis and intracellular killing defects have been variously described. These changes are most common during severe hyperglycaemia or keto-acidosis. Impairment of lymphocyte function, particularly cell-mediated immunity, has also been reported. These abnormalities may correlate with the increased incidence of some infections such as group B streptococci, staphylococcal skin infections and mucocutaneous candidiasis in diabetics.

Haemostatic changes

Disseminated intravascular coagulation may complicate diabetic keto-acidosis. Platelet hyper-reactivity leading to increased platelet adhesion and aggregation may be involved in the accelerated rate of atheroma development in diabetics. Elevated fibrinogen and other clotting factors, particularly factor VIIIc, may also play a part in atheroma development.

CARDIAC DISEASE

Congenital heart disease

Right-to-left intracardiac and large vessel shunts lead to cyanosis, impaired tissue oxygen delivery and consequently secondary polycythaemia. This contributes to an increased risk of vascular occlusive events in patients with cyanotic congenital heart disease. Mild-moderate thrombocytopenia associated with moderate depression of fibrinogen and autopsy findings of fibrin clots in the tissues suggest the presence of chronic low grade DIC in these patients. Venesection requires great care as there have been reports of sudden death following this procedure. Thus isovolumic venesection with saline or 5% albumin replacement should be carried out. Venesection, by reducing the red cell mass, improves systemic blood flow and reduces peripheral vascular resistance, leading to improved tissue oxygen delivery.

Valvular heart disease

Severe regurgitant jets may cause chronic low grade intravascular haemolysis by direct mechanical damage to red cells in the turbulent flow. Secondary chronic haemosidinuria may then lead to iron deficiency. Autoimmune haemolytic anaemia and/or thrombocytopenia may occur as part of the post-extracorporeal perfusion syndrome but they resolve spontaneously within the first 1–2 weeks. Intravascular haemolysis is a common minor complication of some types of prosthetic valves, e.g. Star-Edwards' valve. Severe haemolysis may occur if a prosthetic valve develops a leak causing a severe regurgitant jet around the valve base.

Atrial myxoma

Atrial myxoma may cause normochromic normocytic anaemia, elevated ESR with red cell rouleaux formation, polyclonal rise in immunoglobulins and leukocytosis.

Hypereosinophilic syndrome

In this syndrome, which is of undetermined aetiology, there is marked eosinophilia associated with eosinophil infiltration of the tissues, leading to organ dysfunction. The eosinophil count is in the range $5–50 \times 10^9/l$. There is mild-moderate normochromic normocytic anaemia and normal platelet count. Visceral organomegaly accompanies a constrictive cardiomyopathy associated with cardiac failure and arrhythmias. It is unknown whether the widespread tissue damage is caused by the infiltrating eosinophils, or whether some unidentified tissue agent also attracts eosinophils to the areas of tissue damage.

RESPIRATORY DISEASE

Chronic obstructive airways disease

Two main clinical patterns are recognised in patients with chronic bronchitis and emphysema. 'Pink Puffers' develop dyspnoea and over-inflated chests and maintain relatively normal blood gases. 'Blue Bloaters' have better exercise tolerance but develop hypoxaemia associated with oedema, plethora, cyanosis and polycythaemia. The reasons for these differences in response to chronic lung damage are unknown. The conditions may be further complicated by recurrent respiratory infections, cardiac failure, iron deficiency anaemia and reduced oxygen affinity due to elevated 2,3-DPG.

Idiopathic pulmonary haemosiderosis

In this condition recurrent rupture of pulmonary capillaries leads to recurrent haemorrhage into pulmonary alveoli. This results in cough, dyspnoea and haemoptysis. Iron deficiency anaemia consequently develops. A similar pattern of pulmonary haemosiderosis associated with acute glomerulonephritis occurs in Goodpasture's syndrome.

BACTERIAL INFECTION

Acute bacterial infection

Leukocytes

Neutrophilia accompanies most acute bacterial infections. The total white cell count may range from $10–25 \times 10^9/l$ up to $50–75 \times 10^9/l$, the count correlating roughly with the severity and extent of infection. Increased proportions of band neutrophils, metamyelocytes and myelocytes may appear in the peripheral blood, particularly in severe infections. Deeply staining basophilic granules (toxic granulation) are often recognised in the neutrophil cytoplasm in severe infection. Other changes include cytoplasmic vacuolation and the appearance of blue-staining inclusions of $1–2$ μm diameter. These are Dohle bodies, which are lamellar aggregates of rough endoplasmic reticulum. Very high leukocyte counts of $75–120 \times 10^9/l$ with numerous granulocyte precursors present in the peripheral blood, with the result that this condition may be mistaken for chronic myeloid leukaemia. But elevated neutrophil alkaline phosphatase activity and the absence of the Philadelphia chromosome distinguish this leukaemoid reaction from chronic myeloid leukaemia.

Occasionally in severely ill patients an inappropriately poor neutrophil response or a neutropenic response is observed in the presence of serious bacterial infection. This may occur in the presence of a primary haematological disorder, chronic debilitating illness including alcoholism, or for no apparent reason. It may be due to exhaustion of the bone marrow neutrophil pool, but shift from the circulating to the marginating pool may also occur. Usually there is evidence of an adequate neutrophil response manifested by the presence of pus or purulent secretions at the site of infection. Neonates often develop neutropenia in response to infection because they rapidly deplete their limited marrow neutrophil reserve.

The mechanisms underlying the neutrophilia associated with bacterial infections are only partly understood. Infection stimulates increased release of neutrophils from the massive bone marrow storage pool which is at least ten fold greater in size than the normal circulating pool. This may be mediated by interleukin-1. The outpouring of granulocyte precursors is due to augmented stimulation of bone marrow granulopoietic activity. Interleukin-1 stimulates increased production of colony-stimulating factors which promote granulopoiesis.

Neutropenia ($<1.5 \times 10^9$/l) may occur in any bacterial infection as explained above. However, it is most common in salmonellosis, typhoid, brucellosis, pertussis and rickettsial infections. Lymphocytosis ($> 4.0 \times 10^9$/l) is a characteristic finding in the acute phase of pertussis. It is rarely seen in other bacterial or fungal infections. It may occur in tuberculosis, rickettsial infections, syphilis and brucellosis.

Lymphopenia ($<1.0 \times 10^9$/l) not uncommonly accompanies the neutrophilia of acute bacterial infections. Its presence in elderly patients with severe bacterial infection is a poor prognostic sign.

Monocytosis may occur in any acute bacterial infection but most commonly occurs in tuberculosis and brucellosis.

Anaemia

Depression of erythropoiesis with reduced absolute reticulocyte counts occurs within the first few days of onset of serious bacterial infections. Normochromic normocytic anaemia may subsequently develop if the infection becomes protracted. The pathogenesis is that of anaemia of chronic disorders described above. Haemolytic anaemia may occur in a variety of bacterial infections, e.g. streptococcal, staphylococcal, pneumococcal, *Haemophilus influenzae*, typhus. The pathogenesis is usually intravascular fragmentation haemolysis of the micro-angiopathic type due to disseminated intravascular coagulation. Direct red cell membrane damage may occur in *Clostridium welchii* infection due to production of alpha-toxin which acts as a lecithinase and may cause fulminant intravascular haemolysis. Accompanying fulminant DIC is also found in most cases.

On the Pacific coast of South America, Oroya fever (*Bartonella bacilliformis*) causes a clinical syndrome of fever, bone and joint pains, myalgia, generalised lymphadenopathy and severe haemolytic anaemia. A characteristic warty eruption, verruga peruana, is found on the skin. The red cells are phagocytosed by the reticulo-endothelial system due to the presence of the organism on or just within the surface of the red cell membrane. The condition responds well to penicillin if treated early.

Mycoplasma pneumoniae infection is associated with the presence of cold agglutinins in over 75% of affected individuals. However, overt Coomb's positive haemolytic anaemia is rare, with only some 50 reported cases in the literature. The cold agglutinins are IgM antibodies with specificity for the I antigen of the red cell membrane. *M. pneumoniae* may share antigenic determinants with the red cell membrane I antigen, or the organism's peroxidase may alter the I antigen to render it iso-immunogenic.

Haemostastic defects

Disseminated intravascular coagulation is a well-recognised complication of any serious bacterial infection. It is most commonly associated with gram negative septicaemia, in which large amounts of endotoxin are produced. The clinical features may range from the presence of a petechial rash to gross haemostatic failure. Waterhouse-Friderichsen syndrome is the association of meningococcal septicaemia with widespread purpura and severe bleeding into the tissues, especially bilateral adrenal haemorrhage. Purpura fulminans is the presence of large ecchymoses which rapidly become gangrenous, occurring in streptococcal septicaemia. The laboratory characteristics of DIC are described in Chapter 32. Treatment is based on prompt, adequate antibiotic therapy to control the primary condition. Supportive treatment with blood, fresh frozen plasma, cryoprecipitate or platelet concentrates is often required.

Thrombocytopenia may complicate bacterial infection even in the absence of DIC. Platelet destruction by macrophages due to the non-specific binding of immune complexes is probably the most common mechanism. Severe infection causes inhibition of platelet production by the bone marrow.

Thrombocytosis is not uncommonly found during the recovery phase of acute bacterial or fungal infections. The platelet count is usually in the range 500–700 $\times$ 10^9/l. No specific treatment is required.

Chronic bacterial infection

Anaemia of chronic disorders is commonly found in patients with chronic infections. Occasionally patients may present for investigation of anaemia and only after exclusion of malignancy or connective tissue disorders is a chronic sequestered infection considered. Chronic pyelonephritis is the commonest such infection, particularly in females. Brucellosis may cause ACD as well as monocytosis or lymphocytosis.

A variety of haematological changes may occur in tuberculosis (Table 29.12). During active pulmonary tuberculosis there is usually normochromic normocytic anaemia associated with elevation of the erythrocyte sedimentation rate. These changes correlate roughly with the extent and activity of the disease and are re-

Table 29.12   Haematological changes in tuberculosis

Anaemia of chronic disorder
Megaloblastic anaemia – especially intestinal TB
Sideroblastic anaemia – isoniazid
Gross elevation of ESR
Leukaemoid reaction
Leuko-erythroblastic anaemia
Myelofibrosis
Pancytopenia
Thrombocytopenia – rifampicin

versible following adequate treatment. Interestingly, some antituberculous chemotherapeutic agents may cause pyridoxine- responsive sideroblastic anaemia, and this should be considered in patients with persisting severe anaemia despite an otherwise good response to chemotherapy. Folate deficiency due to inadequate dietary intake in debilitated patients may further complicate the anaemia. Disseminated miliary tuberculosis may present due to the manifestations of bone marrow involvement with leuko-erythroblastic anaemia or a leukaemoid reaction. Confusion with myelofibrosis or chronic myeloid leukaemia may occur, particularly in patients with splenomegaly. Bone marrow culture for *M. tuberculosis* should be performed in cases of doubt, or in patients with a history of contact with active tuberculosis. Empirical antituberculosis therapy may be required in patients who deteriorate before culture results are available.

VIRAL INFECTION

Haematological changes commonly accompany viral illness. Some viral infections produce characteristic haematological changes. A discussion of the general haematological changes in viral infections will precede discussion of these more specific syndromes.

White cell changes

Mild neutropenia with relative or mild absolute lymphocytosis commonly occurs in acute viral illnesses, e.g. influenza, hepatitis, rubella, measles, adenoviruses, coxsackie viruses, mumps. However a mild granulocytosis may occasionally accompany the lymphocytosis. The neutropenia is rarely severe enough to predispose to severe secondary bacterial infection. It is the breakdown of local mucosal defences due to the primary viral illness which accounts for the relatively commonly recognised secondary bacterial infections.

Anaemia

Haemolytic anaemia may occur during or following viral

infections such as measles, cytomegalovirus, varicella zoster, herpes simplex, hepatitis, Epstein-Barr or influenza infections. The Coomb's test may or may not be positive. Specificity for anti-i may be recognised. Neuramidase production during viral infections may cause alteration of red cell membrane antigens to render them immunogenic. In other cases passive adsorption of virus particles on to the red cell membrane may provoke an increased rate of clearance of red cells by the reticulo-endothelial system.

Thrombocytopenia

Mild-moderate thrombocytopenia is a frequent observation in patients with acute viral illnesses. Purpura may result from the combination of changes in local vascular integrity and mild thrombocytopenia. In addition viral infections may induce impaired platelet function by unknown mechanisms. The mechanisms causing thrombocytopenia are variable and also poorly understood. Some recognised mechanisms are as follows: the thrombocytopenia may occur as part of a DIC syndrome. Some viruses cause direct infection of megakaryocytes causing impairment of their function, e.g. measles, rubella, CMV, EBV.

Passive adsorption of immune complexes on to platelet membrane may lead to increased clearance by the reticulo-endothelial system.

Haemostatic changes

DIC is an occasional serious complication of common acute viral infections, and a common complication of infection with the arboviruses causing viral haemorrhagic fevers. Haemolytic uraemic syndrome or thrombotic thrombocytopenia purpura may follow acute viral illnesses.

Infectious mononucleosis

This condition has characteristic clinical and haematological changes due to acute infection with the Epstein-Barr virus. The syndrome most commonly occurs in late adolescence or early adulthood in individuals who did not acquire the infection in earlier life.

Clinical features

The incubation period is 4–8 weeks. Initially a flu-like illness with sweats, chills and fever is accompanied by general malaise, headache and anorexia. Within 1–3 days the individual develops a sore throat and generalised tender lymphadenopathy. About 10% of patients develop a transient erythematous or macular rash. Clinical examination shows an ill patient with fever of 38–40°C and either accompanying bradycardia or a normal heart rate rather than tachycardia. The throat is inflamed and oedematous and a tonsillar exudate is commonly seen. Small purpuric lesions on the soft palpate may occur. The lymph nodes are palpable as discrete, mobile tender nodes in the neck, supraclavicular fossae and axillae. Half the patients have a palpable spleen. Hepatomegaly with or without jaundice may occur. The acute illness is self-limiting in 1–2 weeks in the majority of individuals. This may be followed in some patients by a protracted period of lethargy and fatigue.

Complications. Table 29.13 lists the possible complications of acute infectious mononucleosis. Complications are rare but some of them are serious.

Table 29.13 Complications of infectious mononucleosis

Thrombocytopenia	Immune complex adsorption to platelet membrane
Haemolytic anaemia	Anti-i antibody (detectable in 50% patients) but titre high enough to cause haemolysis in only 1–2% patients
Aplastic anaemia	Very rare
Ruptured spleen	2nd–3rd week – Rare
Hepatitis	Transient jaundice in up to 10% More serious hepatitis in small proportion
CNS complications	Encephalitis, meningo-encephalitis, meningitis, Guillain-Barré syndrome, peripheral neuropathy, Bell's palsy
Myocarditis	Rare; transient ECG abnormalities not uncommon

Laboratory features

During the first week the white cell count is usually normal or only slightly elevated. By the end of the second week it has usually risen to 10–$30 \times 10^9/l$. Over 70% of the leukocytes are large, atypical lymphocytes (Plate 29). They are variable in shape and size and have an irregular cytoplasmic outline. The nucleus is large with a coarse chromatin pattern and occasional nucleoli may be seen. The cytoplasm is basophilic with occasional eosinophilic granules. Mild neutropenia and thrombocytopenia may accompany the lymphocytosis.

The diagnosis can be confirmed by demonstrating the presence of heterophile antibodies which react with antigens from a variety of species. The antigens are glycolipids present on red cells and in tissues of a variety of animals, bacteria and plants. Heterophile antibodies

may be detected by the Paul-Bunnell test or a rapid system, the Monospot. These heterophile antibody tests are positive in 75–80% of patients during the acute illness with relatively good specificity and a low false-positive rate. Specific serological tests to detect antibodies to various EBV antigens are also available.

Treatment

There is no specific treatment for the acute illness and none is usually necessary, since it is self-limiting. Corticosteroids have been used for serious complications such as encephalitis, Guillain-Barré syndrome, hepatitis, and so on.

Pathogenesis

The infection is probably transmitted in infected saliva. The infectivity is relatively low and thus requires close contact such as kissing. The virus passes via the oropharyngeal mucosa to B-lymphocytes of the tonsils and the tissues of Waldeyer's ring. Subsequently it passes into lymphoid tissue throughout the body. Infection of B-lymphocytes causes their proliferation and a state of polyclonal B-cell activation, with further production and shedding of virus. A specific immune response against the EBV viral antigens follows. The atypical lymphocytosis of the peripheral blood represents proliferation of T-cells in an aggressive cell-mediated immune response directed against the infected B-cells.

Heterophile antibody-negative infectious mononucleosis

An acute clinical syndrome of sore throat, fever, generalised lymphadenopathy and splenomegaly may occur in individuals who remain seronegative for heterophile antibodies. Agents proven to cause this form of 'seronegative infectious mononucleosis' include cytomegalovirus, *Toxoplasmosis gondii*, rubella virus, adenovirus, human immunodeficiency virus and occasionally EBV itself.

The frequency of development of the full clinical syndrome due to primary infection with these agents is much lower than for EBV and incomplete clinical patterns are fairly common. The specific diagnosis can often, but not always, be made by demonstrating a rising titre of antibody to the relevant infectious agent.

Cytomegalovirus infection

This virus causes clinical illness in a variety of settings. In the normal population primary infection is commonly subclinical. Some individuals develop a mononucleosis-like syndrome which is self-limiting. The situations in which CMV infection are most serious are in the unborn fetus and in immunosuppressed patients.

Clinical features

A self-limiting acute illness with many similarities to infectious mononucleosis (IM) may occur in adolescents or adults who acquire CMV. The constitutional upset parallels IM but lymphadenopathy and pharyngeal involvement are usually less severe. A similar pattern of atypical lymphocytosis is seen. The complications are listed in Table 29.14; all are rare.

Table 29.14 Complications of primary CMV infection

Pneumonitis
Myocarditis
Polyneuritis
Inner ear damage
Hepatitis
Polyarthritis
Cold agglutinin haemolytic anaemia

A similar clinical illness may appear 4–12 weeks after a blood transfusion in susceptible individuals who receive blood or blood products from a CMV-positive donation. The condition is largely avoided, however, by transfusing blood that is greater than 2 days old, since CMV will not survive longer than this in stored blood.

Congenital CMV infection. About 1% of neonates are positive for CMV but only rarely does it cause clinical illness. Anaemia and thrombocytopenia may persist for several weeks. Jaundice, hepatosplenomegaly, chorioretinitis, microcephaly and pneumonitis may occasionally be recognised. The diagnosis is confirmed by positive CMV cultures from urine or other body secretions such as throat swabs. Alternatively, typical CMV intranuclear inclusion bodies may be identified in cells of the CSF or in urinary casts.

CMV infection in immunosuppressed patients. Rapidly progressive pneumonitis, hepatitis, renal failure and damage to other tissues may occur due to reactivation of latent CMV, primary acquisition of CMV from blood or blood products, or from a transplanted organ. The disease is rapidly fatal in a high proportion of cases. There are no specific laboratory findings and the atypical lymphocytosis is not seen. The diagnosis is confirmed by direct CMV isolation from body secretions or biopsies. The characteristic inclusion bodies may be identified. Treatment with a specific antiviral agent, e.g. gancyclovir, along with hyperimmune CMV-specific immunoglobulin, although still experimental, appears to improve the prognosis when administered in the early

stages. However, prevention is obviously most important. Patients requiring severe immunosuppression for organ transplantation should be screened for the presence of CMV-specific antibodies. Patients who are found to be antibody-negative should receive blood and blood products from CMV-antibody-negative donors. Unfortunately there is no method of preventing reactivation of infection in individuals who have previously acquired the virus.

Parvovirus B19 infection

The human parvovirus B19 (HPV B19) was initially identified serologically in blood donors. In otherwise healthy children it causes the acute exanthematous illness known as fifth disease. A similar illness may occur in susceptible adults but the rash is less prominent and generalised arthralgia more frequent. HPV B19 is highly contagious and intermittent pandemics occur. The majority of adults have subclinical infection. Virus is shed from the throat and urine and also contaminates donated blood.

The most serious consequence of HBV B19 infection is that it causes the transient aplastic crisis of sickle cell disease, hereditary spherocytosis and other severe haemolytic disorders. Reticulocytopenia is an almost inevitable consequence of HPV B19 infection. This may go unnoticed in individuals with normal red cell survival, but provokes a precipitous fall in haemoglobin in patients with haemolytic anaemia. The virus has a cytotoxic effect on erythroid progenitor cells, causing abrupt inhibition of erythropoiesis. Severe red cell aplasia may occur in immunocompromised individuals. Less commonly HPV B19 infects granulopoietic or megakaryocytic cell lines, causing transient leukopenia or thrombocytopenia, usually associated with reticulocytopenia.

Hepatitis viruses

The hepatitis viruses, hepatitis A virus, hepatitis B virus and non-A non-B hepatitis viruses only rarely cause serious haematological complications. In the majority of cases moderate neutropenia with a relative or absolute lymphocytosis are the only haematological findings. The red cell survival is shortened in up to 70% of patients but overt haemolytic anaemia occurs only occasionally. In most cases of haemolytic anaemia the Coomb's test is positive. Acute severe intravascular haemolysis may occur in patients with glucose-6-phosphate dehydrogenase deficiency. The most serious haematological complication of hepatitis virus infections is aplastic anaemia. Fortunately this complication is rare, occurring in <0.3% of cases of acute viral hepatitis. Hepatitis A virus is most commonly implicated. The majority of patients are adolescents or young adults. The onset is within 10 weeks of the onset of the hepatitis. The mortality is 90% or higher, even with bone marrow transplantation. In survivors full haematological recovery occurs between 3 and 24 months after the onset.

Viral haemorrhagic fevers

A variety of arboviruses and arenaviruses may cause acute haemorrhagic illnesses in different parts of the world. These viruses are transmitted by blood-sucking arthropods or through close contact with secretions or excreta of infected rodents. A simplified classification is outlined in Table 29.15.

Table 29.15 Classification of viral haemorrhagic fevers

Arboviruses (transmitted via infected mosquitoes)	
Togaviruses	Africa, India, Thailand
Dengue-virus group	SE Asia
Flaviviruses	Yellow fever – Africa
	S America
Arenaviruses (transmitted via infected rodents)	
Argentinian haemorrhagic fever	S America
Bolivian haemorrhagic fever	S America
Lassa fever	W Africa
Others	Central and S America
	W Africa

The clinical features range from a mild dengue-like illness with headache, fever, myalgia, rash, leukopenia and thrombocytopenia, to a severe haemorrhagic illness with respiratory symptoms and severe bleeding diathesis associated with severe constitutional symptoms. Bleeding is manifested by purpura and ecchymoses, mucous membrane and gastrointestinal bleeding, and frequently fatal bleeding into major organs. The bleeding diathesis is characterised by generalised fibrin deposition, severe thrombocytopenia, prolongation of in vitro coagulation tests and deficiency of various clotting factors such as V and VII. Thus the pathogenesis is essentially that of a severe form of disseminated intravascular coagulation. Early administration of heparin leads to a dramatic clinical improvement in some forms of viral haemorrhagic fever. Treatment is otherwise based on intensive support measures including blood and blood-product therapy. Convalescent plasma, containing neutralising antibodies, may be of value in some forms such as Lassa fever, Marburg-Ebola virus disease and Argentinian and Bolivian haemorrhagic fevers.

Human retrovirus infections

Two main forms of retrovirus are known to cause serious illness in humans: human T-cell leukaemia/lymphoma virus I (HTLV-I) and human immunodeficiency virus (HIV); see Chapters 15, 16 and 22.

These viruses have several common properties. They have tropism for the CD4 antigen expressed on helper/inducer T-lymphocytes, the CD4 molecule acting as the viral receptor. On gaining entry to the cell they are able to incorporate their RNA genetic material into the DNA of the cell's nucleus by the activity of a unique enzyme, reverse transcriptase. Subsequently, after a protracted period of latency, they induce clinical disease in a variable proportion of individuals. The two viruses are contrasted in that HTLV-I induces transformation of T-cells, causing a lymphoproliferative disorder, whereas HIV produces a cytolytic effect, leading to helper T-cell depletion and immunodeficiency. The modes of transmission are identical, i.e close sexual contact, mother to fetus, and blood borne from contaminated instruments, needles, etc., or blood and blood products. HTLV-I has been recognised as the aetiological agent of adult T-cell leukaemia in Japan and other parts of SE Asia and also in parts of the Caribbean. Sporadic cases are recognised worldwide. HTLV-I may also cause a slowly progressive myelopathy. HIV is the aetiological agent of the present pandemic of the acquired immune deficiency syndrome (AIDS). Another retrovirus, closely related to HTLV-I, and termed HTLV-II, has been implicated as the aetiological agent of T-cell hairy cell leukaemia in two case reports.

PROTOZOAN INFECTIONS

Toxoplasmosis

Primary acquired *Toxoplasma gondii* infection produces a clinical syndrome very similar to infectious mononucleosis in otherwise healthy individuals. Fever, malaise, generalised lymphadenopathy and hepatosplenomegaly are accompanied by an atypical lymphocytosis or occasionally monocytosis. Myocarditis is a rare complication. In healthy individuals subclinical infections are not uncommon. However, immunosuppressed individuals are at risk of life-threatening disseminated toxoplasmosis. Generalised tissue involvement occurs with free organisms and cysts present in brain, heart, lungs, kidneys and other organs. Congenital infection may cause hydrops fetalis, or a syndrome of generalised lymphadenopathy, hepatosplenomegaly, rash and severe occular and neurological damage. The diagnosis is confirmed by identifying the organism or its cysts in tissue biopsy specimens or by a rising titre of specific antibody. Treatment for neurological or eye infection in immunosuppressed patients is with a sulphonamide plus pyrimethamine.

Malaria

Malaria is caused by four different species of *Plasmodium* transmitted by the bite of the female anopheline mosquito. A variety of haematological changes may occur depending on the type and circumstances of infection. Anaemia occurs in all types of infection. The pathogenesis is complex and includes direct red cell disruption by parasite infection, haemolysis due to splenic sequestration, immune complex adsorption to red cell membranes, and adverse effects of drugs on parasitized red cells. Secondary folate deficiency and transient episodes of erythroid hypoplasia may also occur.

Severe fulminating intravascular haemolysis (Blackwater fever) leading to a precipitous fall in haemoglobin, with haemoglobinuria and acute renal failure, is a well-recognised complication of *P. falciparum* infection. It is often provoked by initiation of treatment with quinine. Severe disseminated intravascular coagulation is a frequent accompanying complication.

Leukocyte changes in acute malaria infection are common. Mild-moderate leukopenia is most common. Falciparum malaria may be accompanied by marked neutropenia with shift to the left and relative or absolute monocytosis. Mild thrombocytopenia with platelet counts in the range 60–120 $\times 10^9$/l are also frequently observed. This may be due to DIC, splenic sequestration or macrophage destruction of platelets with passively adsorbed immune complexes.

The diagnosis depends on examination of well-prepared thick and thin blood films to identify the erythrocytic phase of the infection. Ring forms, trophozoites, schizonts and gametocytes may be recognised in Vivax, Malariae, and Ovale infection. Falciparum infection is characterised by the presence of many ring forms with double or multiple infections of erythrocytes, double chromatin dots in the ring forms and crescent shaped gametocytes; trophozoites and schizonts are are rarely seen.

Treatment requires prompt administration of anti-malarial chemotherapy with supportive measures. Falciparum infection may be rapidly fatal and should be considered as a medical emergency. Chloroquine remains the first choice treatment in areas in which chloroquine-resistance has not occurred. In chloroquine-resistant areas (e.g. S America, NE India, E Africa and SE Asia) quinine is administered for severe infections.

Leishmaniasis

Visceral leishmaniasis (Kala Azar) is caused by *Leishmania donovanii* transmitted by the bite of infected sandflies. The clinical features include episodic fever, malaise, weight loss, lymphadenopathy and hepatosplenomegaly. Accompanying pancytopenia commonly occurs. The condition may mimic a variety of primary haematological disorders. There may be gross splenomegaly which, associated with pancytopenia, may be mistaken for myelofibrosis. The bone marrow and spleen, as well as other tissues, may be heavily infiltrated with parasite-laden macrophages. The diagnosis is confirmed by identifying Leishman-Donovan bodies in the bone marrow or spleen. Serological tests may also be useful. Treatment is with antimonial agents such as stibogluconate, meglumine antimoniate or with pentamidine or amphotericin.

Trypanosomiasis

African trypanosomiasis is caused by *Trypanosoma rhodesiense* and *gambiense* transmitted by the bite of the tsetse fly. The clinical features include fever, headache, peripheral oedema, lymphadenopathy and splenomegaly. Severe infection – with CNS involvement – is rapidly fatal. The diagnosis is confirmed by identification of the organism on a well-prepared blood film. Treatment with suramin, pentamidine or melarsoprol may be curative if administered before cerebral involvement begins.

American trypanosomiasis is caused by *Trypanosoma cruzi* transmitted by the faeces of reduviid bugs, which enters skin abrasions or mucosal surfaces such as the conjunctiva. Severe conjunctivitis with gross oedema of the eye is followed by development of generalised lymphadenopathy, hepatosplenomegaly and subsequently severe brain, cardiac and gastrointestinal complications. Parasites are identified during the acute febrile episodes on a well-prepared blood film. Treatment with nifurtimox is curative in the majority of cases. Elimination of the reduviid bugs with gamma benzylhexachloride from houses may prevent recurrences.

HELMINTHIC INFECTIONS

The characteristic haematological finding in helminthic infections is the appearance of eosinophilia. This is most prominent during the early systemic phase of these illnesses. Persistent eosinophilia usually accompanies the more chronic gastrointestinal complications. In the investigation of a patient with eosinophilia it is important to note that these parasites may not be recognised in stool samples for many weeks or months and repeated examination over a protracted period may be required to make a positive diagnosis.

Hookworm infestation of the intestine is probably the commonest cause of iron deficiency anaemia worldwide. The adult worms directly utilise iron and may also cause chronic gastrointestinal blood loss.

BIBLIOGRAPHY

Bagby J C 1987 Haematologic aspects of systemic disease. Haematology/Oncology Clinics of North America 1 (no. 2)
Bunch C, Weatherall D J 1982 The haematological manifestations of systemic disease. In: Hardisty, R M, Weatherall D J (eds) Blood and its disorders, 2nd edn. Blackwell Scientific Publications, ch. 33
Lee G R 1983 The anaemia of chronic disease. Seminars in Haematology 20: 61–80
Lew D P 1988 Haematological aspects of infectious diseases. Parts 1 and 2. Seminars in Haematology 25 (nos. 2 and 3)

Haemostatic disorders

30. Platelets

C. A. Ludlam   H. H. K. Watson

The integrity of the vascular system is dependent upon the presence of adequate numbers of functional platelets. These interact with plasma coagulation factors and elements of the vessel wall in a complex sequence of reactions to prevent bleeding (Fig. 30.1). The individual biochemical mechanisms leading to adhesion of platelets to vessel walls and aggregation of platelets to form a primary haemostatic plug are well characterised. As the structure and function of normal platelets are well understood, it has been possible to identify the underlying biochemical defect in many of the more common congenital platelet disorders.

Platelet stucture

After their release from megakaryocytes (Fig. 30.2) in the bone marrow platelets circulate in the blood for 8–10 days as biconvex discs with a normal concentration in the range $150-350 \times 10^9/l$. For the purpose of describing the structure of the platelet, it can be conveniently divided into distinct areas (Fig. 30.3).

The peripheral zone comprises the plasma membrane with an associated glycocalyx on the exterior surface and an underlying circumferential band of microtubules. The phospholipid bilayer of the membrane plays an integral part in the events of coagulation, providing an environment which facilitates interaction with plasma coagulation factors. The surface-connected open canalicular system represents invaginations of the membrane and provides a channel for the uptake of substances and the discharge of granule contents during the platelet release reaction. In the resting state platelets are maintained in their discoid form by the microtubules and their associated microfilaments (Fig. 30.3). During aggregation platelets assume a spherical form and extend pseudopods from the surface membrane to facilitate platelet-platelet contact. The glycocalyx is rich in glycoproteins (GP), some of which function as receptors for various agonists transmitting signals to the interior of the platelet. Many of the glycoproteins have been well

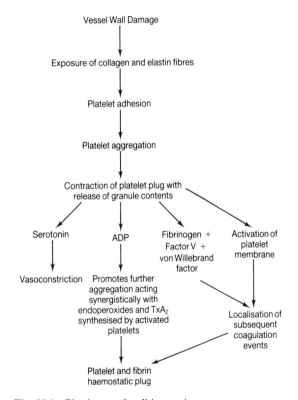

Fig. 30.1   Platelet vessel wall interaction.

characterised but their roles as receptors are still poorly understood. However, it is well established that GpIb together with plasma von Willebrand factor mediates platelet adhesion to the subendothelium whilst the GpIIb-IIIa complex acts as a receptor for fibrinogen during platelet aggregation (Fig. 30.4). A thrombin receptor on the platelet surface has been identified as GpIb.

The cytoplasm of the platelet contains organelles. The smallest and most abundant of these are the glycogen

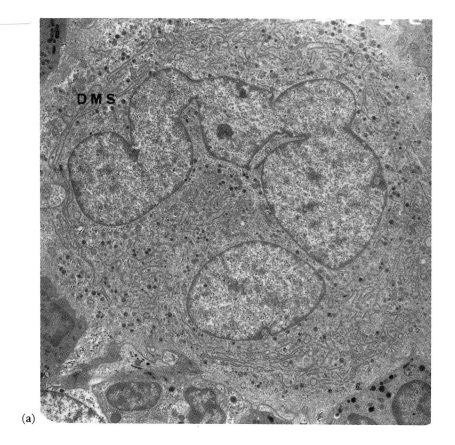

(a)

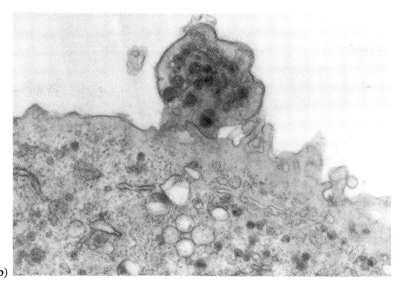

(b)

Fig. 30.2 Electronmicrograph of megakaryocyte with multilobed nucleus. Numerous alpha granules occupy the cytoplasm. A complex membrane system is present (**a**). Platelets form at the periphery by fusion of the demarcation membrane system (DMS) by budding (**b**).

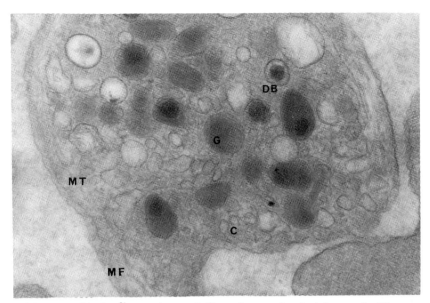

Fig. 30.3 Platelet electronmicrograph illustrating cytoplasmic alpha granules (G), dense bodies (DB) and open canalicular system (C). Microtubules (MT) and thin microfilaments (MF) are aligned in a circumferential manner.

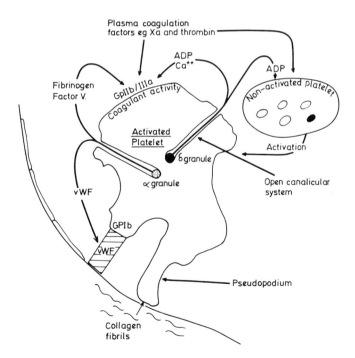

Fig. 30.4 Diagrammatic representation of platelet adhesion, and activation and development of surface coagulant activity.

storage granules and their presence, together with that of mitochondria, indicates that platelet metabolic energy is derived from glycolysis. The cytoplasm is also rich in microtubules and microfilaments; actin is the major protein component of the microfilaments and together with myosin controls platelet shape. Following stimulation actin and myosin interact, inducing the platelets to become spherical and extrude long pseudopodia; storage granules are moved to the centre of the cell before discharging their contents to the exterior via the open canalicular system.

In addition to the open canalicular system platelets possess a second membrane system located in the cytoplasm, the dense tubule system. This system appears to be derived from the smooth endoplasmic reticulum of the megakaryocyte and in addition to storing Ca^{2+} and providing arachidonic acid it may be involved in the maintenace of platelet shape.

Three major types of storage granules have been described in platelets (Table 30.1). The dense or δ-granules are the principal storage site for amines and calcium, whilst the α-granules contain a variety of proteins, some of which are unique to platelets. The lysosomal granules store acid hydrolases. Substances liberated from the dense granules during the release reaction, e.g. ADP, cause neighbouring platelets to aggregate and release; this is observed during the second phase in platelet aggregation studies in vitro. It is generally believed that α-granule proteins are involved in the promotion of coagulation, haemostasis and tissue repair.

Table 30.1 Platelet granule constituents

α-granules	δ-granules	lysosomes
Fibrinogen	Serotonin	Glucuronidase
Factor V	ADP/ATP	Galactosidase
von Willebrand factor	Ca^{++}	Elastase
Plasminogen	Mg^{++}	Collagenase
Fibronectin		
α_2-antiplasmin		
β-thromboglobulin		
Platelet factor 4		
Thrombospondin		
Platelet-derived growth factor		

Metabolism

The ability of the platelet to respond to an agonist is dependent on the efficient operation of a complex sequence of biochemical events initiated by activation of phospholipase C. Calcium appears to behave as an intracellular mediator linking the external stimulus to the ob-

served platelet responses, whilst cAMP promotes inhibitory response within the platelet (Fig. 30.5).

In the resting state most intra-platelet Ca^{2+} is located within the dense granules and the dense tubular system. Stimulation of the platelet results in an increase in the availability of free Ca^{2+} in the cytosol where it binds to calmodulin which activates the light chain of myosin.

The ability of Ca^{2+} and cAMP to act as messengers within the platelet, regulating stimulation and inhibition of aggregation respectively, is dependent on their potential to influence arachidonic acid metabolism within the platelet. Arachidonic acid is released from membrane phospholipid, particularly that of the dense tubule system, by Ca^{2+}-stimulated phospholipase A_2. In the normal platelet arachidonic acid is converted to the endoperoxides PGG_2 and PGH_2 by the action of cyclooxygenase. Both of these possess pro-aggregatory activity and are further metabolised to another pro-aggregant, TXA_2 by thromboxane synthetase (Fig. 30.6). The net effect of the production of TXA_2 is to stimulate the release reaction in activated platelets. Substances so liberated, e.g. ADP, induce the activation of further platelets, thus enhancing the process. The effect of the release reaction is observed as the second phase of aggregation and is irreversible. Aspirin acetylates and irreversibly inhibits cyclo-oxygenase. The subsequent impairment of arachidonic acid metabolism is responsible for the inability of the affected platelet to respond normally to aggregating agents. Similarly, inhibition of the thromboxane synthetase redirects the endoperoxides PGG_2 and PGH_2 into the formation of PGE_2 and PGD_2, which are inhibitors of platelet aggregation. Endoperoxides may also diffuse out of platelets and be converted by the endothelial cells to PGI_2 which is also a potent inhibitor of platelet aggregation.

CLINICAL PRESENTATION OF PLATELET DISORDERS

Mucocutaneous bleeding with easy bruising, epistaxis and gastrointestinal haemorrhage are characteristic of platelet disorders. Purpura is usually only observed with thrombocytopenia, and is only rarely seen with qualitative platelet disorders. Individuals with myeloproliferative disorders, e.g. essential thrombocythaemia, may on the other hand present with major arterial occlusion or digital ischaemia due to the production of hyperactive platelets. Of the congenital disorders many are recessively inherited. Important aspects of the history and clinical examination of a patient suspected of having a platelet disorder are given in Chapter 8. A full and careful drug history is essential, for many medicines either inhibit platelet function or cause

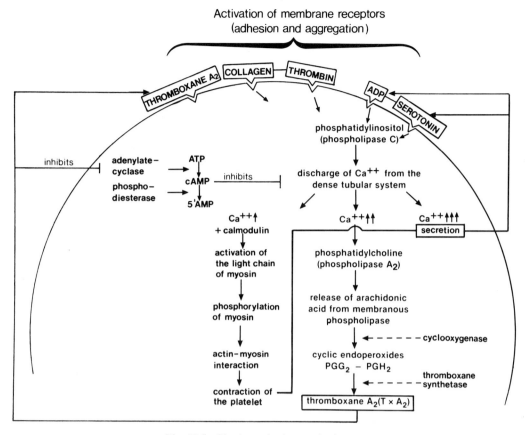

Fig. 30.5 Platelet activation mechanisms.

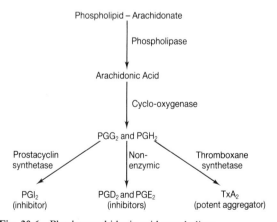

Fig. 30.6 Platelet arachidonic acid metabolism.

thrombocytopenia. A drug with mild antiplatelet activity may cause clinically significant bleeding by unmasking a previously undiagnosed platelet disorder.

A full general examination is necessary with particular attention to the documentation of purpura and bruising, or evidence of vascular ischaemia. Apart from attempting to exclude previously undiagnosed medical disorders care should be taken in assessing whether the patient has palpable splenomegaly or an enlarged liver. Rare congenital syndromes are associated with skeletal abnormalities or albinism and these, if present, are important clues to the diagnosis.

Initial investigation should include a platelet count, blood film and bleeding time (provided the platelet count is greater than $50 \times 10^9/l$), as well as a prothrombin time, APTT, fibrinogen and factor VIII activities, to exclude a coagulation disorder and von Willebrand's disease. Only then should specific tests of platelet function be undertaken. It is usual to undertake platelet aggregation assessment in vitro initially and to base further investigation upon the pattern of results obtained. In thrombocytopenic patients, a bone marrow is an essential investigation and an autologous platelet survival

Table 30.2   Causes of thrombocytopenia

Marrow disorders

Congenital thrombocytopenias Table 30.9

Hypoplasia
Infiltration   Leukaemia
                      Myeloma
                      Carcinoma
                      Myelofibrosis
                      Osteopetrosis

B_{12}/folate deficiency
Iron deficiency

Haemolytic anaemias

Micro-angiopathic anaemias
Evans' syndrome

Immune thrombocytopenias
See Table 30.6 and 30.7

Hypersplenism

Lymphomas
Congestive splenomegaly
    e.g. portal hypertension

Infections   Kala azar
                      Malaria

Storage disorders   Gaucher's disease
                      Niemann-Pick disease

Infections
Viral   Epstein-Barr virus
                      Cytomegalovirus
                      Human immunodeficiency virus
                      Rubella
                      Measles
                      Mumps
                      Herpes zoster (chicken pox)
                      Influenza

Rickettsial   Typhus
                      Rocky Mountain spotted fever

Bacterial   Gram negative septicaemia
                      Meningococcal septicaemia
                      Typhoid
                      Sub-acute bacterial endocarditis
                      Congenital syphilis
                      Brucellosis

Protozoa   Malaria
                      Toxoplasmosis
                      Trypanosomiasis

Other

Disseminated intravascular coagulation
Drugs – Table 30.7
Liver disease
Uraemia
Collagenoses, e.g. SLE
Vascular neoplasms, e.g. giant cavernous haemangioma
                      (Kasabach-Merritt Syndrome)
Extra-corporeal circulation
Massive blood transfusion
Heat stroke
Burns
Cyanotic congenital heart disease
Eclampsia
Hyperthyroidism

study often helps elucidate the mechanism causing the reduced platelet count.

THROMBOCYTOPENIA

In the majority of instances thrombocytopenia is but one manifestation of either a haematological disorder involving additional cell lines or a systemic disease (Table 30.2). Thus for most patients the cause of the reduced platelet count is easy to discern. Several mechanisms may contribute to the thrombocytopenia and in some patients it may be difficult to define the dominant cause. In alcoholics, for example, thrombocytopenia may be due to liver disease, depression of the bone marrow by alcohol, disseminated intravascular coagulation, splenic pooling or folate deficiency.

Isolated thrombocytopenia, in which the platelets appear morphologically normal, is relatively uncommon and the causes are listed in Table 30.3. Unless the patient has evidence of mucocutaneous bleeding it is often unwise to investigate a patient extensively until the thrombocytopenia has been confirmed by a repeat blood sample to enumerate the platelets. The causes of spurious thrombocytopenia are given in Table 30.4; a careful examination of the blood film will allow these to be identified. A coagulation screen should be undertaken in all patients to assess whether the thrombocytopenia is part of a generalised coagulopathy. Some of

Table 30.3   Causes of isolated thrombocytopenia with normal platelet morphology

Normal or increased megakaryocytes

Acute ITP
Chronic ITP
Neonatal ITP
Iso-immune neonatal thrombocytopenia
Drug-induced immune thrombocytopenia – Table 30.7
Infections – Tables 30.2 and 30.6
Post-transfusion purpura
Thrombotic thrombocytopenic purpura (TTP)
Haemolytic uraemic syndrome (HUS)
Disseminated intravascular coagulation (DIC)
Hypersplenism
Congenital thrombocytopenias — Table 30.9

Reduced megakaryocytes

Drugs   Cytotoxics – alkylating agents
                         – antimetabolites
             Non steroidal anti-inflammatory agents
             Chloramphenicol
             Thiazides

Alcohol

Cyclic thrombocytopenia
Thrombocytopenia with absent radius (TAR) syndrome
Idiopathic aplastic anaemia in evolution

Radiotherapy

Table 30.4   Causes of spurious thrombocytopenia

Platelet aggregates
   Inadequate sample collection – poor venepuncture

Platelet agglutinins
   Cold agglutinins
   EDTA-dependent agglutinins

Macrothrombocytes

Platelet satellism – platelets adhere to neutrophils

Table 30.5   Disorders associated with large or small platelets

Disorder	Other features
Macrothrombocytes	
May-Hegglin anomaly	White cells contain Döhle bodies
Bernard-Soulier syndrome	Ristocetin aggregation absent
Epstein's syndrome	Renal failure and nerve deafness
Montreal platelet syndrome	Spontaneous aggregation
Grey platelet syndrome	Large amorphous platelets without α granules
Myeloproliferative disorders	Polycythaemia, leukocytosis and splenomegaly
Microthrombocytes	
Wiscott-Aldrich syndrome	Eczema
	IgM deficiency
	Recurrent infections
Iron deficiency	

the congenital platelet syndromes, particularly those with large platelets (macrothrombocytes), can be diagnosed from the blood film (Table 30.5). If thrombocytopenia is associated with normal platelet morphology, a bone marrow aspirate will be required to assess the number and morphology of the megakaryocytes.

A bone marrow possessing normal or increased numbers of megakaryocytes indicates that the thrombocytopenia is either due to increased destruction or abnormal pooling of platelets within the circulation or spleen or that platelet production is ineffective, as in megaloblastic anaemias. A decreased number of megakaryocytes implies reduced production of platelets as the cause of the thrombocytopenia. Furthermore, the

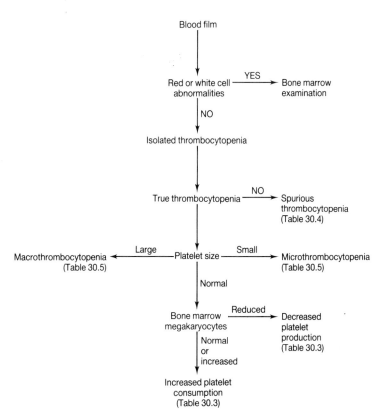

Fig. 30.7   Investigation of apparent thrombocytopenia.

marrow aspirate may allow diagnosis of an underlying disorder, e.g. leukaemia or carcinomatous infiltrate. A scheme for investigating thrombocytopenia is given in Fig. 30.7. and this forms the basis for the classification of thrombocytopenia in this chapter.

THROMBOCYTOPENIA WITH NORMAL PLATELET SIZE

In the majority of cases of thrombocytopenia platelet size appears normal on a well-spread peripheral blood film. In such instances, to assist in the elucidation of the mechanism and possible cause, a bone marrow examination is required. Although a smear from an aspirate will give a quick estimate of megakaryocyte numbers as well as morphology, a trephine biopsy allows a more reliable assessment. Such a biopsy may also provide crucial information about other cell lines or evidence of infiltration by non-haematological cells; this may not be readily discernible on a marrow smear.

Normal or increased numbers of megakaryocytes in bone marrow

Thrombocytopenia with normal or increased megakaryocyte (Fig. 30.8) numbers signifies:

1. increased platelet consumption
2. splenic pooling
3. ineffective platelet production

For splenic pooling to result in significant thrombocytopenia the spleen is usually palpable but marrow examination is still useful, however, to confirm that there are a reasonable number of megakaryocytes and that marrow hypoplasia is not contributing to the

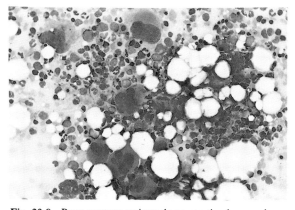

Fig. 30.8 Bone marrow aspirate demonstrating increased numbers of megakaryocytes.

thrombocytopenia. When reasonable numbers of megakaryocytes are present it is sometimes difficult to know whether platelet production is effective. Hypersegmented megakaryocytic nuclei, which may be multilobed, indicate a primary megakaryocyte defect as the cause of the thrombocytopenia. Evidence of dysplasia in the myeloid or erythroid cell lines, particularly the presence of megaloblastic or sideroblastic change, would further indicate failure of marrow platelet production as the cause of thrombocytopenia.

In conditions of thrombocytopenia with normal erythroid and myeloid precursors and normal numbers of megakaryocytes of either normal morphology or cells with large, poorly defined immature nuclei, it is reasonable to assume that there is increased consumption or sequestration of platelets within the circulation (Table 30.3). In some instances measurement of autologous platelet survival will assist in discerning the mechanism of the reduced platelet count.

Idiopathic thrombocytopenic purpura (ITP)

Idiopathic thrombocytopenic purpura is due to the premature removal by the reticulo-endothelial system of platelets coated with antibody. These auto-antibodies may either be idiopathic or drug-induced and react with a platelet membrane component. Alternatively, circulating immune complexes may adhere via Fc receptors on the platelet membrane. It can be very difficult to distinguish between auto-antibodies and immune complexes because the only techniques that are readily available measure total platelet or membrane-associated immunoglobulin. They do not distinguish between immunoglobulin alone and when it is part of an immune complex. The specificity of most antibodies for the different membrane components is unknown in most instances, although some are directed against the glycoprotein IIb/IIIa complex. Specific immunoglobulins associated with platelets can be quantitated; in most patients IgG can be detected and in some IgM and the C3 component of complement is also present. It is likely that these are true auto-antibodies and are of polyclonal type containing a mixture of immunoglobulin subclasses. Splenic macrophages recognise the Fc portion of the IgG resulting in adherence and phagocytosis. Liver macrophages have receptors for IgM and C3 and this organ may be the site of destruction of platelets which are coated with these molecules. The amount of platelet-associated IgG is inversely related to the platelet count and platelet survival time. Cell-mediated immunity may also be disturbed and contribute to the premature destruction of platelets. Rarely ITP and warm auto-immune haemolytic anaemia present in the same individual either simultaneously or consecutively. This combination has been termed Evans' syndrome and can be particularly resistant to treatment. These two conditions may be viewed as being at opposite ends of a continuum, with Evans' syndrome in the centre.

Although the predisposition to haemorrhage in ITP is related to the degree of thrombocytopenia, the amount of bleeding is often less than would be anticipated for the platelet count. Many individuals have platelet levels of $10–20 \times 10^9/l$ for prolonged periods without any symptoms other than an occasional spontaneous bruise. The lifespan of the platelets is very short, often only a few hours, and most of the circulating cells are therefore recently released from the marrow and are of above average size and are metabolically very active; consequently they are effective in securing haemostasis. In an occasional patient bleeding is noted at a platelet count of $50 \times 10^9/l$ and this may be due to the antibody inhibiting platelet function inducing a storage pool type disorder. There are thus two mechanisms working to opposite effect which modify platelet function in ITP; the young platelets being metabolically more active but the auto-antibody tending to impair functional integrity.

Clinically ITP can be divided into an acute, usually self-limiting, condition, and a more chronic disorder in which the onset of clinical symptoms is often more gradual.

Acute ITP

Purpura, ecchymoses, epistaxis and bleeding gums appear abruptly. This syndrome occurs predominantly in children up to their mid-teens, although it is not infrequently seen in young adults and occasionally in the elderly. It affects both sexes equally in childhood. A history of upper respiratory infection within the previous 2 weeks is common but it may be difficult to assess the significance of this as head colds are common in children. Occasionally thrombocytopenia may be a manifestation of a well-characterised viral infection, e.g. EBV, CMV, HIV, measles, mumps, etc. (Table 30.6). Additional mechanisms may predispose to thrombocytopenia with viral infections. These include damage by virus to endothelial cells, megakaryocytes or platelets, viral-antibody complex coating of platelets with premature phagocytosis by the RES, loss of sialic acid from the platelet surface by viral neuraminidase, or mild viral-induced DIC. Enquiry should be made about a family history of bleeding and platelet counts undertaken on siblings and parents. A scrupulous drug history is mandatory.

Table 30.6 Diseases associated with ITP

Viral infections	Epstein-Barr virus
	Cytomegalovirus
	Human immunodeficiency virus
	Acute childhood exanthemata
Autoimmune disorders	Autoimmune haemolytic anaemia (Evans' syndrome)
	SLE
	Rheumatoid arthritis
	Scleroderma
	Thyrotoxicosis
	Hashimoto's thyroiditis
Lymphoproliferative disorders	Hodgkin's disease
	Non-Hodgkin's lymphoma
	Chronic lymphocytic leukaemia
Miscellaneous	Sarcoidosis

The blood film is usually normal apart from the thrombocytopenia. The platelets may appear a little larger than normal, this being a megakaryocytic response to the thrombocytopenia. A mild eosinophilia may occasionally be observed, as may atypical lymphocytes. A bone marrow aspirate will reveal a marked increase in megakaryocytes.

Course and therapy

Without any specific therapy half of the children will spontaneously remit within 4 weeks, with about 85% being in remission at 4 months; serious or fatal haemorrhage is very rare.

If bleeding is confined to moderate purpura and ecchymoses, it is reasonable to observe the child. Situations likely to lead to trauma should be avoided so far as possible. The place of steroid therapy in children with this condition remains controversial. With steroids haemorrhage stops promptly and after a few days the platelet count increases. The mechanism by which the capillary bleeding ceases before the rise in platelet count is observed is unknown. Steroids are known to decrease synthesis of PgI_2 by endothelial cells, as well as increase fibronectin secretion; both mechanisms would tend to decrease the likelihood of haemorrhage. The steroids will also decrease both the adherence of auto-antibody to platelets, and phagocytosis of antibody-coated platelets by reticulo-endothelial cells. Synthesis of antiplatelet antibody by the spleen is also reduced. If the child has only moderate purpura and ecchymoses, and has no gastrointestinal haemorrhage or prolonged epistaxis, withholding steroids is reasonable. Children with profuse bleeding, especially of the gums, gastrointestinal tract or epistaxis, should receive prednisolone 1–2 mg/kg/day. It should be quickly withdrawn as soon as the platelet count returns to normal.

Failure of the platelet count to remit either spontaneously or with steroids in 2–3 weeks necessitates re-examination of the diagnosis. This should begin with a review of the history. Symptoms which begin gradually, especially those associated with a history of mild bleeding for some time, should raise the suspicion that the thrombocytopenia may have been of longer duration than previously thought. The possibility of a congenital or familial platelet disorder should be considered and platelet counts performed on other available family members. The drug history should be reviewed. The patient should be re-examined very carefully, in particular to seek evidence of any other disease which might predispose to thrombocytopenia, e.g. lymphoma. A recent blood film should be reviewed to seek evidence of other haematological abnormalities, e.g. erythrocyte fragments in thrombotic thrombocytopenic purpura. Likewise, re-inspection of the original bone marrow and possibly a trephine biopsy may be helpful. If after re-assessing the evidence the diagnosis remains that of ITP, then the dose of steroids should be increased to 2 mg/kg/day for 2 weeks.

Failure of the platelet count to revert towards normal at this higher dose of steroids would be an indication for splenectomy. Splenectomy should also be considered for patients who, although initially responding to steroids, relapse on two occasions after stopping or reducing prednisolone. The chance of remission after splenectomy is said to be better if it is carried out within 6 months of the patient's presentation.

Prior to splenectomy an autologous (if possible) radio-isotope platelet survival study characteristically demonstrates a greatly shortened platelet lifespan and strengthens the case for splenectomy. Controversy surrounds the value of assessing the principal site of platelet destruction by measuring the isotope uptake into liver and spleen. Splenectomy is often of value in alleviating the thrombocytopenia, even when the principal site of sequestration appears to be the liver. If the aetiology of childhood ITP were better understood and the mechanisms leading to platelet destruction by the reticulo-endothelial system were more fully identified, it might be easier to design rational therapy.

If clinically significant thrombocytopenia persists after splenectomy, the patient should be treated as for chronic ITP which persists post-splenectomy. In a child it should be borne in mind that the long-term use of cytotoxic drugs may have a very deleterious effect upon development.

Chronic ITP

This condition predominantly affects adults, and females approximately four times more commonly than males. Platelet auto-antibodies, synthesised by splenic lymphocytes, directed against components of the platelet membrane result in premature removal of circulating cells by reticulo-endothelial phagocytosis.

The usual mode of presentation is of gradually increasing purpura, ecchymoses or other mucocutaneous bleeding. Often there may be quite a prolonged history of excessive bleeding, sometimes of several years' duration. Unlike the acute variety, a preceeding viral illness is uncommon. It is still important to enquire about antecedent illnesses, because a subset of patients exists in whom ITP is the initial presenting feature of a more extensive systemic illness (Tables 30.6). Collagen disorders not infrequently present with thrombocytopenia and it is therefore important to enquire about joint, eye and skin complaints.

Examination usually only reveals evidence of purpura or ecchymoses. Buccal and fundal haemorrhage should be sought; if the latter is present, it should be taken very seriously. Splenomegaly is present in less than 5% of individuals. A search should be made for any systemic disorder that might predispose to thrombocytopenia, e.g. SLE, lymphadenopathy, arthritis.

The diagnosis of chronic ITP is usually made by excluding congenital thrombocytopenia and other causes of isolated thrombocytopenia (Table 30.3), together with predisposing systemic disorders. The peripheral blood film is usually normal apart from the reduction in platelets, some of which may appear a little large. Bone marrow aspirate will reveal normal erythroid and myeloid cell lines with a normal or increased number of megakaryocytes. It is important to exclude leukaemia or marrow infiltration by non-haematological cells. The diagnosis can be substantiated by finding increased platelet-associated immunoglobulin and reduced survival of autologous isotope-labelled platelets. These are very specialised investigations not widely available. Other investigations are aimed at identifying any underlying disorder and should include chest X-ray, viral antibody titres to EBV, CMV, HIV, and auto-antibody screens, including anti-DNA and a direct Coomb's test.

Management

A strategy for managing patients with chronic ITP is presented in Fig. 30.9. For patients with only minor haemorrhage, e.g. purpura, ecchymosis, epistaxis or minor gastrointestinal haemorrhage, initial treatment should be with prednisolone 0.5 mg/kg/day. In the

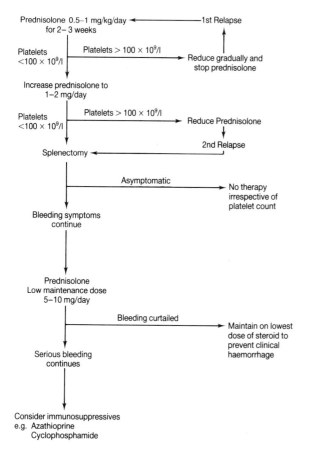

Prednisolone 0.5–1 mg/kg/day ◄──────── 1st Relapse
for 2–3 weeks

Platelets   Platelets > 100 × 10⁹/l
<100 × 10⁹/l ──────────────────────► Reduce gradually and
                                       stop prednisolone

Increase prednisolone to
1–2 mg/day

Platelets   Platelets > 100 × 10⁹/l
<100 × 10⁹/l ──────────────────────► Reduce Prednisolone

                              2nd Relapse

Splenectomy ◄──────────

                Asymptomatic
           ──────────────────────► No therapy
                                    irrespective of
                                    platelet count
Bleeding symptoms
continue

Prednisolone
Low maintenance dose
5–10 mg/day

                Bleeding curtailed
           ──────────────────────► Maintain on lowest
                                    dose of steroid to
                                    prevent clinical
                                    haemorrhage
Serious bleeding
continues

Consider immunosuppressives
e.g. Azathioprine
     Cyclophosphamide

Fig. 30.9 Strategy for treating chronic ITP.

majority of patients, bleeding stops within one to two days, although the platelet count may start to rise only after 5–7 days. The mechanism of action of steroids in immune thrombocytopenia is discussed under acute ITP. In those in whom the platelet count becomes normal the prednisolone should be reduced, but when the daily dose reaches 15 mg/day, further diminution of the dose should be very gradual and spread over 1–2 months. It is often at this time that relapses occur and these may be precipitated by too rapid withdrawal of steroids. If the platelet count falls, the dose of steroids should be increased and maintained at this higher level for several weeks before attempting a reduction. If on the initial dose of steroids the platelet count does not rise above $100 \times 10^9/l$ within 3 weeks, the dose of prednisolone should be raised to 1–2 mg/kg/day. Once the platelets are over $100 \times 10^9/l$ the dose can be reduced and eventually discontinued, provided the platelet count is well maintained.

Splenectomy should be considered for those individuals who relapse twice on steroids, or fail to obtain a platelet count of over $100 \times 10^9/l$ on steroids. Patients who do well on steroids are more likely to respond well to splenectomy. This not only removes a site of platelet destruction but also a source of antiplatelet antibody production. At least 10 days prior to elective surgery pneumococcal vaccine should be given; as the majority of patients eventually require splenectomy it may be better to vaccinate all patients at presentation when steroid therapy is started and before there is too much immunosuppression. Pneumococcal vaccination is more effective given prior to splenectomy. Vaccination in the absence of the spleen results in a lower anti-pneumococcal antibody titre and absence of specific IgM. Despite platelet counts in the region of $20–40 \times 10^9/l$ excessive bleeding is uncommon at splenectomy, particularly if the splenic vessels are clamped early during the operation. If the platelet count is less than $30 \times 10^9/l$, it is prudent to have platelets for transfusion available in the operating theatre, but these should be used only if there is excessive intra-operative haemorrhage. The platelet count usually begins to rise 2–3 days postoperatively and may increase to very high levels; a peak count over $500 \times 10^9/l$ indicates that a favourable longterm result is likely. Following operation the steroids should be tapered and stopped.

All patients are at increased risk of pneumococcal and meningococcal septicaemia following splenectomy. Although children are at greater risk than adults, this sudden catastrophic complication can occur at any age. Phenoxymethyl penicillin 250 mg daily (or erythromycin 250 mg daily for those hypersensitive to penicillin) should be given for life even in those who have received pneumococcal vaccine. Even if an individual has been vaccinated the penicillin must be continued indefinitely, because the vaccine only contains the polysaccharide antigen from some of the virulent strains.

If recurrence of thrombocytopenia occurs after splenectomy, the aim of therapy should be to maintain the patient free of haemorrhagic symptoms rather than render the platelet count normal. Such patients should be screened for the possibility of a remaining splenunculus by examining the blood film to ensure that Howell-Jolly bodies are present. An isotope liver and spleen scan, or [111] In-platelet imaging of the splenic area may also be useful. Many individuals are asymptomatic, with platelets at $20–30 \times 10^9/l$ or less and in this circumstance no therapy is indicated despite the thrombocytopenia. In some individuals a small dose of prednisolone at 5 mg daily is sufficient and this can be continued for prolonged periods without significant side effects. It is very rare for patients not to be rendered free of bleeding by a small dose of prednisolone.

If severe symptomatic thrombocytopenia persists the diagnosis of ITP should be reconsidered and other diagnoses entertained, particularly a congenital thrombocytopenia. If a platelet survival study has not previously been carried out, this should be considered, even if homologous platelets have to be used, in order to demonstrate a reduced lifespan which may be as short as 1 hour. This will confirm that excessive destruction is taking place and that the thrombocytopenia is not the result of ineffective platelet production due to a megakaryocytic maturational defect. The only remaining long-term therapy for symptomatic patients is the use of immunosuppressives such as cyclophosphamide or azathioprine. Vincristine and vinblastine-loaded platelets (to target the phagocytic cells) are occasionally successful. Such therapies are virtually never indicated in the view of the authors and should only be considered for patients who continue to have significant haemorrhagic symptoms; they should never be given merely to raise the platelet count in an asymptomatic patient.

Intravenous immunoglobulin will increase the platelet count in many patients with ITP. Dose regimes vary but large amounts need to be given, e.g. total dose 2 g/kg, usually by daily infusions spread over several days. The platelet count begins to rise after several days and peaks at 5–10 days but remains elevated only for 1–3 weeks in most individuals before declining to previous levels. The mechanism of action is unknown but the immunoglobulin may inhibit endogenous antibody production or produce reticulo-endothelial blockade and inhibit platelet phagocytosis. The decreased platelet destruction may be consequent upon T-cell subset changes. Intravenous immunoglobulin should be considered in any patient with ITP in whom only a temporary rise in platelets is required either to stop haemorrhage (particularly if responsive to steroids) or to cover a surgical procedure. As the effect is only temporary, intravenous immunoglobulin has no place in the long-term management of thrombocytopenia.

Major catastrophic bleeding, e.g. intracranial or massive gastro-intestinal haemorrhage, should be treated with platelet transfusions (12–24 donations), which may need to be repeated at frequent intervals because of their short lifespan. Prednisolone at 2 mg/kg/day should also be given and emergency splenectomy considered. Plasmapheresis, which may need to be repeated daily for several days, may reduce the level of antiplatelet immunoglobulin temporarily while other measures, e.g. steroids, take effect. Such severe bleeding is extremely rare and death from haemorrhage in ITP hardly ever occurs.

Neonatal ITP

See Chapter 34.

Iso-immune neonatal thrombocytopenia

See Chapter 34.

Drug-induced ITP

An increasing number of medicines is being implicated as causing antibody-mediated thrombocytopenia (Table 30.7). Two principal types of mechanism are implicated. The drug may bind to the platelet resulting in the development of a neoantigen, to which the individual develops a specific auto-antibody, with the subsequent antibody coating of the cell causing its premature removal by the reticulo-endothelial system. The second is the 'innocent bystander' mechanism in which the drug binds tightly to a plasma protein, and an antibody is produced which attaches to the drug-protein complex to give an immune complex. This complex binds tightly to the platelet, via the Fc receptor, and is phagocytosed by the reticulo-endothelial system. The mechanism by which most drugs cause apparently immune-mediated thrombocytopenia is unclear and in many instances the presence of an antibody can only be inferred.

Table 30.7 Drugs implicated as causing immune-mediated thrombocytopenia

Carbamazepine
Chlorothiazide
Gold salts
Heparin
Hydroxychloroquine
Methyl DOPA
Phenothiazines
PAS
Penicillins
Quinine
Quinidine
Rifampicin
Sodium valproate
Sulphonamides

The patient is almost always, without exception, taking the drug when the thrombocytopenia is observed. Those coming to medical attention usually present with mucocutaneous haemorrhage, which in the case of quinine can be very severe causing major life-threatening haemorrhage. The bone marrow will exhibit either a normal or increased number of megakaryocytes. Platelet-associated immunoglobulin may be increased and platelet survival reduced. In a few instances, e.g. quinine, addition of the drug in vitro to the patient's platelet-rich plasma, or the patient's serum and control platelets, will result in their aggregation.

On most occasions stopping the offending drug results in the platelet count rapidly returning to normal. If there is severe bleeding, platelet transfusions are indicated and these may need to be repeated frequently because of the reduced platelet lifespan. Steroids should be given to individuals with platelet counts less than 20 $\times$ 10^9/l, particularly in the presence of purpura or other manifestations of bleeding. Recovery of platelet count usually occurs promptly but on the rare occasion when this is not observed splenectomy may be necessary, especially for gold-induced thrombocytopenia because the drug remains in the body for a prolonged period.

Quinine- and quinidine-induced thrombocytopenia

Presentation of patients, who may have been taking this drug for many years, is often dramatic with sudden haemostatic failure resulting in severe purpura, ecchymoses and occasionally gastrointestinal, fundal or CNS haemorrhage. Some foods and beverages, e.g. tonic water, contain quinine which can precipitate profound thrombocytopenia in a previously sensitised person. The mechanism is thought to be of 'innocent bystander' type: the immune complex becomes attached to glycoprotein 1b on the platelet and is then removed by the reticulo-endothelial system. Steroids 1–2 mg/kg/day are indicated because bleeding is commonly observed, but if there is severe haemorrhage repeated platelet transfusions may be necessary.

Gold-induced thrombocytopenia

Gold salts (gold sodium thiomalate, aurothioglucose) used in the treatment of rheumatoid arthritis may cause antibody-mediated thrombocytopenia of abrupt onset. Thrombocytopenia is more likely to be observed in individuals who are HLA DR3 positive, a similar finding to patients with SLE. Some authorities have therefore suggested HLA-typing patients before administering gold salts. Gold can also inhibit megakaryocyte maturation, leading to a bone marrow failure of platelet production. There are also many other mechanisms by which patients with rheumatoid arthritis may develop thrombocytopenia, e.g. hypersplenism or marrow depression by non-steroidal anti-inflammatory drugs, and these must be considered when evaluating an individual patient. Management is to withdraw the drug and treat with prednisolone for a short period. Although dimercaprol will enhance the excretion of gold it does not shorten the period of thrombocytopenia. Occasion-

ally splenectomy is required for steroid-resistant thrombocytopenia and this procedure is often curative.

Heparin-induced thrombocytopenia

Heparin is prepared from either porcine gut or beef lung and the mucopolysaccharide molecules are of varying molecular weight and anti-thrombotic properties. Heparin's anticoagulant effect is mediated by binding to antithrombin III which greatly enhances its activity. As thrombin is a potent aggregator of platelets, heparin by potentiating antithrombin III, has antiplatelet activity, particularly in disseminated intravascular coagulation and venous thrombo-embolism, when considerable amounts of thrombin are formed. Mild persistent thrombocytopenia observed after heparin administration may result from contaminants within the product. Clinically this causes no difficulties; the platelet count rarely falls much below 100 $\times$ 10^9/l. Daily platelet counts should be performed and heparin at full dose continued.

A more severe thrombocytopenia is occasionally seen which begins 7–14 days after starting heparin therapy. It results from generation of a heparin-dependent antibody, and increased IgG and C3 can be detected on the platelets. The antibodies are probably directed at a heparin-platelet complex. The platelet count may fall to quite low levels and further major arterial or venous thrombosis ensues probably due to platelet aggregate formation in vivo. Management is difficult because the heparin will have been given for a primary thrombotic event and the secondary heparin-induced thrombosis may be life-threatening. The heparin should be stopped and an alternative antithrombotic agent considered, e.g. ancrod, streptokinase or warfarin.

Post-transfusion purpura

This rare disorder is seen predominantly in parous women who develop an antibody to a platelet-specific membrane antigen, usually PL^{A1}, as a result of allo-immunisation by a fetus during pregnancy. The antigen PL^{A1} is very common, being found in 98% of the population. At 10 days after transfusion of blood containing PL^{A1}-positive platelets to a PL^{A1}-negative woman possessing anti-PL^{A1}, severe thrombocytopenia develops with resultant mucocutaneous bleeding. This is a most unexpected occurrence, because the patient's platelets are PL^{A1}-negative and the mechanism by which they are removed from the circulation is not understood. One possible mechanism is that the transfused PL^{A1}-positive platelets stimulate an anamnestic response and at 10 days sufficient antibody has been synthesised to react with the donor platelets. These antibody-coated platelets may interact with the patient's own platelets in an 'innocent bystander' mechanism leading to their premature removal by the reticulo-endothelial system.

Clinically profound thrombocytopenia results in severe mucocutaneous haemorrhage and some reports indicate a high mortality. Therapy should initially be with large doses of prednisolone (2 mg/kg /day) but further measures are often necessary to control bleeding. Transfusion of random platelets is contra-indicated because it often exacerbates the bleeding diathesis, but platelets from a PL^{A1}-negative donor may be useful when there is severe haemorrhage. Plasmapheresis to reduce the concentration of anti-PL^{A1} may help but will need to be repeated daily for a number of occasions. Recent reports have demonstrated a dramatic rise in platelet count with intravenous immunoglobulin and this should now perhaps be considered as first-line therapy.

Increased utilisation of platelets of uncertain aetiology

Thrombotic thrombocytopenic purpura (TTP, Moschowitz's syndrome)

In this uncommon disorder thrombi of platelet aggregates occlude small vessels of many organs causing neurological and renal disturbances. The aetiology of the syndrome is unknown. Current evidence suggests that there may be a defect of endothelial cells resulting in decreased production of PGl_2 or the presence of a plasma factor that inhibits its synthesis, or its stability is reduced by lack of a stabilising factor. Until recently this disorder carried a high mortality but following the observation that either plasma infusion or plasma exchange is beneficial, 80% of affected individuals now survive.

Patients present with fever, fluctuating neurological symptoms and signs, uraemia and thrombocytopenic bleeding. Besides thrombocytopenia the blood film exhibits many red cell fragments and spherocytes characteristic of micro-angiopathic haemolysis. A coagulation screen is normal or there may be minor prolongation of the APTT or prothrombin time.

Initial therapy should consist of infusion of 1–2 litres of fresh frozen plasma which should be repeated as frequently as the circulating volume will allow. If there are facilities for plasmapheresis, daily 3–5-litre exchanges should be undertaken; replacement being with fresh frozen plasma. If this is not effective, other forms of therapy include high dose steroids (2 mg/kg/day), vincristine (2 mg i.v.) or antiplatelet drugs (aspirin

300 mg daily and dipyridamole 300–400 mg daily). Occasional remissions have followed splenectomy. Platelet transfusions are contra-indicated, as they tend to worsen the clinical symptoms by causing the formation of further thrombi, but when all else fails and the patient has severe haemorrhage they should be considered.

Haemolytic uraemic syndrome

This is very similiar to TTP except that it is often preceded by an antecedent viral infection and is most commonly seen in young children. Renal failure is often severe due to preferential formation of thrombi in renal arterioles and glomerular vessels of the kidney, whilst neurological features are rare. The peripheral blood changes are similiar to TTP. The coagulation screen is normal or only reveals slight prolongation of the APTT or prothrombin time. As for TTP, therapy is controversial. General medical ·support of the patient is most important and dialysis should be started promptly. Steroids are the therapy most commonly used but are of doubtful value, as are heparin, fibrinolytic therapy and antiplatelet drugs. Infusion of PGl_2 has been tried; it may be of additional value as a vasodilator in reducing the blood pressure.

Ineffective platelet production

In a thrombocytopenic patient without splenomegaly but with both normal platelet lifespan and numbers of megakaryocytes in the bone marrow it is reasonable to suspect that there is ineffective platelet production by abnormal megakaryocytes. It is very difficult to quantify the efficiency of thrombopoiesis because of lack of a megakaryocyte-specific metabolic marker to quantify platelet production. Ineffective platelet production most commonly occurs in megaloblastic anaemias but it is also seen in paroxysmal nocturnal haemoglobinuria and some leukaemias. Congenital thrombocytopenias may masquerade as acquired ineffective platelet production (because of the presence of megakaryocytes in the bone marrow) unless a careful history is taken, family platelet counts undertaken, or platelet survival measured.

Thrombocytopenia due to 'hypersplenism'

In a normal individual without splenomegaly approximately 30% of the body's platelets are pooled within the spleen but they are in dynamic equilibrium with those in the circulation. In the presence of a grossly enlarged spleen up to 90% of the platelets may reside in the spleen, leaving only 10% in the circulation. In most instances the marrow can increase platelet production markedly to cope with the extra demand for platelets but clearly at some point output cannot be increased and the platelet count falls. Thrombocytopenia in a patient with splenomegaly may also be due to other mechanisms which concomitantly predispose to the enlarged spleen, e.g. liver disease.

THROMBOCYTOPENIA WITH REDUCED NUMBER OF MEGAKARYOCYTES

Thrombocytopenia accompanied by reduced megakaryocytes in the marrow indicates failure of megakaryocytic development as the cause of the reduced platelet count. A reduction in megakaryocytes may be seen in a marrow that is:

1. Hypoplastic with a panmyelopathy, i.e. with a reduction in all cell lines, as in aplastic anaemia
2. Hyperplastic, as with an infiltrative disorder such as leukaemia, lymphoma or carcinomatosis
3. Apparently normal except for the reduction in megakarocytes due to disorders in Table 30.3.

In infiltrated marrows it is tempting to assume that the megakaryocytes are squeezed out by the malignant cells; however it is more likely that megakaryocyte development is suppressed by unidentified humoral factors. Having assessed the overall degree of marrow cellularity and abundance of megakaryocytes it is essential to determine whether the erythroid and myeloid cell lines are maturing normally and are present in normal proportions. It is important to exclude, on morphological grounds, a myelodysplastic syndrome as well as a frank leukaemic process. The discussion hereafter assumes that the only abnormality in the bone marrow is apparently confined to the megakaryocytes.

Drugs

Many cytotoxic drugs used to treat leukaemias, lymphomas and solid tumours induce thrombocytopenia in a dose-dependent manner (see Chapter 23). With increasing number of cycles or pulses of chemotherapy thrombocytopenia tends to become more profound and persistent. For the majority of drugs, thrombocytopenia and leukopenia are the dose-limiting toxicities, although for mithramycin thrombocytopenia alone may limit its further use. Alkylating agents, antimetabolites and anthracyclines give immediate dose-related reduction in platelets and white cells with prompt recovery. Nitroureas, e.g. BCNU and CCNU, cause a gradually progressive and prolonged depression of counts. With all these drugs it is usual to note reduction of all cell lines, although if marrow is sampled just at the point of

recovery it will appear very active, possibly leading to confusion in interpretation. This recovery process will become obvious in the subsequent days as peripheral blood counts increase. A wide range of drugs occasionally appear to inhibit platelet production and some of these are listed in Table 30.3. Thiazide diuretics induce a selective thrombocytopenia which is presumed to be due to their toxicity on megakaryocytes. Occasionally the fetus of a mother on such a diuretic will be thrombocytopenic due to placental transfer of the thiazide; recovery occurs spontaneously after birth.

Alcohol

Binges of alcohol, especially in an alcoholic, may cause profound thrombocytopenia. Cessation of drinking will be followed within 1–2 weeks by the platelet count returning to normal. Sometimes during recovery the platelet count may temporarily overshoot, resulting in a a mild thrombocytosis, before returning to normal. During recovery the blood film may reveal platelets of larger than normal size. Ethanol is not only directly toxic to megakaryocytes but it may also inhibit platelet function, thus exacerbating the potential haemorrhagic state.

Cyclic thrombocytopenia

In this rare disorder of unknown aetiology the individual often becomes severely thrombocytopenic every 20–40 days. It is thought to be due to failure of megakaryocyte maturation, as their numbers are reduced at the nadir of the platelet count. Treatment with hormones, steroids and splenectomy are without effect.

Idiopathic

In some individuals a combined reduction in platelets and megakaryocytes is seen without any apparent cause. Such patients may be in an early stage of aplastic anaemia; some will develop a myelodysplastic syndrome or leukaemia; a few may be exposed to marrow toxins at work or with hobbies and these should be assiduously enquired about.

Thrombocytopenia with absent radius (TAR) syndrome

This uncommon autosomal recessive disorder presents at birth with skeletal abnormalities, usually bilateral absence of radii, and bleeding due to thrombocytopenia (Fig. 30.10). There may also be abnormalities of the heart and kidneys. As platelet survival is normal and

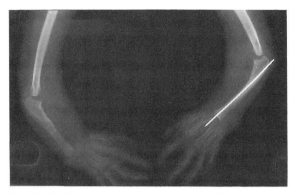

Fig. 30.10 Thrombocytopenia with absent radius syndrome (TAR) illustrating lack of radii and the presence of an intramedullary pin in a baby to correct radial deviation at wrist on the left side.

megakaryocytes are reduced in number, it is assumed that there is a megakaryocytic maturation defect. The syndrome often results in a severe haemorrhagic disorder and, even in those who do not bleed spontaneously, platelet transfusions will be needed to cover the multiple orthopaedic operations necessary to correct skeletal abnormalities. It is reported that as many as a third of babies affected may die but that in those who survive bleeding becomes less as the child grows up.

THROMBOCYTOPENIA WITH LARGE PLATELETS (MACROTHROMBOCYTOPENIA)

These are a small group of rare congenital platelet disorders, and it is very important to distinguish them from other much more common acquired causes of thrombocytopenia. In these conditions the platelets are obviously large, sometimes with a diameter equivalent to that of erythrocytes. Several acquired conditions may be associated with platelets which appear slightly larger than normal, e.g. ITP, but these have been considered for the purposes of this chapter as being of normal size.

May-Hegglin anomaly

In this dominantly inherited disorder, moderate thrombocytopenia with large platelets is associated with Döhle-like bodies in the leukocytes, and thus the diagnosis can be made from the blood film (Fig. 30.11). The Döhle-like bodies are present in the granulocytes, eosinophils, basophils and monocytes, and although similar by light microscopy to true Döhle inclusions found in normal neutrophils during infection, they are probably structurally different in the May-Hegglin

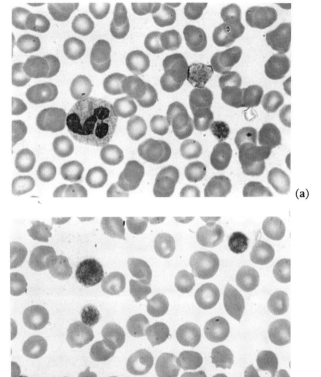

(a)

(b)

Fig. 30.11 Blood film of May-Hegglin anomaly showing giant platelets and Döhle bodies in leukocytes (a) and Bernard-Soulier syndrome illustrating large platelets and post splenectomy red cell changes (b).

anomaly. The bleeding time may be normal or slightly prolonged but it is shorter than anticipated for the platelet count. The consensus of evidence is that, although the platelets are large, they are structurally and functionally normal, as is their survival within the circulation. The total circulatory platelet mass is probably normal and the fundamental defect is one of abnormal megakaryocytic fragmentation, although the biochemical basis for this is unknown. The shorter-than-anticipated bleeding time probably reflects a normal total circulating platelet mass and that indicates the large platelets are individually more haemostatic than normal-sized ones.

Often the patients present only with excessive postoperative bleeding. Severely affected individuals may have purpura, epistaxis or menorrhagia. As the bleeding disorder is usually clinically mild, specific therapy is only occasionally required, usually after trauma. If the bleeding time is normal, no specific therapy may be required for minor surgery. Patients with external bleeding, e.g. epistaxis, or undergoing extraction should receive cyclokapron. Platelet transfusion should be avoided if possible because of the rapidity with which allo-immunisation may develop. There is no good evidence to indicate that splenectomy is helpful.

Bernard-Soulier syndrome

In this autosomally recessive condition with giant platelets (Fig. 30.11) the principal abnormality is a marked reduction in the membrane content of sialic acid. This reduction in sialic acid probably causes the platelet lifespan to be short, resulting in thrombocytopenia. The functional defect is mainly related to the reduction in the membrane glycoprotein 1b(GpIb). This is the platelet receptor for von Willebrand factor (vWF). All vWF-dependent reactions are therefore reduced and this accounts for the prolonged bleeding time (disproportionate for the degree of thrombocytopenia), reduced adhesion and ristocetin- and bovine factor VIII-induced platelet agglutination. There is also a reduction in glycoprotein V, and this may add to the functional impairment of the platelets.

Bleeding in Bernard-Soulier syndrome therefore results both because platelets are reduced in number and because their function is defective.

The clinical expression is very variable with minor cutaneous haemorrhagic symptoms; recurrent epistaxis, bruising and menorrhagia may be particularly troublesome. Some individuals have very frequent bleeding episodes which may prove difficult to treat effectively. In a young person it is important to distinguish this syndrome from immune thrombocytopenia.

Diagnosis depends on finding large platelets on an otherwise normal blood film. Aggregation to ristocetin or bovine factor VIII is greatly reduced or absent due to a reduction in GpIb. To substantiate the diagnosis the amount of this glycoprotein can be measured by polyacrylamide gel electrophoresis.

Patients with a severe form of this syndrome can be difficult to treat. For external bleeding, e.g. epistaxis, cyclokapron may prove useful, while menorrhagia may respond to hormone therapy. Platelet transfusions should be avoided except during severe haemorrhagic episodes because antibodies against GpIb are liable to develop, thus seriously reducing the efficacy of subsequent transfusions. Splenectomy may raise the platelet count temporarily, but it has no place in the conventional management.

Grey platelet syndrome (α storage pool deficiency)

In this very rare, autosomally recessive disorder the platelet count is usually only mildly reduced. Morphologically some of the platelets are very large with a rather amorphous appearance due to the lack of α granules. The platelet content of granule constituents, e.g., β-thromboglobulin, platelet factor 4, fibrinogen and thrombospondin, is decreased. The plasma concentration of β-thromboglobulin is high, presumably reflecting the inability of the megakaryocytes to package the α granule proteins. One other interesting feature of this disorder is that fibrosis develops in the bone marrow. This may be due to an additional granule component, platelet-derived growth factor, leaking out of the marrow megakaryocytes and stimulating fibroblast proliferation.

The underlying platelet defect in this rare disorder is unknown. The aggregation response to ADP, adrenaline, collagen and thrombin may be reduced due to the reduction of releasable thrombospondin or fibrinogen. The contents of the dense bodies, e.g. ADP and 5HT, are normal, although their release is impaired in response to the usual agonists. It would therefore appear that α granule constituents promote dense body release but the details of how this takes place remain obscure.

In the few reported cases bleeding has been severe from early childhood. Most haemorrhage is mucocutaneous, including purpura, although, unusually for a platelet disorder, haemarthroses have also been observed.

Experience of therapy in this disorder is limited because of its rarity. Platelet count increments have been achieved with both steroids and splenectomy but neither can be routinely recommended. Platelet transfusions are effective in arresting severe or intractable haemorrhage.

Macrothrombocytopenia deafness and renal disease (Epstein's syndrome)

This is a rare familial disorder of uncertain inheritance pattern with only a moderately reduced platelet count. A blood film reveals large platelets but no other abnormalities are observed until the erythrocyte changes of uraemia develop as renal function deteriorates. Some patients have reduced platelet aggregation responses to ADP, adrenaline and collagen, whereas others appear to be normal. Bleeding is usually clinically mild. Hearing impairment of sensorineural type progressively causes deafness. Renal manifestations include non-progressive proteinuria and an acute glomerulonephritis-like syndrome which may result in the development of uraemia. This disorder appears distinct from Alport's syndrome, in which there is deafness and haematuria but platelet number and morphology are normal.

Antiplatelet drugs should be avoided. Steroids and splenectomy are of unproven value. Platelet transfusions should be avoided and used only for serious haemorrhagic episodes.

Other causes of thrombocytopenia with macrothrombocytes

There are other reports of rare platelet syndromes associated with large platelets and thrombocytopenia. Many reports describe only single cases or families, and functional abnormalities, severity of clinical manifestations, inheritance and response to treatment seem very variable.

The Montreal platelet syndrome is dominantly inherited with macrothrombocytopenia, prolonged bleeding time and impaired platelet function in vitro.

Mediterranean macrothrombocytopenia is characterised by only a moderately reduced platelet count and cells that appear to function normally.

THROMBOCYTOPENIA WITH SMALL PLATELETS (MICROTHROMBOCYTOPENIA)

Recognition, by visual inspection of a blood film, of small platelets is much harder than the identification of macrothrombocytes. With increasing use of automated particle counters the ability to size platelets is becoming more precise and the presence of microthrombocytopenia easier to quantify. A variety of reports indicate that there may be a spectrum of familial disorders characterised by microthrombocytopenia and X-linked inheritance, but the Wiscott-Aldrich syndrome is the most severe and therefore best characterised. Several acquired conditions are associated with small platelets and these are listed in Table 30.5.

Wiscott-Aldrich syndrome

This X-linked syndrome consists of a triad of eczema, recurrent infections and microthrombocytopenia. Bleeding can be marked and may lead to death. The haemorrhagic manifestations are more severe than expected for the degree of thrombocytopenia, suggesting platelet functional impairment. Because of the severe thrombocytopenia platelet function assessment is difficult, although several reports have suggested that it is defective on in vitro testing. The bleeding time is longer than would be anticipated for the degree of thrombocytopenia. The immunological deficiency results in recurrent infections. The primary underlying abnormality is unknown but IgM production is impaired and isohaemagglutinins are absent from the serum. The increased incidence of lymphomas is further evidence of immune impairment. Diagnosis depends upon finding

marked microthrombocytopenia and absent isohaemagglutinins in a child with eczema.

Until recently splenectomy has been considered too hazardous but, with pre-operative pneumococcal vaccination and prudent use of antibiotics, this procedure should be contemplated, particularly in the absence of a bone marrow transplant donor. Post-splenectomy the platelet count and size both increase, with a consequent dramatic reduction in bleeding manifestations. When function is assessed in vitro this appears to be normal. Thus the mechanism causing the thrombocytopenia is obscure, although it may, in some individuals, have an autoimmune basis as a reflection of the altered immune status. The mechanism by which platelet size increases post-splenectomy remains obscure. Allogeneic bone marrow transplantation, however, is probably the treatment of choice as this rectifies both the platelet and immune abnormalities.

THROMBOCYTOSIS

An explanation must be sought for any patient having a platelet count persistently over $400 \times 10^9/l$. In the majority of individuals an elevated count reflects a serious underlying disorder. In a symptomatically ill patient, thrombocytosis is an incidental observation when it is usually secondary to the underlying pathology. The causes of such a reactive thrombocytosis are listed in Table 30.8. Occasionally asymptomatic individuals are found to have a raised platelet count. It is then necessary to determine whether the thrombocytosis is secondary to an undisclosed pathology or whether the true diagnosis is essential thrombocythaemia or another myeloproliferative disorder due to an autonomous malignant proliferation of megakaryocytes. Important details in the history and examination of the patient are considered in Chapter 8.

To a large extent the diagnosis of essential thrombocythaemia is made by excluding secondary causes of the

Table 30.8 Causes of a raised platelet count

Malignant thrombocytosis (thrombocythaemia)	Reactive thrombocytosis
Essential thrombocythaemia	Chronic inflammatory disorders
Primary proliferative polycythaemia	Malignancy
Myelofibrosis	Tissue damage
Chronic myeloid leukaemia	Haemolytic anaemias
	Post-splenectomy
	Rebound post-thrombocytopenia
	Post-haemorrhage
	Drug-induced, e.g. vincristine

thrombocytosis. A careful history is necessary with particular emphasis on ascertaining whether there is underlying inflammation or malignancy; the presence of fever, weight loss or gastrointestinal symptoms clearly suggest underlying pathology. On the other hand, a patient with essential thrombocythaemia may present with extensive venous thrombosis precipitated by the elevated platelet count, and they may have spent a few days in bed because of the thrombosis and developed bronchopneumonia. In such circumstances it can sometimes be difficult to determine whether the high platelet count caused the thrombosis or whether the platelet count is raised secondary to the chest infection.

In the asymptomatic patient, clinical examination should be particularly thorough to search for clues that might lead to the diagnosis of an inflammatory disorder. The finding of splenomegaly strongly favours essential thrombocythaemia, although it might reflect an underlying lymphoma. Evidence of digital ischaemia or gangrene in the presence of peripheral pulses suggests either essential thrombocythaemia or one of the causes of small vessel occlusion, e.g. diabetes or vasculitis. The presence of bleeding, e.g. epistaxis, in the face of a raised platelet count favours the diagnosis of essential thrombocythaemia, as the platelets clearly are less haemostatic than normal.

Investigation of suspected reactive thrombocytosis should be directed to ascertain the underlying cause. In a patient without symptoms and with normal erythrocytes and leukocytes the film should be carefully inspected. The presence of bizarre giant platelets favours essential thrombocythaemia. Additionally in this condition features of hyposplenism may appear at presentation due to gradual asymptomatic infarction of the spleen, and the film should be scrutinised for Howell-Jolly bodies and other evidence of reduced splenic activity. To a large extent the diagnosis of essential thrombocythaemia is made after exclusion of secondary causes and therefore it is important to investigate such patients fully. Tests of platelet function may be helpful for a prolonged bleeding time or reduced or enhanced aggregation favour a diagnosis of essential thrombocythaemia.

Post-splenectomy thrombocytosis

After splenectomy for any cause, the platelet count increases, usually reaching a peak after 1 or 2 weeks. Occasionally levels exceed $1,000 \times 10^9/l$ and concern is expressed about the possibility of thrombo-embolism developing. Unless the patient has an underlying myeloproliferative disorder there is no unequivocal evidence that high post-splenectomy platelet counts are associated with an increased incidence of thrombo-embolism. It is, however, prudent to ensure that standard anti-thrombolic treatment, e.g. subcutaneous heparin, is given and mobilisation is actively encouraged. Patients in whom the platelet count does not eventually return to normal levels do have an increased incidence of venous thrombo-embolism. This is particularly likely following splenectomy for warm autoimmune haemolytic anaemia, where the haemolysis continues post-operatively.

ESSENTIAL THROMBOCYTHAEMIA

Malignant proliferation of megakaryocytes leads to a high platelet count and in many instances the platelets will be functionally impaired. Essential thrombocythaemia is part of the myeloproliferative spectrum that includes primary proliferative polycythaemia, chronic myeloid leukaemia and myelofibrosis. Patients may present with clinical and laboratory features intermediate between these syndromes. Additionally, essential thrombocythaemia may 'transform' into either primary proliferative polycythaemia, myelofibrosis or acute leukaemia. The cause is unknown, although occasional cases are associated with chromosomal abnormalities, eg $21q^-$.

Clinical presentation is varied: spontaneous bruising, epistaxis or gastrointestinal haemorrhage represent the haemorrhagic spectrum of symptoms. Thrombosis of major arteries, e.g. femoral, as a result of the high platelet count will present with the acute symptoms of arterial occlusion. Ischaemia of the toes (and occasionally fingers) with palpable peripheral pulses indicates occlusion of small vessels either by platelets, diabetes or a vasculitis due to one of the collagenoses. Platelet counts around $2000 \times 10^9/l$ result in hyperviscosity which contributes to the thrombotic potential. Except at these very high levels there is a poor correlation between the count and thrombotic or haemorrhagic tendency; e.g. a count of $400 \times 10^9/l$ may cause ischaemic symptoms which resolve when the platelet count is reduced to normal.

On examination evidence of bleeding and thrombosis should be noted. Palpable splenomegaly may be present, although some patients have splenic atrophy. Hepatomegaly is sometimes noted. When first seen most patients have platelet counts over $1000 \times 10^9/l$ but an increasing number of patients are being recognised at counts only just about $350 \times 10^9/l$. Occasionally a routine blood count in an apparently well person reveals a high platelet count. The morphology of the cells may be bizarre with giant forms being prominent. Often the haemoglobin and white count are at the upper end of the normal range. A high platelet count along with a normal haemoglobin with microcytosis may indicate that the true diagnosis is of iron-deficient primary proliferative polycythaemia. Evidence of hyposplenism, e.g. Howell-Jolly bodies, spherocytes or target cells, should be searched for on the blood film.

Assessment of the platelet function may aid in the diagnosis. The bleeding time is usually normal but may be prolonged. Absent second phase platelet aggregation to adrenaline is characteristic, although not always observed, and may be due to an abnormality of α receptors on the membrane surface. Other functional defects have been described but there is no universal agreement as to their significance. Despite many studies there is no good relationship between in-vitro abnormalities and thrombotic or bleeding tendencies.

Treatment is aimed at reducing the platelet count to normal and inhibiting platelet function. Aspirin, 300 mg daily, often dramatically relieves the symptoms of digital ischaemia and transient ischaemic attacks. A patient presenting with a platelet count in the region of 2000 × 10^9/l and an arterial thrombotic episode should have the platelet count promptly reduced. Platelet phoresis is one possible therapy but this procedure will have to be repeated daily. As the spleen acts as a large reservoir for platelets, apheresis in the presence of splenomegaly is usually ineffective in reducing the platelet count quickly. Alternative therapy is mustine 10 mg i.v. on alternate days. The nausea and vomiting associated with this therapy may cause the patient considerable distress and the benefits must be weighted carefully against the patient's condition. For individuals with moderate symptoms, e.g. bruising, epistaxis or digital ischaemia, the platelet count can be reduced more gradually. Radiophosphorus (^{32}P) at a dose of 112 MBq/m^2 is probably the initial treatment of choice for older patients and hydroxyurea for those less than 50 years. The phosphorus is taken up by the bone, and the alpha emissions irradiate the marrow to suppress megakaryocyte proliferation. The platelets begin to fall after 1–2 weeks and reach a nadir at 6–8 weeks. The count will stay within the normal range for a variable time, ranging from 2–3 months up to many years, before relapsing.

It is often difficult to know when to give further therapy. Any patient who develops symptoms due to the thrombocythaemia, even although the platelet count is only mildly elevated, should receive further radiophosphorus. The platelet count should not be allowed to rise to the level at which the patient originally presented with symptoms. In an asymptomatic patient the platelet count should probably not be allowed to exceed 1000 × 10^9/l. Repeated injections of ^{32}P can be safely given, usually at 1–3-yearly intervals. The interval between in-

jections may decrease as the disease becomes more active and a modest increase in dose to 130 MBq/m^2 can be given. The total maximum recommended dose of ^{32}P is 700–750 MBq.

When the platelet count becomes unresponsive to radiophosphorus, oral chemotherapy can be considered, in the form of busulphan 4 mg daily until the platelets reach 300 × 10^9/l, after which maintenance therapy should consist of small doses, e.g. 2 mg on alternate days, to keep the platelets less than 500 × 10^9/l. Other alkylating agents, e.g. melphalan or cyclophosphamide, can also be used instead; these can be given as single doses or as short courses at monthly intervals.

Essential thrombocythaemia can range from being a very benign disorder requiring infrequent treatment to an aggressive condition becoming resistant to radiophosphorus or alkylating agents. The disease may transform to any of the other myeloproliferative disorders; the most usual transformations are to myelofibrosis or primary proliferative polycythaemia. In some patients the condition progresses to a form of acute myeloid leukaemia that is particularly resistant to chemotherapy.

QUALITATIVE PLATELET DISORDERS

Qualitative platelet disorders, or thrombopathies, may arise from either a congenital metabolic abnormality of the cell (Table 30.9) or secondary to a variety of acquired diseases or drugs. Leukaemias and myeloproliferative disorders are commonly associated with defective platelet function which may predispose to bleeding or thrombosis. Some medicines, e.g. non-steroidal anti-inflammatory drugs, may inhibit platelet function, whereas others cause thrombocytopenia by

Table 30.9 Congenital disorders of platelet function

Disorders of primary aggregation
Thrombasthenia
Bernard-Soulier syndrome

Disorders of secondary aggregation
Defects of arachidonic acid pathway
    Phospholipase
    Cyclo-oxygenase
    Thromboxane synthatase

Storage pool disorders (SPD)
α-granule SPD (Table 30.10)
δ-granule SPD (Table 30.10)

Miscellaneous
Some familial thrombocytopenias
May-Hegglin anomaly
Epstein's syndrome
Platelet-type von Willebrand's disease
Montreal platelet syndrome

depressing their production by megakaryocytes.

Clinically thrombopathies may produce a haemorrhagic diathesis ranging from mild post-operative bleeding to severe recurrent bruising, epistaxis and menorrhagia. Purpura can occur with a normal platelet count but it is an uncommon symptom.

The possibility of a qualitative platelet disorder should be considered in any patient with a history strongly suggestive of a bleeding disorder, particularly with mucocutaneous haemorrhage, in which the APTT, prothrombin time, fibrinogen and factor VIII and von Willebrand factor are normal. It is important to exclude von Willebrand's disease before investigating platelet function. Although the bleeding time is characteristically prolonged, a normal time does not exclude a thrombopathy.

Apart from a peripheral blood platelet count and bleeding time an initial screen should include careful inspection of the blood film. Platelet morphology should be assessed; many congenital disorders with macrothrombocytes also have thrombocytopenia and these are listed in Table 30.5. A scheme for investigating patients with a possible thrombopathy is outlined in Figure

30.12. Platelet aggregation is the first in vitro functional investigation that should be undertaken. The response of the patient's platelets to a variety of aggregating agents, including ADP, adrenalin, collagen, ristocetin and arachidonic acid is assessed. This is achieved using an instrument known as a platelet aggregometer which measures the transmission of light through a sample of platelet-rich plasma. When coupled to a chart recorder an increase in light transmission is observed following the addition of an aggregating agent to the sample under test; this reflects the formation of platelet aggregates and a corresponding decrease in the optical density of the sample. In the ensuing description of the various thrombopathies they have been grouped into those that principally affect primary or secondary aggregation.

DISORDERS OF PRIMARY PLATELET AGGREGATION

Afibrinogenaemia

Lack of available fibrinogen to interact with its platelet membrane receptor, GpIIb/IIIa, exposed by aggregating

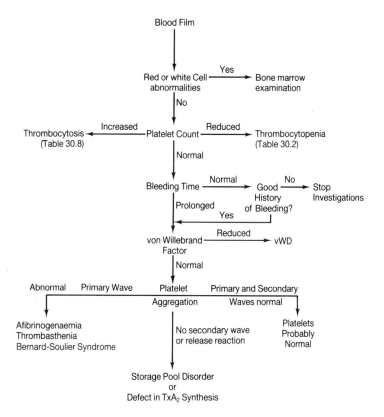

Fig. 30.12 Investigation of possible thrombopathy.

agents, results in reduced platelet activity. Additionally the reduction in plasma fibrinogen concentration, particularly to levels less than 500 mg/l, causes a coagulation disorder which may exacerbate the bleeding manifestations. The bleeding time is prolonged and aggregation to ADP, adrenaline and collagen is depressed.

The clinical severity of this rare disorder is very variable but in its severe form may be associated with joint and muscle haemorrhages.

Treatment of acute bleeds is to raise the plasma fibrinogen concentration by the use of cryoprecipitate.

Thrombasthenia (Glanzmann's disease)

The platelet count and morphology are normal but the bleeding time is prolonged in this rare recessively inherited disorder.

The platelets are deficient in the membrane glycoproteins IIb and IIIa as well as in fibrinogen stored in the α granules. The platelet-specific antigens PL^{A1} and PL^{A2} are also reduced or absent, suggesting that these are an integral part of this glycoprotein complex. During normal platelet aggregation to ADP or adrenaline, fibrinogen binds to a specific membrane receptor which is probably GpIIb/IIIa. In thrombasthenia the lack of this receptor and releasable fibrinogen are presumably the cause of the failure of aggregation in vitro and the haemorrhagic symptoms in the patients.

The clinical haemorrhagic manifestations are very variable. In its most severe form, frequent recurrent mucocutaneous haemorrhage is common in the form of epistaxis, spontaneous bleeding, purpura and gastrointestinal haemorrhage. The diagnosis is usually straightforward because the platelets fail to aggregate in response to ADP, adrenaline and thrombin.

Individuals with a severe form of the disorder with frequent bleeds from a young age can be very problematic to treat. Platelet transfusions should be avoided if possible because antibody to GpIIb/IIIa may develop, rendering further transfusions less efficacious. Faced with this acquired inhibitor and a patient with a severe bleed, plasmapheresis may offer a way of increasing the efficacy of transfused platelets. Menorrhagia can be troublesome and should be treated by hormonal therapy.

Uraemia

The cause of the platelet malfunction in uraemia is unknown but is presumed to result from the accumulation of 'toxins' (e.g. urea, guanidino succinic acid, phenols). Other studies have proposed abnormalities of prosta-glandin synthesis or von Willebrand factor as the cause of the defective function.

Bleeding can be a distressing complication of renal failure. Clinically it is of platelet type, with gastrointestinal haemorrhage often being life-threatening. The bleeding time is prolonged and aggregation to ADP and adrenalin or collagen may be greatly reduced.

Bleeding can often be markedly reduced by dialysis; peritoneal dialysis is reported to be more effective than haemodialysis, possibly because platelets may be further damaged on the dialysis membrane. Transfusion of red cells to raise the haemoglobin may help prevent bleeding. Cryoprecipitate and DDAVP are sometimes useful therapy but their mode of action is uncertain.

Paraproteinaemias

Haemostatic failure in most patients with myeloma and related disorders is approximately correlated with the level of the paraprotein. A polyclonal increase in immunoglobulin concentration is not usually associated with clinically significant platelet dysfunction. The coagulation mechanism may be impaired by a variety of mechanisms (Ch. 20 and 32) and platelet function is also reduced due to coating of the cell by the paraprotein. Hyperviscosity may also predispose to haemorrhage. When myeloma causes renal failure, platelet function will be further impaired by the ensuing uraemia. Clinically the patients usually present with platelet-type bleeding, epistaxis and purpura being most common; fundal haemorrhages may be seen in those who are hyperviscous. On investigation the bleeding time may be prolonged and platelet aggregation to ADP, adrenaline and collagen reduced.

Treatment should be aimed at reducing the level of paraprotein, this often being achieved most satisfactorily by plasmapheresis.

DISORDERS OF SECONDARY PLATELET AGGREGATION AND THE RELEASE REACTION

For the secondary wave of aggregation to be observed the platelet requires intact granules as well as a competent mechanism which brings about the release of their contents. This process requires an intact metabolic pathway for the release of arachidonic acid to its conversion to thromboxane A_2. In addition, intracellular calcium must be released from storage sites for the secretory mechanism to function normally. Details of the metabolic pathways are to be found on page 329. If either the α or δ granules lack constituents then clearly the amount of these substances liberated is reduced, resulting in a haemorrhagic state.

Abnormalities of the platelet arachidonic acid pathway

Phospholipase pathway

Arachidonic acid is liberated from membrane phospholipids by phospholipases A_2 and C; defects in these enzymes may result in mild bleeding symptoms. This group of disorders is ill characterised at present.

Cyclo-oxygenase deficiency

The enzyme cyclo-oxygenase catalyses the conversion of arachidonic acid to the endoperoxides PGG_2 and PGH_2, which are subsequently metabolised to thromboxane A_2. Its formation is essential for a normal release reaction and hence in cyclo-oxygenase deficiency secondary aggregation to ADP and adrenaline and aggregation to collagen are impaired.

As aspirin acetylates cyclo-oxygenase and irreversibly inhibits its activity, it is essential to ensure that the individual has not taken this medicine, in any of its guises, during the 10 days preceding aggregation studies. Clearly it may be very difficult to be certain that a patient with an apparent congenital cyclo-oxygenase deficiency is not taking the occasional aspirin. Unlike aspirin other non-steroidal anti-inflammatory drugs, e.g. indomethacin and phenylbutazone, are reversible inhibitors of cyclo-oxygenase.

As the bleeding disorder is clinically mild, treatment is only occasionally necessary. As with other platelet disorders it is good practice to avoid platelet transfusion so far as possible. Excessive bleeding can sometimes be avoided after dental extraction and other minor surgery by the use of cyclokapron 50 mg/kg/day in four equally divided doses.

Thromboxane synthetase deficiency.

This is a very rare disorder in which the enzyme that converts endoperoxides PGG_2 and PGH_2 to TxA_2 is defective. This metabolic block results in redirection of the metabolic pathway towards PGD_2 and PGI_2, both of which are inhibitors of aggregation.

Storage pool disorders

In this group of conditions there is a reduction in the contents of either α or δ granules or both (Table 30.10). For a list of granule constituents see Table 30.1. The deficiency can be either congenital or acquired.

Table 30.10 Storage pool deficiencies

Disorder	Inheritance	Other characteristics
Delta (δ) granule disorder		
Congenital		
Familial	Dominant	May have decreased δ-granule contents as well
Hermansky-Pudlak	Recessive	Tyrosinase-positive Oculocutaneous albinism Pigment accumulation in macrophages
Chediak-Higashi	Recessive	Oculocutaneous albinism Recurrent pyogenic infections Large abnormal granules in polymorphs
Wiscott-Aldrich syndrome		Small platelets on blood film Thrombocytopenia IgM deficiency Recurrent infections Eczema
TAR Syndrome	Recessive	Thrombocytopenia with absent radius
Acquired		
Immune thrombocytopenia Leukaemias DIC		
Alpha (α) granule disorder		
Congenital		
Grey platelet syndrome	Recessive	Large amorphous 'grey' platelets Fibrosis in marrow
Acquired		
Post-cardiopulmonary bypass		

Delta-granule storage pool deficiencies (δ-SPD)

Several well-characterised congenital and acquired syndromes have been described in which the concentration of the δ- granule constituents are reduced (Table 30.10). Clinically these patients have mucocutaneous bleeding of variable severity. In the congenital form most patients have no associated metabolic or skeletal abnormalities and the disorder is dominantly inherited. Investigation reveals a normal or prolonged bleeding time and absence of the second wave of aggregation, although both investigations may be normal. Diagnosis is made by finding a reduced platelet content of ADP and ATP; an increase in the ATP/ADP ratio is said to be the most sensitive indicator of the disorder.

Management of these individuals should be the same

as for all other platelet disorders. Platelet transfusions should be avoided so far as possible to minimise the risk of allo-immunisation. One study has demonstrated that cryoprecipitate may promote haemostasis by an unknown mechanism and another that DDAVP may be useful.

Alpha-granule store pool deficiency (α-SPD)

In some individuals with a storage pool deficiency, there is a combined reduction of α-and δ-granules. The grey platelet syndrome (described earlier in this chapter) is a very rare congenital entity in which there is a selective reduction in α-granules.

An acquired form of α-SPD is found in patients who have been on cardiopulmonary bypass; the δ-granule contents are well preserved. This SPD contributes to the potential bleeding state in the patients following surgery.

DRUGS INHIBITING PLATELET FUNCTION

Many drugs have been shown to possess anti-platelet activity (Table 30.11) and amongst these the non-steroidal anti-inflammatory agents are the principal inhibitors of the release reaction. Some, e.g. aspirin, irreversibly suppress platelet function by non-competitive inhibition of cyclo-oxygenase. The effect persists for the duration of the platelets' survival in the circulation. Others, e.g. indomethacin and phenylbutazone, are reversible inhibitors of the enzyme and their effect is consequently short-lived. Phenylbutazone is a relatively weak inhibitor of platelet activity. Indomethacin, in addition to its effect on cyclo-oxygenase, may affect platelet function by inhibiting phospholipase activation.

Sulphinpyrazone is also a competitive inhibitor of cyclo-oxygenase but it may possess other antiplatelet activities which are not yet understood and may be important in vivo. In addition it has been postulated that sulphinpyrazone may have a protective effect on the endothelium, whilst its ability to normalise a reduced platelet survival is well known.

Some drugs, most notably dipyridamole, inhibit platelet function by inducing an increase in platelet cAMP levels. Dipyridamole may do this by blocking phosphodiesterase activity and stimulating cAMP production by adenylate cyclase. The anti-thrombotic effect of dipyridamole and its ability to prolong a reduced platelet survival time appear to be enhanced in the presence of aspirin. The exact mechanism by which this synergism is produced is not known.

Heparin has been shown to both inhibit and promote platelet aggregation and it is likely that this dual effect is related to the molecular weight heterogeneity of the mucopolysaccharide. Thus high molecular weight heparin from porcine intestinal mucosa appears to be more active than low molecular weight fractions in aggregating platelets. The anti-platelet activity of heparin, mediated by its effect on thrombin, is widely recognised but another mechanism may involve the induction of a refractory state following partial activation of the platelets by heparin.

Prolongation of the bleeding time has been observed as a side effect of dextran infusion. The inhibitory effect of dextran on platelets appears to be dose-related and may be associated with the ability of platelets to absorb the polysaccharide. This process produces a change in the electrophoretic mobility of the platelet and it has been postulated that platelet membrane function may be altered as a consequence.

Benzyl penicillin, carbinicillin and ticarcillin, in high doses, inhibit platelet function in an unusual manner and by an ill-understood mechanism. Bleeding manifestations only become apparent several days after starting the drug and may persist for some time after its withdrawal. The drugs inhibit platelet aggregation to ADP, adrenaline, collagen and ristocetin, possibly due to coating of the membrane by the penicillin. In general medical practice bleeding manifestations are rare unless the patient is also thrombocytopenic due to myelosuppression in association with the use of cytotoxic drugs. Management consists of withdrawing the drug and the use of platelet transfusions, which may be particularly necessary because of the prolonged effect of the drug in vivo.

Table 30.11   Drugs inhibiting platelet function

Non-steroidal anti-inflammatory agents
   Aspirin
   Indomethacin
   Phenylbutazone
   Sulphinpyrazone

Antibiotics
   Penicillins
   Cephalosporins

Dextran
Heparin
Calcium channel blockers
Furosemide
Phenothiazines
Tricyclic antidepressants
Antihistamines
β-blockers
Monamine oxidase inhibitors
Hydroxychloroquine

NON-THROMBOCYTOPENIC PURPURA

A wide range of hereditary and acquired disorders result in purpura with a normal platelet count. The hereditary disorders, e.g. Ehlers-Danlos, are probably due to the presence of defective collagen failing to support vessel walls and activating primary haemostasis. The acquired syndromes range from the very benign, e.g. senile purpura and purpura simplex, to catastrophic purpura fulminans.

Ehlers-Danlos syndrome

This variably inherited disorder presents with hyperextendable skin and hypermobile joints. Bleeding occurs into the skin and also the gastrointestinal tract. In some individuals the bleeding can be severe and may be associated with a platelet defect.

Marfans syndrome

The arachnodactyly and long limbs make this an easy condition to recognise. In addition there may be defects in the aortic wall as well as the eye, resulting in dislocation of the lens. A collagen defect is probably the underlying abnormality.

Purpura simplex (simple easy bruising)

This presents in young women with small bruises or purpura on the arms, thighs, buttocks and breasts. It is a harmless, self-limiting condition that is not associated with serious bleeding. Some cases may be associated with platelet functional abnormalities. Aspirin should probably be avoided.

Senile purpura

Large subcutaneous bruises on the dorsum of the hands, and forearms of the elderly are characteristic and result from atrophy of tissue supporting the blood vessels. The reddish-blue discoloration persists for a long time and usually leaves a stain in the skin. The condition is harmless.

Factitious bleeding

This is induced by the patient on accessible parts of the body either by sucking the skin (like a Hess test) or by hitting or rubbing the skin. Occasionally serious bleeding results. The condition may be difficult to diagnose. Some individuals may be psychologically disturbed and help with this may be of great benefit.

Non-accidental injury

This is usually observed in children when there is a discrepancy between the history (cause of the bruising) and examination. Often the bruises are of varying ages and on occasions may have a definite pattern, e.g. impression of fingers and hand.

Hereditary haemorrhagic telangiectasia

This dominantly inherited condition presents with increasing numbers of flat, round, reddish lesions on lips, face, hands and gastrointestinal tract (particularly visible in the mouth). The small telangiectasia blanch on pressure and the underlying defect is probably an abnormality in the elastic fibres supporting the vessels. Arteriovenous fistulae may develop in the lungs and there is an association with hepatic cirrhosis and hepatomas. Iron deficiency is a common presentation from occult bleeding into the gastrointestinal tract, although young people may present with troublesome recurrent epistaxis. Occasional patients also have low grade disseminated intravascular coagulation or platelet functional abnormality. Treatment is with local measures, e.g. nasal cautery.

Giant cavernous haemangiomas (Kaṣabach-Merritt syndrome)

This benign tumour of blood vessels can occur at any age in the skin or internal organs. The sluggish circulation in the dilated thin-walled vessels results in activation of the coagulation cascade and platelets with resultant low grade disseminated intravascular coagulation. Occasionally this may be exacerbated with acute episodes which may respond to heparin.

Embolic purpura

This is seen with sub-acute bacterial endocarditis, prosthetic heart valves, atrial myxomas and carcinomas. The splinter haemorrhages are usually seen in the nails due to occlusion of small vessels.

Henoch-Schonlein purpura (allergic vasculitis)

This clinical disorder may be precipitated by drugs, foods, insect bites and bacterial infections, especially β-haemolytic streptococci. The purpura tends to present over the extensor surfaces of the arms and thighs, although it may occur in any part of the body. Biopsy reveals a perivascular inflammatory reaction. Other common presenting symptoms are arthropathy, glomerulonephritis, gut disturbances, pleurisy and pericarditis.

Drugs

Many drugs have been associated with non-thrombocytopenic vascular purpuras. The incriminating medicines are mostly the same ones that have been associated with inducing immune thrombocytopenias (Table 30.7).

Scurvy

Vitamin C is required for normal collagen synthesis and a dietary deficiency may lead to perifollicular haemorrhages. Subperiosteal bleeds may be observed and serious haemorrhage into the gut and brain can occur. Diagnosis is by finding a reduced level of leukocyte ascorbic acid.

Purpura fulminans

This severe disorder has recently been noted to occur in patients with protein C deficiency (Ch. 33), although it is uncertain at present whether all cases are due to this disorder. Presentation is usually in children with crops of necrotic skin lesions which are observed on the limbs, buttocks, nose and ears. Biopsy reveals occlusion of small vessels and subcutaneous haemorrhage. The blood film reveals micro-angiopathic changes and disseminated intravascular coagulation is common. In the later stages respiratory, hepatic and renal failure may develop. Treatment is symptomatic and fresh frozen plasma may be beneficial, but careful haemostatic monitoring is necessary with appropriate blood products as necessary.

BIBLIOGRAPHY

Byrnes J J, Moake J 1986 Thrombotic thrombocytopenic purpura and haemolytic uraemic syndrome: evolving concepts of pathogenesis and therapy. Clinics in Haematology 15: 413–442

Clemetson K J 1988 Membrane glycoprotein abnormalities in pathological platelets. Biochemical Biophysical Acta 947: 53–73

Harker L A 1987 Acquired disorders of platelet function. Annals of the New York Academy of Sciences 509: 188–204

Karpatkin S 1985 Autoimmune thrombocytopenia. Seminars in Haematology 22: 260–288

Kelton J G, Levine M N 1986 Heparin-induced thrombocytopenia. Seminars in Thrombosis and Haemostasis 12: 59–63

Murphy S, Iland H, Rosenthal D, Laszlo J 1986 Essential thrombocythaemia: an interim report from the Polycythaemia Vera Study Group. Seminars in Haematology 23: 177–182

Rao A K, Holmsen H 1986 Congenital disorders of platelet function. Seminars in Haematology 23: 102–118

White J G 1987 Inherited abnormalities of the platelet membrane and secretory granules. Human Pathology 18: 123–139

31. Congenital coagulation disorders

R. A. Sharp   C. D. Forbes

Haemostasis is the process by which loss of blood from the vascular compartment is stopped after injury. This is a complex mechanism which consists of a platelet component, a vessel wall reaction and an intact coagulation mechanism. In this chapter we consider the clinical consequences of a defective coagulation mechanism due to genetic abnormalities of the individual factors.

The coagulation mechanism in the human is the result of evolution and is a complex series of reactions which

are accelerated and have biological feedback mechanisms in-built. The end product of this complex mechanism is the fibrin meshwork which forms from an inert soluble precursor in plasma fibrinogen and which enmeshes the red cells, white cells and platelets to form a stable plug which prevents further blood loss at the site of injury.

For descriptive purposes it is usual to divide the reactions into a series of steps, the first of which involves the contact of blood with a foreign surface which is not

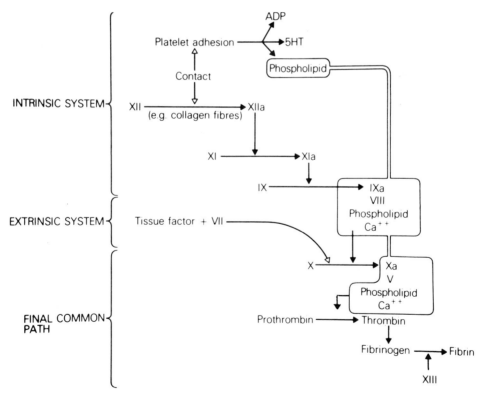

Fig. 31.1 Coagulation cascade showing the intrinsic system, extrinsic system and the final common pathway which leads to fibrin formation. There is evidence that factor VIII is altered by thrombin generation and that the structural alteration greatly accelerates the subsequent steps.

normally present, e.g. subendothelial collagen, elastic fibres, cut skin, muscle, etc. This contact activation step (Fig. 31.1) involves at least four factors present in plasma as inactive precursors. The first, Hagemann factor (factor XII), is activated to a serine protease (XIIa) which has a role not only in activation of coagulation but also in activation of fibrinolysis, kinin generation, complement activation and formation of permeability factors. In coagulation, activated Hageman factor requires two additional plasma factors (prekallikrein and high-molecular-weight-kininogen) to activate factor XI to its active form (XIa) which in turn activates factor IX to IXa. This series of sequential activation products is common to many plasma enzyme reactions and is called a cascade or waterfall sequence. Activated factor IX is adsorbed onto platelet phospholipid micelles which also adsorb factor VIII (antihaemophilic factor) and this complex then activates factor X to factor Xa. The platelet phospholipid is produced when platelets are disrupted as they adhere and aggregate at the site of vessel injury. Activated factor Xa is adsorbed to phospholipid with factor V and calcium ions to produce a complex which converts prothrombin to thrombin. Thrombin has multiple functions. It is a powerful accelerator of the whole system and by a direct action on factor VIII it produces a conformational change in the molecule which accelerates the reaction many-fold. In addition, thrombin is a powerful and irreversible aggregator of platelets and rapidly causes more platelets to aggregate at the site of vessel injury, hence accelerating the formation of platelet phospholipid micelles which enhances later stages of coagulation. Thrombin cleaves fibrinopeptide fragments from the fibrinogen molecule allowing polymerisatian of fibrin. In addition, thrombin activates factor XIII which in turn induces covalent cross-linking of fibrin polymers. This system is known as the intrinsic system, as all its components are in plasma (i.e. intrinsic to plasma). In addition damage to tissues releases a factor that activates factor VII, which in turn activates factor X. This is the extrinsic system. The importance of the balance between these two systems can only be guessed at from our knowledge of the patients who have been defined as having deficiencies.

A variety of inhibitors of the activation process and of activated factors have been described. These include C_1 inactivator, antithrombin III, and proteins S and C. Their biological function is to ensure that activation does not occur in vivo and if it does to rapidly remove activated factors.

Congenital coagulation disorders are rare and affect only 1–2 persons per 10 000 of the population. The most common is factor VIII deficiency (classical haemophilia or haemophilia A) and this affects about 1 per 10 000 males in the UK, with approximately 5500 persons having been identified. There is a great variation internationally, with an incidence ranging up to 9 per 10 000 of the male population in South America. The second most common disease is deficiency of factor IX (haemophilia B or Christmas disease) and this is approximately one-tenth as common as haemophilia A, although there are great local variations in incidence which depend on factors such as geography (cf. the incidence in the Tenna Valley in Switzerland), social factors (cf. the inbreeding in the Amish community in Ohio and Pennsylvania) and religion (large families).

It is suspected that the incidence of von Willebrand's disease approximates to that of haemophilia A but in most countries only the severely affected patients are well documented and nationally registered, and many mildly affected patients remain incompletely documented.

The other defects are rare and for practical purposes the majority of this chapter will refer to the problems of haemophilia A and B and von Willebrand's disease.

FACTOR VIII AND IX DEFICIENCY

These defects are inherited as X-chromosome-linked disorders and therefore are usually only found in males. There is a range of disease severity from mild to moderate to severe. The classification depends on the clinical observation of the degree of excess bleeding. This will usually run in parallel with the measured level of factor VIII or IX biological activity in plasma, although this is not always the case. In severely affected patients (usually with a factor level of <1%) bleeding occurs spontaneously, often without any apparent trauma. Usually the first bleeds start at about 6 months when the child starts to become more mobile in his cot and often these are superficial bruises and haematomas. Many parents and their medical attendants worry about the possibility of child abuse if the disease is undiagnosed in the family. It is uncommon for the newly born baby to bleed excessively from the umbilical cord but if surgery (such as circumcision) is carried out early then excess bleeding may occur. Spontaneous bleeding remains a lifelong problem in this group, with every organ being affected; in particular the joints are frequently involved. There has been a clinical suggestion that with advancing years the number of bleeding episodes declines in the severely affected patient (with no recordable change in factor level) but it would seem probable that patients look after themselves better with advancing years.

Moderate severity is an intermediate group in which

excess bleeding usually requires a degree of trauma or may be associated with surgery. The measured level of plasma factor ranges from 1–5% of normal. Such patients have significantly fewer bleeding episodes than the severely affected and require significantly less blood products. They may bleed into or out of any part of the body and may have chronic joint disease like the more severely affected. Often, after injury, a joint may become the target of recurrent bleeds due to synovial hypertrophy and hyperaemia and on occasion the moderate patient may behave as a more severely affected patient with recurrent joint bleeding. The mild patient may have few bleeding problems and may only bleed when severely challenged by trauma or surgery. The measured level of factor ranges from 5–50%. For this reason it is believed that many such patients escape accurate diagnosis and registration and may present only later in life and as elderly individuals when major surgery is required, and presumably a large number are never diagnosed.

Approximately 20% of patients are 'severe', 20% are 'moderate' and 50–60% are 'mild'. It is of interest that this ratio of severe to mild varies even within the UK and in a recent survey the west of Scotland had a greater percentage of milder patients than any other region.

In individual families with haemophilia and Christmas disease, the severity of the defect runs true and this has been well documented in several generations with measurements of factor VIII and IX levels. Individual families may of course be more prone to problems and consume significantly more concentrate than others. The reason for this is not really clear.

In haemophilia A the defect is in the level of factor VIII as measured in a biological (activity) assay. As seen in Fig. 31.1, the factor VIII molecule plays a key role in the blood coagulation cascade. It is synthesised in the liver, as well as in other organs, and is bound non-covalently to von Willebrand factor (vWF) which acts as a carrier. The plasma half-life of factor VIII is approximately 12 hours. The normal level ranges from 0.5–2.0 μ/ml but it may be elevated by stress, increasing age, exercise, pregnancy and oral contraceptive use. Factor VIII is activated by thrombin and acts as a co-factor in the activation of factor X by factor IXa.

There is a statistically higher level of factor VIII in people with blood group A than O. The reason for this is not clear but it has been suggested that it might be used to enhance harvesting of factor VIII for therapeutic use by donor selection. This may also be a factor in the increased incidence of thrombosis in blood group A patients.

Factor IX is one of the vitamin-K-dependent factors and is a glycoprotein containing carboxyglutamic acid residues which confer on it calcium-binding activity. The concentration in normal plasma is about 3 μg/ml and the biological activity ranges from 0.5–1.5 u/ml. The half-life of infused factor IX is approximately 18–24 hours. The molecular weight of factor IX is approximately 55 000 and it is a single chain glycoprotein. It is activated by factor XIa in the presence of calcium ions in two steps: in the first, slow reaction an arginine-alanine bond is cleaved giving rise to a two-chain intermediate joined by a disulphide bond. This inert intermediate is then cleaved at an arginine-valine bond to give rise to activated factor IX (IXa) and a polypeptide residue. The activated material has a molecular weight of approximately 54 000 and consists of a heavy chain (MW 38 000) and a light chain (MW 16 000) joined by a disulphide bridge. It is probable that this activated factor IX is then adsorbed onto phospholipid micelles (produced from disrupted platelets) to which factor VIII is also adsorbed. In the presence of calcium ions this complex initiates activation of factor X. There is a powerful positive feedback mechanism, with thrombin altering the structure of factor VIII and accelerating the reaction many hundred-fold.

CONSEQUENCES OF BLEEDING

Arthritis in haemophilia

Chronic degenerative arthritis is the external stigma of most severely affected haemophiliacs. This may involve single joints but most often involves several weight-bearing joints, especially the knees, elbows, ankles and shoulders. The chronic slow progression of the joint degeneration is brought about by more dramatic episodes of acute haemarthrosis which induce long-term changes in the joint, some of which target that individual joint for further acute bleeding episodes. It is therefore common to find that the arthropathy is asymmetrical and the clinical features vary greatly from time to time.

Acute haemarthrosis

Joint bleeding is the most important cause of morbidity in haemophilia and may be the presenting feature in more severely affected patients. The incidence of acute bleeds tends to be greatest in childhood and diminishes in later life. The reason for this has never been fully understood but it may be related to undisclosed childhood trauma to the joint or a peculiarity of the growing articular surfaces and their vascularity. No matter the cause, most patients declare that the sites, extent, frequency and duration of acute bleeds diminish with age. In most studies of young haemophilic children the majority of the severely affected have had acute bleeding and many have permanent residual defects by the age of puberty.

Clinical features

In the severely affected patients there is usually no history of prior trauma. Many patients have premonitory symptoms such as a feeling of warmth or a 'prickling' feeling over the joint. No signs are usually present but if it is the patient's experience that these feelings precede a full blown bleed, then they should be encouraged to treat at this stage as a preventive measure despite the absence of scientific proof of efficacy. Pain is the most commonly recorded symptom of the acute bleed. It is usually extremely severe to excruciating and affects the whole joint which rapidly becomes swollen and warm and is held immobile in a flexed position. On examination the features are those of an acute inflammatory process, exquisite tenderness to touch, increased heat, swelling and limitation of movement (Fig. 31.2.). The patient resents examination of the joint and at this time requires adequate amounts of analgesia and factor replacement to halt further bleeding. In patients who have experienced multiple previous bleeding episodes there may already be altered articular surfaces with synovial hypertrophy, as well as fibrosis of the joint capsule and atrophy of the surrounding muscle cuff, and

the features of acute bleeding are not as obvious; however pain remains the dominant presenting symptom.

Investigations

The majority of patients require no further investigation of the joint. There is little evidence that joint aspiration adds anything to the diagnosis. In well-controlled studies of aspiration versus conventional management of the acute bleed there was no observable difference in outcome at 6 weeks, with only a slight reduction in the amount of pain experienced in those joints which were aspirated. X-ray of the joint adds little to management (Fig. 31.3). There is usually obvious soft tissue swelling, the synovium may be easily seen as a result of previous haemosiderin deposition and there may be evidence of chronic degeneration. The only justification is to fully document the extent and rate of onset of articular changes.

Thermography plays no part in routine management but does have research applications. It is of value in determining the extent of the inflammatory process and on using both infra-red and microwave thermograms a

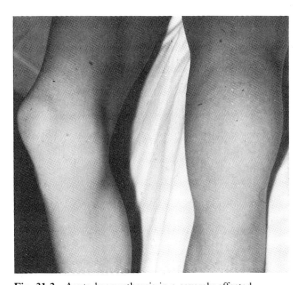

Fig. 31.2 Acute haemarthrosis in a severely affected haemophiliac. The left knee suddenly became acutely swollen and exquisitely painful and walking was impossible. The dominant features are extreme tenderness, swelling, slight flexion and an increase in temperature.

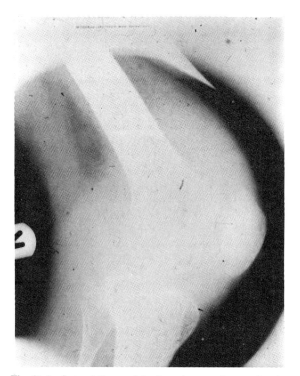

Fig. 31.3 Lateral X-ray of the knee in acute haemarthrosis which shows the soft tissue swelling and the outline of the synovium which had had haemosiderin deposited from previous acute haemarthrosis.

rise in joint temperature can be found. This may be +5°C and provides an objective assessment in the measurement of therapies. Despite the rapid resolution of most acute joint bleeds from the clinical point of view, the joint temperature may remain abnormal when all the other features have resolved. Similarly radio-nuclide joint scans have no place in routine evaluation of the joint but they are being developed as a method of quantitation of blood flow and of inflammation in the synovium. For this purpose the most valuable is ^{99m}Tc-pertechnate, which reflects synovial hyperaemia. These scans, which can be quantitated, remain abnormal for up to 3 months after the acute bleed and like objective tests of temperature reflect the ongoing joint changes which result in the degenerative process.

Pathology

Very little is really known about the evolution of the pathological changes in the human joint after bleeding. Most of the knowledge of early changes has been derived from studies of intra-articular injection of blood in experimental animals and this has been supplemented by clinical, radiological, operative and a small number of post-mortem studies.

Bleeding into the joint probably originates from the synovium, which after the first episode of bleeding becomes hypertrophied and hyperaemic. As a result of joint action the synovium is injured and the resulting haematoma in the synovium rapidly expands and ruptures into the joint with the production of symptoms similar to those of acute inflammation. A rapid migration of inflammatory cells into the synovium occurs and there is an increase in numbers of synovial living cells. Synovial hyperaemia and hypertrophy occur rapidly and frond-like processes of synovium rapidly grow. Histologically they are stuffed with lymphocytes, histiocytes and polymorphs, many of which contain haemosiderin from degraded red cells. There is some evidence that the presence of tissue-bound iron stimulates the production of cathepsins which produce destruction of cartilage and hence degeneration of the articular surfaces. In addition there is fibrosis of the joint capsule and as a result of immobility and probably also hyperaemia there is rapid atrophy of the surrounding muscles.

Management

The keystones of management are replacement of factor and control of pain. Enough concentrate should be given to bring the level to about 30 per cent of normal and this can be predicted. Administration of this alone may rapidly diminish pain but in addition large amounts of

analgesia may require to be given. Repeat doses of concentrate may be required for 4–5 days. In addition significant benefit in pain control results from immobilisation in a splint. This does not inhibit the giving of physiotherapy in an attempt to preserve muscle function. There is some evidence of improvement of symptoms from steroids but these are not routinely used and may now be contraindicated in HIV positive patients. Many patients also claim significant benefit from the use of ice packs and these may be used to speed the resolution of the joint.

Chronic haemophilic arthritis

Chronic degenerative changes appear after a succession of acute bleeds. The main joints affected are the large weight-bearing joints such as knees, elbows, ankles and shoulders. It is rare for the smaller joints to be affected. The changes tend to be progressive with age and are most marked in the more severely affected.

Clinical features

Most of the joints affected become deformed with fixed flexion deformities, resulting from muscle contractures; atrophy of muscles around, above and below the joint tend to accentuate the changes. This is compounded by the imbalance of muscle groups which may result in valgus and rotational deformities. In younger patients hypertrophy of the bone ends results from the marked hyperaemia and this compounds the unusual appearances.

Pain may not be present in even severely deformed joints; however, as the joint destruction progresses, this may become a dominant clinical feature and lead to escalating demands for analgesia and, on occasion, analgesic abuse. As the movements of joints become more limited by pain and ankylosis, more patients require mobility aids such as sticks, crutches and wheelchairs.

Pathology

The appearances of the joint are similar to those of villonodular synovitis, with extensive areas of brown pigment (haemosiderin) in the synovium and articular cartilage. There is often gross synovium hypertrophy with production of finger-like fronds which are extremely vascular and may have collections of varicose veins on their surfaces. The cartilage loses its sheen and becomes irregularly pitted; it may flake off in the centre of the articulation and at the periphery may be replaced by ingrowth of synovium. The thickness of the cartilage

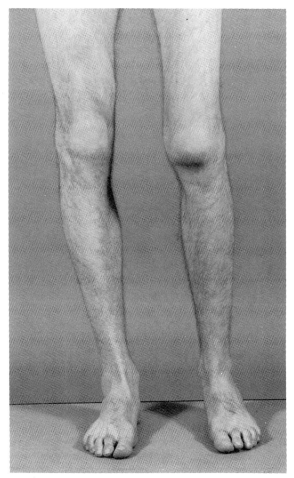

Fig. 31.4 Typical chronic degenerative joint disease in haemophilia with associated muscle cuff atrophy.

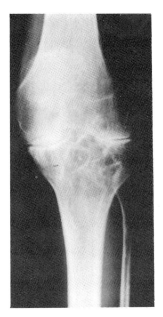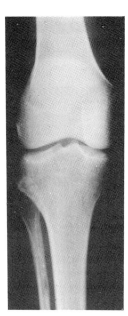

Fig. 31.5 Chronic haemophilic joint disease of the knee which shows loss of the joint space, loose body formation, extensive sub-chondral cyst formation and both hypertrophy of lower end of femur and flattening of the tibial lobule.

is generally less than normal and in areas it may be totally deficient. Haemorrhage beneath the cartilage layer leads to the formation of bone cysts (Fig. 31.4 and 31.5).

Radiology

The radiological findings are characteristic of the disease and tend to be progressive. As a result of hyperaemia there is usually osteoporosis in relation to the affected joint and soft tissue shadowing due to synovial iron deposition. As there is progressive loss of articular cartilage, the joint space is reduced and eventually subchondral cysts form as the adjacent bone is resorbed. Ankylosis may occur in the long term and this may be associated with formation of osteophytes. Associated with hyperaemia there may be local bone overgrowth, e.g. of femoral condyles following knee joint bleeds.

Management

Despite recent advances in control of bleeding problems these chronic joints are managed conservatively with control of pain, enhancement of mobility by physiotherapy and simple orthopaedic correction of deformities using lightweight splints or manipulation. Reconstructive surgery may be required when conservative means have failed or when pain control proves ineffective. Most surgeons will attempt a variety of intermediate procedures such as synovectomy before reconstruction, as there remains doubt about long-term results in this group of patients. To date there is extensive experience with hip and knee joint replacement (Fig. 31.6) and this has been shown to be of value in pain relief particularly, as well as in facilitating improved mobility.

During surgery haemostatic levels of factor must be maintained to prevent bleeding and this must be continued until healing is complete – up to 3 weeks. Physiotherapy can be started immediately after surgery and should be given after the infusion of concentrate. As synovial tissue is rich in fibrinolytic activators, most centres use a fibrinolytic inhibitor such as tranexamic acid.

It is important that all joint surgery in haemophilia is

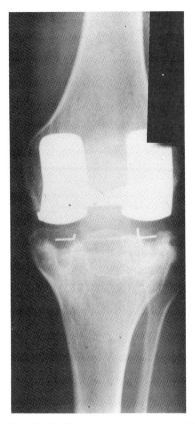 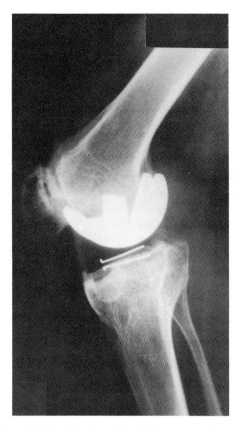

Fig. 31.6 Knee joint replacement carried out in a patient with chronic arthropathy with recurrent pain and deformity. The major positive result was total relief of pain.

done in designated centres which have the surgical and haemostatic expertise.

Neurological problems due to bleeding

Intracranial bleeding remains one of the most serious and common complications of the bleeding state. Bleeding may be spontaneous or a result of minor trauma only and may occur into any part of the brain, spinal cord or its meninges. The presentation is usually dramatic with rapid development of headache, loss of consciousness and other features of intracranial pressure rise. Subdural haematoma is frequent and the evolution of the signs is rapid and not usually associated with the fluctuating conscious levels seen in other patients. Patients may occasionally present with a grand mal fit. It is mandatory to initiate haemostatic treatment early in all haemophilic patients who have a head injury or in whom there is an acute symptom or sign suggesting an intracranial bleed. Investigations such as CT scanning can then be done and if necessary appropriate surgery planned to evacuate the haematoma. Despite introduction nationally of this policy many patients still succumb, such is the rapid progression of the bleeding.

It has been our policy to ensure haemostasis by giving a massive dose of concentrate sufficient to raise the levels above 1 μ/ml (100%). Therapy must be continued until all neurological signs have resolved or, if surgery has been done, until complete healing is obvious. About 15% of patients who survive such episodes will have epilepsy subsequent to the resultant fibrosis and these should be considered for long-term anticonvulsant therapy. It has been our policy to continue this for 2 years after the event.

Bleeding into the vertebral canal is rare but is usually catastrophic when it occurs. Because of the rigid confines of the vertebral bodies bleeding rapidly leads to cord compression and loss of function. Urgent replacement therapy and surgical decompression are necessary. Bleeding in this site carries a high morbidity and mortality.

Damage to peripheral nerve function is normally a

result of compression and this usually is best treated conservatively. The most common lesion is bleeding into the iliopsoas muscle with compression of the femoral nerve. This presents with severe lower abdominal/groin pain, with the patient usually lying with the hip and knee flexed. There is exquisite tenderness in the lower quadrant of the abdomen and also loss of sensation in the anterior aspect of the thigh and loss of the knee jerk. Treatment consists of replacement therapy, analgesia and rest of the leg with an appropriate plaster of Paris splint.

Therapy must be continued until the patient is fully mobile and active physiotherapy must start soon after the bleed to try to preserve the function of the affected muscle groups.

Compression damage may be seen of other peripheral nerves such as radial, ulnar, peroneal and the brachial plexus. Treatment should be conservative following the above guidelines.

Renal bleeding

Haematuria has always been a common feature in bleeding disorders and has usually been thought to be of minor significance. However, there has been some recent evidence suggesting that recurrent bleeding may be associated with long-term renal impairment and hypertension resulting from clot obstruction. Such obstruction may follow an overt episode of bleeding or be associated with episodes of microscopic haematuria. As haemophilic patients are liable to the same spectrum of renal disease as non-bleeders, it is important to investigate bleeding as in any other patient group. This will include urine culture, creatinine clearance, isotope renography, intravenous urogram, retrograde urograms and cystoscopy, as indicated.

Individual episodes of haematuria should be managed with concentrates and analgesics if clot colic occurs. In addition a high fluid intake is of value to wash out small clots which do form. There has been a vogue for the use of fibrinolytic inhibitors but these may cause clots present to become unlysable, and clot presence in the long term may affect renal function and viability.

A range of other renal pathologies has been reported. These include nephrotic syndrome, analgesic nephropathy, pyelonephritis, carcinoma and perirenal haematoma.

Renal failure from a variety of causes is also well described and requires to be managed as for any other patient group. Due to the development of other haemostatic abnormalities resulting from renal failure, treatment with dialysis may need to be introduced

earlier than normal and in selected patients renal transplantation may be necessary.

Gastrointestinal bleeding

Upper gastrointestinal bleeding used to be a major problem in bleeding patients due to the apparently high incidence of peptic ulceration and the fact that such patients appeared to bleed at an earlier stage of disease than non-bleeders. The advent of H_2-blocking agents has, however, produced a dramatic fall in this complication and it is rapidly becoming a rarity, with resultant surgery for ulcer now virtually non-existent.

Acute erosions are still seen in patients taking aspirin and alcohol, despite warnings to the contrary. Such patients should be handled as all other groups of patients, with a diagnosis being made by endoscopy (after appropriate concentrate) and if necessary by biopsy. H_2-blockers should be given and continued for at least 6 weeks. It has been our policy to stop H_2-blockers when the symptoms abate; however, in those with persistence of symptoms, long-term therapy, perhaps even life-long, may be required. From mortality figures available it is clear that use of concentrates over the past 30 years has reduced the death rate but H_2-blockers have controlled the rate of recurrence of ulceration and dramatically reduced the need for surgery.

Bleeding into the bowel wall remains an infrequent but difficult diagnostic problem. This condition usually presents acutely with severe abdominal pain and features of obstruction, and mimics a large number of acute abdominal emergencies such as perforation of an ulcer, acute appendicitis and cholecystitis. Despite new imaging techniques, the diagnosis remains difficult and may only be resolved by the response to adequate replacement therapy. Barium meal and follow-through has been used but carries a risk in the presence of obstruction; CT scanning and ultrasound are of little value due to the small size of the lesion.

Fresh bleeding from the rectum is a common problem and usually of trivial importance. The usual causes are haemorrhoids and anal fissures. As in all patients a definitive diagnosis is required by proctoscopy and rectal examination. Local measures are usually successful but surgery may occasionally be required. If bleeding is obviously from a more distant source, barium enema, colonoscopy and biopsy are required (after appropriate therapy).

Muscle bleeding

Spontaneous and traumatic muscle bleeding is one of the

most common problems in haemophilia and rivals joint bleeding as the main cause of limitation of movement. When bleeding results from direct trauma there is usually superficial bruising and extravasation of blood. When bleeding starts within the muscle belly the first symptoms are pain, swelling and inability to use the muscles because of pain. On examination the features are dominated by tenderness and the patient will hold the part in a neutral position to protect it, usually with the adjacent joints flexed. Bleeding into the muscle belly usually leads to an expanding haematoma which is retained within the muscle attachments. Blood tracks with the muscle fibres and produces anoxia and death of these; this can be shown by measurement of muscle-related enzymes and also anatomically by ultrasound. Resolution of the haematoma is a slow process and may take several months to occur. Damaged muscle is replaced extensively by collagen, as there is no effective replacement of muscle fibres. The result is a shortened muscle lacking in power.

Occasionally an expanding haematoma of muscle will compress adjacent nerves and blood vessels to produce a compression syndrome, which may require to be relieved surgically.

The diagnosis is usually easy to make on clinical grounds and may be confirmed by estimation of muscle enzymes, e.g. creatine kinase (CK) and aspartate aminotransferase (AST), and by ultrasound. Haematoma in muscles in the abdomen and thorax may present a more difficult problem but this can be resolved with ultrasound or CT scanning.

The treatment is conservative at all times with infusion of adequate amounts of factor concentrates and adequate analgesia. Surgery may very occasionally be required if there is evidence of compression and this continues despite factor infusion. In addition, pain relief may be achieved by use of a cold pack (e.g. 3 M packs) and by splinting of the part. Aspiration of the haematoma has no part to play and carries a risk of inducing a chronic sinus.

Pseudotumours

This is a rare complication of muscle bleeding in haemophilia and with the advance to more effective concentrates should disappear completely. There is however a legacy of patients from the past. The common sites of formation are thigh and pelvis, calves, feet, arms and hands (Fig. 31.7). The lesion starts as a haematoma which does not resolve fully and recurrent bleeding results in progressive expansion with pressure in surrounding structures which become eroded. In the past these swellings could become enormous and erode through bone, producing pathological fractures, and even through skin, which resulted in infection within the cavity, septicaemia and death.

The diagnosis is usually obvious from the clinical history and examination. Special investigations such as radiology, ultrasound and CT scanning are necessary to define the size and extent of the swelling and to pinpoint which tissues have been eroded.

It is to be expected that active treatment of muscle haematomas will prevent the occurrence of pseudotumours in the future. If such a chronic haematoma develops, it should be actively treated with long-term concentrate infusion and, if necessary, with immobilisation of the part. It is likely that with improvements in management early surgery is now to be recommended, especially for peripheral lesions of arms and legs.

Radiotherapy has been used in a last ditch attempt to sclerose a lesion but no properly controlled studies have been reported. Some individual cases have claimed success and would suggest that it might be used.

Extensive mutilating surgery such as hindquarter amputation should now be in the past, as these lesions should be treated effectively early in their development.

Dental bleeding and its implications

Dental bleeding has always been a common presenting feature in bleeding disorders and in the past has represented a serious cause of morbidity and mortality. Usually little bleeding occurs until the natural shedding of the 'milk' teeth and the first indication of the defect may occur only after an elective dental extraction. Often such extractions are associated with an infected socket and it is a clinical impression that bleeding in this situation is more likely to occur and be more severe. It is also an impression that bleeding is more severe after extraction of teeth with multiple large roots. The bleeding characteristically occurs after several hours, presumably as the immediate response to the injury platelet plugging and vaso-constriction require some time to wear off. The oozing starts and this may be intermittent in nature as some local coagulation occurs. The end result is a continuously forming fibrin clot in the socket with bleeding occurring at the base – the so-called 'haemophilic clot'. It is probable that haemostasis is also impaired by the local fibrinolytic action of saliva which may digest away haemostatic fibrin strands.

Local applications of a large range of 'haemostatic' materials have been applied (silver nitrate, topical

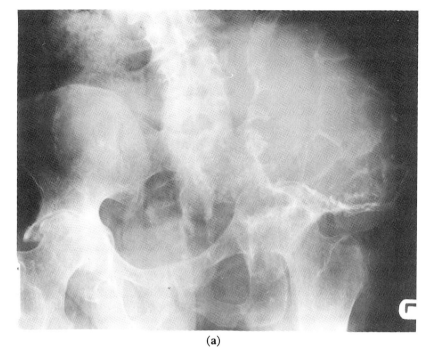

(a)

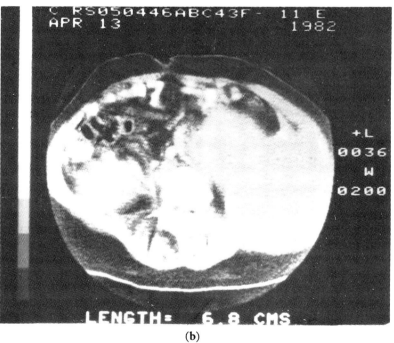

(b)

Fig. 31.7 Pseudotumour of pelvis. This shows the effects of progressive enlargement of bilateral pseudotumours of pelvis. Erosion of the wing of the ileum is far advanced on the left side. The CT scan shows the extent of organ displacement by the bilateral tumours in the pelvis.

thrombin, etc.) with little evidence of efficiency. In addition, physical protection of the socket with a pre-formed dental plate has been shown to be of some value but in severely affected patients bleeding may continue under the plate with massive clot formation. Suturing of the socket probably has some value in the patient who has been made haemostatic with appropriate plasma replacement therapy and also may be effective in patients who are only mildly affected. If this treatment is used when a patient is severely affected and untreated with concentrates, then bleeding may occur into the surrounding soft tissues and tracks along the jaw with resultant cutting out of the sutures and eventual rebleeding.

Routine extractions are best done on an out-patient basis with the patient investigated and prepared in advance. This includes screening for hepatitis B and HIV status and determination as to whether an inhibitor is present. In addition, a prophylactic broad spectrum antibiotic (e.g. ampicillin) is often used if the gum is obviously infected. There are, however, no scientific studies which have proven this, but it seems a sensible precaution. A fibrinolytic inhibitor should also be given, e.g. tranexamic acid (cyclokapron) 1.0 g four times per day. It is probably best to start therapy orally before extraction so that the inhibitor is incorporated in any fibrin thrombin which forms at the time of extraction.

As healing occurs rapidly in dental sockets, elevation of the deficient clotting factor levels is usually only necessary for a few days. In some selected mild/moderate factor VIII-deficient haemophiliacs this may be achieved by infusion of desmopressin (DDAVP des-amino-d-arginine vasopressin). In this situation a trial dose should be given the previous week and the response of factor VIII noted. This is then repeated in a dose of up to 0.3 μg/kg body weight prior to elective procedure and continued for 3–5 days. The response is variable and subject to tachyphylaxis.

It is best to monitor responses to ensure that a haemostatic response is maintained. It is also important to inhibit the fibrinolytic response to DDAVP with concomitant therapy with a fibrinolytic inhibitor. In the more severely affected patients or in a more major procedure, therapy with plasma concentrates is required and therapy must be continued until the socket is healed, otherwise recurrent bleeding may be found several days later.

When measures to ensure haemostasis are taken, as in the above procedures, suturing is advocated and this may include a variety of haemostatic plugging materials, e.g. surgical, calgitex, etc.

If bleeding occurs several days after the cessation of therapy, the same process of local and systemic measures is required.

TREATMENT OF HAEMOPHILIA A AND B

Haemostasis is secured in these deficient states by the intravenous infusion of adequate amounts of factor VIII or IX concentrates. The requirement of concentrate depends on:

1. The severity of the defect
2. The type of injury or the extent of surgery
3. The site at which haemostasis is required
4. The possible presence of inhibitors.

As already stated the half-life of factor VIII is approximately half that of factor IX and for this reason infusion of factor VIII may be required twice per day to maintain a haemostatic level. Additional factors which require to be considered are:

1. The normality of other components of haemostasis
2. The plasma volume of the patient
3. The potency of material to be used.

It is possible, knowing these factors, to accurately calculate the amount of concentrate which is required to give a predicted rise in the factor level. In some patients this predicted value may not be achieved and this presumably indicates that some material has been sequestered.

Different levels of factor may be required for haemostatic control according to the extent of the challenge, e.g. in a spontaneous bleed into a muscle or joint, a predicted value maintained at approximately 0.3 u/ml is often suitable, whereas with major surgery or a major internal bleed a value of 1 u/ml should be aimed for. It is important to limit excess use of concentrates and there is some evidence that excess use was common in the past. The best clinical indicator is the patient, who will often be able to indicate subjectively that internal bleeding is controlled. It is mandatory that haemostatic values of concentrate be maintained until the wound or injury has totally healed and this may require 10–14 days of continuous therapy.

Haemophilia A therapy

A variety of different blood products is available to treat haemophilia A and B; further details are given below and in Chapter 35.

Whole blood

This was once the major standby for bleeding but its use should be discouraged except where acute bleeding continues and circulatory support is required. It would then be used in conjunction with concentrates.

Plasma

Fresh plasma and fresh-frozen plasma is now rarely used as it is an inefficient way of administering adequate amounts of factor VIII. The volume required in an adult per infusion is 1–1.5 litres and repeated use rapidly leads to circulatory overload despite use of diuretics. The only possible value is in limiting recipient exposure to a small number of donors but it is an inefficient way of using resources.

Cryoprecipitate

Therapeutic use of cryoprecipitates still continues for selected patients. The disadvantages of low activity and labour of reconstitution are offset by the small donor exposure and this, may be particularly important in young children, especially in those recently diagnosed in which the dangers of hepatitis are an important consideration. In the UK cryoprecipitate is now rarely used because evidence is accumulating that the heat or chemical treatment of factor VIII concentrates may render them safe from transmitting non-A non-B hepatitis. It is important to stress that all new patients should be immunised against hepatitis B as soon as possible. Various ways have been sought to increase the yield of cryoprecipitate from donors. These include exercise prior to donation and infusion of des-amino-D-arginine vasopressin. Each donor unit should contain about 70–100 u of factor VIII and this should form the basis of the dose calculation. However, the great variability in recovery must always be remembered and if assays of the post-infusion levels are not done, then careful clinical monitoring is necessary.

There is also good evidence of the value and effect of cryoprecipitate in the management of von Willebrand's disease. It has been suggested that in addition to the known correction of the factor VIII level there may be factors present which stimulate the endogenous production of factor VIII and also correction of the bleeding time. It has been suggested that this might be vWF.

Cryoprecipitate has also been advocated as safer from the point of view of transmission of HIV infection due to the small number of donors in each pool and attempts have been made to heat treat it. This has not found favour due to technical problems in the UK but is used in the Netherlands.

Intermediate and high purity factor VIII concentrates

Major efforts have been made to educate the medical profession about the importance of efficient use of blood and its fractions. As a result of this more than half of the blood donations in the UK are now used for frac-

tions, in particular for harvesting plasma for collection into large pools for use as the starting materials for production of concentrates. The first step is production of cryoprecipitate which is then further purified by a series of adsorption and precipitation steps or by selective adsorption to a column containing a specific factor VIII antibody. Subsequent elution produces a highly pure material.

All concentrates are now heat treated by a variety of techniques, with temperatures in excess of 60°C for periods ranging from 24–72 hours. There is now evidence that these higher temperatures do inactivate HIV and have made the products safer. However, there is still evidence of hepatitis transmission, especially non-A non-B hepatitis although the risk is reduced. In addition, there is concern that heat treatment at higher temperatures may alter protein structure and produce neo-antigens, which in turn may alter the immunity of the recipient. Although it has been possible to demonstrate new high-molecular-weight protein complexes (probably of factor VIII, fibrinogen and fibronectin), no clinical sequelae have been documented. Some concentrates are treated with chemicals instead of heat.

Factor VIII infusion in haemophilia

All factor VIII products require to be given intravenously. There is no evidence that they can be given orally, even if coated with lipid, and subcutaneous or intramuscular injection is of little value. After infusion there is a rapid rise in the measured factor VIII level. This may not reach the value predicted from knowledge of the dose given, the patient's baseline level and the plasma volume. It is probable that some may be adsorbed to vascular endothelium and some may move into the extravascular compartment. This rapid rise is followed by a rapid fall with an exponential decay. The biological half-life of the active coagulant activity varies from 8–10 hours and this is similar no matter how the material is produced or how it is heat-treated.

A variety of complex formulae have been devised to attempt more rational administration. These involve knowledge of the patient's weight (and hence calculated plasma volume), the rise of factor VIII required and the dose of the factor VIII in the vial. In most situations this is unnecessary and imparts a spurious accuracy, and dosage is usually assessed with a 'best guess' system in which a standard number of ampoules is used followed by a clinical assessment as to whether bleeding has been controlled or not. However, in major surgery and in severe trauma it is critical to know exactly the dose required to achieve haemostasis and then to check with post-infusion assays that it has been achieved. Infusions are then given twice per day and a haemostatic level maintained until healing has occurred. This may involve therapy for 10–14 days on a reducing scale.

The question arises as to how much factor VIII is haemostatic. We know that haemophilic patients with above 5% of normal levels lead a reasonably normal life but by clinical experience we feel that higher levels must be achieved therapeutically. For minor bleedings and trauma these should be of the order of 30% normal and for major bleeding or major surgery 100% values should be attempted and maintained.

Treatment of Christmas disease (factor IX deficiency)

Factor IX is much more stable than factor VIII and remains active when stored in plasma at $-20°C$ for many months. A variety of factor IX concentrates have been made and employ the supernatant plasma from the production of cryoprecipitate. This is usually adsorbed by DEAE-cellulose which removes factors II, IX and X, which are subsequently eluted with a citrate buffer. Factor IX concentrates are stable in the freeze-dried situation for many years.

Infusion of factor IX concentrates produces a rapid rise in plasma factor IX levels and a decay curve which is biphasic. The rapid first decay has a half-life of 5 hours and the slower second phase a half-life of 24 hours. As with haemophilia the dose to be used can be calculated using weight-based formulae but these are often not used and a dose based on clinical experience is used instead. In major trauma or major surgery it is mandatory to ensure that haemostasis is achieved and post-infusion levels are necessary. Because of the longer half-life it is usual to give therapy only once per day.

Self treatment and prophylaxis

With the advent of stable concentrates of factors VIII and IX it has proved possible to use these products for self-therapy. Most severely affected patients are now encouraged to learn the techniques of self-venepuncture and infusion. In some severely arthritic patients who have limitation of arm movements this may not be possible technically and an alternative is to train a near relative. Self-therapy programmes have now been established for 10 years and have transformed the lives of patients. They can treat bleeds early, and they have mobility and control of their destiny. This has led to significant improvement in lifestyle, better educational achievement and better employment prospects. Readier access to concentrates has led to higher consumption per

head per year of factor VIII (about 35 000 units per head per year).

Prophylaxis is the ultimate aim of all those concerned with haemophilia treatment but this must await the advent of a safe product. In some circumstances this may be used to provide long-term haemostasis, e.g. in a patient with recurrent haemarthrosis or muscle bleeds. The concerns are cost of treatment, the exposure to huge amounts of plasma and possible long-term side effects of the protein load.

Adverse effects of plasma concentrates

Hypervolaemia

This was a common complication of repeated use of fresh frozen plasma which was used in a volume of 1–1.5 l once per day. Even concomitant use of an effective diuretic allowed therapy for only 2–3 days.

Allergic reactions

Minor allergic reactions are common with all plasma products and may involve only slight shivering or a minor skin rash which responds to an antihistamine. However, on occasion severe allergy with acute skin and laryngeal oedema and severe bronchospasm may occur. Such cases are extremely rare and require intravenous hydrocortisone and antihistamines. Occasional fatalities have been recorded.

Allo-antibodies

Very occasional episodes of haemolytic anaemia have been recorded in hemophiliacs treated with concentrates over a prolonged period. Many concentrates contain large amounts of isohaemagglutinins, e.g. anti-A and anti-B, which accumulate due to their long half-life in plasma.

Anti-factor VIII antibodies arise in 5-10% of patients, with the result that factor VIII infused for therapeutic purposes is rapidly neutralised and treatment is thus relatively ineffective (see below).

HIV infection in haemophilia

Very soon after the initial description of AIDS in homosexuals in 1981 it was appreciated that the same disease was being seen in intravenous drug abusers and in patients with haemophilia and those who had received other blood products. It is now appreciated that contamination of factor VIII and IX concentrates occurred in late 1980 and 1981 and as they were prepared from donor pools of up to 25 000 donors for international use, the disease was transported rapidly round the world. Although there is clear evidence of contamination of the American product with HIV initially, there have been documented instances of local products also being involved. From figures collected by the World Federation of Haemophilia there is evidence of transmission of the virus to over 80 countries with tens of thousands of haemophiliac patients being infected.

In most countries the chances of being infected were greater in those treated with factor VIII rather than with factor IX, suggesting that the method of factor IX production destroyed the virus. In the United Kingdom studies of seroprevalence of HIV infection in haemophilia show about 40% of patients to be antibody-positive. This figure ranges from 15% in the west of Scotland to 60% in Newcastle and London. If only a population of severely affected patients is looked at, the figure is approximately 90%. There is country to country variation in Europe but in America, where the amount of factor VIII used per patient per year has always been much greater, the seroprevalence figures are proportionately much higher. In contrast, in Christmas disease the UK figure for infected patients is 6% and this figure is mirrored in European countries in which the factor IX process is similar. The exception is France, where the figure is 40%, reflecting the difference in the method of factor IX concentrate production. In von Willebrand's disease a figure of approximately 5% HIV antibody positively reflects the use of small pools of locally produced cryoprecipitate.

As with the other risk groups a small number of patients have been described with a glandular fever-like illness 1–3 months after infusion of concentrate subsequently shown to be contaminated with virus. There may be fever, rash, myalgia, arthropathy and lymphadenopathy. These features rapidly settle down. The rate and scale of progression of infected patients into the diagnostic categories of ARC and AIDS is not yet clear. Initially it seemed that this was going to be different from other risk groups, in particular from the homosexuals. In 1986 in the UK study about 13% of positive patients had developed clinical symptoms, of which about 3% fell into the AIDS category, and the rest had a range of signs including lymphadenopathy, skin rashes, candidiasis, etc. This figure is now changing and our initial optimism is waning with (in 1988) an incidence of AIDS of approximately 10%. The number of patients with haemophilia and AIDS has remained surprisingly constant when considered as a percentage of the total AIDS figures and represents 1–4 per cent of the total in most countries who report accurate figures.

The spectrum of opportunistic infections in haemophilia is identical to that in other risk groups, with *Pneumocystis carinii* pneumonia being the commonest cause of death. In addition, psychiatric and behavioural problems due to direct viral invasion of brain cells produces major problems in management in haemophilia. Surprisingly, one major difference is the highly significantly lower incidence of Kaposi's sarcoma, which has been diagnosed in only 3 haemophilic patients with AIDS compared to at least 50% in all the other risk groups. The significance of this fact is unknown but may represent the possibility of two separate viruses causing AIDS, one of which (causing Kaposi's sarcoma) is killed during factor VIII preparation.

Serendipitous studies of immune function carried out prior to accidental HIV infection in haemophilia suggested alteration of tests usually associated with immune disturbance, i.e. alteration of T_4/T_8 ratios and also loss of skin reactivity to antigenic stimuli. It has been suggested, but not proved, that these patients were immune-suppressed before infection with HIV, perhaps by some component in the huge amounts of injected foreign protein in the concentrate. If this is so, it is in line with the suspicion in other groups that immune alteration (by repeated viral infections, malnutrition, i.v. drugs) may have predisposed the patient to infection.

Despite intense research it has not been possible to identify the factors which seem to protect some patients infected with virus from progression to a clinical problem. There are as yet no studies of drugs being used to modify the disease at this stage. Perhaps when less toxic drugs are available this may become possible.

The major problem faced by the Haemophilia Director is to ensure that all the other bleeding problems of his haemophiliac patients are coped with in the light of this new disease. The effect of HIV infection on patients and their families has been devastating and has produced major psychiatric and social difficulties in every aspect of the families' social and personal life. The implication of a positive HIV antibody test is that patients are not able to obtain life insurance and hence a mortgage for house purchase. In addition, society generally has spurned the positive patient, both at school and at work. Major programmes of education may alter these attitudes.

There has been concern about spread of HIV within the haemophiliac's family. In the UK the evidence is that about 10% of wives are already infected by sexual contact and a small number of babies have been infected transplacentally.

Since 1985/86 attempts have been made to heat treat concentrates and early evidence suggests that a variety of heating procedures is effective. The temperatures used range from 60°C to 80°C in the dry and wet state for periods ranging from 8 hours to 72 hours. This has resulted in loss of activity (up to 50%) at the higher temperatures maintained for longer periods. Unfortunately as yet no product is free from transmission of hepatitis-B and non-A non-B hepatitis.

For those patients who are free of HIV infection the outlook would seem to be good, with provision of heated concentrates at this time and the imminent arrival of recombinant factor VIII.

Hepatitis after use of plasma concentrates

It is now over 50 years since it was realised that hepatitis was transmitted by therapeutic plasma infusions. There has been an explosion of knowledge with regard to both hepatitis B and non-A non-B hepatitis, and vaccination is now available against hepatitis B.

The incidence of clinical jaundice varies greatly in reported studies from 1–20% of recipients of concentrates. However, this is purely the tip of the iceberg as serial biochemical measurements of liver-specific enzymes may be found in up to 90% of patients after treatment. These measurements (ALT) indicate infection of the liver with viruses with different incubation times.

Measurement of markers of hepatitis B in blood samples of multiply-transfused haemophiliac patients indicates that over 90% have antibody to hepatitis B surface antibody (HB_sAb). In a small number of patients (1–5%) there is evidence of persistence of hepatitis B surface antigen (HB_S-Ag) and this may be associated with persistent biochemical markers of liver impairment. It is now possible to immunise patients and their immediate families with an effective and safe recombinant vaccine and this should be done in all patients who are antibody negative.

In addition to hepatitis B there has been evidence of other transmissable agents causing liver disturbance – perhaps more frequently than hepatitis B virus. No specific serological markers are yet available and for this reason the name non-A non-B hepatitis is used. It is possible that two viruses are involved, one with a short (4–6 weeks) and the other with a long (20–30 weeks) incubation time. This may present with clinical jaundice but is more likely to be picked up on biochemical screening of patients' serum as elevation of levels of alanine aminotransferase (ALT).

Up to 50% of all regular users of concentrates have persistent liver abnormalities on testing and a small number have developed clinical evidence of liver decompensation with stigmata associated with cirrhosis. Studies in selected centres of such patients have shown that over half have evidence of structural liver damage, ranging from chronic active and chronic persistent hepatitis to frank multilobular cirrhosis. There is little correlation between abnormalities of biochemical tests and histological diagnosis. Repeat liver biopsy has shown progression of the hepatic pathology in most cases and it would seem clear that chronic liver disease is going to be a major problem in haemophiliac patients in the future.

There seems little that can be done to alter the course of the liver disease. To date no concentrate has been shown to be consistently free of viruses but it is to be hoped that newer methods of heat treatment and sterilisation of concentrates may make this possible. Alternatively, identification of the non-A non-B viruses may provide an effective vaccine or the availability of recombinant concentrates may be accelerated.

Other treatments in haemophilia

Use of des-amino D-arginine vasopressin (DDAVP) in haemophilia A

The plasma levels of factor VIII in normal people may be raised by infusion of the vasopressin analogue DDAVP intravenously. This also stimulates release of plasminogen activator and prostacyclin from the vascular endothelium. It has also been suggested that the drug will, in addition, enhance haemostasis by increasing platelet adhesion to damaged vascular endothelium. Moreover, DDAVP has a powerful anti-diuretic action and may be used in the control of diabetes insipidus.

In mild and moderate haemophilia and in von Willebrand's disease, it can be used in the elevation of the baseline levels of factor VIII and should slowly be given intravenously in a dose of up to 0.3 μg/kg body weight. In this situation a five-fold rise in baseline levels is to be expected in good responders and this is often sufficient to allow minor surgery to be carried out. It is always best to administer the dose well in advance of the operation to monitor the effects by factor VIII assays, as the result is unpredictable. Therapy may be continued for several days but there is usually a rapid fall-off in response, with little effect by day 5. Factor VIII produced by stimulation by DDAVP has the same half-life as plasma concentrates.

Most clinicians would use concomitant treatment with a fibrinolytic inhibitor to neutralise the action of the released plasminogen activator. There are few side effects of note. There may be generalised facial flushing, which is thought to be due to prostacyclin release. In addition continued use may cause fluid retention, with elevation of the blood pressure and weight gain.

Fibrinolytic inhibitors

The role of fibrinolysis in enhancing bleeding in haemophilia has long been debated. Routine use of fibrinolytic inhibitors has been tried but in clinical trials no significant benefit has been proved. However, in certain selected circumstances there is undoubtedly a local fibrinolytic state, e.g. post dental extraction. In these circumstances use of aminocaproic acid (EACA) or tranexamic acid (AMCA) is of proven value to protect against thrombus dissolution by activators in saliva. A similar situation also applies in the kidney where urokinase probably potentiates renal bleeding. However, use of inhibitors of fibrinolysis should be guarded due to the dangers of production of clot in the kidney and subsequent renal failure. In recurrent haemarthrosis the situation is not clear. Histologically it is possible to show plasminogen activator in the hyperaemic synovium; for this reason many clinicians use inhibitors but the results are anecdotal.

Analgesics

Pain from bleeding into the joints, muscles or body cavities is a major problem in haemophilia care. The most common problem is chronic joint disease where the pain is of low intensity and constantly present. Acute exacerbations are frequent as further bleeding occurs. Use of paracetamol or codeine derivatives is useful in low level pain but severe pain requires pethidine or morphine. Non-steroidal anti-inflammatories are potentially dangerous due to inhibition of platelet function which potentiates the bleeding defect.

Steroids

Trials of steroids have been tried in a range of haemophilic bleeding situations, especially in haemarthrosis and renal bleeding, but they have been shown to be of little value.

HAEMOPHILIA A – INHERITANCE AND GENETIC COUNSELLING

Haemophilia is inherited in an X-linked recessive fashion. It is the classical example of a genetically determined disorder of this kind where only males are affected and the abnormal gene is transmitted by unaffected carrier females (Fig. 31.8). It is now known that the factor VIII gene is located on chromosome Xq 2.8. The mutation rate (which has been estimated at $1-4 \times 10^{-5}$) is relatively high, as up to one-third of cases are apparently sporadic with the absence of any family history.

Genetic counselling encompasses a wider range of objectives than simply to advise on genetic probabilities. Counsellees may require information as to the general nature of haemophilia, the treatment required, with its potential complications, and advice as to any modification in lifestyle of affected offspring. A neutral stance is best, as parents or prospective parents may resent advice to restrict reproduction. The counsellees are usually either the parents of a known haemophiliac child (in which case the mother is of course an obligate carrier) or potential parents who know of a family history of haemophilia. The first step is always to confirm the diagnosis in the index case. Thereafter an assessment of probability of carriership is required before being able to inform individuals of the risks to offspring and what can be done to modify the outcome in terms of antenatal diagnosis.

Carrier detection

The first step is the construction of as full a pedigree as is practicable. Initial estimates as to the probability of carriership are made from knowledge of the pedigree, using the fact of the X-linked recessive nature of inheritance to identify obligate carriers and also by assessment of 'prior' probabilities. Further information from a variety of laboratory investigations is then considered.

VIII and vWF in carrier detection

In the female only one X chromosome of the pair is 'active' in any one cell (the Lyon hypothesis); hence carriers will have on average 50% of normal VIII levels. This fact on its own is, however, of poor discriminant value on account of the wide range of normal levels. If VIII and vWF (which is under autosomal control) are both measured on several occasions and the VIII:vWF ratio calculated, this provides a much more useful discriminant function, as carriers of haemophilia A have disproportionately high levels of vWF compared to VIII. If the VIII:vWF ratio is less than 0.7 on three occasions, then the estimated probability of carriership is 80%.

DNA analysis

The advent of the new methods of DNA analysis has, in some cases, allowed more precise predictions of carriership. Restriction enzymes can be used to cut DNA at specific base sequences into DNA fragments of varying length, which can be separated according to molecular weight by electrophoresis. The restriction fragment pattern will obviously be identified from the DNA of any one chromosome of a homologous chromosome pair.

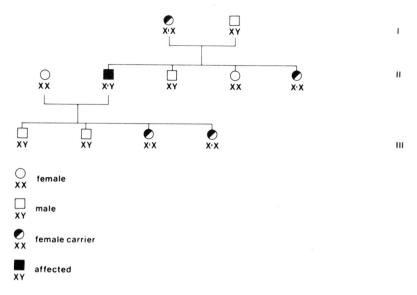

Fig. 31.8 Genetic transmission of haemophilia. The defective gene is transmitted as a sex-linked recessive characteristic.

However, during evolution non-coding intergenic DNA sequences are less well conserved than genomic DNA. These changes may lead to the creation or loss of a specific restriction enzyme cutting site or a change in the distance between two sites. The restriction fragment pattern may, therefore, be different for each of the two chromosomes of any one homologous pair. Should the haemophilia be inherited along with certain restriction fragment patterns, the disorder can be tracked through families.

In a minority of cases of factor IX deficiency there is deletion of the factor IX gene, the absence of which can be detected by the use of the appropriate gene-specific probe.

Antenatal diagnosis

Fetal sexing is possible from karyotypic analysis of amniotic cells obtained by amniocentesis at approximately 18 weeks of gestation, with a view to selective abortion of males, if this is what the parents desire, bearing in mind that there is a 50% chance that a male child would be unaffected.

Fetal blood sampling from umbilical vessels is now possible under ultrasound control at around 18–20 weeks' gestation. The reliable measurement of factor VIIIc content from such samples is not really feasible in view of sampling difficulties and the resulting effect on bio-assay results. The advent of an immuno-assay for factor VIIIcAg permits the more reliable detection of haemophilia from this source. There are risks of inducing abortion from such procedures, and these are very much higher if the fetus is affected.

Fetal materials can be more reliably assayed for content and structure of DNA rather than for gene products. Chorionic biopsy early in pregnancy is now possible as a source of fetal DNA and its analysis as described above may be informative.

PSYCHOLOGICAL PROBLEMS IN HAEMOPHILIA

As with all chronic, painful, disabling diseases, major psychological problems occur which determine the outcome of the patients, social, personal and professional life. Numerous studies have been carried out in haemophiliacs and it is apparent that as medical management has improved, the nature and variety of these problems has altered. Not only is the patient himself involved but also his parents, siblings, friends and workmates.

The major problems occur early after diagnosis with the overwhelming emotions of guilt, recrimination, anxiety and anger. The result is that major stress forms the constant background of the child's life with parental friction and often separation. Other siblings may be neglected in the effort to ensure the affected child is looked after. Constant, recurrent admissions to hospital accentuate the problem and these episodes are often ex-aggerated by failure of the hospital services to cater for the special needs of the family.

With the advent of more organised care and better prophlylaxis, attendance at school has improved and the recent generations of patients now have the same opportunity for educational achievement as their peers. This is reflected in the increased numbers who now go on to higher education, including university, and into apprenticeships. Employability in this group is vastly improved as a result. We are still, however, left with the vast number of older patients who, because of loss of educational opportunity, are able only to do manual or semi-skilled jobs, most of which are totally unsuitable for persons with disabilities such as chronic arthropathy, etc. The end result is a rate of unemployment several times the national average. In this group unemployment compounds the background stresses and there is good evidence of significant depression, anxiety states, loss of social standing and resultant physical illness.

In addition, psychiatric syndromes are well recognised, with an additional incidence of alcoholism, drug dependence (often with analgesics given for arthritic pain) and suicide.

To this background of stress are now added the difficulties of HIV infection, which produces major problems including anxiety about self, family, education and employment (see later). Remarkably, patients and their families have coped with this new catastrophe and its advent has at least resulted in more counselling being made available for the old as well as the new problems.

COAGULATION FACTOR INHIBITORS AND THEIR MANAGEMENT

Inhibitors to VIII are found in 6–12% of severe haemophiliacs; these are thought to be iso-antibodies which have developed as a consequence of exposure to 'foreign' transfused VIII. Acquired 'haemophilia' due to the development of auto-antibodies has also been described in association with autoimmune disorders, following pregnancy and occasionally spontaneously in elderly subjects with no obvious underlying disorders.

A variety of other acquired inhibitors of coagulation have been described. These include the 'lupus' anticoagulants and heparin-like anticoagulants which have been reported in association with myeloma (Ch. 32).

Factor VIII inhibitors in haemophiliacs

These are usually IgG antibodies of restricted class (most frequently IgG_4 kappa), although other IgG classes and occasionally IgM antibodies have been reported.

Most have high affinity and specificity for VIII, neutralising it completely when present in excess in a reaction that is temperature-, time- and pH-dependent. Their presence may be suspected if a haemophiliac develops increased frequency and severity of bleeds with apparent failure to respond to conventional doses of therapeutic concentrates. Post-dose assays will demonstrate poor 'recovery' of factor VIII levels. Simple screening tests involve measuring the APTT of mixtures of patients and normal plasma before and after incubation at 37°C. When an inhibitor is present in significant amount, the addition of normal plasma will fail to or only partially correct the prolongation. Quantitative assay of antibody, however, is less straightforward and usually based on the periodic assay of residual VIII after incubation of known quantities of test plasma, with normal substrate plasma as a source of VIII. One such assay is the Bethesda assay. The accuracy and reproducibility depend upon the reaction kinetics of the antibody present.

Management of haemophiliacs with inhibitors

Management is difficult. In the recent past factor VIII replacement therapy was withheld for all but the most serious, life-threatening bleeds in the hope that, in time, antibody titres would decline and, when necessary, increased doses of concentrates would achieve, albeit temporarily, therapeutic levels before an anamnestic response led to excess antibody production. Obviously the success of this approach depends on the baseline antibody levels and the briskness of immunological response. In some cases there is a 5–7 day therapeutic 'window' before titres rise significantly, permitting successful haemostasis with the use of usual therapeutic materials. Some clinical response may be seen even in those patients with high antibody titres even in the absence of a demonstrable rise in VIII. The use of 3–4 times the conventional doses of therapeutic concentrates is therefore a reasonable initial approach for significant bleeding episodes. Therapeutic options for cases refractory to human factor VIII include:

1. Porcine factor VIII. This is available in a polyelectrolyte fractionated form (Hyate-C, Speywood Labs). Activity of inhibitors is less for this animal product and useful therapeutic response can be achieved.
2. Activated prothrombin complex concentrates. These are thought to act by bypassing VIII in the coagulation cascade. The two commercially available products are Autoplex (Travenol) and FEIBA (Factor VIII inhibitor bypassing activity–Immuno). They are expensive and potentially thrombogenic but have

been reported as useful in controlling bleeding in difficult cases. The 'non-activated' factor IX concentrates used in Christmas disease patients have also been used.

3. Plasmapheresis. This can be tried to remove sufficient antibody to allow successful treatment with human factor VIII. Usually marked rebound of antibody levels occurs, however.

Attempts to reduce the level of inhibitor over the longer term have been made. Current strategies include the use of immunosuppressive drugs, sometimes as an adjunct to plasmapheresis, and attempts to induce immunological tolerance with the chronic administration of variable doses of factor VIII. The latter approach has been successful in some cases.

Inhibitors to factor IX do occur infrequently in Christmas disease patients and have also been reported in association with autoimmune disorders. Indeed there have been very occasional reports of acquired inhibitors to most of the other coagulation factors.

VON WILLEBRAND'S DISEASE

Erich von Willebrand first described a familial bleeding disorder in inhabitants of the Aland Islands in 1926. Mucous membrane bleeding and bleeding following minor injuries was common. In contrast with haemophilia both sexes were affected and joint bleeding was rare. The skin bleeding time was prolonged and at the time the disorder was thought to be due to a platelet and/or vascular defect. However, it is now known that the characteristic defect found in the group of disorders we now call von Willebrand's disease is defective platelet adhesion to the subendothelium due to various quantitative or qualitative abnormalities of the factor VIII complex and its components.

Factor VIII is found in the plasma as a complex of two proteins:

1 Factor VIII, the procoagulant portion which is deficient in haemophilia A
2. von Willebrand factor, which has a much higher molecular weight, exists as a series of multimers of varying size and is synthesised within the endothelial cell and the megakaryocyte. It is found in both the plasma and platelets and is required for successful adhesion of platelets (to exposed subendothelial collagen) by specific receptors. It is also thought to act as a transport and stabilising molecule for factor VIII. This protein is abnormal or deficient in von Willebrand's disease.

These component parts of the factor VIII complex are measured using a variety of laboratory methods, which

has at times led to rather confusing terminology. The international Committee on Thrombosis and Haemostasis has recommended the following nomenclature.

FVIII/vWF – Factor VIII procoagulant/von Willebrand factor complex.

FVIII Act – (formerly referred to as VIIIc) procoagulant activity usually assayed. using clotting methods.

FVIII Ag – (Formerly VIIIcAg) factor VIII antigen measured using various immunological methods with homologous antisera. This measurement normally correlates closely with FVIII Act.

vWFRCo – von Willebrand factor is required for the platelet aggregation induced in vitro by ristocetin and hence ristocetin cofactor activity can be used as an indirect method of quantitation.

vWFAg – (formerly factor VIII RAg or 'related antigen') von Willebrand factor antigen measured by immunological methods using heterologous antibodies to FVIII/vWF. This measurement correlates with vWFRCo activity.

Clinical features

Inheritance is typically autosomal dominant, although some variants are inherited in recessive fashion. When severe the disease may present in early childhood with apparently spontaneous bleeding from mucous membranes, e.g. epistaxes. Haemarthroses are rare. More often patients present with protracted bleeding following surgical procedures, particularly dental extractions. In women menorrhagia is fairly common.

Diagnosis and classification

Diagnosis is usually fairly straightforward with typical family history, prolonged skin bleeding time (using a template method increases sensitivity) and prolongation of the APTT with a normal prothrombin time. Specific assays of components of the factor VIII complex reveal uniform reduction in VIII Act, vWFRCo and vWFAg in the typical case. In contrast, in haemophilia the bleeding time is normal and although the VIII Act is reduced, vWFAg and vWFRCo are normal or even increased.

Further subclassification of von Willebrand's disease requires more detailed analysis of vWF multimers using two-dimensional immuno-electrophoresis and polyacrylamide gel electrophoresis (PAGE). The various types are briefly outlined below, although it must be remembered that there is considerable heterogeneity even amongst the individual types listed.

Type I–   all the various sizes of vWF multimers are found in the plasma either simply uniformly decreased in quantity (IA) or with a relative decrease in those of larger size (IB). This latter group may show higher vWFAg than vWFRCo levels.

Type II–   large and intermediate-sized multimers are usually absent. Numerous subtypes have been described according to pattern of inheritance, structural abnormalities of the vWF, discordance between platelet and plasma patterns, responsiveness of platelets to ristocetin, etc.

Type III–   typically severe and inherited in recessive fashion, these patients have only trace amounts of vWF.

Management

Fresh frozen plasma, cryoprecipitate and intermediate purity factor VIII concentrates all contain both VIII and von Willebrand activity and will correct the coagulation defect and the bleeding time in von Willebrand patients. The higher purity factor VIII therapeutic concentrates have less vWF and may be less effective in correcting the bleeding time. Transfusion of these products not only produces an immediate rise but also leads to a secondary rise in VIII Act which is maximal at 18–24 hours. This is due to increased release of endogenously produced factor VIII Act in response to the vWF infused. Indeed early experiments demonstrated similar rises when plasma from severe haemophiliacs was infused into vWD patients.

Doses of therapeutic concentrates required are estimated in the same way as those required in the management of haemophilia A. Monitoring of plasma levels is also carried out along similar lines. Local measures to effect haemostasis are particularly important in von Willebrand's disease. Epistaxes, which are common, may require packing or cautery. Therapeutic levels of factor VIII have to be achieved to cover removal of packing. Anti fibrinolytic drugs such as tranexamic acid can be useful adjuncts to other therapy, although they are contra-indicated if there is any suggestion of bleeding from the urinary tract. Dental extraction should be managed much as it is in haemophilia, with a single, adequate pre-operative dose of factor VIII concentrate along with tranexamic acid,

which should be continued for 7 days. Good local haemostasis should be effected with splinting and suturing as required. Menorrhagia can be a problem and may require hormonal therapy. Factor VIII levels are increased by oral contraceptives and also during pregnancy, which might explain why there are relatively few problems with postpartum bleeding.

As in mild or moderate haemophilia A, DDAVP will increase factor VIII levels, particularly in type I von Willebrand's disease, and although the effect is transient it can be used to achieve therapeutic levels avoiding the potential complications of blood product usage. It should not be used in severe von Willebrand's disease and may be ineffective in the other subtypes.

Von Willebrand's disease is generally a less severe bleeding disorder haemophilia with a good prognosis, although severely affected individuals can have catastrophic haemorrhagic episodes.

OTHER FACTOR DEFICENCIES

Contact factor deficiencies

Factor XII

Factor XII (Hagemann factor) is the key protease in the intrinsic coagulation pathway. Contact with various negatively charged surfaces (e.g. subendothelial collagen, glass or kaolin) leads to its activation, with subsequent activation of factors XI, IX and so forth. Although deficiency states lead to gross prolongation of the whole blood clotting time and the APTT in vitro, patients rarely have any clinically significant bleeding tendency. Indeed an increased propensity to thrombotic episodes has been suggested. The fact that factor XI can be activated in the absence of XII in a platelet-dependent system and that XII is also involved in fibrinolysis may help to explain this apparent paradox.

Factor XII deficiency was first documented in the Hagemann family in 1955, hence the eponym. The pattern of inheritance follows an autosomal recessive fashion. Most patients are asymptomatic. Occasionally a mild bleeding tendency has been reported but more frequently an association with increased thrombotic episodes has been suggested. Affected subjects have grossly prolonged WBCT and APTT. Factor XII activity in bio-assays is usually virtually undetectable, although immuno-assays have identified cross-reacting material in some cases.

Fletcher factor (prekallikrein) and Fitzgerald factor high-molecular-weight kininogen.

These are also important in the contact system of coagulation. Kallikrein, derived from prekallikrein, liberates kinins from kininogens activating both the intrinsic system and fibrinolysis. Congenital inherited deficiency states of both have been described, albeit infrequently, but affected subjects are rarely symptomatic. The APTT is prolonged but in Fletcher deficiency this prolongation is correctable by prolonging the activation phase (contact with kaolin) of the test. There is some heterogeneity of these disorders in that several kindred have been reported with a variety of defects of the kininogen system. Most are inherited like Hagemann deficiency in autosomal recessive fashion.

Factor XI

Deficiency of factor XI is also transmitted in an autosomal recessive fashion. It appears to occur more frequently in Jewish families. Affected individuals usually have a mild but clinically significant bleeding tendency. Post-operative bleeding can be troublesome, although it is easily prevented or controlled with modest amounts of fresh frozen plasma. Predictably the APTT is prolonged and the diagnosis established by specific bio-assay.

Fibrinogen

Conversion of circulating fibrinogen to fibrin is a complex process and involves the proteolytic cleavage of fibrinogen, the subsequent polymerisation of the residue and stabilisation of the polymer. Thrombin cleaves the fibrinogen molecule at the arginyl-glycine bonds of the amino-terminal end of the Aα chain, with the production of an acidic peptide, fibrinopeptide A, and subsequently thrombin cleaves the Bβ chain, with the production of fibrinopeptide B. Both these peptides may be detected in plasma using a radio-immuno-assay and are a reflection of thrombin generation, and as such may be used as markers of thrombosis.

The residuum of the molecule which has undergone conformational change forms end-to-end associations with similar molecules (soluble fibrin) and side-to-side polymerisation rapidly occurs. In this state the fibrin is soluble in 5M urea. Cross-linking of the polymer now occurs under the action of factor XIIIa which has also been activated by thrombin and this cross-linked fibrin is soluble in urea. Some fibrin monomer may also form complexes with circulating fibrinogen and high-molecular-weight FDP's, and this may be used as another marker of intravascular thrombin generation.

Congenital afibrinogenaemia

This is a rare genetic disorder which is inherited as an autosomal recessive trait. To date under 200 cases have

been recorded, with more males than females being found. Despite the low levels of fibrinogen in the plasma it is rare to have a major bleeding problem. Bleeding may occur at the umbilicus at birth and following trauma, surgery and childbirth. The condition may be diagnosed by assay of fibrinogen in plasma, which is extremely low as measured either immunologically or chemically. In addition, there may be minor changes in tests of platelet function, i.e. aggregation and adhesion, but platelet products are normal (BTG, PF$_4$). There may also be a modest prolongation of the bleeding time.

Treatment is to replace the deficient fibrinogen by infusion of plasma, cryoprecipitate or fibrinogen concentrates. As the infused fibrinogen has a long half-life (4–6 days), an infusion once per week may be all that is required for prophylaxis in the very severely affected and this may only be necessary in the majority of patients when they are injured. As all fibrinogen-containing blood products are especially able to carry hepatitis virus, it is worthwhile actively immunising against hepatitis B early in life and continuing this protection (cDNA-prepared vaccine is now available).

Dysfibrinogenaemia

This disorder implies a qualitative defect in the fibrinogen molecule which results from a genetic abnormality. Many such defects have now been described and are usually named after the city of origin of either the patient or the research group. It is important that these molecules be comprehensively and centrally investigated and a proper biochemical and genetic classification be obtained.

The result is a fibrinogen which is functionally defective and this may be found as a long thrombin time, one stage prothrombin time, or activated partial thromboplastin time. In most patients the amount of fibrinogen is normal as measured by immunological or chemical means.

Paradoxically, thrombo-embolism is a common presenting feature of these cases rather than bleeding. The reason is not clear but it has been suggested that this is due to deficiency in the normal antithrombin properties of fibrin. Treatment is usually not needed.

Factor XIII.

Factor XIII (fibrin stabilising factor) is present in plasma as an inactive precursor which, when activated either by factor Xa or by thrombin, forms the enzyme transglutaminase which covalently bonds fibrin polymers. The reaction is biphasic, the first step being removal of a small peptide of MW 4 000 from the A chain, followed rapidly by dissociation with an active dimer of modified α chains and inactive dimer of β chains. The active enzyme catalyses a reaction between the γ-chains of fibrin γ-γ dimers and between α-chains to form an α polymer.

The defect is rare and only about 200 cases have been described in the literature. These all tend to be severely affected and it is probable that many milder cases are missed because of failure to perform routinely a simple screening test. The mode of inheritance is not always clear. There is a male preponderance which may suggest sex linkage. There is an incidence of consanguinity in the parents, particularly in the females, and this may suggest an autosomal recessive trait.

The homozygote is usually severely affected and has a major life-long bleeding tendency, which may present at birth as bleeding from the umbilical cord. The pattern of bleeding is similar to haemophilia, with the additional feature that haemorrhage at the central nervous system seems commoner and also wound healing is delayed, perhaps due to deficiency of a fibroblast activity which is factor XIII-dependent.

The diagnosis of *severe* deficiency of factor XIII is simple and should form part of the routine haemostatic screen. Plasma is clotted by addition of calcium chloride and the resultant clot is tested for solubility in 5M urea or 1% monochlorocetic acid.

Factor XIII when infused has a long half-life in plasma (up to 7 days) and provides haemostasis at very low levels. It is therefore only necessary to infuse plasma weekly.

Factor V deficiency

Inherited factor V deficiency is extremely rare and was first described in 1943. Inheritance is autosomal with homozygotes affected with a bleeding disorder of variable severity, although heterozygotes are occasionally symptomatic. Associated congenital renal, cardiovascular and skeletal abnormalities have sometimes been described. Bleeding after dental extraction is fairly common, as is mucosal bleeding. This feature and the observation of prolonged skin bleeding time in 30% of patients may be related to the fact that factor V is found in platelets as well as plasma. Laboratory investigation reveals prolonged PT and APTT. Assays based on the one stage PT using factor V-deficient substrate plasma will confirm the diagnosis.

Combined deficiency of factor V and VIII occurs more frequently than can be explained by chance association. It is interesting to note that factors V and VIII have structural and functional similarities. It has been postulated that deficiency of inhibitor to protein C (protein C inactivates activated forms of factors V and VIII) could explain this associated deficiency, but more recently this hypothesis has been refuted and the mechanism is still open to question. Clinical features and inheritance are as described for isolated factor V deficiency.

Inherited deficiencies of factors II, VII and X

These factors (along with factor IX) require vitamin K for synthesis of their active forms and vitamin K deficiency must be excluded before considering the possibility of an inherited deficiency.

Factor II

Inherited deficiency of prothrombin is extremely rare. True deficiency states (hypoprothrombinaemia) do occur, with immuno-assay and bio-assay levels of prothrombin being similarly reduced. Several dysprothrombinaemic states have also been reported where abnormally functioning molecular variants have been described. These disorders are inherited in an autosomal recessive fashion. Affected individuals usually have a bleeding disorder of mild to moderate severity and may have trouble with mucosal bleeding, bruising, postoperative bleeding or menorrhagia. Laboratory investigation reveals a prolonged one stage PT and APTT. Prothrombin assay is required for a definitive diagnosis. Clinically significant bleeding problems can be managed with prothrombin complex concentrates or fresh frozen plasma.

Factor VII

This deficiency is rare, occurring in <1 in 500 000. Affected individuals may or may not have a clinically significant bleeding disorder, the severity of which does not necessarily directly relate to the measurable factor VII levels. There is thought to be considerable genetic heterogeneity. Inheritance is autosomal recessive. Laboratory investigation reveals prolonged PT and APTT. The RVV time test (which uses Russell's viper venom to activate factor X directly) will be normal. This can help differentiate factor VII deficiency from deficiencies of II, V or X when substrate plasmas for specific assays are not available.

Hereditary factor X deficiency

This is thought to have considerable genetic heterogeneity, with both true deficiency states and abnormal variants being described. Inheritance is autosomal recessive and bleeding of similar severity to that seen in VII deficiency may occur. Affected individuals have prolonged PT, APTT and RVVT (see above). The skin bleeding time is also occasionally prolonged, possibly because of the interaction of factor Xa with platelets.

Acquired isolated factor X deficiency has also been described in association with amyloid.

Combined deficiency of factors II, VII, IX and X

Inherited deficiency of these vitamin K-dependent factors has been described. They are structurally similar and all require vitamin K for the gamma carboxylation of constituent glutamic acid residues, which is necessary for their activity. An inherited defect of this process is thought to be responsible.

BIBLIOGRAPHY

Bloom A L 1987 Inherited disorders of blood coagulation. In: Bloom A L, Thomas D P (eds) Haemostasis and thrombosis. Churchill Livingstone. Edinburgh, pp 394–396

Brettler D B, Forsberg A F. O'Connell F D et al 1985 Long term study of hemophilic arthropathy of the knee Joint. American Journal of Haematology 18: 13

Forbes C D 1984 Clinical aspects of the hemophilias and their treatment. In: Ratnoff O D, Forbes C D (eds) Disorders of hemostasis. Grune & Stratton. pp 177–239

Holmberg L, Nilsson I M 1985 Von Willebrand disease. Clinical Haematology 14: 461

Jones P 1984 Living with haemophilia. MTP Press, Lancaster

Levine P 1987 Clinical manifestations of therapy of hemophilias A and B. In: Colman R W, Hirsh J. Marder V J, Salzman E W (eds) Hemostasis and thrombosis. Lippincott, pp 97–111

Lusher J M 1984 Hemophilia. Desmopressin acetate (DDAVP): its use in disorders of haemostasis. Thrombosis and Haemostasis 6: 385

Petricciani J C, Gust I D, Hoppe P A, Krignen H W 1986 AIDS – the safety of blood and blood products. John Wiley, New York

Smith P S, Levine P H 1984 The benefits of comprehensive care of haemophilia: a five year study of outcomes. American Journal of Public Health 74: 616

32. Acquired coagulation disorders

C. D. Forbes

Acquired defects of blood coagulation have three main causes:

1. Increased consumption of coagulation factors and platelets, e.g. in acute and chronic disseminated intravascular coagulation and in cardiopulmonary bypass.
2. Failure of synthesis of coagulation factors due to malabsorption state, administration of anticoagulants or in renal failure.
3. Endogenous production of inhibitors.

DISSEMINATED INTRAVASCULAR COAGULATION

Normal haemostasis is maintained by a balance between fibrin deposition, resulting from activation of the coagulation cascade, and fibrin removal by activation of a normal fibrinolytic enzyme system. The mechanism by which a fine balance is maintained is not clearly understood despite detailed knowledge of the factors concerned and their interaction.

Disseminated intravascular coagulation occurs when the coagulation cascade is activated, with the resultant deposition of fibrin and platelets in the arterial and venous trees. Fibrin deposition in excess of normal stimulates fibrinolysis as a secondary phenomenon in an attempt to maintain vascular patency. The end result is depletion of platelet numbers, consumption of coagulation factors and loss of haemostasis.

A large number of conditions have now been shown to produce both acute and chronic DIC and these are shown in Table 32.1. In all patients a search must be made for such factors, as treatment usually depends on their identification and removal (or neutralisation).

Much of our knowledge of the mechanisms of DIC induction have been produced from experimental studies and these may not correlate directly with the clinical conditions described below. Experimentally DIC may be induced by infusion of animal tissue

Table 32.1 Disorders causing DIC

Infections and infectious diseases	Bacterial, viral, protozoan
Obstetric	Amniotic fluid embolism, abruptio placentae, dead fetus, abortion, pre-eclampsia and eclampsia
Cancers	Lung, pancreas, ovary, prostate Acute leukaemias
Shock	Traumatic, cardiac arrest, blood loss
Intravascular haemolysis	Mismatched blood transfusion
Envenomation	
Vasculitis	Haemolytic uraemic syndrome, thrombotic thrombocytopenic purpura
Burns	
Extracorporeal circulations	
Haemangiomatous lesion	Kasabach-Merritt syndrome, Klippel-Trenauney syndrome
Infusion of factor IX concentrate	
Head injury	

homogenates, in particular brain, erythrocyte stroma, thymus, testis and liver. The result of such infusions is to activate the coagulation cascade with production of fibrin on the endothelium. There is also reduction of the levels of the coagulation factors and the appearance of their activation products. Occlusive thrombi are not usually produced, as fibrinolysis is simultaneously activated and the growth of fibrin controlled. In addition, a normally active reticulo-endothelial system is important for fibrin removal. If this is blocked by prior injection of thorium dioxide, occlusive thrombi are more likely to be formed. A similar phenomenon is found during pregnancy and treatment with corticosteroids.

There are four factors to be considered in the aetiology of DIC. These are endothelial injury, platelet activation, coagulation cascade activation and fibrinolysis.

In free-flowing blood platelets rarely adhere to the endothelium, presumably due to the continuous generation and release of prostacyclin, and thrombosis does not occur on normal endothelium.

A variety of factors are known to damage endothelium. These include viruses, bacteria, endotoxins, antigen-antibody complexes and toxins. In addition, it is likely that anoxia and pH changes have a similar effect. Following the loss of endothelium, the supporting structures, collagen and elastic fibres, are exposed. Platelets readily adhere to these structures, undergo viscous metamorphosis and cause local aggregates to form. Platelet activation also causes generation of thromboxanes which cause local vasoconstriction and this reduces flow at the site of the thrombus. In parallel, coagulation is activated and fibrin deposited on and between platelet aggregates. Platelets may also be directly activated by viruses and endotoxins. In some instances thromboplastins may directly activate coagulation at various levels in the coagulation cascade and these may be absorbed directly into the circulation from damaged tissue. In addition, exposure of plasma to collagen from which the endothelium has already been shed may also initiate coagulation via the factor XII pathway.

Fibrinolysis is probably a secondary phenomenon in most instances. Tissue plasminogen activator is released from damaged endothelial cells or via collagen-factor XII interaction.

Clinical aspects

Acute DIC presents as a dramatic illness with predominantly haemorrhagic manifestations and occasionally with thrombosis. The patient is usually extremely ill, and may have fever, acidosis, hypoxia and hypotension. These features may be compounded by hypovolaemia associated with major blood loss. Bleeding may occur into any tissue or out of any part of the body. There are usually multiple petechiae or blood-filled bullae, and these may be localised due to associated trauma, e.g. over boney prominences, under a blood pressure cuff or at the sites of injections. There may be evidence of bleeding from the alimentary tract (haematemesis or melaena), the lungs, vagina or renal tract. Occasionally there may be clinical evidence of digital or skin gangrene and there may be dysfunction of heart, lungs, kidneys or brain due to disseminated thrombosis.

There may in addition be other clinical evidence of the primary disease process (see Table 32.1).

Infections and Infectious diseases (Table 32.2)

Meningococcal septicaemia was the first infection in which DIC was described and it is estimated that approximately 70% of all cases of DIC are associated with infections. A wide range of bacterial and viral infections may be implicated. The disease presents very acutely with profound shock, ecchymosis, visceral bleeding and death – the classical Waterhouse-Friderichsen syndrome of meningococcal septicaemia.

A group of patients at particularly high risk are those who have lost splenic function due to either congenital abnormality, surgical removal or atrophy. The most common bacterial infection is with *Streptococcus pneumoniae* which rapidly leads to a Waterhouse-Friderichsen-like syndrome with death. So common is this in asplenic patients that routine prophylaxis with pneumococcal vaccination is strongly advised.

The mechanism of DIC induction is not known. It is possible that the infecting organisms induce endothelial damage directly, but there is also some evidence that endotoxins from gram negative organisms directly activate Hagemann factor and platelets, and such activated factors induce endothelial damage, white cell activation and release of toxic metabolites.

Treatment is supportive, with control of acute hypotension, anoxia and bleeding. The main thrust of management should be aimed at the primary infection and a range of antibiotics given. There is little evidence that anticoagulants or antiplatelet agents have any place in management and indeed may enhance bleeding.

A local variant of this syndrome is purpura fulminans

Table 32.2 Organisms causing acute disseminated intravascular coagulation

Bacteria	*Neisseria meningococcus*	
	Escherichia coli	
	Pseudonomas aeruginosa	
	Klebsiella	
	Streptococcus pneumoniae	
	Staphylococcus aureus	
	Clostridium perfringens	
	Neisseria meningitidis	
	Haemophilus influenzae	
Viral	Varicella	Herpes simplex
	Hepatitis A, B, NANB	Dengue
	Cytomegalovirus	
Fungi	*Aspergillus*	
	Candida albicans	
Protozoa	Malaria	
	Schistosoma	

which usually follows an uncomplicated viral infection such as varicella, rubella or measles. The lesions follow 2 to 3 weeks later and appear dramatically as gangrenous skin patches over the extremities, buttocks and face, coinciding with hypotension, fever and collapse of the patient. The prognosis is poor with a high mortality and morbidity. Amputation of limbs or grafting of skin is often necessary. There is some evidence that heparin may be of value but no trial evidence has been produced due to the rarity of the condition. The mechanism of tissue damage is probably that already described.

Pregnancy complications

Complications of pregnancy and delivery represent the second most common cause of DIC. During the course of pregnancy there is a progressive rise in blood coagulation factors, especially fibrinogen and factor VIII, a decrease in fibrinolytic activity and a reduction in the levels of reticulo-endothelial clearance of activated coagulation factors.

Amniotic fluid embolism. This is an unusual complication of pregnancy occurring in about 1:50 000 deliveries. It is important, as there is clear evidence of causation. As a result of damage to the membranes or uterine trauma, amniotic fluid gets into the maternal circulation and embolises. An immediate effect on the lung may induce respiratory arrest and death. If the patient survives this, acute DIC ensues with all the features of acute haemostatic failure and shock. A common site of massive uncontrolled haemorrhage is the uterine bed in which the coagulation abnormality compounds uterine atony. Amniotic fluid embolism can be confirmed by the finding of fetal epithelial cells in the mother's buffy coat and occasionally lanugo hairs. This material is intensely thrombogenic, activating both platelets and the coagulation mechanism. There is some evidence that the coagulation cascade is activated at factor X level.

Mortality is very high (75–85%) and treatment should be aimed at supportive measures and control of the uterine bleeding by direct manual pressure or by packing.

Abruptio placentae. This is a relatively frequent complication of pregnancy. DIC usually is a problem in situations in which a large retroplacental blood clot has formed. The main problem is hypofibrinogenaemia which is present in a quarter of patients. The cause of this is probably two-fold: (a) the loss of fibrin into the clot, and (b) the absorption of thromboplastins from the placenta. The patient usually presents with abdominal pain and is found to be hypotensive. Her coagulation tests are usually grossly abnormal. Renal cortical-necrosis remains a common complication. The management consists of support of the patient's circulation, replacement of red cells and emptying the uterus. Once this stimulus has been removed the fibrinogen rapidly rises. There is some evidence that infused fibrinogen concentrates may precipitate further renal damage and they are rarely required.

Dead fetus syndrome. Retention of a dead fetus results in DIC usually within 3 weeks. The mechanism is probably the absorption of necrotic fetal material which has a thromboplastin-like action. About 1 in 4 of such patients exhibits the features of DIC. The most appropriate treatment is to expedite the emptying of the uterus and this may on occasion necessitate a Caesarean section. There is some evidence that infusions of heparin stop the progressive consumption of fibrinogen. These can be stopped when labour is induced.

Abortion. Septic abortion has now become a rarity due to recent legislation. However, in the past attempts to induce abortion illegally often resulted in the introduction of infection, especially *Clostridium perfringens*. Acute DIC often resulted (see above) and the mortality and morbidity was high. The initiating factors were probably both placental and fetal thromboplastins absorbed into the maternal circulation, as well as septicaemia.

Treatment should be directed towards the infection and shock. Appropriate concentrates containing fibrinogen are of value but have a risk of hepatitis B transmission.

With regard to modern methods of inducing therapeutic abortion with hypertonic urea or saline or with prostaglandins, minor changes are often seen in platelet function and coagulation tests but only rarely is DIC found.

Pre-eclampsia and eclampsia. Pregnancy-induced hypertension has now been widely investigated and there is extensive evidence that platelet function is activated and there are changes in the coagulation cascade which are similar to those in DIC. Whether these are cause or effect is still problematical but patients with severe hypertension who develop fits (eclampsia) may show clear clinical, laboratory and histological evidence of frank DIC.

Treatment consists of control of the blood pressure by appropriate therapy with either β-blockers or combination α- and β-blockers. Prostacyclin has also been claimed to be successful. Delivery of the fetus rapidly results in resolution of the BP and the disappearance of proteinuria.

Malignancy

Clinical presentations of DIC are uncommon in malignancy, although on objective testing there is frequently some evidence of coagulation activation. DIC is more likely to occur when the cancer is far advanced, particularly when it has significantly replaced the bone marrow. The common types of cancer usually associated with DIC are lung, pancreas, stomach, prostate and ovary. All the leukaemias may also be involved, especially promyelocytic leukaemia. A variety of factors has been implicated – particularly a thromboplastin from the mitotic cells — but in addition fibrinolytic activators have been described and in some situations hypofibrinogenaemia may be found in isolation. Rarely is treatment necessary due to the low grade nature of the process and this should be directed at the primary disease. There are anecdotal reports of heparin use in acute DIC to prevent coagulation activation and also of use of inhibitors of fibrinolysis such as cyclokapron (AMCA – amino methyl cyclohexane carboxylic acid). Transfusion of whole blood and plasma concentrates may be necessary as well.

Trauma and shock

Shock from whatever cause may be associated with DIC but this is especially true if it is linked with trauma which is often complicated by infection. A variety of stimuli are then implicated, with vascular damage being induced by tissue anoxia, infection, endotoxins, immune complexes, changes in pH and activation of the complement system. The prime event in this situation appears to be activation of platelets, with platelet consumption and deposition of platelet microthrombin in the vascular tree, particularly that of the lungs. The role of the white cell in this respiratory distress syndrome complex is not understood but some of the pulmonary features are consistent with white cell activation and liberation of leukotrienes and lipoxygenases.

Treatment is supportive, with control of hypotension, anoxia and infection. Regimens of platelet-modifying drugs and anticoagulants have been used in a wholly uncontrolled fashion.

Acute intravascular haemolysis

The syndrome is uncommon in clinical practice and may follow mismatched blood transfusion, freshwater drowning, favism and paroxysmal nocturnal haemoglobinuria. Experimentally, injection of red cell stroma has been used to induce acute DIC and in clinical practice transfusion of as little as 100 ml of mismatched blood may induce activation of platelets and of coagulation. The clinical situation is complicated by shock, hypotension, hyperpyrexia and anoxia. There has been a suggestion that blockage of the reticulo-endothelial function is a prerequisite for DIC in acute haemolysis.

Treatment consists of removal of the stimulus and treatment of the primary cause, then ensuring adequate renal function by support of the blood pressure and correction of anoxia and of the changes of acidosis. Some physicians advocate the use of heparin but there is little clear evidence of benefit.

Envenomation

This is an uncommon problem in the western world but remains on a world-wide basis a common cause of morbidity and mortality. Snake venoms contain many different types of enzymes which may activate coagulation and platelets, activate fibrinolysis, damage the endothelium and lyse red cells. Venom of members of the *Viperidae* particulary contains procoagulant enzymes, some with unique actions which selectively activate different components of the coagulation cascade, and these have been used to produce diagnostic tests for coagulation screening, e.g. Russell's viper venom activates Factor X, Malayan pit viper venom activates fibrinogen and the saw-scaled viper venom converts prothrombin to thrombin.

Most snake venoms have specific anti-venoms which rapidly inhibit the DIC process. Support may be required to correct anaemia and replace essential coagulation factors.

Vasculitic disorders

A variety of disorders are lumped together under this heading and these include collagen vascular disorders, haemolytic-uraemic syndrome and thrombotic thrombocytopenia.

The haemolytic-uraemic syndrome is an acute onset disease with fever, vomiting, rapid onset of renal failure, and laboratory features of thrombocytopenia, haemolysis and a micro-angiopathic blood picture. The disease may follow an acute respiratory or alimentary infection. The disease seems to be self limiting in children but is more severe in adults, particularly in pregnant women and in those taking oral contraceptives. In renal biopsies the picture is of glomerular infarction with platelet-fibrin thrombin in arterioles. There is growing evidence that endothelial damage is the prime effect and this in turn reduces the endothelial cells' ability to generate or release prostacyclin. Combinations of antiplatelet drugs and anticoagulants have been used widely but no controlled trials of different therapies have been mounted.

Thrombotic thrombocytopenic purpura (Moschowitz's syndrome) is an apparently related condition in which the target organ is the central nervous system. It is of acute onset, with rapidly changing neurological features. It is rapidly fatal. The laboratory features are those of thrombocytopenia, haemolysis, a micro-angiopathic red cell picture and renal impairment. There may be increased fibrinogen turnover but there are usually no other laboratory or clinical features of DIC. Because of the rarity of the condition little work has been done but, as with haemolytic uraemic syndrome, it has been suggested that a defect of prostacyclin release from injured endothelium is involved. The trigger for the disease is unknown and treatment with antiplatelet agents and anticoagulants is empirical, as is the attempt to remove the presumed toxin by plasmapheresis.

Extensive burns

Extensive severe burns may on occasion be associated with DIC, with haemorrhagic complications due to thrombocytopenia and coagulation factor consumption. The cause is not fully known but is probably a combination of thromboplastins released from injured tissues and from damaged red cells which produce acute haemolysis. In addition, there is often severe hypotension due to fluid loss and plasma infusions, anoxia due to smoke inhalation and infection of the burnt sites. Treatment consists of support of the patient generally and correction of the metabolic abnormalities. There is little evidence that antiplatelet agents or anticoagulants are of any value.

Extracorporeal circulations

Exposure of blood to any foreign surface leads to protein adsorption, platelet adhesion and aggregation, and activation of coagulation. The extent of the problem depends on the type of surface to which blood is exposed and the duration. Additional factors are the presence of filters, the type of pump used to maintain the circulation and the need to oxygenate the haemoglobin. This problem arises usually in cardiodpulmonary bypass which is prolonged. Rarely is it now seen as a clinical problem in haemodialysis or in haemoperfusion.

The associated factors which may enhance bleeding are the concomitant use of heparin, antiplatelet agents and large volumes of plasma or blood transfused. In addition there may be anoxia, acidosis and infection. Surprisingly, despite all these potential stimuli this is not a common problem due to the advent of shorter surgical procedures.

Haemangiomatous lesions

A range of haemangiomatous lesions may be associated, with platelet and coagulation factor consumption.

Originally this was described with a giant cavernous haemangioma in an infant who presented with thrombocytopenia and coagulation factor consumption (Kasabach-Merritt syndrome), but it has now been described in a variety of other vascular tumours, e.g. Klippel-Trenauney syndrome, and haemangiomas of liver and spleen.

The changes seem to be associated with sequestration and activation of platelets and coagulation factors in the abnormal vessels of the lesion which are associated with a low flow and a low shear.

Treatment should be directed at the vascular abnormality, with either surgery, radiotherapy or microembolisation techniques. If DIC is severe, then heparin may be used to control the process until definitive measures are effective.

Infusion of factor IX concentrates

Infusion of concentrates of factor IX are accepted treatment for genetic deficiency of factor IX and may also be used when an acquired inhibitor of factor VIII is present (p. 369). These have been prepared in a wide variety of ways and usually contain small amounts of factors II, VII and X. During early development of these concentrates some activation of these factors probably was inevitable and infusion of them resulted in DIC as well as local thrombosis. The use of newer products which contain small amounts of heparin and anti-thrombin III are much safer and produce only minimal shortening of coagulation times on objective testing.

Head injury

Penetrating head injury with extensive brain trauma may be followed by acute DIC. The mechanism is presumably absorption of thromboplastic materials. Extensive clinical features may develop in such patients and the haemostatic defect may induce further brain damage due to haematoma formation. Treatment consists of plasma or concentrate transfusion in association with triage of the primary lesion.

Laboratory investigation of DIC

Investigations should be aimed at evidence of platelet activation, coagulation activation and fibrinolysis. As will be appreciated, there is no hard and fast pattern of changes which can be applied across the board and this is a reflection of the different aetiologies.

Simple screening tests can easily be done and a rapid result obtained. These include the thrombin time, prothrombin time and activated partial thromboplastin time, all of which may be prolonged. Fibrinogen is usually reduced and fibrinogen-fibrin degradation products increased. The platelet count is usually reduced.

The above screening tests usually allow a diagnosis of DIC to be made. More sophisticated tests are available which will help to more accurately define the extent of the haemostatic defect (Table 32.3) but these are used only occasionally if there is doubt about the diagnosis, or as research investigations.

Table 32.3 Laboratory investigation of suspected disseminated intravascular coagulation

Investigation	Result
Screening investigations	
Haemoglobin	Often low due to bleeding
Blood film	Presence of micro-angiopathic features
Platelet count	May be reduced in acute DIC
Thrombin time	Prolonged due to presence of FDPs
Prothrombin time	Prolonged due to factor
Partial thromboplastin time	consumption and presence of FDPs
Fibrinogen	Decreased amount quantitatively – macroscopically small clot in tubes
FDPs (D dimer)	Increased
Specialised tests	
Factors	
V and VIIIC	Often decreased
VIIIC and VIII:RAg	Discrepancy in values
XIII	Decreased
XII, HMW-kininogen, and prekallikrein	May be decreased
Fibrinopeptide A/B	Increased
Antithrombin III	Decreased
Platelets	
Aggregation	Defective
B-thromboglobulin	Increased due to platelet release reaction
Platelet factor 4	
Fibrinolysis	
B-β 15–42	Increased
Plasminogen	Decreased
α_2 antiplasmin	Decreased
Activator	May be increased
Plasmin/antiplasmin complexes	Present

Additional test

Reptilase time. This test is dependent on the action of certain snake venoms (*Agkistrodon rhodostoma* and *Bothrops jararaca*) directly on fibrinogen to convert it to fibrin. This reaction is independent of heparin presence. The time compared to a control is prolonged if fibrinogen is depleted and also if fibrin polymerisation is inhibited by high levels of FDP5.

Factor assays. These are of value to demonstrate activation of the coagulation cascade. Of particular importance is the measurement of levels of factors V and VII, which are extremely sensitive indicators. In addition, measurement of the difference between the level of coagulant factor VIII and the immunological level reflects thrombin generation. Other factors, such as XIII, XII, high-molecular-weight kininogen and pre-kallikrein, may also be consumed but are rarely measured and are of little clinical value.

Measurement of the released peptide fragments from fibrinogen proteolysis (FPA and FPB) is a reliable and sensitive indicator of thrombin generation. Consumption of antithrombin III may also be found as the complexes with thrombin are rapidly cleared.

Platelets and platelet activation. As platelets adhere and aggregate to the endothelium, the count falls. Local production of prostacyclin may, however, cause platelet aggregates to disperse and the result is that the platelet count may be normal. These platelets, however, show defective aggregation patterns to ADP, collagen and adrenaline. The tracings are not diagnostic and rarely of relevant clinical value. Measurement of β-thromboglobulin (β-TG) platelet factor IV provides evidence of platelet factor aggregation and release.

Fibrinolysis

Activation of fibrinolysis as either a primary or secondary phenomenon results in plasminogen consumption, increased levels of activator, decreased inhibitor (α_2-antiplasmin) and the presence of plasmin/antiplasmin complexes. Digestion of fibrin monomer by plasmin results in elevation of levels of B β 15–42 peptide levels.

Treatment

The keystones of treatment are:

1. Support of the patient
2. Treating the initiating factor
3. Replacement therapy
4. Controlling the thrombotic process.

Patient support

Patients with acute DIC are usually severely ill either because of the primary disease and its consequences or because of the results of DIC. Such patients are often best managed in an intensive care situation in which constant nursing supervision is possible. Most will require good venous access for infusion of drugs and plasma factor concentrates and for measurement of central venous pressure. This is most effectively done by insertion of a central venous line. This must be done with great care due to the liability to bleed at the insertion site and for this reason the femoral vein may most safely be used.

Anoxia and hypotension are invariable consequences of acute disease and are synergistic. High flow oxygen is necessary but may not be very effective due to concomitant adult respiratory distress syndrome. Severe hypotension may be difficult to remedy and require a combination of drug and fluid replacement.

Initiating factors

As these triggers are so variable it is mandatory to identify them and specific treatment as set out above rapidly instituted. Often the result of removing the stimulus is a dramatic improvement in the course of the disease.

Replacement therapy

Large volumes of crystalloids, plasma substitutes, plasma and blood may be required to deal with shock. Fresh frozen plasma may be used to replace coagulation factors depleted by consumption but these should be reserved for severe bleeding in patients where either the trigger factor has not been identified or cannot be adequately treated. Cryoprecipitate is an effective way of elevating the plasma fibrinogen rapidly. It is also rich in factor VIII. Each bag of cryoprecipitate contains approximately 0.5 gm of fibrinogen. All blood products do, however, carry the risk of virus transmission and they should be used with caution.

Because it is now established that antithrombin III levels are lowered in DIC due to consumption, it has been suggested that AT III concentrates could be of value in decelerating the consumption by inhibiting factor Xa. New concentrates are now being evaluated and double-blind controlled trials will be necessary to resolve this issue.

If it is considered that a platelet defect is compounding the bleeding (i.e. either in absolute numbers or the platelets are defective) a platelet transfusion may be of value. Transfusion of 5–10 packs of platelets may rapidly terminate bleeding. These platelets have a shortened half-life and transfusion may be necessary again in a matter of hours. However, it is possible to buy enough time to allow treatment of the primary disease to be effective.

Control of thrombotic process

There is little agreement of the use of heparin in DIC. Theoretically heparin should enhance the activity of anti-Xa in the form of heparin-AT III complex. However the risk is that heparin may enhance bleeding. Initial enthusiasm for its use has worn off and it tends to be reserved for a situation that has not responded to the above measures. If used it should be given i.v. in a bolus of 5 000 μ stat 1000 μ/hr. The fibrinogen level and platelet counts should be performed to monitor the effect.

DISORDERS OF VITAMIN K METABOLISM

Deficiency of vitamin K in the diet, or its malabsorption, or the presence of drugs of the coumadin group lead to deficient hepatic synthesis of prothrombin, factor VII, factor X and factor IX. Vitamin K serves as a cofactor for a hepatic enzyme system required for the carboxylation of glutamic acid present on these molecules. The resultant molecules synthesised in the absence of vitamin K cannot bind calcium and remain functionally deficient. In addition, vitamin K is also responsible for γ–carboxylation of protein C, the function of which is to inhibit activated factors V and VIII and stimulate fibrinolysis.

Vitamin K cannot be synthesised by humans and must be taken in the form of vegetables and fruit. Vitamin K is fat-soluble and its absorption from the intestine depends on the presence of normal amounts of bile and normal intestinal function.

Deficiency of the vitamin K-dependent clotting factors may then occur due to:

1. Reduced availability in the diet
2. Malabsorption
3. Failure of utilisation, e.g. due to anticoagulant drugs or hepatic disease.

Haemorrhagic disease of the newborn

Synthesis of vitamin K-dependent factors starts late in fetal life and at birth the levels are significantly lower than adult levels. This is especially so in the premature or immature infant. Following a term birth there is a fall in the levels of factors for a few days, after which there is a gradual rise towards normal levels. However, in some babies this may not occur and levels fall and haemostasis is impaired. Bleeding may occur on the third or fourth days, usually into the gastrointestinal tract, skin or internal organs. The disease may be prevented by routine administration of vitamin K parenterally (1 mg). This condition is more likely to occur in breast-fed babies rather than those fed with cow's milk, due both to the endogenous levels of vitamin in the milk (cow's milk contains four times the amount of vitamin K) and to differences in the intestinal flora found in babies fed on cow's milk preparations. In addition, the disease is more common in mothers who take anticonvulsant therapy during pregnancy.

Treatment of bleeding consists of administration of vitamin K parenterally and if necessary transfusion. (This topic is more extensively covered in Chapter 28).

Malabsorption states

Defects of vitamin K absorption are only a small facet of the widespread metabolic consequences of malabsorption. This may result from:

1. Intestinal disease – usually affecting the general handling of fat – e.g. coeliac disease, intestinal surgery, ulcerative colitis, prolonged use of broad spectrum antibiotics.
2. Hepatobiliary diseases – in which production or release of bile salts is defective. Bile salts are required to emulsify dietary lipid, e.g. obstructive jaundice, hepatic failure.
3. Dietary deficiency – this is a relatively rare problem and may only be seen in association with other severe deficiencies.

In many such patients other disorders may predominate and the haemorrhagic tendency may only be found on routine screening of the blood for a defect. Occasionally severe bleeding may occur from the gastrointestinal tract, skin and other mucous membranes. Such a bleeding defect may be compounded by co-incidental deficiency of vitamin C with resultant endothelial and platelet defects.

Management should be directed towards the prime disease and replacement of multiple vitamin deficiencies may be required. Vitamin K, 10 mg per day, is usually sufficient to correct a long-standing deficiency.

Therapeutic use of oral anticoagulants

The indications and control of anticoagulants are more extensively covered in Chapter 33. The most commonly used agent in the UK is warfarin but all the coumadin group act by inhibiting the regeneration of the active hydroxyquinone form of vitamin K, with resultant failure to γ-carboxylate glutamic acid residues on the molecules of factors II, VII, IX and X. The result is production of non-functional molecules. Depending on dose of warfarin and duration of therapy the levels of these functional factors are progressively depressed and

by use of laboratory tests a close degree of anticoagulation may be maintained. However, such therapy carries a major hazard of bleeding. Reversal of action can be achieved by stopping the drug, giving vitamin K (either orally or intravenously) and in extreme cases by transfusion (plasma or plasma concentrates). Unfortunately these plasma concentrates have been responsible for transmission of hepatitis B and should be used only in extreme situations.

Many drugs given to patients interfere with the activity of oral anticoagulants and may be responsible for haemorrhage by a variety of actions, e.g.

1. Displacement from albumin-binding sites, e.g. mefenamic acid, phenylbutazone, ethacrynic acid
2. Decrease in warfarin metabolism, e.g. cimetidine, cotrimoxazole, metronidazole
3. Receptor-site affinity, e.g. glucagon, thyroxine
4. Concomitant haemostasis inhibitor, e.g. aspirin and related non-steroidal anti-inflammatories.

Liver disease

It has been recognised by clinicians for many years that severe liver disease is associated with a variety of disorders of bleeding and it has been shown that the majority of coagulation factors are produced in the liver. These include the vitamin K-dependent factors (factors III, VII, IX and X), as well as factors XII, XI, VIII, V, XIII and fibrinogen. In addition, components of fibrinolysis (plasminogen, activators, inhibitors), complement, kinins and permeabilty factors are produced. Diseases of the liver which interfere with cell function or excretion are therefore associated with a variety of disorders exhibiting a wide range of abnormalities, both clinical and laboratory.

Spontaneous bleeding may be found from mucosal or serosal surfaces and from the genito-urinary and gastrointestinal tracts. Impaired haemostasis may exaggerate haemorrhage from varices, peptic ulcers or surgical incisions.

The following mechanisms may alone or in combination produce haemostatic defects.

Failure of synthesis of coagulation factors

Vitamin K-dependent factors. As already described, disease of hepatocytes or failure to produce or excrete bile salts leads to defective production of factors II, VII, IX and X. Such defects are associated with prolonged prothrombin and activated portal thromboplastin times. If the basic disease is in the hepatocytes, then administration of vitamin K is ineffective.

Factor V deficiency. Chronic and acute liver disease is associated with decreased synthesis of factor V. This compounds the haemorrhagic tendency associated with vitamin K-dependent factor depletion and this can be demonstrated by prolongation of the prothrombin time and by specific assays. In some patients activation of fibrinolysis with production of plasmin may further deplete factor V by direct degradation of the molecule.

Fibrinogen. Fibrinogen is exclusively synthesised in the liver and in severe hepatic cell necrosis there may be a severe fall sufficient to produce a haemostatic effect. However, in less severe disease the levels may be normal or supranormal. Changes in fibrinogen may be coincidentally found because of associated consumption due to disseminated intravascular coagulation, increased fibrinolysis, haemorrhage or massive transfusion. When low levels of fibrinogen have been implicated in the causation of haemorrhage, infusion of fibrinogen (either as cryoprecipitate or as a concentrate) may be undertaken.

Other factors. Factors XII, XI, XIII and Fletcher factors may be reduced in acute and chronic liver diseases. The clinical significance of these changes is probably of little importance.

Disseminated intravascular coagulation and abnormal fibrinolysis

Acute disseminated intravascular coagulation associated with fibrinolytic activation is common in acute liver diseases. It has been postulated that thromboplastins from necrotic hepatocytes may activate coagulation. There is probably a series of additional factors that is necessary for the full-blown syndrome to develop. This includes:

1. Reduction of clearance of activated factors due to reticulo-endothelial or hepatic cell dysfunction
2. Reduced clearance of plasminogen activator
3. Reduction in synthesis of α_2-antiplasmin and anti-thrombin III.

Disorders of platelets and platelet function

A fall in the platelet count is very common in liver disease patients but usually this is not low enough to cause bleeding. There may, however, be other factors which induce a qualitative platelet defect in the remaining platelets.

Causes of a fall in platelet number include:

1. Sequestration in the spleen due to associated portal hypertension. This is associated with a significant reduction in platelet lifespan.
2. Folate deficiency – this is particularly true in the alcoholic due to dietary deficiency of folate or increased metabolism.
3. Direct effects of alcohol – many chronic alcoholics have a low platelet count which is thought to be due directly to alcohol. The platelets which are produced are qualitatively abnormal and have a shortened survival.
4. Platelet consumption – platelets may be consumed as part of a generalised DIC syndrome.

In addition to quantitative defects in platelets, a wide range of qualitative defects may be found. These include failure of platelets to aggregate to adenosine, diphosphate, collagen, adrenaline and ristocetin, failure of platelets to induce clot retraction and failure to adhere to foreign surfaces. Production of fibrinogen-fibrin degradation products by a DIC process may also interfere with platelet function.

Treatment

The majority of patients with liver disease require no specific treatment and the defects are of a minor nature. If prolongation of the prothrombin time is due to vitamin K deficiency, then it is a sensible precaution to correct this with a course of vitamin K (10 mg) given parenterally or orally.

If active bleeding is present it is important to define the laboratory profile of abnormalities and the clinical source of the blood loss, e.g. varices, duodenal ulcer, gastric erosion, etc. While these tests are done the patient may be supported with blood transfusion, the blood pressure maintained and if necessary platelet transfusions given. Fresh frozen plasma is particularly valuable as it contains most of the factors which are possibly deficient. Depending on the results of tests concentrates of various factors may be given – fibrinogen, factor VIII, factors II, VII, IX and X. If laboratory tests show evidence of fibrinolysis there is little evidence that inhibitors such as tranexamic acid (cyclokapron) are of value. Treatment should be aimed at the primary disease.

If a particular bleeding source can be identified, then local measures should be employed. These include the use of a Sengstaken tube or laser cautery for varices or surgery for a bleeding peptic ulcer.

CIRCULATING INHIBITORS (ANTICOAGULANTS)

Defects of haemostasis may arise from the formation of auto-antibodies which are directed against a single factor or enzymatic step. They may arise as a result of plasma therapy given for a specific defect, or spontaneously in otherwise healthy individuals, or in association with a range of systemic disorders. Of this group of inhibitors the most common is that occurring in haemophiliacs who have been treated with concentrates of plasma products (Ch. 31).

Factor VIII inhibitors in non-haemophiliacs

These patients are extremely rare. Inhibitors against factor VIII have been described in post-partum women, following drug reactions (especially penicillins), in autoimmune disorders and neoplastic diseases, and in totally healthy individuals. The usual presentation is a haemorrhagic tendency and quantification of the inhibitor is required as described above. In this group of patients the course is extremely variable. Post-partum the inhibitor diminishes in titre over many months and may disappear; subsequent pregnancies may be totally normal. In some patients with autoimmune disease, such as systemic lupus or rheumatoid arthritis, the inhibitor may persist and increase in titre.

If treatment is required, then corticosteroids, immunosuppression with azathioprine or cyclophosphamide and treatment with high dosage of factor VIII concentrates may be required.

Factor IX inhibitors

The occurrence of inhibitors in factor IX-deficient patients is rare and accordingly knowledge is sketchy. They occur in 1–2% of deficient patients and exceptionally rarely in non-deficient patients. The presentation of the clinical problems is similar to that already described for haemophilia A. Treatment consists of immune suppression and the use of activated concentrates of factor IX.

Inhibitors against other factors

Inhibitors are rarely found in von Willebrand's disease. The antibodies which have been described are all polyclonal IgGs directed against the factor VIII: C-von Willebrand factor complex. In addition, antibodies have been found in patients with autoimmune and lymphoproliferative disorders who develop an acquired von Willebrand's disease. These inhibitors may disappear with treatment of the basic pathology.

Inhibitors to factor V are also extremely rare and usually have appeared in deficient patients, but they may occur in post-surgical patients or in those treated with tetracyclines or streptomycin. The inhibitors have been IgG or IgM and have produced a profound bleeding tendency associated with a high mortality. Steroids and immunosuppression have both been used but it is difficult to evaluate the results of these anecdotal reports, as the natural history of the inhibitor is to gradually decline in titre.

In addition, very rarely have inhibitors been described against factors X, XI, XIII, II and fibrinogen. They have been in patients with genetic deficiencies of the factors or with autoimmune disorders such as SLE. Treatment has usually been given with steroids and immunosuppression.

Lupus anticoagulant

This inhibitor was originally described in systemic lupus erythematosus and is said to occur in up to 10% of such patients. In addition it may be found in other autoimmune disorders, in patients with haematological malignancy and also in otherwise normal patients. The action of the inhibitor is against reactions in the coagulation cascade which are dependent on the presence of phospholipid micelles, especially involving factors VIII and V. However, they may also rarely inhibit a wide range of other reactions, both in coagulation, fibrinolysis, prostacyclin generation and platelet reactivity. When bleeding does occur it tends to be troublesome and only controllable when the basic disease is controlled either with steroids or immunosuppression. Of great interest is the large number of patients who present with thrombotic problems and also with recurrent abortion.

RENAL DISEASE

Both acute and chronic renal failure may be associated with haemostatic defects. These are usually of a minor nature, with excess bruising and epistaxis, and it is only rarely that a life-threatening haemorrhage occurs. Care must, however, be taken if a patient requires a renal biopsy or a major surgical procedure. A variety of defects have been reported involving coagulation factor deficiencies, DIC and platelet abnormalities.

Coagulation factor deficiencies.

These are rare in renal failure. In nephrotic syndrome, where there is persistent massive proteinuria, there may be a selective loss of factor IX and also occasionally of factor XII.

In a severely ill patient with renal failure who is not eating and who is treated with multiple courses of broad spectrum antibiotics, deficiency of vitamin K may appear. Many such patients also have defects of hepatic function which compounds the problem.

Disseminated intravascular coagulation

This is an uncommon manifestation of renal impairment but may be found in association with acute renal failure induced by infection, following acute glomerulonephritis and as part of the spectrum of acute rejection of a transplant.

The bleeding syndrome of renal failure is most often seen in severe acute renal failure associated with infection and presents with diffuse mucosal bleeding, anaemia and generalised systemic upset. Cause and effect are usually not clear but laboratory studies show generalised ischaemia of tissues due to microvascular thrombosis. As well as DIC there may be uraemia, haemolytic anaemia, a qualitative platelet defect and disturbed generation of prostacyclin.

Platelet abnormalities

Quantitative and qualitative defects in platelets are common in acute and chronic renal failure. A variety of mechanisms have been postulated and it is likely that in most patients a number of factors apply, e.g.

1. Renal failure depresses megakaryocyte production, leading to a low platelet count.

2. Consumption of platelets may be an integral part of the disease process, e.g. thrombotic thrombocytopenia purpura (TTP), haemolytic-uraemic syndrome (HUS) and pre-eclampsia. There is some evidence of a defect in prostacyclin-stimulating factor.

3. Thrombocytopenia may follow use of heparin given during haemodialysis.

There is some evidence that accumulation of metabolic products such as phenols, urea and guanidosuccinic acid may induce the qualitative defect. Following dialysis platelet function may temporarily return to normal.

In the majority of patients no treatment of the haemostatic defect is necessary and renal biopsy may be undertaken even in the presence of minor disorders. If necessary dialysis may be required to correct the defect before a surgical procedure. In severe cases the patient requires general medical support and treatment of any primary disease. Administration of cryoprecipitates or DDAVP may correct the bleeding time to allow a surgical procedure.

BIBLIOGRAPHY

Bailton F E, Letsky E A 1985 Obstetric haemorrhage. Causes and management. Clinics in Haematology 14: 3

Beck R L 1985 Haemostasis defects associated with cardiac surgery, prosthetic devices and other extracorporeal circuits. Seminars in Thrombosis and Haemostasis 249: 11

Bick R 1981 Disseminated intravascular coagulation. A clinical/laboratory study of 48 patients. Annals of the New York Academy of Sciences 370: 843–850

Brozovic M 1987 Acquired disorders of coagulation. In: Bloom A L, Thomas D P (eds) Haemostasis and thrombosis. Churchill Livingstone, Edinburgh, pp 519–520

Goldsmith G H 1984 Haemostatic disorders associated with neoplasia. In: Ratnoff O D, Forbes C D (eds) Disorders of haemostasis. Grune & Stratton, New York, p 351

Hirsh J 1986 Mechanisms of action and monitoring of anticoagulants. Seminars in Thrombosis and Haemostasis 12, no. 1

Prentice C R M 1985 Acquired haemostatic disorders. Clinics in Haematology (Coagulation disorders) June 1985: 414

Preston F E 1982 Disseminated intravascular coagulation. British Journal of Hospital Medicine 28: 129

Verstraete M, Collen D 1986 Thrombolytic therapy in the eighties. Blood 67: 1529

White G C, Morder V J, Colman R W, Hirsh J, Salzman E W 1987 Approach to the bleeding patient. In: Colman R W, Hirsh J, Morder V J, Salzman E W (eds) Haemostasis and thrombosis, 2nd edn. Lippincott, Philadelphia, pp 1048–1060

Wilde J T, Roberts K M, Greaves M, Preston F E 1988 Association between necropsy, evidence of disseminated intravascular coagulation and coagulation variables before death in patients intensive care units. Journal of Clinical Pathology 41: 138–142

33. Thrombotic disorders

G. D. O. Lowe

The assessment of patients with suspected thrombo-embolism was considered in Chapter 9. The present chapter considers the diagnosis of thrombosis, the evidence that antithrombotic treatment or prophylaxis is effective, the administration of anticoagulant and thrombolytic treatment, and some of the prothrombotic disorders.

ARTERIAL THROMBO-EMBOLISM

Myocardial ischaemia and infarction

Recent necropsy and angiographic studies suggest that the majority of patients with acute myocardial ischaemia or infarction have acute thrombosis in the related coronary artery. Most of these thrombi are superimposed upon a pre-existing atherosclerotic plaque which is frequently stenotic and fissured, sometimes associated with intra-intimal haemorrhage. Acute myocardial ischaemia is currently considered as a dynamic series of vessel-blood interactions. Plaque rupture initiates formation of platelet-fibrin thrombus, which may propagate to a completed thrombotic arterial occlusion, or which may embolise to the myocardial microcirculation. Release of vasoconstrictor substances (thromboxane A_2, serotonin) from platelets may also trigger coronary artery spasm. The prevalence of occlusive thrombus in acute myocardial infarction decreases with time from the onset of symptoms, possibly due to endogenous fibrinolysis or to haemodynamic dislodgement.

Acute myocardial ischaemia may present clinically in several ways:

Sudden death, with or without preceding chest pain

This usually is ischaemia-induced ventricular fibrillation. Some patients are successfully resuscitated and admitted to hospital, where subsequent investigations may or may not show myocardial infarction.

Unstable angina

Definitions of this syndrome vary, but a practical one is prolonged ischaemic chest pain, without evidence of myocardial infarction on serial electrocardiograms or cardiac enzyme estimations.

Myocardial infarction

Prolonged ischaemic chest pain, with evidence of infarction on serial electrocardiograms and/or cardiac enzyme estimations, is the clinical presentation of this condition. The electrocardiogram may show that infarction is local and transmural: 90% of such patients have acute thrombus in the relevant coronary artery at early angiography or necropsy. Alternatively, infarction may be subendocardial: at angiography or necropsy such patients usually have diffuse atherosclerosis, but a lower prevalence of acute thrombosis.

Treatment of myocardial ischaemia and infarction

Symptomatic treatment of acute myocardial infarction and ischaemia and their complications is considered in standard textbooks of cardiology. The recent rediscovery of the central importance of acute thrombosis has reawakened interest in specific antithrombotic therapy, in both the acute and the chronic phase.

Sudden death

Following resuscitation, such patients are at increased risk of recurrent acute myocardial ischaemia and sudden death. They usually have severe atherosclerotic stenoses, and the findings of platelet aggregates in the myocardial microcirculation, high fibrinopeptide A levels in the plasma, and mural coronary thrombi at necropsy all suggest that acute thrombosis plays an important role. At present there is no evidence for benefit of prophylactic antithrombotic therapy in such patients following resuscitation, but it seems reasonable to consider treatment as for unstable angina or acute myocardial infarction, as appropriate.

Unstable angina

Two recent randomised controlled trials have each shown that aspirin significantly reduces the risks of subsequent myocardial infarction or death, by about 50%, in patients with unstable angina (Harker, 1986). This may reflect the effect of aspirin in reducing irreversible platelet aggregation, and hence extension of platelet thrombo-embolism on fissured coronary arterial plaques; it might also reflect inhibition of thromboxane A_2-induced vasospasm. Recent angiographic studies have confirmed that a substantial percentage of patients with unstable angina have non-occlusive coronary thrombi; hence it is possible that aspirin might reduce the risk of subsequent completion of the occlusion by platelet deposition or by platelet-mediated spasm. One study used 325 mg of aspirin for 12 weeks; the other used 1300 mg of aspirin for a mean duration of 19 months. At present there is little evidence that anticoagulant or thrombolytic therapy is effective in prevention of further coronary events. Nitrates, beta-adrenergic blockers, calcium antagonists and coronary artery bypass grafting are frequently administered, but again there is little evidence that they prevent further coronary events. For this purpose aspirin currently appears the drug of choice.

Myocardial infarction

The total published evidence suggests that acute thrombolytic therapy with intravenous infusion of streptokinase reduces acute mortality by about 20%. Such treatment has not been widely adopted, presumably due to the financial cost, the extra work and the adverse effects of bleeding and allergic reactions. A recent, large study of high-dose, short-duration intravenous streptokinase – a more practicable regimen – confirmed a reduction in short-term mortality, which was most impressive in younger patients with their first, anterior infarct, without heart failure, and who were treated within a few hours of onset of symptoms. Intravenous streptokinase should, therefore, now be seriously considered as routine management in such patients (see Appendix I). Further studies are required to determine whether or not the reduction in early mortality is maintained in the following months and also to determine the relative efficacy, safety and cost of newer thrombolytic agents such as acylated plasminogen-streptokinase activator complex (APSAC), tissue plasminogen

activator (tPA), urokinase and pro-urokinase (Mitchell, 1986). Intracoronary infusion of streptokinase and other thrombolytic agents has also been performed, but the expense and logistics of such treatment preclude its use as routine therapy. Similar problems apply to acute coronary angioplasty and acute coronary bypass grafting as for routine therapy for acute myocardial infarction. However, such treatment may be appropriate in selected patients, e.g. those with acute coronary thrombosis complicating coronary catheterisation.

At present, the evidence that anticoagulation reduces mortality in acute myocardial infarction is controversial (Meade, 1984). Anticoagulation should, however, be considered following thrombolytic therapy, to prevent re-occlusion, which is common; and also in patients prone to venous or systemic thrombo-embolism, i.e. those with previous venous thrombo-embolism, large infarcts, heart failure and slow mobilisation. There is no evidence that antiplatelet therapy is beneficial in acute myocardial infarction, nor is there reason to think that such treatment would affect an occlusive thrombus.

Secondary prophylaxis after myocardial infarction

The total evidence suggests that aspirin, 1300 mg/day, reduces the risk of cardiovascular death by about 16% in the subsequent 1–3 years. However, no single study has been large enough to show a statistically significant reduction in mortality; nor is it likely that such a large study will be performed. The presumed mechanism is the prevention of further platelet-mediated coronary thrombi. The prophylactic effect of aspirin may be additive to the prophylactic effect of beta-adrenergic blockers. At present, it seems reasonable to consider secondary prophylaxis with aspirin and/or beta-blockers for 1–2 years following myocardial infarction, unless contra-indicated. The benefit of other antiplatelet drugs (dipyridamole, sulphinpyrazone, clofibrate) is controversial or unproven. Current large clinical trials are evaluating the combined effects of the three most promising therapies following myocardial infarction (intravenous high-dose streptokinase, aspirin, and beta-blockers).

The benefits of long-term anticoagulation after myocardial infarction are controversial. Conflicting results of clinical trials may partly reflect different intensities of anticoagulation: studies with high intensity anticoagulation (International Normalised Ratio 2.5–5) have shown reductions in recurrent myocardial infarction and death of about 50%, whereas studies with less intensive or unreported degrees of anticoagulation showed less benefit. Such high-intensity anticoagulation carries appreciable bleeding risks (4–20% incidence of bleeding per patient-year), and requires a highly-organised, intensive anticoagulant control service. This may explain why physicians prefer less toxic and less expensive secondary prophylaxis with aspirin and/or beta-blockers.

Limb ischaemia and infarction

It is likely that thrombosis on atherosclerotic plaques also plays a central role in acute-onset leg ischaemia (intermittent claudication, rest pain, ulceration) and in acute leg infarction (gangrene). Further systematic angiographic and necropsy studies are required to prove this. Cardiac embolism is also an important cause of acute leg infarction, and a search for cardiac sources of thrombo-embolism (atrial fibrillation, valve disease, myocardial infarction, endocarditis) should always be made. Arterial occlusion may sometimes be due to aortic aneurysm, arterial trauma (including inadvertent arterial injection by drug abusers) or a 'paradoxical' embolus from venous thrombosis which traverses a patent foramen ovale.

Intravenous heparin is the conventional treatment for acute limb ischaemia, pending surgical assessment for emergency catheter embolectomy or reconstructive surgery. Its use is logical, to prevent further thrombotic extension or embolisation, but there are no controlled studies to confirm its efficacy. Thrombolytic therapy with streptokinase has been used in acute leg ischaemia; while aspirin, prostaglandin infusion, oral anti-coagulants, defibrinating agents (e.g. ancrod) and thrombolytic therapy have each been used in chronic leg ischaemia. However, there is as yet little evidence of clinical benefit in controlled trials. One controlled study of aspirin and dipyridamole showed reduction in the progression of angiographic peripheral arterial disease; however, the clinical benefit of such long-term anti-platelet therapy has yet to be shown. Patients with peripheral arterial disease have a greatly increased risk of ischaemic heart disease and stroke; hence antithrombotic prophylaxis should aim to reduce myocardial and cerebral events, as well as reducing further limb arterial disease.

Cerebral ischaemia and infarction

Conventionally, clinical episodes of focal neurological dysfunction attributed to ischaemia or infarction of the brain are classified by their time course:

Transient ischaemic attacks (TIAs). These usually last a few seconds or minutes, but may last up to an arbitrary limit of 24 hours. The extent of disability may be major or minor. They may recur, and may herald the occurrence of completed stroke, particularly in the following few weeks.

Completed strokes. These last for over 24 hours. They may resolve in a few days (reversible ischaemic neurological deficit, RIND), become progressively severe (progressing stroke, stroke-in-evolution) or remain stable in extent. The extent of disability may be major or minor. Although transient ischaemic attacks are usually attributed to ischaemia, and completed strokes to infarction, computerised axial tomography (CAT scanning) may show infarction in patients with TIAs, and no evidence of infarction in patients with clinical completed strokes (Warlow & Morris, 1982).

Transient ischaemic attacks

These are diagnosed by a history of transient focal neurological dysfunction or visual loss, which may be recurrent, and by the exclusion of other diagnoses, such as epilepsy, migraine, hypertensive or metabolic encephalopathy, hypoglycaemia or intracranial tumour. CAT scanning may be indicated to exclude the latter, which may present as a classical clinical 'transient ischaemic attack'.

Platelet-rich thrombo-embolism from neck arteries or from the heart is currently believed to account for many of these ischaemic episodes; however, in about 25% of patients investigations show no source of embolism in the neck or heart. Patients with TIAs are at increased risk of both completed stroke and of coronary artery events. There is little evidence that oral anticoagulants reduce these risks. However, in patients with a cardiac source of embolism, long-term anticoagulants should be considered (see below). CAT scanning should be performed prior to anticoagulation to exclude cerebral haematoma or tumour as the focal lesion. There is better evidence that aspirin (900–1300 mg/day) reduces the risk of completed stroke, myocardial infarction or death. Many physicians currently prescribe a smaller dose of aspirin, e.g. 300 mg/day, but there is no basis for such practice in published clinical trials. The situation will be clarified by the results of a large controlled study of aspirin (300 mg/day or 1200 mg/day) which will be reported shortly (the UK-TIA study). At present, the effect of aspirin appears more marked in men than in women. The basis for this prophylactic effect of aspirin is presumably the same as in unstable angina: reduction of irreversible platelet aggregation and hence extension of platelet thrombo-embolism on fissured arterial plaques in the neck or coronary arteries.

The value of surgery (e.g. carotid endarterectomy) is controversial: a randomised trial of surgical versus medical management of TIA is in progress. At present, local expertise and enthusiasm determines the extent to which evaluation by ultrasound and angiography with consideration for surgery is pursued.

Completed strokes

Of patients in a community study with a clinically definite first stroke who underwent CAT scanning or necropsy, 83% had 'cerebral infarction', 9% had intracerebral haemorrhage, 6% had subarachnoid haemorrhage, and 2% had subdural haematoma or intracranial tumour. In only 50% of patients with 'cerebral infarction' did CAT scanning show an infarct: the other 50% showed normal appearances or atrophy, and infarction was presumed from the lack of other pathology. Angiographic studies show that 80–90% of patients with stroke have atherothrombotic stenoses or occlusions in the appropriate artery in the first 12 hours. The prevalence of occlusive thrombosis decreases with time from onset of symptoms. The situation is, therefore, similar to acute transmural myocardial infarction, and may again reflect endogenous fibrinolysis or haemodynamic dislodgement. Necropsy studies have shown that embolism from the heart may account for up to 50% of fatal cerebral infarctions, but the proportion of non-fatal cerebral infarctions due to cardiac embolism is not known with certainty.

The symptomatic treatment of completed stroke and its complications is considered in standard textbooks. As regards specific antithrombotic treatment, thrombolytic therapy is still undergoing cautious evaluation and is not recommended at present. Some doctors prescribe anticoagulants for patients with acute cerebral infarction in whom cardiac embolism is thought likely. This is rational, to prevent thrombotic extension or recurrent embolism which is common in the subsequent few weeks. However, CAT scanning is required prior to anticoagulation, to exclude primary intracranial haemorrhage or haemorrhagic infarction: 15% of patients with atrial fibrillation and completed stroke had such lesions at CAT scanning in one series. Even if CAT scanning excludes such lesions, anticoagulant therapy may still promote bleeding into softened, initially non-haemorrhagic, cerebral infarcts. The risks, benefits and timing of early anticoagulation in cardio-embolic stroke are still controversial (Meade, 1984).

There is no evidence that antiplatelet agents are beneficial in completed stroke, either in the acute stage, or as secondary prophylaxis of further thrombotic events. Reduction in blood viscosity, by haemodilution or defibrination, may increase cerebral perfusion in acute stroke, and is currently being evaluated in large controlled studies. Haematocrits over 0.48–0.50 are as-

sociated with increased mortality in acute stroke, possibly because of increased blood viscosity, and it seems sensible to prevent dehydration by adequate fluid administration, intravenously if required.

Retinal thrombo-embolism

Transient retinal ischaemic attacks (amaurosis fugax) should generally be managed as are TIAs. Temporal arteritis must be considered immediately (headaches, temporal artery thickening and tenderness, neck and shoulder stiffness and tenderness, high erythrocyte sedimentation rate or plasma viscosity) in older patients, and high-dose steroids started if this diagnosis is likely. Central retinal arterial occlusion and retinal vein thrombosis show characteristic features at fundoscopy, and require immediate referral to an ophthalmologist. A head-down tilt and haemodilution with dextran infusion should be given immediately in central retinal arterial occlusion, but visual recovery is usually poor. Patients with retinal vein occlusion require fluorescein angiography and observation for several months to detect capillary non-perfusion and its sequelae of neovascularisation and post-thrombotic glaucoma, which require laser photocoagulation. Antithrombotic drugs have no proven value.

Primary prevention of arterial thrombosis

On general health grounds it appears sensible to persuade smokers to stop smoking and overweight persons to lose weight. However, there is at present little evidence that reduction in smoking, weight, blood pressure or blood lipids reduces heart attacks and strokes, with the exception that treating severe hypertension reduces the risk of stroke, and that lowering moderately raised blood pressure in the elderly reduces heart attacks. As regards primary prevention with antithrombotic drugs, a study of aspirin is currently being conducted in Britain. Oral anticoagulants are obviously unsuitable for primary prevention, in view of their bleeding risks and the very low risk of thrombosis.

Prevention of thrombotic occlusion of arterial bypass grafts

Published trials of anticoagulants or antiplatelet drugs in prevention of thrombotic occlusion of vein or prosthetic bypass grafts have shown conflicting results. However, a recent, large study has shown that dipyridamole before surgery followed by dipyridamole plus aspirin after surgery significantly improved the patency rate of aortocoronary artery vein bypass grafts in the year following surgery. No adequate studies of antiplatelet drugs in prevention of thrombotic occlusion of peripheral arterial bypass grafts have been reported.

CARDIAC THROMBO-EMBOLISM

It is conventional to consider prophylactic long-term oral anticoagulant therapy in patients with rheumatic heart valve disease, artificial heart valves or other cardiac disorders with increased risk of systemic thrombo-embolism (e.g. non-rheumatic atrial fibrillation). However, as with prevention of arterial thrombosis, when anticoagulation is sufficiently intense to succeed in preventing thrombo-embolism, the price to be paid is a ten-fold increase in bleeding complications, including intracranial bleeding which is usually rapidly fatal. Unfortunately, the published studies were not adequately designed and therefore do not allow a confident assessment of risks and benefits of anticoagulation. The doctor must therefore guess the balance of risk and benefit for the individual patient.

VENOUS THROMBO-EMBOLISM

Deep leg vein thrombosis

Only 50% of patients presenting with clinical features suggestive of deep leg vein thrombosis (acute pain, swelling, tenderness, distended veins, change in colour or temperature) have thrombosis confirmed when venography is performed routinely. The other 50% of patients may have a popliteal cyst (Baker's cyst), which may or may not have ruptured, calf muscle strain or haematoma, erysipelas or cellulitis, lymphoedema, or unknown pathology. Since differential diagnosis is not possible on clinical grounds, it is important to confirm the diagnosis objectively. Ascending venography is currently the method of choice in the UK: it can be performed as an out-patient procedure in patients presenting to hospital casualty departments.

Follow-up studies have confirmed that patients with negative venograms who are not given anticoagulant therapy rarely experience pulmonary embolism, nor do they usually require hospital admission. Patients in whom venography shows thrombosis confined to veins below the knee have a low incidence of pulmonary embolism at lung scanning. Whether such patients require anticoagulant therapy is controversial, but anticoagulants should certainly be considered as prophylaxis against extension of the thrombus in patients who are immobile or who have other thrombotic risk factors. Impedance plethysmography is a non-invasive alternative to venography: it is a sensitive and specific test for thrombosis above the knee, but frequently misses thrombus below the knee. There is recent evidence that patients with negative impedance plethysmography who are not given anticoagulant therapy rarely experience pulmonary embolism. This again suggests that thrombi confined to veins below the knee have a low risk of pulmonary embolism. It is likely that plethysmography and other non-invasive techniques (ultrasound, thermography) will become more widely available for diagnosis of deep vein thrombosis in the future. Leg scanning after injection of ^{125}I-fibrinogen is not recommended for diagnosis of suspected deep vein thrombosis, since this method is insensitive to thrombi above the mid-thigh, and may take 3 days to give a positive result.

Patients with thrombi above the knee have a high risk of pulmonary embolism, and also of the long-term post-phlebitic syndrome which follows destruction of venous valves. It is therefore rational to consider antithrombotic therapy in such patients, and most physicians would give conventional anticoagulant therapy (intravenous heparin followed by oral warfarin) unless contra-indicated (see Appendix II). Unfortunately, no randomised controlled trials have been published; hence relative risks and benefits of anticoagulant therapy are unknown. Thrombolytic therapy with streptokinase has also been advocated: a review of six randomised trials of streptokinase versus heparin showed a significantly higher rate of thrombolysis with streptokinase, but a similarly higher rate of bleeding. Since there is not yet good evidence that thrombolytic therapy reduces the incidence of either pulmonary embolism or the post-phlebitic syndrome, the routine use of thrombolytic therapy in deep vein thrombosis does not appear justified, in view of its adverse effects and cost. Streptokinase should, however, be considered in the uncommon syndrome of impending venous gangrene, since limb viability is threatened and impressive benefit of thrombolytic therapy has been reported anecdotally. Venous thrombectomy may also be considered in this situation, but recurrent thrombosis after surgery is common.

In patients with proximal deep vein thrombosis in whom anticoagulants are contra-indicated, or in whom pulmonary embolism occurs despite anticoagulant therapy, interruption of the inferior vena cava should be considered to prevent pulmonary embolism, for example by insertion of a Greenfield filter. All patients with proximal deep vein thrombosis should be fitted with full-length elastic stockings to wear all day long-term, to reduce the development of the post-phlebitic syndrome (two stockings should be prescribed, so that each can be washed alternate weeks).

Pulmonary thrombo-embolism

Only 30% of patients presenting with clinical features suggestive of pulmonary thrombo-embolism (acute chest pain, breathlessness, fainting, shock, cough, haemoptysis) have embolism confirmed when pulmonary angiography is performed routinely. Indeed, such symptoms occur as frequently in patients without pulmonary embolism as in patients with pulmonary embolism. Since differential diagnosis is not possible on clinical grounds, it is important to confirm the diagnosis objectively. Isotope lung scanning is the most useful initial test: with normal or low-probability results it is reasonable to withhold anticoagulant therapy, and with high-probability results to give anticoagulant therapy unless contra-indicated. Pulmonary angiography should be considered if lung scanning shows intermediate-probability appearances, or if clinical suspicion does not accord with lung scan results. If pulmonary angiography is not available or not feasible in such patients, bilateral leg venography should be considered, since if this shows leg vein thrombosis it seems reasonable to give anticoagulants. However, negative venograms are seen quite frequently in the presence of pulmonary embolism. One reason for this combination may be that the entire leg thrombus has embolised. Pulmonary angiography should be considered urgently as the primary investigation in patients with suspected massive embolism, who may be candidates for thrombolytic therapy or surgical embolectomy. Pulmonary angiography has a 5% morbidity and 0.2% mortality, death being practically confined to patients with high right ventricular end-diastolic pressure (over 20 mm Hg). Follow-up studies have shown that normal pulmonary angiography almost always excludes patients with clinically significant pulmonary embolism

While most physicians would give conventional anticoagulant therapy (intravenous heparin followed by oral warfarin) unless contra-indicated, there are no adequate controlled trials in the literature, hence the relative risks and benefits of anticoagulant therapy are unknown. Thrombolytic therapy with streptokinase has also been advocated: controlled trials of streptokinase versus heparin have shown significantly increased lysis, but also significantly increased bleeding, and no reduction in mortality. The routine use of streptokinase in pulmonary embolism does not appear justified, in view of its adverse effects and cost. Streptokinase should, however, be considered in massive pulmonary embolism confirmed at pulmonary angiography, in view of anecdotal benefit. In patients in whom anticoagulants are contra-indicated, or in whom embolism recurs despite anticoagulant therapy, interruption of the inferior vena cava should be considered.

Prevention of venous thrombo-embolism

While most patients with clinically suspected deep vein thrombosis or pulmonary thrombo-embolism do not have the disease, most patients with objectively-diagnosed thrombo-embolism do not have clinical signs or symptoms (Lowe & Prentice, 1985; Goldhaber, 1985). Most patients dying of pulmonary embolism do so suddenly, without preceding symptoms of deep vein thrombosis or minor embolism. Therefore, even if antithrombotic treatment of established thrombo-embolism is effective, it can never make an impact on the disease. Prevention in all patients at risk of venous thrombo-embolism is the only effective approach. Such patients include all who are confined to bed for more than a few days after surgery or in medical wards: the risk increases with age, obesity, varicose veins, previous venous thrombo-embolism, malignancy, paralysis, and surgery or fractures in the pelvis, hip or lower limb. There is good evidence that fitted elastic stockings, sequential calf compression or low-dose heparin (5000 units subcutaneously 12-hourly until mobile) significantly reduce the incidence of deep vein thrombosis, and reasonable evidence that they reduce the incidence of pulmonary embolism. Low-dose heparin causes minimal prolongation of clotting times and minimal increased bleeding; it does not usually require laboratory control. However, stockings or calf compression may be preferred to heparin in patients at high risk of bleeding (e.g. neurological or ophthalmic disease or surgery; retroperitoneal surgery). Such routine prophylaxis is relatively ineffective in patients undergoing hip surgery; carefully-controlled warfarin therapy, adjusted-dose subcutaneous heparin or subcutaneous injections of ancrod are effective in such patients.

ADMINISTRATION OF THROMBOLYTIC AND ANTICOAGULANT THERAPY

The contra-indications to thrombolytic and anticoagulant therapy are considered in Chapter 9. An outline of administration of thrombolytic therapy is given in Appendix I, and an outline of anticoagulant therapy in Appendix II. When given as prophylaxis of deep vein thrombosis to immobilised patients, oral anticoagulants can be discontinued when the patient is fully mobile. When given for treatment of acute venous thrombo-embolism, oral anticoagulants can be stopped after 6–12 weeks, unless there is a continuing prothrombotic risk factor or history of recurrent venous thrombo-embolism. It should be remembered that many drugs interact with oral anticoagulants: a list is given in the British National Formulary, which should always be consulted with any change of therapy in anticoagulated patients.

PROTHROMBOTIC DISORDERS

Prothrombotic clinical and laboratory risk factors were outlined in Chapter 9. A brief discussion of the haematological aspects of some of these states is now given.

Polycythaemia (Chapter 26)

There is good evidence that in patients with primary proliferative polycythaemia the risk of both arterial and venous thrombosis increases with the haematocrit, which should be maintained at less than 0.45 by venesection, ^{32}P therapy or cytotoxic drugs. Possible mechanisms for thrombosis include increased platelet adhesion and aggregation produced by physical and chemical effects of red cells, and increased blood viscosity. Aspirin and other antiplatelet agents are contra-indicated, since they increase the risk of bleeding. Persons with high haematocrits who do not have primary proliferative polycythaemia also have an increased risk of arterial disease, but the benefit of reducing the haematocrit in such persons is unknown. In patients with thrombosis or arterial disease it seems reasonable to maintain the haematocrit at less than 0.50 by regular venesection. In some patients this can be achieved by reducing smoking or by regular blood donation.

Thrombocytosis (Chapter 30)

Some patients with thrombocytosis have a bleeding tendency, due to platelet dysfunction. However, others develop episodic peripheral or neurological ischaemia, often associated with increased tendency to platelet aggregation ex vivo. Such episodes may respond to aspirin therapy.

Chronic renal failure

The increased risk of arterial disease in patients with chronic uraemia has been attributed to their hypertension and hyperlipidaemia. Whether treatment of these disturbances reduces the risk is not known. They have a decreased risk of pulmonary thrombo-embolism at necropsy.

Nephrotic syndrome

Nephrotic patients have an increased risk of venous thrombosis, including renal vein thrombosis. Whether their risk of arterial disease is increased is controversial. Possible reasons for the increased incidence of venous thrombosis include increased plasma levels of high-molecular-weight clotting factors such as fibrinogen and factor VIII; increased levels of fibrinogen and other high-molecular-weight proteins which increase plasma and blood viscosity; and decreased plasma levels of the low-molecular-weight coagulation inhibitor, antithrombin III, which is excreted in the urine. It seems reasonable to consider anticoagulant therapy in such patients unless contra-indicated, especially if the antithrombin level is low (less than 70% of normal; see below).

Hyperlipoproteinaemia

Such patients have an increased risk of premature arterial thrombosis, and conventional treatment involves reduction in plasma lipids by diet and drugs. However, results of controlled primary and secondary prevention studies have been disappointing (Hampton, 1986).

Lupus anticoagulant (Chapter 32)

This is an antibody directed against phospholipid: it therefore prolongs the activated partial thromboplastin time (APTT), which depends on the interaction of several clotting factors upon a phospholipid surface. The screening test for a coagulation inhibitor is positive, i.e. the test plasma prolongs the APTT of normal plasma after mixing. The anticoagulant is distinguished from specific inhibitors of clotting factors by adding an excess of phospholipid, whereupon the APTT is normalised. It is common in systemic lupus erythematosus (hence the name) and may also occur in other autoimmune diseases. In recent years it has been recognised that patients with lupus anticoagulant have an increased risk of both venous and arterial thrombosis, as well as recurrent abortion. These risks may reflect an association with diminished synthesis of prostacyclin. The anticoagulant effect may respond to steroid therapy, but the exact roles of steroid and antithrombotic therapy are not yet known. If not recognised by the administration of a baseline APTT, the prolonged APTT may complicate heparin therapy.

Factor XII (Hagemann factor) deficiency (Chapter 31)

These patients also have a prolonged APTT: factor XII deficiency is confirmed by specific assay of factor XII. They also appear to have an increased risk of arterial and venous thrombosis, possibly due to deficiency of the factor XII-dependent pathway of fibrinolysis. The original patient, Mr Hagemann, died of pulmonary thrombo-embolism. As with the lupus anticoagulant, the benefits of antithrombotic therapy are unknown, and the prolonged APTT may again complicate heparin therapy.

Dysfibrinogenaemia (Chapter 31)

Some of these patients have an increased risk of thrombosis rather than of bleeding, possibly because the molecular abnormality interferes with plasmin-mediated fibrinolysis. The benefits of antithrombotic therapy are again unknown.

Antithrombin III deficiency

Congenital deficiency of the coagulation inhibitor antithrombin III (plasma level less than 70% of mean normal) is inherited as an autosomal dominant characteristic, and has an estimated prevalence of about 1 in 4000 in the population, as does haemophilia. It is found in 2–5% of patients screened because of idiopathic, recurrent or premature venous thrombo-embolism; hence screening of such patients appears worthwhile. The risk of venous thrombosis is increased by pregnancy (in which the incidence is 50%), surgery, illness or immobility. Prophylactic anticoagulation should be given, either temporarily at such times, or long-term. Antithrombin III concentrates from pooled plasma can be used to cover surgery or the post-partum period, but they carry the risk of viral transmission.

Deficiency of protein C, protein S or heparin cofactor II

These are recently discovered coagulation inhibitors, congenital deficiency of which also appears to be autosomal dominant and associated with increased risk of venous thrombo-embolism. Screening of patients with idiopathic, recurrent or premature venous thrombo-embolism will probably be worthwhile, but at present testing is not widely available in hospital laboratories. As with antithrombin III deficiency, prophylactic anticoagulation may again be indicated. Protein C deficiency has been associated with coumarin-induced skin necrosis, and with fatal thrombosis in homozygous neonates.

Plasminogen deficiency

A small number of patients with premature venous thrombo-embolism have recently been found to have decreased levels of plasminogen activity in plasma. Treatment with anabolic steroids may increase plasminogen levels into the normal range.

Plasminogen activator deficiency

Patients with premature venous thrombo-embolism or myocardial infarction have a higher prevalence of reduced response of tissue plasminogen activator (tPA) to stimuli such as venous occlusion or intravenous infusion of the vasopressin analogue desmopressin (DDAVP). Plasma plasminogen activator levels, measured as the euglobulin clot lysis time or the lysis area of a fibrin plate produced by the euglobulin fraction of plasma, normally increase markedly following such stimuli, due to release of tPA from venous endothelial stores. About 8% of the general population show a reduced response, but about 30% of persons with premature venous thrombo-embolism or myocardial infarction show such a response. Most of these persons release tPA from endothelium normally, but its activity in plasma is masked by high levels of plasminogen activator inhibitors. These inhibitors are associated with general acute-phase protein reactions, and high levels may be partly a consequence of recent thrombosis; high levels are also associated with hypertriglyceridaemia. Whether high tPA inhibitor levels promote thrombosis by reducing lysis of fibrin in vivo is unknown. Levels of tPA-inhibition can be reduced by anabolic steroids, such as stanozolol or ethyloestrenol, and there is evidence that such therapy may be beneficial in recurrent superficial or deep venous thrombosis. However, such treatment interacts with oral anticoagulant therapy and should be carefully monitored for side effects.

High-normal fibrinogen levels

Several recent studies have shown that a high-normal plasma fibrinogen level is a strong primary risk factor for ischaemic heart disease and stroke. Whether this association is causal is unknown, but fibrinogen might promote arterial disease by infiltration of the arterial wall, increasing platelet aggregation or increasing plasma and blood viscosity. There are currently no drugs which can safely reduce fibrinogen levels in the long term.

High-normal factor VII levels

One study has shown that a high-normal factor VII activity level is also a primary risk factor for ischaemic heart disease, possibly because it increases thrombin generation. Oral anticoagulants will reduce factor VII activity, but as discussed above there is little evidence that they are effective in primary or secondary prevention of heart attacks.

APPENDIX I: ADMINISTRATION OF THROMBOLYTIC THERAPY

If patient is on heparin therapy, stop immediately prior to thrombolytic therapy.

Give hydrocortisone 100 mg intravenously.

Have further hydrocortisone and adrenaline available for allergic reactions.

In acute myocardial infarction, give 1 500 000 units streptokinase in 100 ml normal saline intravenously over 60 minutes.

In venous thrombo-embolism, give 250 000 units streptokinase in 50 ml normal saline intravenously over 30 minutes, then 100 000 units/hour by intravenous infusion in normal saline for 24–72 hours. Confirm lytic state by prolongation of APTT or prothrombin time or thrombin time: if not achieved, increase rate of infusion, or consider urokinase (4400 units over 10 minutes, then 4400 units/hour by intravenous infusion in normal saline).

After thrombolytic therapy, give heparin infusion without a loading dose, when APTT is approximately twice control time.

APPENDIX II: ADMINISTRATION OF ANTICOAGULANT THERAPY

Heparin

Give initial bolus of 5000 units intravenously: continue with 1000 units/hour by intravenous infusion in normal saline.

Reduce dose if baseline APTT or prothrombin time prolonged, or if patient less than average weight.

Check APTT at least daily, and adjust infusion rate to maintain between 1.5 and 2.5 times control time.

Warfarin

Give 10 mg daily for 3 days when starting heparin therapy.

Reduce dose if baseline prothrombin time prolonged, abnormal liver function, cardiac failure, parenteral feeding, less than average weight, or older than 70 years.

Check prothrombin time daily initially and adjust dose to maintain between 2.0 and 4.0 times control time. The Internationalised Normal Ratio, INR, is the ratio of the patient's prothrombin time to the control prothrombin time, when the thromboplastin reagent used to measure the prothrombin times is calibrated against the International Reference Thromboplastin. Recommended therapeutic ranges are as follows:

Prevention of venous thrombo-embolism	
Prevention of cardiac thrombo-embolism in peri-operative period	2.0–3.0 × control
Treatment of venous thrombo-embolism	2.0–4.0 × control, depending on risks: thrombosis/bleeding
Prevention of cardiac or arterial thrombosis	3.0–4.0 × control

Stop heparin when prothrombin time in therapeutic range.

Reduce frequency of prothrombin time testing with stabilisation.

Arrange anticoagulant booklet and supplies, anticoagulant clinic follow-up, and education of patient before discharge.

BIBLIOGRAPHY

Davies M J, Thomas A C 1985 Plaque fissuring – the cause of acute myocardial infarction, sudden ischaemic death and crescendo angina. British Heart Journal 53: 363–373

De Wood M A, Spores J, Notske R et al 1980 Prevalence of coronary occlusion during the early hours of transmural myocardial infarction. New England Journal of Medicine 303: 897–902

Del Zoppo G J, Zeumer H, Harker L A 1986 Thrombolytic therapy in stroke: possibilities and hazards. Stroke 17: 595–607

Goldhaber S Z 1985 Pulmonary embolism and deep venous thrombosis. W B Saunders, London

Gruppo Italiano per lo Studio della Streptochinasi nell'Infarcto Miocardio (GISSI) 1986 Effectiveness of intravenous thrombolytic treatment in acute myocardial infarction. Lancet i: 397–402

Hampton J R 1986 Routine medical therapy for the prevention and treatment of heart attacks. Current Opinion in Cardiology 1: 531–540

Harker L A 1986 Antiplatelet drugs in the management of patients with thrombotic disorders. Seminars in Thrombosis and Haemostasis 12: 134–155

Lowe G D O, Prentice C R M 1985 Thrombosis. In: Bowie E J W, Sharp A A (eds) Haemostasis and thrombosis. Butterworth, London, pp 284–318

Lowe G D O, Small M 1987 Stimulation of endogenous

fibrinolysis. In: Kluft C (ed) Tissue type plasminogen activator (t-PA): physiological and clinical aspects. CRC Press, Boca Raton

Meade T W 1984 Anticoagulants and myocardial infarction. A reappraisal. Wiley, Chichester

Meade T W, Mellows S, Brozovic M et al 1986 Haemostatic function and ischaemic heart disease: principal results of the Northwick Park Heart Study. Lancet ii: 533–537

Mitchell J R A 1986 Back to the future: so what will fibrinolytic therapy offer your patients with myocardial infarction? British Medical Journal 292: 973–978

Sandercock P, Molyneux A, Warlow C 1985 Value of computed tomography in patients with stroke: Oxfordshire Community Stroke Project. British Medical Journal 290: 193–197

Warlow C, Morris P J 1982 Transient ischemic attacks. Marcel Dekker, New York

Winter J H, Fenech A, Ridley W et al 1982 Familial antithrombin III deficiency. Quarterly Journal of Medicine 51 (New Series): 373–395

Yusuf S, Collins R, Peto R et al 1985 Intravenous and intracoronary thrombolytic therapy in acute myocardial infarction: overview of results on mortality, reinfarction and side-effects from 33 randomised controlled trials. European Heart Journal 6: 556–585

34. Haemostasis in the neonate

E. A. Letsky

Normal haemostasis is determined by the interaction between the vessel wall, platelets, coagulation and anticoagulant factors and fibrinolysis. Constant changes occur in the components of these systems in the healthy neonate over the first few weeks of life and the haemostatic mechanisms are not mature by adult standards until 6–9 months of age. To complicate matters further, these changes are dependent not only on the post-natal age of the infant, but also on the gestational age.

Although the healthy term infant can maintain haemostatic competence, profound physiological and pathological stimuli may tip the balance in the direction of either thrombosis or haemorrhage. The alterations in the haemostatic system in the sick term and premature infant can only be interpreted with a knowledge of normal physiology in the developmental and prenatal periods.

Developmental haemostasis

Platelets

Platelets are present in the fetal circulation from 11 weeks' gestation onwards. There appears to be little difference between platelet counts in term and preterm infants as long as they are healthy. Sick preterm infants often develop moderate, and sometimes severe, thrombocytopenia depending on the cause. The normal neonatal platelet count lies in the adult range. Although platelet function tests in vitro are impaired due, it is thought, to a basic developmental defect in membrane, the bleeding time in normal term and preterm infants is the same or slightly shorter than in adults or older children.

Clotting factors

Visible evidence of clotting of fetal blood has been observed as early as 12 weeks' gestation. For practical clinical purposes concentrations of clotting factors have

Table 34.1 Coagulation levels as a percentage of normal adult values

	Preterm (27 weeks)	Term
Factor XIII	50	50
Contact factors XI, XII	20	20–50
Vitamin K-dependent factors		
II, VII, IX, X	30	50
Factors V and VIII	100	100
Fibrinogen	100	100

A prolonged thrombin time in the healthy neonate is presumed to be due to the presence of fetal fibrinogen.

been studied in cord blood of term and preterm infants at the time of delivery (Table 34.1). There are profound changes in the neonate during delivery and the levels obtained will be affected by these changes. Factor VIIIC levels are 30–50% higher in vaginally delivered infants than in those delivered by Caesarean section. Fibrinogen, factor V and factor VIII levels are within the normal range in term and preterm infants. Cord plasma shows a prolonged thrombin and reptilase time, suggesting an altered function of fibrinogen, but there is still controversy regarding the existence of a structurally distinct fetal fibrinogen.

Studies on the factor VIIIC-von Willebrand factor (vWF) complex show that the newborn factor VIII complex is elevated in both term and preterm infants. In addition vWF levels remain elevated until 3 months of age, suggesting that this elevation is not just a reaction to the process of delivery.

Concentrations of factors II, VII, IX and X, the Vitamin K-dependent procoagulants, are reduced in both term and preterm infants. Compared to adult levels the percentage increases from approximately 30% at 24 weeks' gestation to 50% at term. There is also a quantitative defect of the γ carboxylation of the glutamic acid residues caused by the deficiency of vitamin K (see below).

Factors XI, XII – prekallikrein (PK) and high-molecular-weight kininogen (HMWK) – are the so-called contact factors. These are reduced by adult standards, with concentrations of 20–30% in the preterm infant and 20–50% at term. These levels are not associated with significant haemorrhage in adults, but may be a major cause of prolonged in vitro partial thromboplastin time (APTT) in the normal newborn.

Anticoagulants

The four major naturally occurring anticoagulants are α_2 macroglobulin, antithrombin III, protein C, and protein S.

α_2 macroglobulin depends upon reticulo-endothelial clearance to exert its physiological role rather than inactivation. It complexes with serine proteases including the procoagulants thrombin, Xa, IXa and kallikrein. Although there are normal levels by adult standards in the newborn, the effect may be reduced because of the immaturity of the reticulo-endothelial system.

Antithrombin III levels are reduced in the newborn. They rise from levels of below 30% of adult values in preterm infants to 60% at term. However, these low levels, which can be associated with a thrombotic tendency in adults, are balanced by the lower levels of vitamin K-dependent procoagulants which antithrombin III inhibits. The newborn is thought, therefore, not to be at thrombotic risk because of the low levels of antithrombin III. On the other hand, the vitamin K-dependent anticoagulants protein C and its cofactor protein S are both reduced by adult standards in the newborn infant. The role of these factors is to inactivate factors V and VIII – two of the major rate-limiting steps in blood clotting. These factors are at normal adult or increased concentrations in both term and preterm infants. The physiological imbalance between factors V and VIII and protein C may be a cause for the thrombotic tendency in the newborn infant.

Fibrinolytic system

The newborn infant, whether mature or preterm, demonstrates an overall increased fibrinolytic activity which lasts for several hours, probably due to increased activator activity. This is in spite of levels of plasminogen ranging from 25% for preterm to 50% in term infants. Sick infants, with the additional stress of DIC or respiratory distress (RDS), frequently deplete their fibrinolytic potential. In healthy infants plasminogen reaches normal adult levels by approximately 2 weeks of age. Because newborn plasminogen has been demonstrated to be defective in its function, it has been suggested that infusions of plasminogen may help in reducing the severity of RDS. Normal infants do not show increased levels of FDPs if the blood is collected properly. Elevated levels of FDPs are seen frequently in sick infants.

Haemostasis screening tests in the newborn

The laboratory investigation of many haemostatic defects in the newborn is limited by the lack of normal reference values and also by difficulties in obtaining adequate samples for testing, uncontaminated with tissue thromboplastin or heparin. Suitable venous samples can usually be obtained with persistence, but the haematologist is dependent on the skills of the bedside neonatologist to obtain such samples for testing, whereas in the investigations of coagulation in the older child and adult they can collect the samples themselves and deal with them immediately if necessary. Peripheral venous samples are preferable to capillary, arterial or indwelling catheter samples, as all of these may give rise to significant artefacts. Care must be taken to correct the volume of anticoagulant in presence of a raised haematocrit. Microtechniques must be instituted because the investigations are usually repeated and are only part of various other parameters which have to be measured in the sick newborn with its comparatively small blood volume.

Every laboratory will have its own normal ranges for the various screening tests, but a rough idea of the deviation from adult results of such tests in the newborn is given in Table 34.2.

Table 34.2 Neonatal haemostasis – screening tests

Test	Pre-term infant ≃ 27–30 weeks	Term infant	Adult
	Bleeding time (Min)		
Bleeding time (Min)	Within adult range	Within adult range	2–10
Activated partial thromboplastin time (APTT) (sec)	70–110	40–60	35–45
Prothrombin time (PT) (sec)	17–29	12–20	12–14
Thrombin time (TT) (sec)	20–28	18–24	15–19

HAEMORRHAGIC DISEASE OF THE NEWBORN

Although some controversy remains as to whether all newborn infants require vitamin K prophylaxis, there is little doubt that haemorrhagic disease of the newborn is virtually non-existent in infants given a parenteral dose of vitamin K at birth. Three patterns of vitamin K deficiency have been described:

Early

Bleeding during delivery or in the first 24 hours is seen in infants whose mothers have taken drugs which affect vitamin K metabolism, e.g. warfarin, anticonvulsants or rifampicin and isoniazid. Rare idiopathic cases occur for which there is no apparent explanation. Bleeding manifestations are variable, ranging from skin bruising or umbilical oozing to devastating intracranial, intrathoracic or intra-abdominal haemorrhage.

Classic

This occurs at 2–5 days of age. A previously normal infant may develop generalised bruising, gastrointestinal bleeding and, less frequently, intracranial bleeding. All infants are relatively vitamin K-deficient at birth and also have low prothrombin levels, partly due to immaturity of the liver.

Human milk contains one-fifth of the vitamin K found in cow's milk, therefore it is not surprising that breast-feeding plays an important part in its pathogenesis. It is thought that bleeding manifestations occur when the prothrombin level drops to 25% of normal adult levels.

Late

This remains an important cause of both morbidity and mortality in infants greater than one month of age. The vast majority present with acute intracranial haemorrhage; those who survive are often left with severe neurological handicap. Although some cases occur as a secondary manifestation of chronic diarrhoea treated with antibiotics, cystic fibrosis or other malabsorption syndromes, many are idiopathic and usually occur in breast-fed infants who did not receive prophylaxis at birth.

Controversies continue but a recommended sensible regime of prophylaxis is as follows:

- All healthy term infants should receive vitamin K 0.5–1 mg orally as soon after delivery as possible.
- All preterm infants should receive parenteral vitamin K.
- All infants who require prolonged intravenous therapy or parenteral nutrition should be supplemented with vitamin K regularly.
- Any infant with chronic diarrhoea, cystic fibrosis, biliary atresia or other cause of malabsorption should have regular supplementations with vitamin K.

- Infants born to mothers who have been taking anticonvulsants, rifampicin or isoniazid should receive parenteral vitamin K as soon as possible after delivery. (It is to be hoped that no infant will be born where a mother is taking warfarin!).
- Exclusively breast-fed infants who develop diarrhoea of more than a few days should be given parenteral vitamin K.

DISSEMINATED INTRAVASCULAR COAGULATION IN THE NEONATE

Disseminated intravascular coagulation (DIC) is always a secondary phenomenon (Ch. 32).

Laboratory evidence and clinical expression of DIC are frequent findings in the sick newborn infant, because triggers of the process such as hypoxia, acidosis, hypothermia, poor tissue perfusion and hypotension quickly develop in the course of neonatal disease whatever its origin, particularly in the preterm infant. The severity of clinical expression is compounded by immaturity, limiting the ability to produce coagulation factors to replace those consumed and the fact that the poorly developed reticulo-endothelial system is unable to clear the products of coagulation, such as FDPs, efficiently.

DIC in the neonate is frequently associated with maternal hypertension and shock, abruptio placentae, placenta praevia and also with a dead twin fetus. Post-delivery associations include both bacterial and viral infection, respiratory distress syndrome, erythroblastosis fetalis, necrotising enterocolitis and hyperviscosity.

The most practical and useful tests for diagnosis and day-to-day management of DIC in the newborn are the platelet count and prothrombin and thrombin times with fibrinogen titre and FDPs. The management must depend on successful elimination of the trigger and will vary accordingly, but it is sometimes necessary to replace coagulation factors with fresh frozen plasma and occasional exchange transfusion is indicated. Platelets are rarely severely depressed except in association with sepsis, and platelet transfusions are almost never required in this situation. Indeed their use may be harmful in providing free thromboplastin and a continuing trigger for DIC.

THROMBOSIS IN THE NEWBORN INFANT

The preterm and term infant are particularly susceptible to acquired thrombotic lesions, in both the presence and absence of indwelling catheters. It is difficult to know whether the apparent increasing incidence is due to the use of more searching and accurate diagnostic methods or due to changing modes of therapy and support in the special care baby unit.

Risk factors for neonatal thrombosis

Three major factors contribute to the formation of thrombin according to Virchow's postulates:

1. Abnormalities of vessel wall
2. Disturbances of blood flow
3. Changes in blood coagulability.

Only those factors of particular significance in the newborn infant will be considered.

Abnormalities of the vessel wall

Abnormal chorion vessels. A wide variety of maternal disorders, including hypertension, may result in thrombin formation in fetal placental veins. Chorion thrombi are of importance because they may embolise to fetal vessels.

Defective closure of the ductus arteriosus. If the ductus does not undergo its normal involutional change, thrombin may form within the vessel and provide a source of emboli to both systemic and pulmonary circulations.

Intravascular catheters both provide a foreign surface and may injure the vessel wall in which they are placed, exposing collagen and releasing thromboplastin. They are frequently associated with thrombo-embolism (see below).

Shock and infection. Endothelial damage provoked by localised or generalised hypoxaemia may well initiate thrombosis, as will the endothelial damage occurring in the course of septicaemia. These are well-known triggers of DIC, but may also cause localised thrombosis.

Disturbances of blood flow

The development of hyperviscosity in the neonate is due mainly to an abnormally high haematocrit. Please refer to the section on polycythaemia for infants at particular risk. Hypotension and venous stasis will also contribute to the risk of developing venous thrombosis in the sick infant with or without pathological polycythaemia.

Changes in blood coagulation and fibrinolysis

Normal physiological changes in neonatal haemostasis, as described above, do not seem to predispose the healthy infant to thrombotic complications. Low levels of antithrombin III are balanced by low levels of procoagulant factors, against which antithrombin III is

directed. However, there is a discrepancy between the low levels of protein C in the neonate and the normal to high levels of factors V and VIII. Hereditary protein C deficiency in its heterozygous form is associated with a thrombotic tendency later in life (see Ch. 33). Severe or homozygous protein C deficiency is associated with massive thrombo-embolism and recurrent purpura fulminans in the neonate. Although successful management with fresh frozen plasma followed by warfarin therapy has been reported, this genetic condition is usually rapidly fatal.

It is not established whether or to what degree any of the special features of normal neonatal haemostasis contribute to the thrombotic tendency in the sick newborn infant. In contrast, convincing demonstrations of the role of vascular damage and disturbances of blood flow in the development of thrombosis have been made by several groups.

Thrombosis associated with the use of indwelling cathethers

There is a potential risk of initiating thrombosis by use of indwelling catheters in the neonate irrespective of the vessel catheterised.

Umbilical artery. Umbilical artery catheterisation is common in the sick newborn and has been associated with severe thrombo-embolic phenomena requiring aggressive intervention in 1% of cases. The incidence of subclinical thrombosis is much higher and can be detected in 20–95% of infants with umbilical artery catheters using arteriography. Sequelae of clinically evident thrombosis include renal hypertension, necrotising enterocolitis, peripheral gangrene and even paraplegia. Follow-up studies in small groups of children up to the age of 4 years have not revealed any sequelae of clinically silent catheter-induced thrombosis.

Prevention of catheter-related thrombosis is an important but controversial issue. It is current practice to use heparin at the rate of 1–10 units or more per hour in many SCBUs. Although catheter patency has been shown to improve when heparin is given in doses of 100–200 μ/kg per day, the effect on incidence of catheter-related thrombosis is still not established. There is also the hazard of bleeding when heparin is given in doses of 5–10 μ/kg/hour in the very-low-birth-weight infant.

Umbilical vein. It is generally believed that umbilical vein catheters carry a greater risk of thrombosis than arterial catheters but this has never been demonstrated in a prospective trial.

Misplacement of the catheter and rapid infusion of hyperosmolar solutions increase the incidence of thrombosis. The incorrect placement of the catheter in the portal or hepatic vein may lead to hepatic necrosis. Portal vein thrombosis resulting in portal hypertension has also been described. Splenic vein thrombosis has been described as a late complication of umbilical catheterisation. The patients present with splenomegaly and gastric and oesophageal varices.

Immediate clinical signs of thrombosis associated with umbilical vein catheterisation are slight or absent, in contrast to those associated with umbilical artery catheterisation.

In order to reduce the risk of hepatic necrosis and portal vein thrombosis, the tip of the catheter should be placed correctly in the inferior vena cava and its position checked by ultrasound before hyperosmolar fluids are infused.

Superior vena cava thrombosis and central venous catheters. This condition is nearly always iatrogenic and induced by central venous catheters. It usually presents with oedema of the scalp, face, neck, arms and chest and may be accompanied by chylothorax.

Specific sites of thromboses in the newborn infant

Renal vein thrombosis (RVT). This syndrome may be encountered at any age, but up to 73% of reported cases occur in the first month of life. RVT may develop in utero. The small calibre of the renal vessels and the low renal blood flow in the perinatal period are thought to contribute to the relatively high incidence in newborn infants. The triad of haematuria, thrombocytopenia and enlarged kidney or kidneys is not invariably present. The infant may present with oedema and cyanosis of the lower limbs if the inferior vena cava is involved. RVT should always be included in the differential diagnosis of either haematuria or large kidneys. Sequelae of RVT include hypertension, renal tubular defects and non-functioning kidneys. Confirmation of diagnosis usually depends on venography. Investigations should include ultrasound and a renal perfusion scan. Management includes peritoneal dialysis if necessary.

The thrombotic lesions originate in small intrarenal vessels not accessible to vascular surgery, but in selected cases of bilateral thrombosis with involvement of the inferior vena cava thrombectomy may be justified.

Peripheral arteries. Obstruction of peripheral arteries is easily recognised because it results in pulselessness, discoloration of skin and fall in skin temperature. The lower limbs are most often affected and the condition is not confined to infants who have arterial catheters.

Cerebral arteries. Thrombosis of the middle cerebral artery seems to be predominantly involved in neonatal autopsy findings of cerebral infarcts in the arterial distribution. Thrombosis may occur in situ following internal ruptures in severe birth trauma; patent ductus arteriosus or the placental fetal vessels are both potential sources of thrombo-emboli.

Clinically, cerebral thrombosis may present with generalised hypotonia, convulsions or prolonged apnoea. Ultrasound scanning is useful in screening for the lesions but the diagnosis should be confirmed with computed tomography.

Pulmonary artery thrombosis. Pulmonary thrombo-embolism may rarely be the cause of neonatal respiratory distress and should be considered in the infant who has persistent pulmonary hypertension and does not respond well to tolazoline infusions. Diffuse pulmonary microthrombi can be found at autopsy.

A neonate who suddenly develops tachypnoea, tachycardia and cyanosis while on total parenteral nutrition through a central venous catheter may well have suffered a pulmonary embolism, but this is usually a post-mortem finding.

Coronary arteries. Myocardial infarction, though rare, may occur in the newborn, even in the absence of congenital heart disease or coronary vascular anomalies. There are typical ECG findings, but there is a more than 90% mortality rate in the few reported cases.

Renal arteries. Thrombo-embolic occlusion of the renal arteries may occur with umbilical artery catheterisation (see above), but it has occasionally occurred spontaneously.

Principles of treatment of neonatal thrombosis

There is no generally accepted protocol for management of neonatal thrombosis. The actions will be influenced by the site and the size of the thrombus and the time elapsing between the occlusion of vessels and restoration of blood flow, either by vessel recanalisation or by establishment of efficient collaterals.

Heparin

Heparin in adult practice is used either in primary prevention of thrombosis or in the secondary prevention of thrombus extension (Ch. 33). Objective evidence of the beneficial role of heparin in treatment of neonatal thrombosis is largely anecdotal. The haemostatic system of the newborn infant is unique and it is not certain whether the rules for efficient heparinisation in adults can be applied. Laboratory monitoring is difficult because the in vitro coagulation times are already prolonged and rapidly become infinite with very small doses of heparin. The generally accepted guidelines are based on individual experience and have not been substantiated by controlled trials. The actual loading dose recommended is 50–100 μ/kg. Maintenance levels of 0.3–0.5 μ/ml are achieved by doses of 16–35 μ/kg per hour and this should be administered by continuing infusion. Duration of therapy depends on clinical state and may vary between a few days and several weeks.

Mild to moderate occlusion can probably be managed with heparin alone, but in the case of extensive thrombosis with critical impairment of blood flow, many centres would attempt to lyse the clot with fibrinolytic agents, and the drug of choice in the neonate is urokinase.

Urokinase

Confirmation of large vessel thrombosis by angiography or ultrasound is a prerequisite for the use of fibrinolytic therapy. Absolute contra-indications are pre-existing severe bleeding or previous major surgery up to 10 days prior to the development of thrombosis. Arterial punctures and invasive procedures should be avoided during therapy.

Treatment is most likely to be successful if established within hours of signs and confirmation of major venous or arterial occlusion. Considerably higher dosage may be tolerated and needed in the neonate than in adults.

A loading dose of 4000 μ/kg given intravenously over 10 minutes should be followed by a continuous infusion of 4000–6000 μ/kg/hour but should be increased if necessary within hours until improved perfusion of the affected part is achieved. It is obvious that such treatment should only be given in a fully equipped SCBU with 2D ultrasound, Doppler facilities and appropriate laboratory back-up. The duration of useful therapy in newborns is as uncertain as the dosage, but treatment may be continued for more than the usual 72 hours. If the thrombin time is not prolonged by the generation of FDPs, then heparin may also be added to prevent extension of the thrombus. The degree of thrombolysis will be determined by the age of the thrombus, its location and plasminogen content.

Laboratory testing should be performed prior to administering urokinase to establish base-lines. Thereafter regular monitoring is required. Suitable rapid tests are measurement of FDPs and fibrinogen levels. Very low fibrinogen levels would indicate urgent readjustment of the dose.

Surgery

In adult arterial thrombosis, if the clot is not removed by endarterectomy the thrombosis tends to recur. This is not so in neonatal thrombosis. In addition, the very small size of vessels in this age group will com-plicate surgical intervention. Surgery in this situation is usually reserved for resection of non-viable tissue. Amputation should be delayed as long as possible by strenuous efforts to prevent secondary infection, but if this ensues then amputation cannot be avoided.

NEONATAL THROMBOCYTOPENIA

Many of these conditions (Table 34.3) are dealt with in detail in other parts of this book (Ch. 30). The most usual mechanism for decreased platelets in the newborn is increased destruction and consumption, as seen in DIC, particularly associated with infection and immunological disorders.

Immune thrombocytopenias (Table 34.4) in the neonate are relatively acute and transitory and depend on transplacental passage of maternal IgG antiplatelet antibodies. They will, therefore, be dealt with a little more fully here.

Table 34.3 Causes of neonatal thrombocytopenia

Inherited	Absent radii TAR syndrome
	Megakaryocytic hypoplasia
	Fanconi's pancytopenia (occasionally in newborn period)
	Myeloproliferative disease (Down's syndrome)
	Osteopetrosis
	Wiscott-Aldrich syndrome and variants
	Bernard-Soulier syndrome
	May-Hegglin anomaly
Immune disorders	Maternal ITP SLE
	Drug-Induced
	Allo-immune
Consumption disorders	DIC
	Large vessel thrombosis
	Necrotising enterocolitis
	TTP
	Postmature and SGA infants (maternal eclampsia)
	Giant haemangioma
	Hyperviscosity syndrome
Infection	Bacterial: sepsis, congenital syphylis
	Viral: CMV, herpes simplex, rubella
	Other: toxoplasmosis
Drugs	Maternal: Tolbutamide, thiazide diuretics
	Infant: Intralipid, tolazoline
Other	Congenital leukaemia
	Post-exchange transfusion
	Metabolic disorders
	Neonatal cold injury

Table 34.4 Immune thrombocytopenia in the neonate

Category	Pathogenesis	Maternal platelet count
Auto-immune	Transfer of non-specific IgG platelet antibody to fetus	May be normal, especially post-splenectomy
Allo-immune	Specific IgG antibody produced by mother against paternally derived fetal platelet antigens – usually Anti PL^{A1}.	Normal

The management of immune thrombocytopenias in the newborn is different for each type and therefore the pathogenesis must be clearly established so that the correct and optimum therapy can be instituted. With autoimmune thrombocytopenia (AITP) the maternal platelet count can vary from normal to profound thrombocytopenia depending on activity of disease, response to therapy and whether or not the spleen has been removed.

Severity of thrombocytopenia in the fetus is difficult to assess, but a direct correlation has been shown between platelet-associated IgG and affected infants. The hazard to the infant is that of intracerebral haemorrhage, usually sustained during delivery; therefore management is aimed towards the most atraumatic delivery possible. In most units the obstetricians feel that Caesarean section is the delivery of choice.

The widely recommended fetal scalp platelet counts are not to be encouraged. These can be obtained only when the cervix is softened and effaced and the woman may be committed to a vaginal delivery by this stage. If the baby is severely thrombocytopenic, serious haemorrhage can occur over which the operator has no control. If it is essential to know the fetal platelet count before delivery, a fetal cord sample can be taken trans-abdominally much more safely under ultrasound guidance before labour is imminent or embarked upon and the mode of delivery planned accordingly. If the mother is thrombocytopenic, conventional treatment with steroids in the first instance should be tried, reducing to the lowest dose possible to maintain a safe platelet count. There is a theoretical hazard in using high dose steroids in the days immediately pre-delivery because of dissociation of IgG antibody from platelets and encouraging free IgG to cross the placenta and therefore cause more severe thrombocytopenia in the fetus. Paradoxically, other authors recommend the use of steroids 10–14 days before delivery to ITP mothers,

saying that these may be helpful in producing higher platelet counts in the neonate and protecting against haemorrhage during delivery.

Certainly, post-delivery, prednisone 2–4 mg/kg b.d. given to the infant may be helpful in raising the platelet count and reducing the tendency to bleed. The use of intravenous IgG immunoglobulin may be necessary if there is no maternal response to steroids and the platelet count is dangerously low. Theoretically the immunoglobulin should also help to protect the fetus.

Allo-immune thrombocytopenia is a much less common disorder and is due in the vast majority of cases to maternal antibodies directed against the platelet antigen PL^{A1} (cf. rhesus haemolytic disease), the mother being PL^{A1} negative and her fetus carrying paternally-derived PL^{A1} antigens on its platelets. In this condition the mother's platelet count is normal but she has free identifiable antiplatelet antibodies in her serum. These antibodies fix to the glycoprotein receptor areas of the platelets and seriously interfere with platelet function. It is probably for this reason that serious spontaneous intracranial haemorrhage may occur in utero prior to delivery and as early as 28–30 week's gestation.

Allo-immune purpura can occur in the first pregnancy and recur in subsequent pregnancies. The first affected pregnancy cannot be predicted but it is important to identify the couple at risk if an otherwise healthy infant is born with thrombocytopenia so that future pregnancies can be managed optimally. Pre-delivery an affected fetus can be identified by finding the specific antibodies in the mother's serum and thrombocytopenia in a fetal cord blood sample. In this situation intravenous IgG immunoglobulin administered to the mother may have a beneficial effect, although only one or two cases have been so treated. It is thought to block the passage across the placenta of specific IgG platelet antibodies. If intravenous immunoglobulin does act by Fc blockade, then all the antibody is free and the immunoglobulin is not in competition with platelets on the maternal side of the circulation.

Some fetuses have been treated by PL^{A1}-negative platelet transfusions prior to delivery. These should not be given unless it can be established that the fetus has not sustained any serious bleeding in utero before treatment is instigated.

Delivery should be by the most atraumatic route possible. There is a high mortality rate in this condition and those who survive may have serious long-term morbidity if appropriate measures have not been taken. The treatment of neonatal allo-immune thrombocytopenia is donor PL^{A1}-negative platelet concentrates or washed maternal platelets. Occasionally other platelet-specific antibodies are responsible, e.g. ZW[6],

Ko^A, Ko^B and PL^{E1}, and either washed maternal platelets or platelets of the appropriate group should be administered.

Paradoxically, immune thrombocytopenia may become worse in the first few days post-delivery in both allo-immune and autoimmune types, although the source of antibody has been cut off. This is probably due to the development of the reticulo-endothelial circulation, particularly in the spleen. The splenic circulation is not established at delivery, but after a few days it will more effectively remove coated platelets from the circulation. Mild thrombocytopenia may continue for several weeks, although normal platelet counts are usually achieved by the end of the first month of life. Active treatment is rarely required after the first week or so of life. The greatest hazard is passed once delivery has been successfully negotiated.

HEREDITARY COAGULATION DEFECTS

Newborn infants with hereditary coagulation defects have surprisingly few problems with bleeding in the first weeks of life, although later they may suffer considerable morbidity and even death resulting from the deficiency (Ch. 31). Only clinical manifestations which have special relevance for the newborn period will be highlighted here.

Bleeding manifestations during the newborn period

Hereditary coagulation defects may present rarely during the first weeks of life.

Clinical manifestations of these defects include:

Cephalhaematoma
Perirenal haematoma
Splenic haematoma
Intracranial haemorrhage
Umbilical oozing
Haematemesis and malaena
Puncture wound bleeding
Post-circumcision bleeding

From 5 to 35% of haemophiliacs and approximately 7% of individuals with other coagulation deficiencies may have symptoms during the neonatal period. Post-circumcision bleeding is the most common manifestation but haemophiliacs have been circumcised without unusual bleeding.

Umbilical haemorrhage is classically associated with factor XIII deficiency, but it has been reported with deficiency of fibrinogen, factors V, VIII and X. The more frequent use of invasive screening, monitoring and prophylactic devices such as scalp electrodes, vitamin K injections, thyroid and PKU screening have increased the identification rate of neonates with congenital coagulopathies.

Factor VIII deficiency – haemophilia A

5–10% of patients with severe classical haemophilia have bleeding manifestations in the neonatal period, following fetal scalp sampling, from the umbilicus or post-circumcision.

Subdural intracerebral and subarachnoid haemorrhages have been described following atraumatic vaginal delivery but the incidence of intracranial bleeding is very low. Subgaleal and cephalohaematomata are more common.

In the normal fetus and neonate factor VIII coagulant activity is within the high normal range, so that a deficiency is easily identified in the laboratory.

Von Willebrand's disease

Von Willebrand's syndrome is more prevalent than classic haemophilia; the homozygous state can be very severe but is rare. Bleeding in a patient with severe von Willebrand's disease may be more difficult to control than that with haemophilia because the abnormal bleeding time is not easily corrected. Bleeding is rare in the neonatal period. The diagnosis during the neonatal period may be difficult because the stress of delivery may increase the factor VIII coagulant activity to within normal limits in infants with mild to moderate disease.

Factor IX deficiency, Christmas disease, haemophilia B

The manifestations in the neonatal period are similar to those for severe classical haemophilia A. The laboratory diagnosis of mild to moderate Christmas disease is more difficult than that of haemophilia A because of the low physiological values of factor IX – a vitamin K-dependent factor – in the normal neonate.

Factor V deficiency

Congenital deficiency of factor V is a rare disease. Symptoms in the neonatal period are uncommon. Umbilical bleeding is the most usual manifestation. Approximately one third of patients with factor V deficiency have prolonged bleeding times. Recent investigations have shown decreased factor X platelet-binding sites in patients with factor V deficiency. Reported values for factor V activity are around 100% of adult values in the normal neonate but vary widely in the fetus, making prenatal diagnosis difficult. Many persons with factor V deficiency remain asymptomatic throughout their lives. There is intrafamilial variability in clinical manifestations of deficiency but it is usually a mild defect – even if combined with factor VIII deficiency.

Factor X deficiency

This is a very rare defect in its homozygous form, with less than 30 patients in literature by 1980. There is a prolonged bleeding time as well as a coagulant defect probably due to the effect of lack of factor X coagulant activity on the function of platelet membrane. The clinical manifestations include mucous membrane bleeding, haematemesis, melaena, haematuria and, most devasting of all in the neonatal period, spontaneous intracranial haemorrhage. Although milder deficiencies and dysprotinaemias are only symptomatic with trauma, more severe forms of the defect are very difficult to manage in the neonatal period and infants with severe factor X deficiency have an increased mortality rate during childhood. Spontaneous cerebral haemorrhage is a frequent cause of death in the few documented cases.

Factor II deficiency

This is another rare defect which can present in its severe homozygous form during the neonatal period with umbilical, intramuscular or post-circumcision bleeding. Accurate diagnosis of hypoprothrombinaemia in the fetus and neonate will be difficult because of the low levels found in the healthy newborn infant.

Factor VII deficiency

This deficiency has been reported in approximately 100 cases and has been associated with both thromboembolism and bleeding. Reported neonatal manifestations include spontaneous intracerebral haemorrhage, often fatal, oozing from umbilical stump, post-circumcision bleeding and gastrointestinal haemorrhage. Normal neonatal concentrations of factor VII are usually between 30 and 50% of adult values in most reported series. Patients with severe symptoms associated with the congenital defect have factor VII values of less than 5% of normal adult values.

Fibrinogen deficiency

Afibrinogenaemia is a relatively severe coagulation deficiency which frequently presents in the neonatal period. Hypofibrinogenaemia and dysfibrinogenaemias are usually clinically less severe. Bleeding manifestations include umbilical cord oozing, post-circumcisional bleeding and spontaneous cerebral haemorrhage. Death

in early childhood is common unless the diagnosis is made and prophylactic treatment initiated.

Factor XIII deficiency

Fibrin stabilising factor deficiency was first described in 1960. Factor XIII circulates as a zymogen that, when activated by thrombin, catalyses the formation of bonds between fibrin monomers to form insoluble fibrin and increases clot resistance to lysis, among its most important activities. Classically this defect presents with bleeding from the umbilical stump in over 80% of cases in the first few weeks of life. Perhaps not so widely appreciated is the fact that spontaneous intracranial haemorrhage is also very common. Ecchymoses, post-traumatic bleeding and abnormal scar formation are frequent manifestations. Routine coagulation screening tests will yield normal clotting times but the factor XIII activity can be measured by assessing clot solubility in 5 Molar urea. A commercially produced screening test using factor XIII antibody-coated latex beads is available. Factor XIII levels are approximately 50% of normal adult values in the neonatal period.

Contact factor deficiencies

Clinical manifestations of these deficiencies are rare (Ch. 31) and they usually present as mild bleeding diatheses late in life. In the neonatal period any deficiency will produce a marked prolongation of the in-vitro partial thromboplastin time.

Management of hereditary congenital bleeding disorders in the neonatal period

The principles of management of all patients are the same at any stage of life and are dealt with in Chapter 31. Differences in detail arise from the haemostatic level required and the necessary frequency of transfusion of the missing factor or factors in the newborn period.

The usual hazards of treatment prevail, but administration of prothrombin complex to treat factor IX and factor X deficiencies seems to carry a high thrombo-embolic risk and should be used with caution. The production of less activated concentrates has resulted in an apparent reduction of this problem. Cryoprecipitates or fresh frozen plasma are the replacement therapy of choice if haemostatic levels of the lacking factor or factors can be achieved without volume overload. The possible risk of transmitting HIV or hepatitis in first generation heat-treated concentrates makes the decision concerning which therapeutic material to use one of local clinical judgement.

The possibility of prenatal diagnosis and carrier detection of the more common coagulation defects is dealt with in detail in Chapter 31.

The relatively common haemophilias and homozygous von Willebrand's disease are the conditions for which prenatal diagnosis is recommended or requested most frequently. These can all be diagnosed in the second trimester by acquisition of pure fetal plasma from the fetal umbilical cord. Fetal sexing can be achieved earlier in pregnancy by chorion biopsy analysis at 8 to 10 weeks' gestation.

Some, but not all, cases of factor VIII and factor IX deficiency can be diagnosed by DNA analysis because of partial deletions or associated restricted fragment length polymorphism, but complicated family studies have to be completed before an at-risk pregnancy is embarked upon for these new, aesthetically more acceptable methods to be used to the optimum.

BIBLIOGRAPHY

Andrew M, Kelton J 1984 Neonatal thrombocytopenia. Clinics in Perinatology 11: 359–391
Buchanan G R 1986 Coagulation disorders in the neonate. Pediatric Clinics of North America 33: 203–220
Corrigan J J Jr 1988 Neonatal thrombosis and the thrombolytic system: pathophysiology and therapy. American Journal of Pediatric Hematology/Oncology 10: 83–91
Hathaway W E, Bonnar J 1987 Hemostatic disorders of the pregnant woman and the newborn infant. John Wiley.
Kunicki T J, Beardsley D S 1989 The alloimmune thrombocytopenias: neonatal alloimmune thrombocytopenic purpura and post-transfusion purpura. Progress in Hemostasis and Thrombosis 9: 203–232
Montgomery R R, Marlar R A, Gill J C 1985 Newborn haemostasis. Clinics in Haematology 14: 443–460
Rodgers G M, Shuman M A 1986 Congenital thrombotic disorders. American Journal of Hematology 21: 419–430

Support of patients

35. Management of the immunocompromised and pancytopenic patient

M. J. Mackie

Infection in clinical haematological practice usually occurs in the setting of a known disease, the implications of which as regards the host's defence systems can be predicted (Ch. 22). Thus certain types of infections occur more commonly with particular diseases and the disease process may modify the presentation and progression of the infection. Furthermore, it is well appreciated that organisms which do not cause invasive, life-threatening illness in normal hosts may do so in the immunocompromised. Occasionally a haematologist is asked to undertake the investigation of a patient with recurrent infections in order to determine an underlying diagnosis; the appropriate investigations are discussed in Chapter 4 and the management of such patients is discussed at the end of this chapter. The spectrum of infectious complications in patients with a primary haematological disorder and congenital immunodeficiency will now be considered and this will be followed by a discussion of the characteristics and treatment of the various types of infection. Finally, prophylactic measures to try and reduce the incidence of infection will be reviewed.

THE INFECTIOUS COMPLICATIONS IN HAEMATOLOGICAL DISORDERS

Acute leukaemias

Every patient undergoing chemotherapy to induce remission will develop at least one episode of fever/infection. Infection is now the major cause of mortality; its incidence and severity are determined by the disease-related neutropenia which is exacerbated by chemotherapy. The severity of the neutropenia not only governs the incidence of infection but also results in its ability to disseminate rapidly and the relative lack of local signs normally associated with an infected focus. Fever is usually the first and often the only sign of infection; its rapid evaluation has already been discussed (Ch. 4). In order for this to be practiced it must be made

clear to patients that they have 24-hours-a-day 'open access' to their ward so that they can be admitted directly at the onset of fever/infection. A wide range of bacteria, both gram positive and negative may be responsible (Plates 30, 31). Until recently gram negative organisms were the most prevalent but many units now see a preponderance of gram positive bacterial infections related particularly to an increased use of central lines. In addition to bacterial infection patients with acute leukaemia are prone to fungal invasion. In a recent survey of causes of death in acute leukaemia not only was infection the most common cause but at post mortem fungal infection was found in the majority of cases (Plates 32–35). The diagnosis of the fungal infection was often not made during life. As discussed in Chapter 4, this is because of the well known difficulties in diagnosis – blood cultures may be negative in disseminated infection and serology is unreliable. A high index of suspicion is therefore required. Important clinical clues may be present, such as myositis, skin lesions or endophthalmitis, but these are uncommon. Involvement of vessels by fungi may cause symptoms of pulmonary embolic or cerebrovascular disease. A cavitating lesion on chest X-ray may be fungal in origin. Persistently severely neutropenic patients who have had a number of courses of antibiotics are at particular risk. The most commonly implicated fungi are species of *Candida*, *Aspergillus* and the *Mucoraceae*, in that order of frequency.

Viruses are also a cause of morbidity in patients with acute leukaemia. Up to 60% of patients with a significantly elevated titre to *Herpes simplex* prior to treatment for acute leukaemia will develop reactivation of the virus. This may clinically be a locally troublesome 'cold sore' but the immunocompromised are prone to more extensive lesions. Moreover, it is now apparent that a considerable number of patients with fever and a sore mouth have oral herpes. Unless the mouth is swabbed and herpes sought specifically, the oral appearances may be passed off as secondary to the neutropenia. Thus, a diagnosis of *Herpes simplex* should be sought in febrile patients with a sore mouth and specific treatment given (see below).

Bone marrow transplantation (BMT)

BMT can be complicated by a variety of kinds of infection. Transplant conditioning and the pattern of haematological recovery determine the particular host defence deficit which predisposes to a particular infection. It is not therefore surprising that the prevalence of particular organisms varies temporarily following BMT (Fig. 16.1, p. 130).

Graft-versus-host disease can further influence the rate of immunological recovery and influence and prolong the patient's susceptibility to infection.

During the first month following BMT, whilst the patient is neutropenic, he is particularly prone to bacterial infections. The management of fever and infection at this time is the same as that discussed in the section on fever in the neutropenic patient. Fungal and viral infection (*Herpes simplex*) may also occur. By one month following infusion of marrow most patients will have generated a sufficient neutrophil count, unless graft-versus-host disease is present, to prevent frequent serious bacterial infections. However, cell-mediated immunity is not normal and infection with cytomegalovirus, *Herpes zoster*, and *Pneumocystis carinii* can occur, usually 2–6 months following transplant (Fig. 35.1).

CMV infection is an important cause of morbidity and mortality following BMT. Although CMV has been associated with fever, hepatitis, gastroenteritis, retinitis, cystitis and graft failure, the most serious infection problem is pneumonitis. CMV pneumonitis accounts for up to 50% of cases of interstitial pneumonitis. In some series 15–20% of all patients who die following BMT have CMV as the primary cause of death. CMV pneumonitis usually occurs during the second or third month after transplant and is more common in older patients, those with graft-versus-host disease and recipients of total body irradiation. Infection is thought to be the result of reactivation of virus in patients with an elevated pre-transplant antibody titre to CMV, or be related to the administration of blood products from CMV-positive donors to recipients who are CMV-negative.

Herpes zoster occurs some 4–5 months post-BMT in up to 50% of patients (Fig. 16.1, p. 130). At presentation the disease has its typical dermatome localisation in 85% of cases, the remainder having a generalised rash. The latter may complicate a further 30% of patients and it is these individuals who are at present at particular risk from visceral complications, in particular pneumonia.

Disease caused by *Pneumocystis carinii* is thought to be the result of reactivation of latent infection acquired in childhood. Its reappearance seems to be triggered by vigorous chemotherapy, particularly if steroids are used.

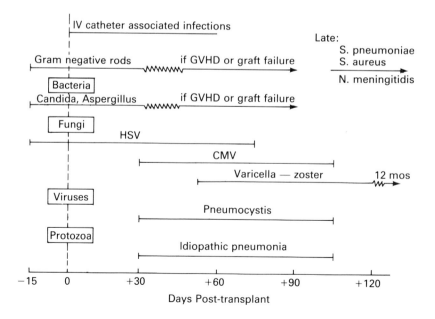

Fig 35.1 Occurrence of infections following BMT (reproduced with permission of Academic Press).

Disease is almost always confined to the lung. Pneumocystis pneumonia can occur in 5% of patients following BMT; although this will be discussed, the incidence can be reduced by using prophylactic cotrimoxazole. The presentaion can be subtle, the majority of patients complaining of dyspnoea and an unproductive cough. The signs on examination in the early stages may be mild – tachypnoea and fever. It is important to appreciate that chest signs may be absent. Thus a high index of suspicion is required when a patient 1–3 months post-BMT develops the above symptomology, and the appropriate investigations as outlined in Ch. 4 should be carried out without delay.

Lymphoproliferative disorders

A variety of infections can complicate lymphoproliferative disorders according to the disease status and the nature of the therapy being given.

During periods of chemoradiotherapy-induced neutropenia the patient is at risk from bacterial, fungal and *Herpes simplex* infection. Another feature of lymphoproliferative disorders predisposing to bacterial infection is an abnormality of immunoglobulins.

Hypoglobulinaemia occurs in chronic lymphatic leukaemia and persistent and recurrent bacterial infection of the chest and sinuses are troublesome complications, especially in the later stages of the disease. Intravenous immunoglobulin replacement therapy reduces the incidence of such infections. The importance of prompt and vigorous treatment of infections in myeloma has recently been emphasised in view of the high incidence of deaths due to bacterial infection. Fever and infection should be treated vigorously using broad spectrum intravenous antimicrobials.

Pneumocystis carinii may complicate acute lymphoblastic leukaemia, non-Hodgkin's lymphoma and chronic lymphatic leukaemia.

Herpes varicella-zoster virus infection may complicate non-Hodgkin's lymphoma, Hodgkin's disease, acute lymphoblastic leukaemia and chronic lymphatic leukaemia. Primary *Varicella* infection occurs especially in children on chemotherapy and after BMT. About 25% of cases will be associated with dissemination, most commonly to the lungs. In immunosuppressed adults *Herpes zoster* is more common, occurring in approximately 15% of cases of Hodgkin's disease and 10% of non-Hodgkin's lymphoma. Up to 30% of localised zoster will disseminate to the lungs, CNS, heart or gastrointestinal tract. Localised and disseminated disease are more frequent in advanced disease and in those receiving combined chemoradiotherapy.

A particular consideration in lymphoma patients is the infectious sequelae of splenectomy. Following this pro-cedure there is overall a 5% risk of sepsis but up to half of the episodes may be fatal. The most frequent organisms isolated are pneumococci, meningococci, *E. coli*, *Haemophilus influenzae* and staphylococci. Children are particularly at risk and splenectomy should be avoided if possible; the incidence of infection is lower following removal of spleen post-trauma compared to its occurrence following splenectomy for haematological indications. Most episodes occur in the first 2–3 years post-surgery but a number of series have emphasised the late occurrence (10–20 years) of serious infection. The progression of the illness may be devastating in its rapidity and be associated with disseminated intravascular coagulation. Various preventive measures have been tried. Prophylactic penicillin V is recommended in children but the length of therapy and its role in adults is controversial. Polyvalent pneumococcal vaccine is now available; it is hoped that this will offer immunisation against most, but not all, strains causing infection, but it does not, of course, offer any protection against the other organisms that may be involved. Response to the vaccine may be poor, probably related to the effects of chemoradiotherapy; it is recommended that the vaccine be given 14 days prior to the start of any such treatment. Although this vaccine has been shown to reduce the incidence of pneumococcal infection in the immunocompetent and in patients with sickle cell disease, its role post-splenectomy is unproven. Certainly patients should be warned to report to their doctor immediately at any sign of infection. Unfortunately, compliance with this advice, and indeed prophylaxis if given, is reduced in the years following splenectomy.

Hairy cell leukaemia with its characteristic pancytopenia is not only associated with bacterial (especially gram positive) infections but also with opportunistic organisms. Numerous reports of mycobacterial infections have been documented. Although *M. tuberculosis* may be involved, infection with atypical mycobacteria, especially *M. kanasii*, is more typical. The lungs may be involved but spleen, lymph nodes or liver may be affected. Conventional antituberculous therapy may be ineffective and treatment may have to be prolonged to be successful. Fungi and toxoplasmosis may also cause infection in patients with hairy cell leukaemia.

Congenital immunodeficiency syndromes

Table 35.1 lists some examples of congenital immunodeficiency diseases but it is appreciated that many other defects have been described. These will usually present because of persistent or recurrent episodes of infection or be identified in a member of a known family.

X-linked hypogammaglobulinaemia described by Bruton usually results in susceptibility to infection commencing in the second year of life. Sinusitis, pneumonia, meningitis and skin sepsis are common, being caused by the organisms shown in Table 35.l; viral infections are dealt with normally. Other complications include arthropathy, malabsorption, a dermatomyositis-like syndrome and neurological problems. Infectious episodes require vigorous antibiotic therapy with physiotherapy as appropriate.

Chronic chest sepsis leads to bronchiectasis. In the past replacement therapy has involved intramuscular injections of immunoglobulin. These are painful and often poorly tolerated. To raise the level of IgG to 200 mg/dl, an untreated patient requires 300 mg of immunoglobulin/kg and monthly maintenance with 100 mg/kg. Fresh frozen plasma can also be used but this has the risk of transmitting infection. More recently intravenous gammaglobulin preparations have become available which are well tolerated. 0.1–0.3 g/kg i.v. is required approximately every 3 weeks; the initial infusion should be as a 3% solution and the infusion rate slowly increased to 50 drops per minute. The patient should be observed carefully for febrile or other reactions but these are uncommon. This therapy is contra-indicated in patients with selective IgA deficiency who have antibodies to IgA. These preparations contain over 90% IgG but do have traces of IgA and IgM. Fortunately it appears that the risk of transmitting HIV infection is negligible. Data suggest that administration of the intravenous preparations results in more easily maintained levels of immunoglobulin and that these result in clinical benefit to the patient.

Various selective immunoglobulin deficiencies occur – low IgA and IgG with normal or elevated IgM; low IgA with normal IgG and IgM; low IgM with normal IgG and IgA. Some of these may be associated with neutropenia which further increases the risk of infection. Furthermore, a transient hypogammaglobulinaemia can occur in infancy. The patient delays manufacturing immunoglobulin until 18–30 months of age. Prior to this there is an increase in susceptibility to infections and replacement immunoglobulin may be required.

Agammaglobulinaemia is also a feature of severe combined immunodeficiency disease. However, not only are these infants prone to bacterial infections, but due to the additional lack of T-cells viral infection can be overwhelming. Pulmonary infection is the rule and mortality occurs from pseudomonas abscesses or *Pneumocystis carinii*. Bone marrow transplantation offers the only hope to those with a donor.

In ataxic telangiectasia IgA deficiency is found in 80% and in Wiscott-Aldrich syndrome IgM is low but IgA and IgG are normal. In the latter the associated thrombocytopenia usually responds to splenectomy but this results in a very high incidence of infectious sequelae. Prophylactic antibiotic should be given, but pneumococcal vaccine should not be expected to be effective. Benefit from transplant has also been recorded. In chronic granulomatous disease neutrophils fail to undergo the respiratory burst following phagocytosis. Organisms such as pneumococci and streptococci which are either catalase-positive or do not make hydrogen peroxide are killed normally. Recurrent abscesses are characteristic

Table 35.1 Examples of congenital immunodeficiency syndromes

Disease	Immunodeficiency	Inheritance	Infections
Severe combined immunodeficiency disease	B-+ T-cell	XL, AR	*Pneumocystis carinii* Candida, bacteria
Wiskott-Aldrich syndrome	B- + T-cell	XL	Pneumococci, *H. influenzae*
Hereditary ataxic-telangiectasia	B- + T-cell	AR	Pneumococci, *H. influenzae*, *S. aureus*
Congenital thymic aplasia (Di George's syndrome)	T-Cell		Candidiasis *Pneumocystis carinii*
Hypogammaglobulinaemia	B-cell	XL	Pneumococcus, *H. influenzae*, *S. aureus*, *P. aeruginosa*
Selective IgM deficiency	B-cell	?	Pneumococci, *H. influenzae*, *E. coli*
Selective IgA deficiency	B-cell	?	Respiratory infections Giardiasis
Chronic granulomatous disease	Leukocyte function defect	XL, AR	*S. aureus*, *S. epidermidis* *E. coli*, *serratia marcesens*, Candida

XL = sex-linked recessive; AR = autosomal recessive; ? = mode of inheritance uncertain in lung and liver. Osteomyelitis may occur. Prolonged antibiotic therapy with penicillinase-resistant antibiotics with good penetrating power is required. Surgical drainage is not to be undertaken lightly, as healing is often prolonged; if a lobectomy is performed, other lobes become infected, with further respiratory impairment.

MANAGEMENT OF FEVER IN NEUTROPENIC PATIENTS

A number of haematological malignancies discussed above are frequently complicated by neutropenia with resultant infection. Fever is usually the first and only sign of infection and thus its management in the presence of neutropenia will now be discussed in detail.

Fever in this group of patients, as in others, may not necessarily always be related to infection. Fever may be related to the disease process itself, to cytotoxic drugs or to infusion of blood products. Such factors should be excluded if possible; this may be difficult (for example in the case of fever secondary to the disease) and if there is any doubt the episode should be managed as an infection.

Table 35.2 shows the frequency with which infection was actually considered to be the aetiology of fever in a series of severely neutropenic patients with fever. It can be seen that even in a series in which fever thought to be related to non-infective causes (drugs, diseases, etc) is excluded, an infection can only be demonstrated in

Table 35.2 Aetiology of fever in severely neutropenic (<1 × 10⁹/l) patients admitted to the Haematology Unit at the Royal Liverpool Hospital

	No	(%)
Indentifiable focus of infection	71	(47)
Clinical/radiological evidence of infection	31	(21)
Conclusive microbiology	40	(26)
Pyrexia of undetermined origin	80	(53)
Total assessed	151	(100)

approximately 50% of cases. The fever in the pyrexias of undetermined origin group may be related to endotoxin or may be due to a subclinical infection with negative or inconclusive microbiology; certainly a high number of these febrile episodes settle satisfactorily with antimicrobial therapy.

Investigations

The investigation of febrile, severely neutropenic patients has already been discussed (Ch. 4 and see Fig. 35.2) and the need for the rapid institution of antibiotic cover before the results of cultures are available emphasised.

Treatment – empiric first line therapy

When considering the type of antibiotic regimen to be used, the efficacy of the agent(s) against the range of

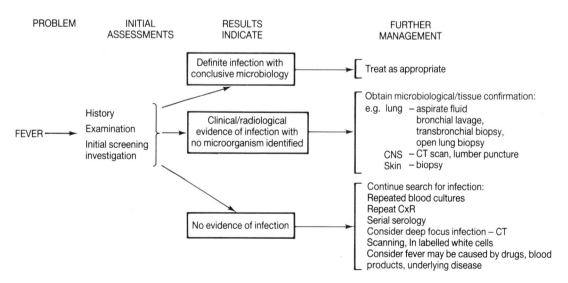

Fig 35.2 Approach to the investigation of fever in immunocompromised patients.

organisms likely to be involved and the toxicity of the antibiotic(s) are the prime considerations; your hospital pharmacist will also remind you of the high cost of most of the current regimens! In determining which drugs will be effective in your unit it is most important to know the local prevalence of individual micro-organisms. Particular organisms may be a problem in one centre but not occur so frequently in another. In addition, the pattern may change; recently there has been an increase in the number of infections caused by gram positive bacteria, reflecting the widespread introduction of central lines. In a recent study at the Royal Liverpool Hospital 50% of organisms cultured from septicaemic neutropenic patients were gram positive. However, as can be seen from the range of bacteria which may potentially be involved (Ch. 4), any antibiotic regimen usually has to cover a spectrum of gram negative and positive organisms. This requirement has led to the widespread use of combinations of antibiotics in this particular clinical situation (Table 35.3). Not only does an appropriate combination give broad antibacterial coverage but combinations of aminoglycoside and semisynthetic penicillins often have a synergistic effect. Combinations have most often contained antibiotics with a wide spectrum of activity including pseudomonas. A typical regimen would contain an aminoglycoside and a semisynthetic penicilin (e.g. piperacillin or azlocillin). The place and advantages of the newer cephalosporins are controversial – only ceftazidime has good antipseudo-monal cover and has been shown in a small number of trials to be effective as monotherapy. However, this antibiotic has relatively low activity against staphylococci. There has been increased use of the vancomycin because of the problem of central line infection with *Staphylococcus albus*. Although the organism may be sensitive in vitro to a number of antibiotics, clinical experience has shown that a response is often only obtained with vancomycin. Because of the increased frequency of gram positive infections the question arises whether vancomycin should be used as part of front-line therapy. Although data are limited they do suggest that there is little to be lost by waiting until a *Staphylococcus albus* has been cultured or there is clinical evidence of catheter exit infection before considering the use of vancomycin. If this drug is then added, most infections resolve and the line can be saved. If resolution does not occur, the catheter should be removed. If such treatment is not successful, the line may have to be removed. New generations and formulations of antibiotics are being produced and they need to be evaluated in neutropenic patients to see if they have an improved efficacy-toxicity ratio.

An awareness of the potential toxicity of antibiotics is essential. The renal effects of aminoglycosides are well known; regular evaluation of renal function (twice weekly at least) and the monitoring of serum levels is required. If such measures are taken and the level of the aminoglycoside varied according to the results, then

Table 35.3 Examples of antibiotics usually used in combination (e.g. any of group A and member group B or C) in febrile neutropenic patients

Drug	Dosage guide	Comments
A. *Aminoglycosides*		
Gentamicin	120 mg i.v. 8-hourly	Nephro- and ototoxic
Tobramycin	120 mg i.v. 8-hourly	Regular serum levels required
Amikacin	500 mg i.v. 12-hourly	
B. *Semisynthetic penicillins*		
Piperacillin	3 g i.v. 6–8-hourly	
Azlocillin	2.5 g i.v. 8-hourly	
Ticarcillin & Clavulanate	3.2 g i.v. 8-hourly	
C. *Cephalosporins*		
Cefotaxime	2 g i.v. 8-hourly	
Ceftazidime	2 g i.v 8-hourly	
D. Others		
Vancomycin	1 g i.v. 12-hourly	Must be infused slowly
		Monitor levels
		Oral administration for *Clostridium difficile* enteritis
Metronidazole	500 mg 8-hourly	For anaerobic infection
		Well-absorbed orally
Erythromycin	1 g i.v. 6-hourly	If mycoplasma or legionella possibilities

NB These dosages are a guide only and will require modification in renal failure.

serious renal impairment is very uncommon. The problem is often compounded, however, by the concomitant use of other nephrotoxic drugs, e.g. amphotericin, cyclosporin. In an attempt to avoid the toxicity of aminoglycosides, combinations of semisynthetic penicillin and a third-generation cephalosporin have been used; there are data to indicate that such a combination is effective but it is extremely costly. In addition, semisynthetic penicillins may affect platelet function and some cephalosporins prolong the prothrombin time.

After a response has been obtained the question of how long to continue treatment arises. Premature cessation of antibiotics, particularly in a severely neutropenic patient, often results in microbiological relapse or re-infection. This problem has led to some authorities recommending prolonged courses of treatment either of a standard length (e.g. 14 days) or until the patient's neutrophil count rises to greater than $0.5 \times 10^9/l$. The benefits of these approaches are not fully proven and the patient's exposure to the toxic effects of antimicrobial therapy is obviously increased. Many units stop antibiotics after a number of days (e.g. 5) of treatment following resolution of fever; others treat until clinical/radiological evidence of infection has gone. Future studies may define parameters, such as the C-reactive protein level, which might help as a guide to the optimum time to stop treatment.

The efficacy of any broad spectrum antibiotic therapy regimen in febrile episodes in neutropenic patients is dependent on two main factors: the aetiology of the fever and a change in neutrophil count during the treatment period. An efficacy rate of 70–80+% can be expected in patients with a pyrexia of undetermined origin. However, if an infection is felt to be the cause of the fever, the success rate falls to around 60%. Within this group, which includes patients with clinically localised infection with and without positive microbiology and septicaemias, there is a variation in response. The latter are difficult to eradicate in neutropenic patients (efficacy 30–60%) and carry a significant mortality (25%). The death rate is higher with gram-negative as opposed to gram-positive organisms, pseudomonas septicaemia being particularly difficult to treat. As might be expected, failure to respond is associated with resistant organisms, and patients who are shocked and/or have relapsed or resistant disease do badly. A number of trials have now demonstrated the importance of a rise in the neutrophil count during antibiotic therapy; even a rise of the order of $0.2 \times 10^9/l$ has been associated with an improved response.

Failure to respond to initial antibiotic therapy

Most clinicians would be concerned if a patient's fever

had not significantly fallen after 72 hours' treatment, especially if clinical deterioration had taken place. Failure of the fever to resolve should result in:

1. Repeated examination of the patient to determine a focus of infection.
2. Repeated blood cultures every 48 hours: repeated chest X-ray every 48–72 hours.
3. Consideration of filling any gaps in the current antimicrobial cover if no microbiological diagnosis is available, e.g. specific therapy for anaerobes, mycoplasma, legionella, viruses, fungi.
4. Revaluation of a possible non-microbiological cause for the fever–review drugs, disease, status and relationship of blood product administration to the fever.

Changes in management may well be indicated by the results of the above. Obviously, if a positive culture is obtained, treatment is guided by the sensitivity of the organism: opacification on chest X-ray often indicates a need for further investigations (see Ch. 4). However, often no clues as to the aetiology of the persistent fever are available after clinical and microbiological revaluation of the patient. In this situation two options are either to use further empiric therapy, most often for fungi, or to consider granulocyte transfusions. If the patient has a central line, even if there is no overt evidence that it is infected, a potent antistaphylococcal antibiotic (e.g. vancomycin) should be tried.

In view of the difficulty in diagnosing fungal infection in vivo and the frequency of the unsuspected fungal infection at post mortem in leukaemics, empiric therapy has been given to febrile neutropenic patients who remain febrile despite antibiotics. One trial added amphotericin (0.5 mg/kg) to the antibiotic regimen if a neutropenic patient was still febrile after 7 days of treatment. The group receiving this combination had fewer infections and in particular less fungal infection than the group who continued on antibiotics alone. Preliminary data from the EORTC Antimicrobial Therapy Project Group also supports a similar empiric use of amphotericin. A fuller discussion on the use of amphotericin will follow in the section on documented fungal infection.

Granulocyte transfusion would appear to be the logical approach to the infection problem in severely neutropenic patients, potentially repairing the major defect in the host defences. However, the logistics of supplying adequate numbers of functional granulocytes has always been appreciated. ABO blood group compatible donors (usually siblings) are most often used and the granulocytes are harvested using a cell separator depending usually on centrifugation. Filtration leukopheresis has largely been abandoned due to the associated incidence of reactions in the recipient and occasional episodes of priapism in the donor.

Between 1975 and 1977 four randomised controlled trials were conducted to determine the therapeutic efficacy of granulocyte transfusions. Three of these reported an improvement in survival when granulocytes were given, benefit occurring particularly in the absence of recovery of the patient's own granulocyte count. These data led to the widespread use of granulocyte transfusions in neutropenic patients who were felt to have had an infection but had failed to respond to antibiotics.

However, several criticisms can be made of the early trials. The numbers involved were small and there were variable levels of neutropenia at entry. The criteria for giving granulocytes did not always require the documentation of infection and different doses of granulocytes were given. In addition, the control groups generally had a poorer response than would now be expected with antibiotic therapy. In 1982 Winston and his colleagues performed a randomised controlled trial involving 95 patients with documented infection. What was felt to be an adequate number of granulocytes was given but the response rate was similar to that in the control group. Because of these data, the practical difficulties of providing granulocytes over a number of days and the complications of transfusion, granulocyte transfusions are now used far less frequently.

Studies are being carried out using growth factors (e.g. granulocyte macrophage colony-stimulating factor) whose administration can shorten the length of neutropenia in animals given cytotoxic drugs. If such an effect can be demonstrated in patients, fewer problems with infection should be experienced; a caveat is that the growth factor may have an effect on the malignant process being treated.

TREATMENT OF SPECIFIC INFECTIONS

Fungal infection

Consideration will now be given to the presentation and treatment of the common fungal infections which affect the compromised host. These are mainly opportunistic infections but may represent reactivation of infections acquired whilst the patient was living in an area where organisms such as *Histoplasma capsulatum*, *Coccidioides immitis and Blastomyces dermatitidis* are endemic.

Candida species

These are the most common cause of fungal infection in compromised hosts (Plate 36). Usually *Candida* *albicans* is involved but *Candida tropicalis* and others may be found. Defects in neutrophil numbers and/or function in the skin, related to the siting of intravenous cannulae, and antibiotic therapy predispose to candida infection. The latter may be of two types, mucocutaneous or systemic. Oropharyngeal and oesophageal candidiasis have a characteristic appearance which can easily be diagnosed microbiologically; topical therapy in the form of nystatin suspension (1–2 million units QDS) swirled in the mouth and then swallowed is usually adequate. Oesophageal candidiasis may be more resistant – ketoconazole 200 mg daily for 10–14 days may be used in resistant cases but the risk of hepatic impairment (significant in 1 in 10 000) has to be considered. Low dose (10 mg) intravenous amphotericin B daily for 7 days is also effective.

Systemic candidiasis most often involves the lungs, kidneys, heart, brain and liver. The potential significance of candidaemia (Ch. 4), particularly its relationship to intravenous cannulae infection, has already been discussed; most clinicians, however, would treat candidaemia in a febrile neutropenic patient who had failed to respond to antibiotics. Biopsy and demonstration of hyphae in the tissues establishes the diagnosis as invasive candidiasis; urgent consideration should then be given to the biopsy of pulmonary infiltrates or skin lesions developing in febrile immunocompromised patients. Intravenous amphotericin B is issued to treat systemic candidiasis; various dosage schedules have been described and there is no agreement as to the total dose which should be given. It is customary to give a 1 mg test dose, the drug being given in 250–500 ml of 5% dextrose and water over 6 hours. If this is tolerated, 5 mg can be given and the dose doubled (every 6–8 hours if the situation is urgent) until 0.5–1 mg/kg has been reached. This therapeutic dose is given every 1–2 days until a total dose of 1–1.5 g has been given.

Immediate problems are fever, rigor and hypotension which can usually be controlled by premedication with oral paracetamol and/or by adding hydrocortisone to the infusion fluid. The latter may help to reduce the tendency of amphotericin to cause phlebitis. The drug is also reno- and hepato-toxic and adjustments to the dosage will have to be made in the face of impairment of kidney or liver function. Particularly troublesome is the effect on the kidney tubule, resulting in hypokalaemia; routine potassium supplements should be given and the potassium level monitored every 1–2 days. Other renal side effects include hyposthenuria, renal tubular acidosis and hypomagnesaemia. Renal problems may be exacerbated by the concomitant use of antibiotics. For intracranial disease amphotericin has to be given by the intraventricular route–0.05 mg initially, then the dosage is increased by 0.05 mg every 12 hours until a dose of 0.5 mg is reached. In candida infection of a heart valve, surgery is usually required to eradicate the infection. 5-fluorocytosine (5FC) can be combined with amphotericin; there is some animal data to suggest this combination has an additive and possibly a synergistic effect against candida. However, clinical benefit of this regimen has not been demonstrated in patients (except for treating cryptococcus). The daily dose of 5FC is 100–150 mg/kg daily, divided into four doses; this drug is metabolised to 5-fluorouracil and there is a suppressant effect on marrow which is not desired in neutropenic patients. Toxicity, however, can be minimised by ensuring that the level is below 80 mμ/ml.

Aspergillus

This fungus is widespread in the environment but local factors, such as contamination of hospital ventilation systems, have led to problems in particular units. *Aspergillus fumigatus* is most commonly involved, and the group is second only to candida in the frequency with which it causes invasive disease in immunocompromised patients. Clinically the most common manifestation is pulmonary disease (Plates 32–35) but 20–30% have disseminated infection (involving brain, heart, kidney, liver, gastrointestinal tract). The patient with lung involvement may have fever, cough and dyspnoea unresponsive to antibiotics; pleuritic chest pain accompanied by a friction rub occurs in 60% of patients and mimics thrombo-embolic disease. Pulmonary infiltration, often with cavitation, is seen on X-ray and bronchoscopy is required to make the definitive diagnosis. Cerebral aspergillosis presents with general signs of lethargy, or focally, depending on the site of the lesion which is often an abscess. The definitive diagnosis depends usually on biopsy: cerebrospinal fluid findings are usually non-specific. The treatment of aspergillosis is with amphotericin B as discussed above. Unfortunately the institution of this therapy does not always ensure a successful outcome.

Mucormycosis

This infection is the third most common fungal infection in compromised hosts, accounting for 5–15% of cases. The species most commonly involved are *Mucor*, *Rhizopus* and *Absidia*. Different patterns of infection occur depending on host factors, e.g. the majority of patients with rhinocerebral mucormycosis have diabetes mellitus, whilst wounds and burns predispose to cutaneous infection. Immunocompromised and especial-ly neutropenic patients usually have pulmonary and/or disseminated disease. Clinically, the symptoms of chest disease are non-specific – cough and fever – but pleurisy may occur, reflecting the tendency of this disease to cause pulmonary infarction. A wide variety of appearances may be found on chest X-ray, the diagnosis requiring biopsy. Treatment is with amphotericin B but the outlook is poor. There have been cases treated successfully with surgical resection of localised lesions.

Treatment of virus infections

Herpes simplex

The drug of choice is acyclovir (acyloguanosine) which is phosphorylated to its active triphosphate form selectively by herpes viruses. It is thus relatively free from host toxicity and in particular is not myelosuppressive. It is excreted by the kidney; nephrotoxicity has been reported. The drug should be given at a dose of 5 mg/kg by slow intravenous infusion over 1 hour every 8 hours for 7 days. If the renal function is abnormal, the dose should be reduced according to the creatinine clearance (25–50 ml/min – 5 mg/kg every 12 hrs; 10–25 ml/min – 5 mg/kg every 24 hrs; 0–10 ml/min – 2.5 mg/kg every 24 hrs or after dialysis). Unfortunately the mean bioavailability of orally administered acyclovir is only 20%; furthermore, in the immunocompromised absorption may be further impaired. Some success has been reported using high oral doses of acyclovir (400–800 mg five times daily) as treatment for herpetic infections in immunocompetent patients, although until more data are available the intravenous route should be used for neutropenic patients with severe infection.

Herpes zoster

10 years ago vidarabine, a purine nucleoside analogue was shown to have a beneficial effect on the healing of local lesions and to prevent dissemination. However, this drug has a long list of side effects including gastrointestinal, neurological and haematological toxicity. Acyclovir in a dose of 500 mg/m^2 i.v. 8-hourly has been shown to retard the spread of local lesions and reduce the frequency of visceral complications.

As might be predicted, post-herpetic neuralgia is not prevented. Although it is obviously desirable to treat *Herpes zoster* as soon as the lesions appear, acyclovir is beneficial even if its institution is delayed. It has been compared with vidarabine in a randomised trial: acyclovir enhanced the clinical and virological clearance of the lesions and reduced dissemination. Furthermore, in view of the lack of toxicity of acyclovir in immunocompromised patients, it is the drug of choice. Preliminary data in immunocompetent patients suggest that orally administered acyclovir in a dose of 4 g daily may be of benefit. However, this requires confirmation before consideration can be given to the evaluation of this route of administration in the immunocompromised.

It is probably advisable to obtain help from an ophthalmologist in the management of ophthalmic herpes because of the risk to the eye and local preventive measures should be taken. Immunocompromised patients in hospital with zoster should be nursed in isolation until existing lesions are dry and no new lesions appear.

Cytomegalovirus (CMV)

A number of antiviral agents have been used in an attempt to treat CMV infection. Acyclovir, interferon and adenosine arabinoside have not proved successful. CMV immunoglobulin (400 mg/kg i.v. on days 0, 4 and 8, and 200 mg/kg i.v. on days 12 and 16) has been reported in one UK study to have benefited six of nine patients with pneumonitis. Early diagnosis and treatment before severe pulmonary damage had taken place were felt to be of prime importance. DHPG (ganciclovir) (9-1,3-dihydroxy-2-propoxmethyl guanine) has been used in a recently reported series of patients with AIDS complicated by CMV infection. This drug inhibits herpes-group virus replication and requires phosphorylation to its effective form. Although this agent appeared to benefit extrapulmonary CMV injections, all patients with pneumonitis died within two months, four of the seven treated succumbing to respiratory failure before completing the course of treatment. A problem with ganciclovir is neutropenia. Initial experience with the antiviral agent foscarnet has also been disappointing.

Other approaches involve attempts to enhance the patient's immune system but these are still under evaluation. However, promising results in the treatment of CMV pneumonitis have been reported with a combination of ganciclovir and CMV immunoglobulin.

Treatment of *Pneumocystis carinii*

Two drugs have been effective in the treatment of pneumocystis: pentamidine isethionate and cotrimoxazole. Pentamidine's main problem is its side effects, which are more pronounced if it is given intravenously. A quarter of patients develop impaired renal function and liver dysfunction; hypoglycaemia, hypotension and haematological abnormalities (megaloblastosis with a low folate) can also occur; approximately half the patients receiving pentamidine experience an adverse effect. It is better tolerated by the intramuscular route but reactions at the injection site may be a problem. The dose is 4 mg/kg intramuscularly daily for 12 to 14 days (total dose should not exceed 60 mg/kg). The drug has to be reconstituted in sterile water. If it is given intravenously, the patient's blood pressure should be monitored closely and glucose given simultaneously. Pentamidine can be given by inhaler which reduces its systemic toxicity. Less toxic therapy is available using cotrimoxazole. Hughes and colleagues established that a high dose (20 mg trimethoprim and 100 mg sulfamethoxazole/kg) given daily was required. They also have compared cotrimoxazole and pentamidine in a randomised cross-over study of children with pneumocystis. Both drugs proved equally effective (78%). Patients who failed on the initial treatment were crossed over to the other drug; 50% of patients crossed over to cotrimoxazole and responded, and one-third of the primary failures on cotrimoxazole responded to pentamidine. In view of the high incidence of side effects associated with pentamidine, high dose cotrimoxazole is the first-line therapy of choice. Many patients respond to the drug given orally but if the patient is very ill intravenous cotrimoxazole can be given; one ampoule is equivalent to one tablet and a recommended intravenous dose is two ampoules every 6 hours. Therapy is usually given for 14 days. Often improvement in terms of resolution of temperature is dramatic but in some patients clinical improvement may take 4–5 days. Patients failing to respond or developing complications of cotrimoxazole therapy should be given a trial of pentamidine. Approximately 15% of patients treated with high dose cotrimoxazole develop side effects: skin rashes and gastrointestinal symptoms are most prevalent but haematological toxicity and liver dysfunction occur. Patients with AIDS, however, given high dose cotrimoxazole have a high incidence (80%) of side effects.

PREVENTION OF INFECTION

Severely neutropenic patients

Patients who are rendered severely neutropenic by aggressive treatment protocols can be predicted, as outlined above, to be at a high risk of developing various types of infection. Approximately 50% of infections in this group of patients are caused by organisms endemic to the host, the remainder being acquired from the environment. Thus, when considering strategies to reduce infection, measures have to be taken to reduce host bacterial flora and to protect the patient from microbes in the environment. In practice both policies (Tables 35.3 and 35.4) are pursued simultaneously to varying degrees.

Table 35.4 shows the measures that can be employed to attempt to reduce the patient's microbiological flora. Gastrointestinal decontamination seems a sensible goal as the bowel is the major source of invasive pathogens. A number of studies in which the use of a non-absorbable antibiotic (NAA) was often combined with measures to reduce exposure to organisms in the environment have demonstrated a reduction in infection. Antifungal agents were added to suppress fungal overgrowth. Although a diminution in infection was seen, few of the trials were able to demonstrate improvements in remission rate or survival. Furthermore, some of the earlier regimens were unpalatable and costly; those containing gentamicin sometimes resulted in the emergence of resistant organisms. More recently described regimens, e.g. NEOCON (neomycin, colistin and oral antifungal agents), are cheaper, easier to administer and better tolerated. They seem to be particularly effective at the lowest levels of granulocyte count.

The aim of administering NAA is to eradicate the

bowel bacterial flora but this renders the gut susceptible to recolonisation with other pathogenic bacteria. An alternative selective approach is to use agents which destroy the gram negative Enterobacteriaceae but leave the anaerobic flora intact. The latter are thought to provide protection against overgrowth. Cotrimoxazole has a selective action on bowel flora and its administration was first shown in 1977, when given primarily as prophylaxis against *Pneumocystis carinii*, to result in a decrease in episodes of bacterial sepsis. Several groups using cotrimoxazole as prophylaxis in adults undergoing remission induction treatment for acute leukaemia have shown a reduction in bacterial infection. Despite a fairly consistent reduction in the number of infections, few of the studies have been able to show an improvement in complete remission rate or survival. Direct comparisons with NAA have shown cotrimoxazole to be equal or superior in efficacy. The incidence of potential problems with cotrimoxazole has varied. In some studies it has appeared to predispose the patient to infection with fungus and cotrimoxazole-resistant bacteria. Skin rashes are relatively common but a more worrying side effect is myelosuppression. Thus, despite considerable experience with cotrimoxazole in neutropenic patients, its role in the prevention of bacterial infection remains controversial. It does, however, as stated previously have a firm role in the prophylaxis against *Pneumocystis carinii*. Ciprofloxacin is currently being evaluated as a further agent for the prophylaxis of bacterial infection.

Table 35.4 Environmental measures to reduce exogenously acquired infection

Laminar air flow
Protective isolation
Avoidance of certain foods, eg salads, dairy produce
Sterile water
Staff hygiene – importance of hand washing

Environmental measures to reduce exogenously acquired infection

The measures that can be taken to reduce the likelihood of the acquisition of pathogens from the environment

Table 35.5 Measures to prevent endogenously acquired infection by reducing patient's organism load/colonisation, augmenting defence mechanisms

Strategy	Regimen	Dosage	Comments
Antibacterial	Non-absorbable antibiotics	Neomycin 500 mg bd	An example of one regimen; see text
		Colistin 1.5 mega uts bd	
	Cotrimoxazole	2 tabs bd	See text
Antivirus	Acyclovir	200 mgs p.o. qds	More data to support efficacy if given i.v.
		5 mg/kg i.v. bd	
Antifungal	Nystatin suspension	1 ml qds	Topical
	Amphotericin Lozenges	10 mg qds	Topical
	Ketoconazole	200 mg po o.d.	Systemic; risk of hepatic complications
Skin cleansing	Triclosan	Daily total body wash	
Prophylactic granulocyte transfusion			See text

are listed in Table 35.3. The provision of a fully protected environment for the patient thus may involve modification of existing accommodation and is time-consuming, particularly from the nursing viewpoint. The provision of laminar airflow, usually combined with a filter, would be expected to be most beneficial if aspergillus were a problem in the unit. Fortunately, relatively low-cost air flow/filter units are now available. It is difficult to separate the relative value of the various components of a protected environment approach, especially as it is usually combined with other forms of prophylaxis, especially non-absorbable antibiotics. The full approach has been shown in a number of studies to reduce the incidence of infection but this has not been consistently associated with a survival benefit.

An interesting recent study from Seattle involving patients undergoing BMT for aplastic anaemia did show a survival advantage and also a reduction in the incidence of graft-versus-host disease in a group randomised to isolation with laminar air flow. However, Schimpff and his colleagues did not demonstrate air filtration to be beneficial. In terms of infection prevention, the type of isolation required is also controversial: simple protective isolation has been compared to standard accommodation and no difference has been noted. Many studies have used small numbers of patients and the associated procedures (hand-washing, food with low microbial content) may well have masked any benefit of the main measure being evaluated. Certainly basic measures can be relatively easily instituted: the microbial load of food should be reduced to a minimum by avoiding fresh, uncooked food (e.g. salads) and making sure the food is thoroughly cooked and preferably microwaved; sterile water/canned drinks should be provided; attention should be given to antiseptic cleansing of the skin; intravenous cannulae sites should be regularly inspected and renewed; particular attention should be paid to the care of the exit site of central catheters; and, most importantly, hand disinfection by the staff with an antimicrobial hand rub should be routine.

Prevention of virus infection

Herpes simplex

As mentioned above, reactivation of *Herpes simplex* occurs frequently in patients undergoing treatment for acute myeloid leukaemia. Similarly, following bone marrow transplantation the majority of patients who are seropositive before the procedure develop infection. This usually affects the mouth. However, before the introduction of acyclovir *Herpes simplex* pneumonia was

the cause of death in approximately 3% of patients undergoing transplantation. Acyclovir at 5 mg/kg (250 mg/m^2) intravenously has been shown in a number of studies, when given twice or three times daily, to markedly reduce the incidence of *Herpes simplex* infection in patients undergoing transplantation or chemotherapy for acute leukaemia. In one study an additional benefit was a reduction in days spent with fever and leukopenia – effects presumably related to the reduction in herpes infection. Less data are available regarding oral prophylaxis. One study from France has demonstrated that simplex infection can be prevented using 200 mg every 6 hours. In agreement with other studies, recurrences were not reduced, however, following cessation of therapy. The same daily dosage was used in a study from Manchester involving patients treated for non-Hodgkin's lymphoma and acute lymphoblastic leukaemia. There was clinical and virological evidence of a significant reduction in infection in the treatment compared to the placebo group. Acyclovir is generally well-tolerated and in particular is not myelosuppressive. A series of patients has been reported from Seattle with neurological problems (altered sensorium, tremor) who were given acyclovir during bone marrow transplantation. The dosage of drug used in all but one of these cases was higher than the above schedules. In addition, it is always difficult to assign cause and effect to a particular drug in a complex situation such as exists post-transplant; however the patients' condition improved following the withdrawal of acyclovir.

Children with no history of exposure to zoster/varicella who have acute lymphoblastic leukaemia or lymphoma should receive zoster immune globulin. The dose (1.25 mg/10 kg; maximum of 6.25 ml) should be given within 72 hours of exposure.

Cytomegalovirus

Attempts have been made both to prevent and treat CMV infection. Three randomised trials of CMV immunoglobulin or immune plasma carried out in the United States were reported during 1982 and 1983. Despite the differing schedules of administration these studies have demonstrated less CMV infection generally in patients receiving prophylaxis. However, a significant reduction in CMV pneumonitis or a survival benefit could not be demonstrated. The benefit in terms of reduction in infection was best seen in patients who were negative pre-transplant for CMV and avoided granulocyte transfusions from CMV-positive donors. The value of administration of blood products from CMV-negative donors has been studied in a trial recently reported from Seattle. Seronegative recipients were randomised in four groups:

1. CMV immunoglobulin and blood products from CMV-negative donors were used.
2. Blood products from CMV-negative donors were used but no immunoglobulin administered.
3. CMV immunoglobulin was given but blood products were obtained from positive and negative donors.
4. No immunoglobulin was administered and blood products were as in 3.

The incidence of CMV infection was 5% in 1; 13% in 2, 24% in 3; 40% in 4. Only six patients of 85 evaluated developed disease associated with CMV infection. It was concluded that CMV immunoglobulin was not useful and that seronegative patients should receive blood products from seronegative donors. The latter does seem the best available approach at present. Most large transfusion centres can supply products from CMV-negative donors to BMT programmes. CMV immunoglobulin is extremely expensive and its prophylactic use could only be recommended if trial data demonstrated clear-cut efficacy in terms of survival advantage.

Antifungal prophylaxis

Topical prophylaxis in the form of nystatin mouth wash often combined with amphotericin lozenges is frequently prescribed to patients undergoing major chemotherapy. The patient is usually instructed to swirl the nystatin around his mouth and then to swallow it, in an effort to avoid oesophageal infection. The efficacy of this approach remains debatable and in particular there is little evidence to suggest that disseminated infection is prevented. Ketoconazole, an imidazole, has a systemic effect and is usually well absorbed orally. Hann and colleagues at the Royal Free Hospital randomised patients undergoing transplantation or chemotherapy to ketoconazole or amphotericin lozenges and nystatin. Evidence of fungal infection was significantly less in patients on ketoconazole. Transplant patients absorbed the drug less well but it still appeared effective. However, in this study there were no biopsy-proven diagnoses of invasive fungal infections and it is still debatable whether ketoconazole prophylaxis reduces invasive candidiasis; it is certainly less effective against aspergillus. Furthermore, there is a danger of hepatic damage with ketoconazole. Some 14% of patients have asymptomatic elevations of hepatic enzymes which are usually transient. However, symptomatic hepatitis has been reported with an approximate frequency of 1 in 10

000. Most patients recover on stopping treatment; the elderly and those with a history of hepatitis or drug idiosyncracy appear to be particularly at risk. It is now recommended that ketoconazole is used with caution for fungal problems which cannot be treated by other therapies. Newer agents such as fluconazole are under evaluation.

Pneumocystis prophylaxis

The ability to prevent *Pneumocystis carinii* infection in high risk groups, e.g. children undergoing treatment for acute lymphoblastic leukaemia and bone marrow transplant recipients, has led to the use of low dose (two tablets twice daily) prophylaxis. Following BMT this is usually instituted at the end of the first month and continued for 3–5 months.

Prophylactic granulocyte transfusions

A number of studies have evaluated the use of granulocytes in an effort to prevent infection. The logistics of giving daily transfusions require considerable organisation and facilities, especially if HLA-matched granulocytes are used. Trials have been performed on patients undergoing bone marrow transplantation and remission induction chemotherapy for acute myeloid leukaemia. A benefit in terms of some aspect of infection control was seen in four of seven trials conducted between 1978 and 1984. However, the dose of granulocytes given and compatibility of the donors varied.

Further problems encountered are exposure to cytomegalovirus and pulmonary complications. Granulocyte transfusion from a positive donor to a recipient initially negative for cytomegalovirus results in a significant risk of seroconversion. The latter, however, did not appear to be associated with increased risk of disease due to cytomegalovirus, although more recently avoidance of cytomegalovirus infection has been achieved by ensuring that all blood products given to patients negative for cytomegalovirus are obtained from negative donors (see below). Pulmonary infiltrates have been reportedly associated with granulocyte transfusion, especially when amphotericin is administered concomitantly. However, such an association has not been a universal finding and pulmonary complications in the setting of therapy with amphotericin and/or granulocyte transfusion therapy have many potential aetiologies. A further potential hazard of granulocyte transfusion is graft-versus-host disease and to prevent this all cellular blood products given to transplant patients should be irradiated with 1.5 Gy prior to their administration.

OTHER ASPECTS OF SUPPORT OF THE IMMUNOCOMPROMISED PATIENT

In the management of compromised patients, who are usually undergoing anti-tumour therapy, there are a variety of problems, in addition to infection, (Table 35.5) which require support.

Table 35.5   Common problems requiring support in the immunocompromised

Anaemia
Bleeding
Side effects of chemotherapy
Metabolic upset
Poor nutrition
Psychological

Anaemia

The patient's haemoglobin should be maintained at around 10 g/l with packed cells or plasma-reduced blood. Repeated transfusions may result in febrile episodes due to recipient antibodies to contaminating white cells. The latter can be removed by filtering, centrifugation or washing of the red cells. If the patient is a bone marrow recipient, red cells and other cellular blood products should be irradiated prior to infusion. If the recipient is cytomegalovirus-negative the blood product should be from a similarly negative donor.

Bleeding

The most common cause of bleeding is thrombocytopenia. There is little doubt that the administration of platelets to a significantly thrombocytopenic ($<50 \times 10^9/l$) patient who is bleeding will arrest the haemorrhage. An adequate dose of platelets (1/10–15 kg body weight) should be given daily for 2–3 days until bleeding is controlled. Patients who are febrile/infected or have splenomegaly may have an increased requirement. Problems arise when the patient becomes sensitised and HLA-matched or HLA-cross-matched compatible platelets may be required. Platelets may be collected from single donors by apheresis; with the latest technology high yields are obtained with reduced white and red cell contamination. This method of collection is particularly suitable if CMV-negative or HLA-matched platelets are required.

The role of prophylactic platelet transfusions in patients undergoing induction treatment for acute leukaemia and BMT remains controversial, although their use is widespread. The studies that have been performed have not shown consistent benefit. The main arguments against prophylactic platelets are that the patient might become sensitised unnecessarily, and a valuable resource is used needlessly. Sensitisation, however, is not universal, even if a prophylactic approach is adopted; in one long-term study of patients undergoing treatment for leukaemia over 50% of the patients who were not initially sensitised never developed lymphocytotoxic antibody. In this trial, as in others, there was no relationship between the number of units of platelets given and allo-immunisation. At present, until there is good trial data, the author uses prophylactic platelet transfusions to keep the platelet count around $30 \times 10^9/l$ in those undergoing major induction chemotherapy for acute non-lymphoblastic leukaemia and following BMT.

Coagulation abnormalities are common and often compound the effects of thrombocytopenia. The underlying mechanisms are often multifactorial and involve increased thrombin formation, fibrinolysis and granulocyte elastase activity. From the practical viewpoint two situations require emphasis. The first is vitamin K deficiency. Patients often are eating poorly, have diarrhoea and are on parenteral antibiotics. Prolongation of the prothrombin and partial thromboplastin times is found and responds to parenteral vitamin K. The second is disseminated intravascular coagulation. In the florid form of thrombocytopenia, prolongation of the coagulation screening tests and elevated fibrin degradation products are found. Vigorous replacement of missing factors with fresh frozen plasma is required but in particular fibrinogen replacement. The fibrinogen should be kept above 1 g/l and cryoprecipitate (2 bags/10 kg initially) is commonly used for this purpose. As consumption is ongoing, repeated clotting studies and appropriate replacement are required until the stimulus to consumption is removed. This usually means that significant chemotherapy-induced reduction of leukaemia cells has been achieved. The role of heparin remains controversial. It has been studied most extensively in acute promyelocytic leukaemia. No concurrently controlled randomised study has been performed, although the available data indicate a trend in favour of heparin usage. The optimal dosage of heparin to be used, its control and schedule of administration are not known. The author uses a continuous 24-hour intravenous infusion of 10–15 000 units of heparin in patients with acute promyelocytic leukaemia; this is combined with daily platelets and replacement therapy. When the marrow has been rendered hypoplastic by chemotherapy, the stimulus activating clotting has been removed and the heparin can be stopped.

Finally, of particular importance is the psychological management of the patient (see Ch. 39); a positive, encouraging attitude is required by all the attending staff, medical and nursing. These patients are often inpatients for long periods of time and are seriously ill, and even the most resilient may lose their determination. It is important to remember that a time may come when it is clear that the patient has resistant or relapsed disease and terminal care is all that is kind and appropriate.

BIBLIOGRAPHY

Bowden R A, Sayers M, Flowmoy N et al 1986 Cytomegalovirus immune globulin and seronegative blood products to prevent primary cytomegalovirus infection after bone marrow transplantation. New England Journal of Medicine 314: 1006–1010

Brown A E 1984 Neutropenia, fever, and infection. American Journal of Medicine 76: 421–428

Pizzo P A, Robichaud K J, Gill F A, Witebsky F G 1982 Empiric antibiotic and antifungal therapy for cancer patients with prolonged fever and granulocytopenia. American Journal of Medicine 72: 101–111

Pizzo P A, Commers J, Cotton D et al 1984 Approaching the controversies in antibacterial management of cancer patients. American Journal of Medicine 76: 436–449

Prentice H G 1984 Infections in haematology. Clinics in Haematology 13: 3

Rubin R H, Young L S 1988 Clinical approach to infection in the compromised host, 2nd edn. Plenum Publishing

Shepp D H, Dandliker P S, Meyers J D 1986 Treatment of varicella-zoster virus infection in severely Immunocompromised patients. A randomised comparison of acyclovir and vidarabine. New England Journal of Medicine 314: 208–121

Winston D J, Ho G, Gale R P 1982 Therapeutic granulocyte transfusions for documented infections. A controlled trial in 95 infectious granulocytopenic episodes. Annals of Internal Medicine 97: 509–515

Yin J A L, Delamore I W 1987 Management of infection in leukaemic patients. In: Whittaker J A, Delamore I W (eds) Leukaemia. Blackwell Scientific Publications, p 239

36. Blood and blood components

G. Galea   S. J. Urbaniak

RED CELL PRODUCTS

Red cell transfusions are given to patients who have become symptomatic from an oxygen-carrying capacity deficit. A number of components are available for transfusion; each has special characteristics and indications. In a stable patient, one unit of red cells will increase the haemoglobin by 1 gm/dl and the haematocrit by 3%. In infants, 3 ml red cells/kg body weight will increase the haemoglobin by 1 gm/dl.

Indications

The patient's clinical condition, not a laboratory test result, is the most important factor determining transfusion needs. Many patients with asymptomatic anaemia do not require transfusion and in most patients loss of approximately 20% of blood volume can safely be corrected by crystalloid solutions alone. There is no evidence that it is necessary to transfuse a patient to a 'normal' haemoglobin prior to surgery. The time-honoured threshold of 10 gm/dl of haemoglobin seems to be based more on theory than on clinical or experimental evidence. It is similarly unnecessary to transfuse post-operatively just to achieve normal haematocrit values.

Fresh whole blood

A unit of whole blood contains the red cells and plasma elements of donor blood plus the anticoagulant. Its total volume is approximately 515 ml with a haematocrit of about 40%.

Use of freshly drawn whole blood less than 24 hours old is a vestige of past transfusion practice when appropriate components were not available. There are no valid indications for specifically transfusing fresh whole blood. For thrombocytopenia appropriate therapy is transfusion of platelet concentrates. For such cases one unit of fresh whole blood would not contain sufficient platelets to be effective. Similarly, fresh whole blood is impractical for replacement of deficient coagulation factors. If the deficit is greater than can be corrected with fresh frozen plasma, specific factor concentrates are preferred.

Whole blood less than 3 days old is the component of choice for exchange transfusion in the newborn. It ensures that electrolyte concentrations, particularly potassium, are within tolerable limits for infants and it also ensures adequate levels of 2,3-diphosphoglycerate and red cell oxygen affinity.

Stored whole blood

Throughout the storage period blood constantly undergoes biochemical, metabolic, morphological and haemorheological changes. This 'storage lesion' is shown in Table 36.1. These storage changes have little significance in most transfusion situations; patients compensate for or reverse them. Blood stored for more than 24 hours at 4°C has few viable platelets and granulocytes. These cells degenerate and, along with fibrin strands, make up the micro-aggregates seen in stored blood. Viable lymphocytes persist through the entire storage period. Although factors V and VIII are

Table 36.1 Biochemical changes in blood during storage (in CPD at 4°C)

	Day of collection	1 week	End of shelf life
RBC viability (%)	100	90	70
RBC ATP (% of initial)	100	95	70
RBC 2,3 DPG (% of initial)	100	90	10
Plasma K$^+$ (mmol/l)	3.5	12	21
Plasma dextrose (mg/dl)	430	370	280
pH	7.2	7.0	6.8
Plasma haemoglobin (mg/dl)	1	13	40

labile at 4°C, the reduced levels are rarely of consequence unless there is excessive consumption (as in DIC) or there is reduced synthesis (as in liver disease).

The supply of whole blood is limited because most units are used for the preparation of components. However, whole blood, which provides both oxygen-carrying capacity and blood volume expansion, is indicated for actively bleeding patients who have lost over 25% of their blood volume. Patients with acute haemorrhage may require transfusion despite normal haemoglobin and haematocrit levels. Acute blood loss of more than one-third of the blood volume is best treated with whole blood. Red cells supplemented by crystalloid and/or colloid solutions are less cost effective than whole blood and the simultaneous use of fresh frozen plasma with red blood cells carries twice the risk of infection transmission. Infusions to restore intravascular volume should be started immediately, beginning with readily available crystalloid or colloid solutions.

Modified whole blood

Platelets and/or cryoprecipitate can be removed from freshly collected blood and the remaining plasma returned to the original bag to reconstitute the red cells to whole blood. The product has virtually the same haemostatic properties as stored whole blood, although it has 30–40% less fibrinogen if cryoprecipitate has been harvested.

Red blood cells

A unit of red cells, also called red cell concentrate, is prepared by removing 200–250 ml of plasma from a whole blood unit. It has a volume of approximately 300 ml and a haematocrit of approximately 70%. Some residual plasma is left with the red cells to ensure their preservation during storage.

Red blood cells are the component of choice to restore or maintain oxygen-carrying capacity. They are most useful in patients with chronic anaemia or congestive heart failure, or in the elderly who cannot tolerate rapid changes in blood volume. The use of red cells for transfusion during surgery is controversial. Losses of 1000 ml or less can be replaced with crystalloid/colloid solutions alone. Frequently (in approximately two-thirds of cases) oxygen-carrying capacity alone is needed and this can be provided by red cell concentrates. If significant volume expansion is also required, whole blood is then the component of choice.

Several 'additive solutions' are in use which are added shortly after phlebotomy to the red cells. These solutions contain varying amounts of saline, adenine and glucose, and some include mannitol. Other compounds, e.g. phosphates or guanosine, are occasionally used, although these are not all licensed in the UK. These additives maintain red cell function without the need for residual plasma and more plasma can therefore be harvested. Moreover, these nutrient solutions give the red cells a greater total volume with a haemotocrit of 55–65% and this less viscous red cell component can be transfused more quickly.

Leukocyte-poor red blood cells

Multiparous women and previously transfused patients may develop antibodies to leukocytes and/or platelets. Patients with leukocyte antibodies may sustain febrile reactions after receiving blood containing incompatible leukocytes. Febrile reactions may also occur, however, in patients without demonstrable white cell or platelet antibodies. Febrile non-haemolytic reactions do not damage red blood cells, but symptoms, such as chills, fever, malaise, etc., may be very uncomfortable. The reactions seem to result from immune damage to donor leukocytes, even those that are non-viable. Some of these symptoms may follow release of C5a when reactions between leuko-agglutinins and leukocyte antigens activate complement. The production of C3a may induce vasomotor instability and lead to hypotension, tachycardia or bronchospasm.

Only a minority of patients (approximately 15%) who experience a non-haemolytic febrile reaction have a similar reaction with the next transfusion. Accordingly, leukocyte-poor blood should probably be offered only after two or more reactions, where leukocyte or platelet antibodies have been demonstrated and there was no response to premedication with steroids or an antihistaminic agent.

Red cells may be modified by centrifugation, washing, filtration or a combination of these techniques, to make them leukocyte poor. By definition, 70% of the leukocytes will be removed and at least 70% of the red cells will be retained, although most methods aim for a minimum residual number of leukocytes to abrogate pyrexial transfusion reactions of $< 0.5 \times 10^9/l$. Saline wash methods are commonly used to prepare leukocyte-poor red cells, but such products expire 12–24 hours from the time of preparation, since the bag containing the red cells has to be opened during the procedure. Recently, micro-aggregate filtration of centrifuged cells has been found to effectively remove leukocytes (to $< 10^8$ WBC). This method does not shorten the expiry date of the product, if in-line filters are used to produce leucocyte-poor cells.

Frozen red cells

Freezing is the ideal form of long-term storage for rare

bloods. Because the extensive washing required to remove the glycerol (which is the most commonly used cryopreservative) also removes leukocytes, platelets and plasma, deglycerolised red cells are suitable for patients with antibodies to these fractions. Frozen blood, however, still has the potential for disease transmission. It has been shown that it can transmit both hepatitis B and non-A non-B hepatitis. Cytomegalovirus (CMV) is usually found in white cells and most workers believe that deglycerolised red cells have a greatly decreased risk of transmitting CMV infection. Freezing was initially thought to kill all nucleated blood cells, eliminating viable lymphocytes and thereby preventing graft-versus-host disease in severely immunodeficient patients. However, viable lymphocytes have been demonstrated after washing, even in blood frozen for several years. Irradiating donor units is the only technique that effectively prevents lymphocyte blastogenesis.

Frozen blood is an extremely expensive product and it is only available in certain specialist centres. It should be used only in specific circumstances after discussing the merits of each case with the blood bank medical staff.

Irradiated blood

Engraftment of donor lymphocytes may occur in severely immunosuppressed or immunodeficient individuals, as well as in premature babies. Indeed it has been described following intra-uterine blood transfusions. Graft-versus-host-disease (GVHD) may be entirely asymptomatic or may consist of a clinical syndrome of fever, skin rashes, hepatitis and diarrhoea, which may progress to a fatal outcome. Pretransfusion irradiation of all blood components containing lymphocytes will prevent GVHD. A radiation dose 1500 cGy renders 95% of all lymphocytes in a unit of blood incapable of replication but the function of the cellular components remains unaffected.

Compatibility testing

Safe transfusion practice depends on accurate ABO and Rh typing of patients and donors, the identification of potentially harmful antibodies in the recipient, and the provision of compatible blood. Donor blood is routinely tested for ABO and Rh(D) grouping. The need for ABO matching is self-evident, due to the invariable presence of anti-A and anti-B in the appropriate groups. Rh grouping is important due to the immunogenicity of the D antigen and the particular need to avoid immunising females during their reproductive years. Although other antigens other than D, e.g. Kell, Duffy and Kidd, are

capable of inducing immune allo-antibodies, this is a much less common occurrence.

The presence of harmful antibodies in the transfusion recipient is routinely sought for in one of two ways. Serum may be screened in advance with a panel of highly selected red cells containing the important antigens (type and screen) or it may be tested directly against donor red cells that are to be transfused (crossmatch). This pre-transfusion testing may take up to 1 hour to perform, depending on the methods used. If a significant antibody is detected during pre-transfusion testing, it is identified and blood negative for that specific antigen is crossmatched. These additional tests take even more time.

When blood is urgently needed before the completion of the above-mentioned tests, a very quick check of the patient's blood group can be performed and blood group-specific (homologous) blood can be issued which will be retrospectively matched. When the need for blood is extremely urgent, uncrossmatched Group O Rh negative blood can be used, particularly if the patient's blood group is not known and the patient is a female of child-bearing age. In males and older females Group O Rh positive may be used. If the patient's blood group is known, blood of the same ABO and Rh group may be used. It needs to be stressed though that the concept of the group O Rh negative 'universal donor' is an outmoded one, since not only does group O whole blood contain anti-A and anti-B which, particularly if present in high titre, can cause haemolysis in A, B or AB blood group individuals, but there is also a definite risk of a haemolytic reaction due to the presence of allo-antibodies other than anti-D, particularly in those previously transfused or pregnant.

Storage of blood in the liquid state

Blood for replacement therapy is stored at 4°C and collected into an anticoagulant. The anticoagulants are designed primarily to prolong the shelf life of the red cells: 21 days in acid-citrate-dextrose (ACD) and 28 days in citrate-phosphate-dextrose (CPD). More recent developments (e.g. the addition of adenine – see above) further extend the viability of red cells during storage to a maximum of 35 days.

Administration

All blood components must be transfused through a filter. This is accomplished by using standard blood infusion sets with in-line filters and drip chambers. Standard filters have a pore size of 127–220 μ; micro aggregate filters have pores of 20–40 μ. The latter need only be used to render the unit of blood leukocyte-poor and their routine use is not indicated.

It is of the utmost importance not to mix drugs of any kind with the blood being given. Simple drugs, e.g. ethacrynic acid, may cause red cell haemolysis, as may 5% dextrose. Normal saline is the only safe crystalloid that may be added to red cell concentrates to speed up their infusion rate.

Reactions

Recipients of blood can experience a number of adverse reactions during transfusion – some troublesome but insignificant, others life-threatening.

These are described in detail in Chapter 38 and therefore a brief classification only is described here.

The more common problems are classified as:

1. Febrile non-haemolytic, due to antibodies in the recipient reacting with donor leukocytes and/or platelets.
2. Allergic, as a result of recipient antibodies reacting with allergens in the donor plasma.
3. Circulatory overload, which may follow giving too much blood too quickly.
4. Haemolytic reactions, which may occur from red cell incompatibilities and can be life-threatening.
5. Anaphylactic reactions, e.g. anti-IgA in the patient reacting with IgA in donor plasma, or unknown factors (idiosyncratic).

The symptoms from transfusion reactions are numerous and non-specific, varying from pyrexia, chest pain, headache, urticaria and wheezing to hypotension and renal failure with DIC. Because symptoms do not confirm the cause, and the treatment and prevention vary with the cause, all adverse reactions must be evaluated in the blood bank and the transfusion stopped until it is clear that it can continue.

PLATELETS

Platelet transfusions are used to treat surgical and medical patients with active thrombocytopenic bleeding or to prevent bleeding in thrombocytopenic patients.

Indications

Predicting who will bleed, especially during surgery, is not easy. Most surgical procedures can be safely completed with platelet counts of $60-70 \times 10^9/l$ and patients with counts of $50 \times 10^9/l$ and a bleeding time less than two times normal usually do not need prophylactic platelet transfusions before surgery. If throm-

bocytopenic bleeding develops in surgery, transfusions to restore the count to $70 \times 10^9/l$ are necessary. These guidelines also apply in massive transfusion settings, where infusions of 15–20 units of blood may significantly dilute platelet counts below haemostatic levels, and to surgical patients with normal platelet counts but with qualitative defects (sometimes associated with myeloproliferative disorders and qualitative inherited disorders).

Prophylactic platelet transfusions are given to non-bleeding patients with rapidly dropping counts or counts below $10-20 \times 10^9/l$ secondary to neoplastic conditions, chemotherapy or aplastic disorders. Significant spontaneous bleeds with platelet counts above $20 \times 10^9/l$ are rare. The level at which prophylactic platelet transfusions are needed must depend on clinical assessment and complicating risk factors such as fever, infection and drug therapy. Because the half-life of platelets is 3–4 days, transfusions may be repeated every 1–3 days until the patient stabilises and recovers bone marrow function.

Unless there is a serious haemorrhage, platelet transfusions are not helpful in treating thrombocytopenia caused by idiopathic thrombocytopenic purpura (ITP), thrombotic thrombocytopenic purpura (TTP), immune-mediated drug purpura and hypersplenism. The factors responsible for the excessive destruction or sequestration of platelets in these conditions affect all platelets, including the ones transfused. Platelet transfusions will not correct problems from post-transfusional purpura or neonatal iso-immune thrombocytopenic purpura, unless Pl^{A1} antigen negative platelets are available for the latter.

Platelet dysfunction caused by extrinsic factors in dysproteinaemia and uraemia are better managed by plasmapheresis and dialysis respectively. Although platelet transfusions are given in disseminated intravascular coagulation (DIC), fibrinogen degradation products interfere with platelet adhesion and aggregation, which makes transfusions less effective.

Source and preparation

Fresh whole blood

Although fresh whole blood (less than 12 hours old) contains approximately 1×10^{11} platelets/donation, there are good reasons why this is an unacceptable therapeutic agent for patients bleeding because of thrombocytopenia: circulatory overload will almost certainly arise before haemostasis is achieved. Moreover, if such blood is issued without doing microbiological testing, the patient will be put at an increased risk of disease transmission, e.g. hepatitis B or HIV.

Platelet-rich plasma (PRP)

PRP should not normally be used as a source of platelets (yield $0.8-0.9 \times 10^{11}$ platelets per 200 ml donation). It is a waste of fresh plasma, which is the exclusive source of factor VIII and has similar problems to whole blood with regard to circulatory overload. Exceptionally, it may be of value where platelets and FFP are required simultaneously.

Random donor platelets

Random donor platelets, known also as platelet concentrates (or simply platelets), are prepared from units of whole blood within 6 hours of collection. They contain a minimum of 0.5×10^{11} and these platelets are suspended in enough donor plasma to maintain the pH within the container above 6.0. This is normally 40–70 ml per platelet concentrate for products stored at 20–24°C. Platelet concentrates contain haemostatic levels of all coagulation factors. Platelets also contain a significant number of leukocytes (approximately 3×10^8) and small amounts of red cells (0.5 ml).

Apheresis platelets

Single donor platelet concentrates are collected by automated methods that return all unneeded portions of the donor's blood to the donor. One unit contains $3-6 \times 10^{11}$ platelets (equivalent to 6–8 units of random donor platelets) suspended in 200–400 ml of fresh donor plasma. Depending on the method of collection this product may also be significantly contaminated with leukocytes and red cells (up to 20 ml). Alternatively, newly developed in-line filters may be used to reduce WBC contamination to $< 10^7$, which delays or abolishes the development of alloimmunisation. Matched single donor platelets are the ideal product for treating patients who have developed HLA- or platelet-specific antibodies and have become refractory or unresponsive to random donor platelets.

Compatibility testing in platelet transfusions

ABO and Rh groups

ABO antigens are present on the platelet surface. Some studies report a slight decrease in recovery of ABO-incompatible platelets over ABO-compatible; others report no change. Because prompt transfusion is more important to patient therapy than waiting for compatible platelet products, patients may be given any ABO type.

There is no D antigen on the platelet membrane. However, Rh negative recipients are at a small risk of becoming sensitised to D antigen by red cells present in Rh positive platelets. For this reason, Rh negative platelets are preferred for Rh negative females who may bear children. If this group must receive Rh positive platelets, one might consider giving Rh immunoglobulin. One standard dose (500 iu) protects against the red cells in approximately 10 platelet concentrates.

HLA compatibility

Platelets manifest HLA antigens whose expression partially results from adsorption of plasma antigens onto the platelet surface. In patients refractory to random platelets, HLA-matching of patient to donor may result in acceptable post-transfusion increments in platelet counts. A single HLA-compatible donor may be able to provide all of the patient's transfusion needs if platelets are obtained by repeated cytapheresis. The most likely source of HLA-identical or -compatible donors would be the patient's relatives.

Additionally, many centres have files of HLA-typed donors. Studies of HLA antigens and survival of transfused platelets indicate that a number of HLA antigens have sufficient serological similarity that platelet survival can be satisfactory even when these antigens are mismatched. Such findings have simplified matching for donors to allo-immunised patients. However, HLA-matching does not guarantee good recovery in allo-immunised patients: no response is seen in 25% of HLA-compatible transfusions. Despite intensive efforts to develop effective crossmatching techniques for platelets, there are no satisfactory tests currently available to determine probable platelet survival in recipients immunised to HLA or other antigens. Patients under consideration for bone marrow transplantation should not receive platelets or other components from family members who are potential marrow donors because pre-transplantation exposure to the donor's antigens increases the likelihood of sensitisation and decreases the chances of a successful transplant.

Calculating the dose and post-transfusion increment

Dose

The required dose of platelets is calculated from body surface area, read off a nomogram using the patient's height and weight. A useful rule of thumb is that one unit of platelet concentrate, with at least 0.5×10^{11} platelets, increases the platelet count 1 hour after transfusion by $5-10 \times 10^9/l$ per sqm of body surface area. The number of units of platelets required (n) can be calculated thus:

$$n = (Pi - Pii) \times BSA/10$$

where Pi and Pii are the desired and initial platelet counts respectively and BSA is the body's surface area in square metres.

Post-transfusion increment

The efficacy of platelet transfusion is estimated by calculating the platelet increment related to the blood volume or body surface area. Many different formulae are in use for the purpose. One commonly used formula is:

$$CI = (Pi - Pii) \times BSA/n$$

where CI is the corrected increment of platelets, Pi and Pii are platelet counts determined 1 hour after and before transfusion respectively, n is the number of platelets ($\times 10^{11}$) transfused and BSA is the patient's body surface area. A CCI (Corrected Count Increment) higher than $7.5 \times 10^9/l$/unit would indicate a successful transfusion of platelets. A CCI lower than that indicates platelet refractoriness in the absence of any other condition that would affect both recovery and survival. A CCI at 24 hours after transfusion of platelets lower than $4.5 \times 10^9/l$ unit would also suggest platelet refractoriness.

Platelet recovery and survival

The recovery of platelets one hour after transfusion in healthy volunteers is approximately 65% of those transfused. Nearly one-third of the transfused platelets are sequestered in the spleen. The survival of autologous fresh platelets is on average 9 days, whereas the survival of platelets from concentrates stored at 20–24°C is only about 4 days. Survival of platelets is affected by a number of factors:

1. ABO and HLA compatibility – see above.
2. Spleen size. Patients with splenomegaly may sequester and destroy in the spleen most of the transfused platelets.
3. Infection, bleeding, DIC. In the presence of any of these conditions, there will be little or no increment in the post-transfusion platelet count.

Storage and handling

Shelf-life for platelets depends on a complex combination of factors: platelet count, plasma volume, pH, temperature, container and agitation. They are normally stored with constant agitation to reduce the physical lesion induced by the interaction of the stored platelets and the container wall. Special platelet packs, either made of polyolefin (PL-732, Fenwal Laboratories) or using a modified plasticiser (CLX, Cutter Biologicals),

are now in common use and allow platelet storage for up to 5 days. Storage at 20–24°C poses a higher risk of bacterial growth, but few problems will be encountered if strict codes are adhered to during production. Platelets may also be stored at 1–6°C with no agitation but they expire 48 hours after collection. Data show, however, that platelets stored at 'room temperature' have superior function and viability and these are the products routinely supplied today.

Administration

Platelet concentrates must be given through a blood filter (170–220 μm). Significant numbers are not lost in the filter, but a substantial loss can occur from the product volume left in the infusion line. To reduce this loss, special component sets are manufactured, with shorter tubing and small filter surfaces and drip chambers. Platelets may be infused as rapidly as the patient tolerates.

Reactions

Reactions associated with red cell transfusions may also be seen with platelets. Acute haemolytic reactions are very rare complications from ABO-incompatible plasma; infants with small blood volumes are at a greater risk. More commonly seen is the development of a positive direct antiglobulin test, which has little effect on the patient's well-being. Febrile nonhaemolytic and allergic reactions are also common. Fever should not be treated with aspirin, which interferes with platelet function.

Of greater concern is allo-immunisation: 60–70% of multiply-transfused patients become sensitised. Therefore, patients should only be given platelets for a defined need and in appropriate minimum amounts. Each individual unit carries a disease transmission risk (e.g. hepatitis, CMV, HIV) equal to whole blood. Rare cases of bacterial contamination have been reported. The leukocytes may also contribute to graft-versus-host disease in immunocompromised patients.

GRANULOCYTES

Granulocytes are used as supportive therapy in neutropenic patients with sepsis. Their value is, however, uncertain. Transfused granulocytes function normally in vivo and migrate to sites of infection. However, because of the cost and time involved in collecting granulocytes, the adverse reactions experienced by both donors and recipients, and their questionable efficacy, the goals of granulocyte transfusions and the criteria for patient selection must be carefully defined.

Indications

Most granulocyte transfusions are given to severely neutropenic patients (absolute granulocyte count less than $5 \times 10^8/l$) with documented infections that have proven resistant to at least 2 days of appropriate aggressive antibiotic therapy. Moreover, patients should have a reasonable chance of recovery. The effect of transfusions is only temporary and the clinical course of the patient will not change unless the marrow recovers.

Although existing neutropenia is an important criterion for selecting candidates for granulocyte transfusions, it need not necessarily be such for septic neonates. There are special reasons for transfusing granulocytes to neonates. Their stem cell reserve is small, even though they are dividing at maximum rate. Moreover, cells take longer to be released from the bone marrow and granulocyte phagocytosis is less efficient than in adults.

A less common use of granulocyte transfusions is in controlling bacterial infections in patients with qualitative neutrophil defects, such as chronic granulomatous disease and severe burns. Prophylactic use of granulocyte transfusions in any patient population is not recommended in view of the high incidence of side effects and its very doubtful efficacy in these circumstances.

Granulocyte collection

Granulocytes are normally collected by single donor cytapheresis. Final products should contain at least 1×10^{10}/bag in approximately 300 ml of plasma. To achieve this number, donors may be pre-treated with corticosteroids and/or a sedimenting agent (hydroxyethyl starch or dextrans). A considerable number of other white cells, e.g. monocytes, platelets $(2-10 \times 10^{11})$ and red cells (10–50 ml) may also be present in the final product depending on the method of collection. Nylon filtration collection does harvest greater numbers of granulocytes, but is no longer used in view of its relatively high incidence of donor and recipient reactions and impaired granulocyte function in the recipient.

Compatibility testing

ABO and Rh antigens are thought not to be present on granulocytes, but because most preparations are heavily contaminated with red cells, ABO-Rh compatibility guidelines parallel those of red cell components. If this is not possible, the red cells in the bag should be ABO compatible with the recipient's plasma. If the product contains more than 5 ml of red cells, it must be ABO-compatible and crossmatched using standard techniques. Rh immunoglobulin may be indicated when Rh positive products are given to Rh negative females who may bear children; one standard dose (500 iu) protects against 5 ml of red cells. Current technology does not provide an effective in vitro compatibility test for granulocytes; although many methods exist, no single one detects all relevant antibodies.

Evaluating effectiveness

Post-transfusional counts, the traditional index of efficacy for other component transfusions, are unreliable for evaluating granulocyte transfusions because the cells rapidly leave the vascular compartment. The best index of efficacy is clinical improvement of the patient.

Storage and handling

Granulocytes should be transfused as soon as possible after collection, and must be infused within 12–24 hours. If storage is unavoidable, granulocyte function is best preserved at room temperature without agitation.

Administration

Granulocyte concentrates are ordinarily given daily for at least 4 to 6 days unless bone marrow recovery or severe reactions supervene. Granulocyte concentrates should be infused through a standard blood administration set with an in-line filter. Potential bone marrow recipients should not receive granulocytes from the potential transplant donor. Concentrates are irradiated (1500 cGy) before administration in immunosuppressed individuals to prevent GVHD from contaminating lymphocytes.

Reactions

Granulocytes are transfused slowly over 2 to 4 hours to minimise transfusion reactions and patients must be closely monitored. Pre-treatment with antihistamines and/or steroids may be necessary to manage reactions.

Haemolytic transfusion reactions are possible with granulocyte transfusions, but they can be avoided by using ABO-compatible blood. Allergic reactions are also common. Febrile non-haemolytic reactions caused by leukocyte antibody-antigen reactions are seen in 5–15% of patients transfused. Patients with lung infections are at special risk of developing severe pulmonary reactions. The aetiology of these reactions is not clear, but contributory factors include fluid overload, localisation of infused granulocytes at the site of infection with granulocyte degranulation, adherence of cells to the endothelium and complement activation. Leuko-agglutinins causing aggregation and embolisation of granulocytes in the lungs present a similar picture and may be the most severe of all. Amphoteracin B, given for fungal infections, increases granulocyte aggregation and exacerbates pulmonary reactions.

Like red cell components and platelets, granulocytes can allo-immunise patients, transmit diseases like hepatitis, CMV and AIDS, and cause GVHD. This is especially important to bone marrow transplant recipients who are at risk from CMV and GVHD and who in the course of their treatment might be considered candidates for granulocyte transfusions.

FRESH FROZEN PLASMA

Plasma is separated from single units of whole blood and is rapidly frozen within 6 hours after donation. The total volume averages 200–250 ml and includes a portion of the anticoagulant. Units of plasma collected by plasmapheresis may have up to 500 ml and paediatric FFP contains 50–100 ml. FFP is stored below $-18°C$ for 6 months or below $-35°C$ for up to 1 year.

Indications

FFP contains normal levels of all the plasma clotting factors including the labile factors V and VIII (see Ch. 32). Few definitive indications for FFP exist, and many patients can be managed more effectively and safely with alternative treatment:

1. Plasma should not be used as a simple volume expander.
2. Plasma should not be used as a source of nutrition.

Situations in which FFP transfusion are considered are as follows:

Specific coagulation factor replacement

It is important to note that aside from factors V and VIII, all the other coagulation factors are stable at 4°C in whole blood. Even in blood stored for 28 days, factor V may be 30% or more, while the level needed for haemostasis may be as little as 10%.

FFP can be used to treat the rare patient with isolated factor V and XI deficiencies, but haemophilia A (factor VIII) and haemophilia B (factor IX) are best treated with heat-treated specific factor concentrates.

Patients deficient in AT III are at risk of thrombosis. Deficiency of AT III may occur congenitally or be ac-quired (liver disease, oral contraceptives, DIC, eclampsia). Acute reduction of AT III levels occurs during trauma, and operative procedures may occasion the need for its replacement. If specific concentrates are not available, FFP is an adequate source of AT III in an emergency.

Multiple clotting factor deficiencies

Severe liver disease. This is among the most common clinical indications for transfusion of FFP. These patients may manifest abnormal bleeding for a variety of reasons (see Ch. 32). Plasma transfusion is indicated if the patient is bleeding, although the ability of FFP to correct plasma factor coagulopathy in these patients is very variable. Need is less clear if the patient is not bleeding, but will be surgically challenged (e.g. liver biopsy). Prothrombin time (PT) and partial thromboplastin time (PTT) are poor predictors of surgical bleeding, and abnormal results are difficult to correct. Stable patients with abnormal coagulation screen not being challenged do not need FFP. Concentrate use is generally contra-indicated in liver disease because of high risk of DIC and thrombosis.

Coumarin drug reversal. Coumarin drugs stop the production of functional factors II, VII, IX and X. Since these drugs have a relatively long half-life (2 days) the effect of their administration may be cumulative. If a patient on coumarin drugs starts to bleed or is scheduled for surgery, the effect of the drugs can be reversed with intravenous vitamin K. This will correct factor deficiency in 6–12 hours. These factors all have different rates of synthesis, which affect the rate of their return to haemostatic levels. Therefore, both the PT and the APTT, tests that adequately assess all factors are recommended following coumarin reversal. If time is pressing, FFP is the treatment of choice, subject to the patient tolerating the volume required.

Massive transfusion. Dilution of coagulation factors in massive transfusion settings (greater than one blood volume in 24 hours) is very uncommon, even when red cells are transfused instead of whole blood. Factor levels may decrease, but they rarely drop below 25–30%. Most factors equilibrate into the extravascular space which serves as a reserve pool and compensates for any potential dilution. Even factor VIII rarely drops below 50%: factor VIII bound to the vascular endothelium is released under stress to provide additional reserve. Unless there is co-existing DIC or another medical condition, factor support is not needed. Platelets, which are largely intravascular, become diluted with massive transfusion and may be needed. The coagulation factors present in platelet concentrates are considerable and help contribute to haemostasis.

Abnormal PT and PTT results are difficult to correct in massive transfusion. If plasma is needed in haemorrhagic shock, large volumes (600–2000 ml) must be given quickly (over 1–2 hours) to effect any significant improvement.

Open heart surgery. In most instances, bleeding episodes associated with by-pass surgery have been related to platelet dysfunction, rather than to deficiency of plasma coagulation factors. Plasma coagulation levels are usually depleted but very rarely to levels which impair haemostasis. Use of FFP would be as for massive transfusion.

Thrombotic thrombocytopenic purpura

Therapeutic plasma exchange with FFP has proven effective in controlling thrombotic episodes. Recent work suggests that TTP may be related to a deficiency of a depolymerase which processes multimeric vWF components of the factor VIII complex. Transfusion of FFP may provide the missing depolymerase activity.

Missing plasma constituents

C1 esterase inhibitor deficiency in hereditary angioneurotic oedema. This condition may be complicated by attacks of laryngeal oedema which accounts for 30% of deaths in this condition. FFP may be used as a temporary life-saving measure, although specific concentrates are now available.

Pseudocholinesterase deficiency may result in suxamethonium apnoea. In addition to applying positive pressure ventilation to the patient, FFP may be used as a source of the missing enzyme.

Serological reasons

FFP may be used to neutralise anti-Lewis prior to transfusion of Lewis-positive blood when Le (a−b−) blood is not available, since it contains soluble Lewis substances that inhibit these weak antibodies.

Compatibility testing

Compatibility testing is not undertaken for plasma transfusions. However, the patient's ABO group must be known prior to product selection to make sure anti-A or B antibodies in the plasma are compatible with the patient's red cells. This is especially important to infants with small blood volumes. If the patient's blood group is not known, AB FFP can be safely given. Rh is not considered in their selection.

Storage and handling

FFP is stored frozen at temperatures below −18°C for up to 6 months from the date of collection (or 12 months at −35°C). Before it can be transfused, FFP is thawed in a 37°C waterbath with gentle agitation. This thawing process takes approximately 30 minutes. After thawing, FFP must be transfused as soon as possible (definitely within 6 hours).

Administration

Standard blood infusion sets or special component infusion sets with in-line 170 μm filters should be used. No added benefit is gained by using micro-aggregate filter sets. Infusion should proceed as fast as the patient can tolerate.

Reactions

Chills, fever and allergic reactions may occur with plasma transfusions, including acute anaphylactic reactions. Severe allergic reactions with pulmonary complications are possible if the donor has antibodies to the patient's leukocytes. Circulatory overload may occur with fast infusion rates. Haemolytic reactions are rare and generally mild, but a positive DAGT may develop if antibodies in the plasma react with the recipient's red cells. Plasma, like all other blood components, has a risk of disease transmission similar to whole blood, with the exception of CMV and HTLV1 that seem to be cell associated viruses. If very large volumes of plasma are transfused rapidly, citrate toxicity is possible, especially in infants and in patients with impaired liver function.

CRYOPRECIPITATE

When FFP is thawed at 4°C, a white cold-insoluble precipitate forms. This material, which is separated from the plasma and refrozen, is the product cryoprecipitate. One bag contains 80–120 units of VIII:C, 40–70% of von Willebrand's factor (vWF) and 20–30% of factor XIII present in the plasma, 150–250 mg of fibrinogen and about 55 mg fibronectin, all suspended in 10–20 ml of plasma.

Indications

The primary use of cryoprecipitate is to control bleeding associated with the deficiency or defect in one of the coagulation factors listed above (see Ch. 31). However, additional applications have been reported. Appropriate uses are as follows:

Haemophilia A

In patients with mild haemophilia A, who are rarely transfused, cryoprecipitate can be used provided DDAVP is not adequate treatment (see Ch. 31). This use of cryoprecipitate is being superseded by virus-inactivated factor VIII concentrates which probably have a lower risk of transmitting viruses.

Von Willebrand's disease

Von Willebrand's disease (vWD) results from a deficiency or abnormality in von Willebrand's factor (vWF), a high-molecular-weight, multimeric glycoprotein that promotes platelet adherence to subendothelium collagen and the formation of the platelet plug. vWF associates with factor VIII in the circulation and may help to stabilise it.

Cryoprecipitate or factor VIII concentrates are the component of choice for treating bleeding episodes in vWD. Patients require both vWF and factor VIII:C for haemostasis, and cryoprecipitate is a concentrate of both in a small usable volume. Some factor VIII concentrates may lose much of their vWF during processing and are not recommended. Cryoprecipitate dose depends on the clinical and laboratory severity of the disease and the nature and severity of the bleed: single doses of 1 bag/10 kg body weight have been found useful. Patient response should be followed clinically and with bleeding times. After cryoprecipitate infusions, vWF levels immediately rise as expected and decline with a half-life of 8–12 hours. The bleeding times may return to baseline values even before, perhaps because of preferential clearance of the larger, more effective vWF multimers.

Factor XIII deficiency

The long biological half-life of factor XIII, coupled with the very low levels required for haemostasis (2–3%) make bleeding episodes easy to treat. Factor XIII is stable in all plasma products, but is concentrated 4–6 times in cryoprecipitate. Doses of one bag of cryoprecipitate per 10–20 kg body weight infused every 3–4 weeks are recommended.

Factor XIII is also decreased in DIC and liver disease, but not sufficiently so to cause symptoms. A heat-treated factor XIII concentrate is available (see below) for treating congenitally deficient patients.

Fibrinogen deficiency

Normal fibrinogen levels are 2–4 g/l. Only 0.7–1 g/l are needed for haemostasis. Decreased levels are found in DIC, liver disease and congenital hypofibrinogenaemia. When these are associated with bleeding, cryoprecipitate should be used. Fibrinogen assays are helpful in calculating the appropriate dose, but to simplify ordering in emergency situations, 8 bags of cryoprecipitate (2 g of fibrinogen) should be given. Cryoprecipitate may also be used in dysfibrinogenaemia associated with liver disease.

Fibronectin deficiency

Fibronectin is a glycoprotein that is involved in cell-to-cell adhesion and helps to remove foreign matter and bacteria from blood by mediating their attachment to phagocytic cells, a process called opsonisation. Some studies show a beneficial effect of cryoprecipitate in patients with surgical trauma and infection, particularly those in septic shock, but this is, as yet, a controversial method of treatment.

Uraemic bleeding

A variety of haemostatic disorders is associated with uraemia. Dialysis has been used to reduce the frequency of bleeding. Platelet transfusions produce only temporary improvement. Neither therapy is uniformly effective. Cryoprecipitate has been used with apparent success. Bleeding times shortened within one to several hours and remained shortened for up to 24 hours.

Storage pool disease

Abnormal bleeding associated with storage pool disease has also been corrected with cryoprecipitate. The mechanism of action, as in uraemia, is unclear.

Compatibility testing

Cryoprecipitate is essentially free from red cells, but it commonly has a very small volume of plasma and therefore ABO antibodies. The plasma of products selected for transfusion should be compatible with the patient's red cells, particularly if the blood volume is small as in neonates. Compatibility testing is not normally done.

Dose calculation

Doses are calculated thus:

Cryo bags needed = total factor VIII units/80 units per bag where total factor VIII units needed = plasma volume × (% desired activity − % initial activity) and plasma volume = (kg body weight × 70 ml/kg)/ (1 − haematocrit).

Storage and handling

After preparation from fresh frozen plasma, cryoprecipitate is stored frozen at temperatures colder than −18°C. Immediately before use, it is thawed in a 37°C waterbath. Thawing occurs rapidly because of the small volume of the product. After thawing, cryoprecipitate may be stored at room temperature for up to 6 hours.

Administration

Cellular material from leukocytes, platelets and red cells, fibrin and amorphous material have been reported in cryoprecipitate. The product must therefore be transfused through a filter. Standard blood infusion sets with an in-line filter (170 μm) are most commonly used. Cryoprecipitate should be transfused as rapidly as the patient can tolerate.

Reactions

When ABO-incompatible cryoprecipitate is given, a weakly positive DAGT may develop, and with very high doses haemolysis may be seen. Febrile and allergic reactions are also possible. The incidence of disease transmission for each unit transfused is similar to that of fresh frozen plasma.

PLASMA DERIVATIVES

Large pools of donor plasma can be fractionated into more purified plasma protein products using the cold ethanol precipitation principle developed by Cohn. The starting product is usually FFP; a cryoprecipitate is separated first from which factor VIII and factor IX concentrates are produced prior to fractionation. This procedure uses the variables of ethanol and protein concentration, ionic strength, pH and temperature to separate three main products: albumin preparations, coagulation factors and immunoglobulins. The main objective is to recover all useful material from the plasma using methods such that techniques employed in the early stages are compatible with those that follow later.

These derivatives contain no cellular elements and are given without regard to ABO or Rh compatibility. No serological testing is done or documented on the patient prior to transfusion.

Albuminoid preparations

Although only 60% of the plasma protein content is albumin, it supplies 80% of the plasma's oncotic activity. It is usually available at either 4.5% or 20% concentration.

4.5% albumin and stable plasma protein solution (SPPS)

These products have a concentration which varies between manufacturers but the most common level is between 4 and 5% by weight (40–50 g/l protein). The salt concentration is usually slightly higher than in normal plasma, ranging from 130–160 mm/l sodium and 100–120 mm/l chloride. The potassium concentration is usually low (<2 mm/l). There is no significant calcium content and minimal citrate (except for SPPS). The manufacturers usually state the degree of purity of the product which is normally >96% albumin for the 5% product. The shelf-life is between 3 and 5 years at room temperature, but albumin should preferably be stored at 4°C. The volume may vary between manufacturers, but 100 ml and 500 ml sizes are commonly available. Because albumin is stored as a liquid, it is readily available for administration with the minimum delay and inconvenience (see Table 36.2).

Table 36.2 Albuminoid solutions

Volume	Variable but 100 ml and 500 ml sizes common
Storage	In liquid state at ambient temperature (5–25°C) for 3–5 years (depends on manufacturer)
Administration	Ready for immediate use No blood group restriction Can be supplemented with electrolytes (K^+ or Ca^{2+}) if required
Potential advantages	No hepatitis risk No fibrinogen or complement (inflammatory mediators) Minimal allergic reactions; 4–5% solution is essentially iso-osomotic and isotonic
Potential disadvantages	Expense (approx £1.50 per gram of albumin). No coagulation factors, immunoglobulins, trace plasma proteins (e.g. enzymes). 20–25% is hyperoncotic and may require dilution with saline. Occasional hypotensive (SPPS) or anaphylactoid (albumin) reactions

20–25% albumin

This is sometimes called 'salt-poor' albumin; it may or may not be genuinely low in Na^+ and/or Cl^- depending on the manufacturer. By and large, there is usually little difference between the electrolyte content of this product and 5% albumin, the only difference being the increased concentration of albumin to 200–250 g/l. The unit volume is usually 100 ml (giving the same total protein concentration as a 400 ml bottle of 4.5% albumin or SPPS). 20% albumin is hyperoncotic and should not be used for plasma exchange unless diluted to 4–5% with an electrolyte solution (Table 36.2).

Indications

Patients receiving 4.5% albumin should be both hypovolaemic and hypoproteinaemic because these products provide fast volume expansion and colloid replacement. The indications for 4.5% albumin solutions include:

1. Hypovolaemia following burns and occasionally after extensive surgery. In such circumstances enough SPPS should be given to maintain an albumin level of approximately 25–30 g/l. The recommended dose for children is 20–30 ml per kg body weight.
2. As a replacement fluid in plasma exchange, and sometimes for priming the pump in cardiopulmonary bypass operations.
3. It may be used initially in haemorrhagic shock whilst awaiting blood. In such instances it is of note that crystalloid solutions are as effective if given in adequate quantities (2–3 times the estimated volume loss). Some studies have shown that albumin solutions may be specifically harmful in the resuscitation of the shocked patient.

The indications for 20% albumin are essentially those where there is hypo-albuminaemia associated with severe peripheral oedema in patients who cannot tolerate the fluid load present in the PPS. It is therefore frequently used in hypoproteinaemic states associated with nephrotic syndrome and liver disease and it is also used as part of the regimes in total parenteral nutrition (TPN), although it must not be used on its own because of lack of some essential amino acids. Because 20% albumin is a hyperoncotic solution it has to be given slowly, particularly in patients who are at risk of circulatory overload and on no account is it to be given undiluted to patients with dehydration.

Administration

Blood administration sets are not needed for infusing albumin. Albumin products must never be allowed to mix with amino acid or protein solutions in the line, since this may cause the proteins to precipitate. 20% albumin must not be mixed with red cells because it is hypertonic.

Reactions

Adverse reactions to albumin products are rare, but allergic symptoms (flushing, urticaria, fever, etc.) have all been reported. Occasionally severe hypotensive episodes have been reported with rapid infusion. This has been attributed mostly to prekallikrein activators, which are precursors of bradykinin. Bradykinin is a potent hypotensive agent that is inactivated in the lungs. Such reactions therefore tend to be more common in situations such as cardiopulmonary surgery, where the lungs are bypassed.

To exclude any risk of transmission of hepatitis or other viral infection, the solution, with caprylate as a stabiliser, is pasteurised for 10 hours at 60°C after bottling. Albumin products have an excellent safety record and there have been no reported incidences of hepatitis or HIV transmission. This is related partly to the pasteurisation process and also to the fractionation process itself.

FACTOR VIII CONCENTRATES

Factor VIII:C can be purified from the cold insoluble fraction of pooled FFP, then lyophilised into a concentrated product that is easy to store and transfuse. Because of their availability, known unitage, ease of use and small volumes, concentrates have replaced cryoprecipitate as the product of choice to control bleeding in individuals with severe haemophilia. Factor VIII concentrates also contain some fibrinogen and vWF, but not enough to warrant their use for these factor deficiencies.

Indications (see Ch. 31)

1. Treatment or prevention of bleeding in patients with haemophilia A.
2. Treatment of bleeding in patients with factor VIII inhibitors.

Patients with antibodies may require very large doses of the concentrate until the antibody is no longer detectable. Simultaneously to treatment with factor VIII concentrates, plasma exchange may be used to 'wash out' the antibody. Alternatively, patients with inhibitors may be treated with porcine factor VIII, factor IX concentrates or with activated products that contain 'factor VIII bypassing activity'.

Calculating dosage

The amount of transfused factor VIII required depends on the nature of the bleeding episode and the severity of the initial deficiency. The same formula as for cryoprecipitate is used (q.v.). Factor VIII has a biological half-life of 8–14 hours.

Storage and handling

Lyophilised factor VIII is stored at 2–8°C for up to 2 years from the date of manufacture. It may, however, also be stored for up to 3 months at room temperature. Like other plasma derivatives stored in glass bottles, it should not be stored frozen. Reconstitution is carried out prior to administration with the addition of sterile pyrogen-free water. Several minutes should be allowed for complete dissolution to occur.

Administration

Factor VIII is given by slow intravenous infusion.

Reactions

Allergic reactions occur infrequently and usually disappear shortly after the infusion is stopped. Because anti-A and anti-B are present in the concentrates, a positive DAT may develop post-infusion and very rarely florid haemolysis may follow large doses.

Factor VIII concentrates currently available are heat or chemically treated. This process is undertaken in an effort to reduce the incidence of viral disease transmission. Heat treatment appears completely to inactivate HIV 1 and may be effective in inactivating non-A non-B hepatitis virus/es also known more recently as hepatitis C.

FACTOR IX CONCENTRATES

These are separated from pooled plasma, lyophilised and bottled into a product similar to factor VIII concentrates.

Non-activated prothrombin complex concentrates (PCC)

Concentrates of the four factors of the prothrombin complex have been available for some time. More recently, several techniques have been developed using ion exchange chromatography to purify factors II, IX and X. Unlike factor VIII, factor IX recovery in vivo is far below expected values.

Activated PCC

Activated factor IX concentrates (e.g. Feiba-Immuno) are derived from the standard factor IX preparations and contain partially activated factors IX, II and X. They are used solely for the therapy of bleeding episodes in patients with factor VIII antibodies.

Indications

The main indications for *non-activated* PCC are:

1. Treatment or prevention of bleeding in Christmas disease.
2. Treatment or prevention of coagulopathy bleeding, caused by severe liver disease or oral anticoagulant overdose, when the patient is unable to tolerate the necessary volume of fresh frozen plasma.
3. Treatment of bleeding in patients with factor VIII antibodies. Both activated and non-activated products have been used in such instances and seem to be equally effective in most patients.

Storage and handling

Factor IX concentrates may be stored for up to 2 years' at 2–8°C, although room temperature storage for up to 1 month is possible without deterioration. Reconstitution of the freeze-dried material is as for factor VIII.

Administration

Factor IX is administered by intravenous injection. As the biological half-life is 18–24 hours, repeat injections are required less frequently than with factor VIII.

Reactions

Rapid infusion rates of PCC have been associated with flushing, tachycardia and hypotension, presumably from the presence of vaso-active substances. These symptoms may disappear quickly when the infusion rate is slowed. Factor IX concentrates carry the same risk of disease transmission as factor VIII and the products available today are all chemical or heat-treated.

Another complication of PCC is the development of serious thrombo-embolic episodes and/or DIC. This may be related to the presence of activated factors or to the presence of platelet activation products in the concentrate. Neonates, patients with liver disease and haemophilia patients receiving large, repetitive doses of PCC are especially vulnerable to these problems. The majority of factor IX concentrates contain small quantities of heparin or AT III to minimise this risk.

Myocardial infarctions have also been reported as a rare complication. It has been proposed that the release of bradykinins following large repetitive doses leads to vascular leakage and myocardial damage.

OTHER FACTOR CONCENTRATES

Factor XIII concentrate

A heat-treated factor XIII concentrate is available for treating congenitally deficient patients.

Factor VII concentrates

These are also available. They are, however, as yet un-licensed in the UK and are only available on a named patient basis. The product is heat-treated but its disease transmission risk (particularly for hepatitis) has not yet been thoroughly evaluated.

Antithrombin III concentrate

This is used for treating thrombotic episodes in patients with congenital antithrombin III deficiency. The suggested dose is 50 u/kg and the infusion should be repeated at 12 or 24 hour intervals. No untoward effects of antithrombin III were noted in a small group of patients treated.

HUMAN IMMUNOGLOBULIN PREPARATIONS

Immunoglobulin preparations are a concentrated solution of gamma globulin made from large pools of human normal plasma. Human normal immunoglobulin (HNI) contains a mixture of immunoglobulins present in the healthy adult population, e.g. antibodies against poliomyelitis, measles, diphtheria, hepatitis, etc., in a concentration that is normally ten times that of the starting pool. When donors with high titre antibodies to a specific disease or vaccine are used in the pool, a hyper-immune product is produced. By comparison with normal immuoglobulins these must have a significantly higher level of antibody against at least one antigen. Because IgG aggregates, and fragments that form during the manufacturing process are capable of activating complement and the kallikrein system and producing anaphylactic shock if given intravenously, standard HNI solutions must be given intramuscularly (see under reactions).

Recently, several techniques have been used to remove IgG aggregates from immunoglobulin preparations and such products can then be given intravenously.

Human normal immunoglobulin (HNI)

This product has been used uncritically in the past. Its main use is in people who are about to travel to areas where hepatitis A is common, although travellers adhering to normal tourist routes may be at no greater risk of exposure than at home. The immunoglobulin gives temporary passive protection and a further dose (1 vial containing 250 mg) may be given after 2–3 months if the patient is staying abroad or travels repeatedly.

For post-exposure prophylaxis to hepatitis A the value of HNI is greatest when given early in the incubation period. It should be given as soon as possible after exposure and is not recommended beyond 2 weeks after exposure. Prophylaxis should be offered to close personal contacts, at schools, and particularly in custodial institutions and hospitals.

HNI may give some protection against icteric non-A non-B hepatitis and it should be considered for protection following needle-stick exposures involving clinical cases of non-A non-B hepatitis.

Replacement therapy with normal immunoglobulin in patients with antibody deficiency syndromes

Replacement may also be required for rare patients with hypogammaglobulinaemia or selective deficiencies of IgG subclasses associated with recurrent infections. When the mainstay of therapy was the intramuscular route, the aim was to maintain an IgG level of about 2 g/l with a dose of 25 mg/kg/week. With the intravenous route it is possible to maintain IgG levels approaching the normal range, i.e. 5 g/l. A dose of 150–300 mg/kg at 3–4-weekly intervals affords better protection against infection than the intramuscular route. It is important to note that the i.v. product is quite distinct from the standard i.m. product and the two must not be interchanged.

During acute infections, immunoglobulin levels usually fall, due either to increased catabolism or secretory loss. The frequency of immunoglobulin administration should be increased: this maintains levels more effectively than increasing the individual dose.

Treatment of idiopathic thrombocytopenic purpura

This use of immunoglobulin represents the application of a new therapeutic principle which has relevance beyond the relatively rare condition of ITP. Recent reports have indicated that in children, and to a lesser extent in adults, the intravenous infusion of high dose immunoglobulin (400 mg/kg daily for 5 days) can provoke a predictable rise in platelet count lasting for days, weeks or even months (see Ch. 30).

It is not known why infused IgG exerts this effect, although it is known that the Fc portion is necessary and reticulo-endothelial blockade may play an important role. The place of this treatment in ITP remains to be defined and its value may be for the control of acute bleeding, for the preparation of steroid-resistant patients for surgery and possibly for chronic ITP.

The effect of high dose IgG may play a role in other autoimmune disorders such as autoimmune haemolytic anaemia or autoimmune neutropenia but further studies are necessary to elucidate this effect.

Storage and handling

Immunoglobulins may be stored at 2–8°C for up to 3 years, depending on the specific product. Freezing may further aggregate IgG molecules and therefore vials must never be frozen.

Administration

Great care must be taken to administer the product by its correct route: standard immunoglobulin must be given intramuscularly, *never* intravenously. Intravenous immunoglobulin should be given at a controlled rate with the infusion rates commencing slowly at 0.01–0.02 ml/kg/min for the first 30 minutes. If no problems occur, the rate may be doubled. The patient should be monitored carefully throughout the infusion and first-line resuscitation equipment, including adrenaline, should be readily available, in case acute anaphylactic reactions develop.

Reactions

The most common reaction to intramuscular immunoglobulin is local tenderness and muscle stiffness at the site of injection. Systemic reactions have occasionally been reported.

Reactions from intravenous products are usually mild and rate-dependent. The most common symptoms are headache, followed by nausea, vomiting and fever.

True anaphylactic reactions are rare and are often associated with a history of severe reactions to other plasma products. Reactions tend to be more common in patients with hereditary hypogammaglobulinaemia to the first few infusions of intravenous immunoglobulin. This is thought to be partly due to immune complexes being formed between the immunoglobulin and bacterial antigens in the recipient.

There does not appear to be any risk of hepatitis and HIV transmission in the intramuscular preparations, even though these products are not heat-treated. Viral elimination seems to be related to the high concentration of antibodies in the products and to the fractionation process itself. Transmission of non-A non-B hepatitis has been reported with various intravenous immunoglobulin preparations that include several different virucidal steps e.g. gel filtration or pH 4/pepsin treatment, in their preparation.

SPECIFIC IMMUNOGLOBULINS

Hepatitis B

Post-exposure prophylaxis

Needle-sticks, damaged skin and mucous membrane exposures are all situations which require prompt decisions about the need for immunoglobulin. The action to be taken is shown in Table 36.3.

Table 36.3 Immunoglobulin prophylaxis for known or suspected acute exposure to hepatitis B

Source of possible infected material	Prophylaxis recommended
Known HBsAg-positive	HBsIg given immediately and first dose of HBV vaccine (at different site)
HBsAg status not known but source is available	
– check HBsAg :	Dose of HBsIg given immediately whilst awaiting results
– if positive :	Commence vaccination
– if negative :	No further action
Source unknown and HBsAg status unknown :	Dose of HBsIg

Materno-fetal transmission

Infants of mothers who are HBsAg-and in particular HBeAg-positive, have a high risk of being infected in the first few weeks of their life, and most of them will become chronic carriers. The common recommendation is to give the newborn immediately (without waiting for the hepatitis results) at birth a single dose of 25–50 iu/kg, followed by a full course of active immunisation.

Regular sexual contacts of carriers and cases of hepatitis B

Active immunisation should be given to contacts who do not possess antibodies (anti-HBs and anti-HBe). If the sexual contact is an isolated incident, the individual at risk should receive anti-HBs immunoglobulin as soon as possible after the exposure.

Varicella (zoster)

Varicella is a severe disease in immunologically compromised individuals. Immunoglobulins containing high levels of antibody to *Varicella zoster* virus are available. The mechanism of protective action of these antibodies is not known, but almost certainly involves the interaction of antibody with the host's effector cells in the attack of the virus-infected cells.

Prophylaxis

Zoster immunoglobulin is used mainly for the passive immunisation of susceptible immunodeficient children and neonates after significant exposure to chickenpox or zoster (Table 36.4).

Table 36.4 Guidelines for the use of varicella zoster immune globulin in the prophylaxis of chickenpox

The following conditions must be satisfied:

1. Underlying condition of recipient:
   (a) Immunosuppressed
   or (b) Infant born to mother who had the onset of chickenpox less than 5 days before delivery or within 48 hours after delivery.
2. Exposure to chickenpox:
   very close, e.g. household, newborn, playschool, etc.
3. No history of chickenpox in the recipient.
4. Younger age group (normally less than 15 years old).
5. Immunoglobulin **must** be given within **96 hours** of exposure.

Individuals older than 15 years are relatively rarely at risk of infection and zoster immunoglobulin is not recommended for routine prophylaxis in non-immunodeficient patients, since the disease is not severe. Pregnant women should not receive zoster immunoglobulin in early pregnancy for post-exposure prophylaxis, as there is no evidence that it prevents fetal infection. It may, however, be indicated in late pregnancy in mothers who have a definite exposure and have no evidence of pre-existing exposure.

Treatment

There is no evidence at present indicating that *Varicella zoster* immunoglobulin plays any role in preventing the dissemination of early infection in immunocompromised hosts.

Measles

Measles may be a severe illness in young infants, and especially in immunocompromised children. In unvaccinated normal infants exposed to measles, especially those under 1 year (when risk of complication is highest), anti-measles immunoglobulin may be given. Exposed immunosuppressed children should be given a dose as soon as possible after exposure.

Rabies

Passive immunisation is of particular value in rabies, be-cause the exact time, source and nature of exposure can usually be identified and there is a long incubation period with persistence of virus in the wound for many days. Human rabies immunoglobulin is available and it should only be given only in association with active rabies vaccination.

Prophylaxis

Human rabies immunoglobulin (20 iu/kg) should be given intramuscularly and by local infiltration round the wound for bites where rabies is considered to be a risk.

Rubella

Immunoglobulin prophylaxis has a very limited role in the prevention of congenital rubella. Maternal infection can lead to serious fetal damage, especially infection occurring during the first trimester. Prevention of maternal viraemia is essential if risk to the fetus is to be avoided.

Prophylaxis

Attempted post-exposure prophylaxis should be strictly limited to non-immunised pregnant women who are exposed to rubella and in whom therapeutic abortion is excluded for any reason. Blood should be taken for rubella antibody assay as soon as possible after exposure, and rubella immunoglobulin given immediately without waiting for the antibody assay results. If the woman is found to be seropositive, she should be reassured immediately that there is no risk. If the initial sample is seronegative, further antibody assays should be done at monthly intervals. A persistent negative rubella IgM antibody indicates successful prophylaxis.

Vaccinia

This is not routinely available, and would only be required in the event of accidental exposure to smallpox virus held in research establishments, or if vaccination is essential in at-risk individuals (see below).

Prophylaxis

Anti-vaccinia immunoglobulin (VIG) should be administered to contacts of smallpox cases 12–24 hours after vaccination, to provide immediate protection while active immunity develops. Eczematous children exposed to smallpox vaccine should be given VIG. It is also indicated with vaccination when the latter is unavoidable but the patient is pregnant or immunosuppressed.

Treatment

For eczema vaccination, generalised vaccinia or localised infections that endanger the eye, VIG should be given.

Cytomegalovirus

Cytomegalovirus (CMV) causes severe infection in immunosuppressed patients and the virus itself also has a profound effect on the host's immune response. CMV is isolated from many patients with fatal interstitial pneumonia after bone marrow transplantation and it is also a cause of death or graft rejection after renal transplants. Infection may result from reactivation of latent infection, reinfection with a different strain or from primary infection.

Passively administered anti-CMV may protect against CMV infection following bone marrow transplantation particularly in patients who have not received granulocyte transfusions.

No firm recommendations on the use of CMV immunoglobulin can yet be given. It is likely that high dose CMV immunoglobulin may prove effective in preventing CMV infection in seronegative immunocompromised patients, where CMV seronegative blood products or organs cannot be supplied.

Tetanus

Prophylaxis

Wounds considered to carry a high risk of tetanus (penetrating, dirty wounds), particularly those present for more than 6 hours before debridement, require protection with anti-tetanus immunoglobulin (250 iu) in patients who are not known to have had previous tetanus toxoid immunisation. Tetanus toxoid should be given at a different site.

Treatment

In established tetanus, large doses (5000–10 000 iu) of anti-tetanus immunoglobulin should be given to bind circulating toxin.

Anti-D immunoglobulin

For most clinical purposes, people may be considered simply as Rh(D) negative or Rh(D) positive, i.e. possessing the D antigen. The administration of D-positive cells to a D-negative individual induces the production of anti-D in a high proportion of cases. The most common cause of this immunisation is a feto-maternal bleed which may occur at any time during pregnancy, especially if bleeding occurs (placenta praevia) or if there is any intervention (amniocentesis, external cephalic version). The principal hazard of anti-D antibodies in women of child-bearing age is the serious risk of haemolytic disease of the newborn (HDN). Anti-D, if given early enough (within 72 hours) following a sensitising episode, has been shown to effectively suppress the antibody response. The practical aspects of anti-D administration are summarised in Table 36.5.

Table 36.5 Prevention of HDN due to anti-D: use of anti-D immunoglobulin

Indication	Dose of anti-D
1. D-positive infant born to D-neg mother	500 iu i.m. within 48 hours
2. Termination of pregnancy or miscarriage	
Before 20 weeks	250 iu
After 20 weeks	500 iu
3. Amniocentesis, version or other possible sensitising episodes*	As per termination
4. Antenatal (depends on local policy)	500 iu at 28 and 34 weeks
All Rh negative women	

Infant's D status should be determined on delivery. Mother's D and anti-D status should be determined during pregnancy or, failing this, immediately after delivery. Fetal cell count in mother's blood should be done to determine if further doses of anti-D are indicated.

*Following procedures done later than 20 weeks, fetal cell count should be assessed: further doses may be needed (100 iu = 1 ml feto-maternal bleed).

BIBLIOGRAPHY

American Association of Blood Banks 1985 Technical manual, 9th edn. Arlington, Va.
Bayer W L 1984 Blood transfusion and blood banking. Clinics in haematology 13(1) Saunders, London
Cash J D 1987 Progress in transfusion medicine. Vols 1 & 2. Churchill Livingstone, Edinburgh
Dacie J V, Lewis S M 1984 Practical haematology, 6th edn. Churchill Livingstone, Edinburgh

Mollison P L, Engelfriet C P, Contreras M 1987 Blood transfusion in clinical medicine, 8th edn. Blackwell, Oxford
Napier J A F Blood transfusion therapy: a problem orientated approach. John Wiley, Chichester
Petz L D, Swisher S M 1981 Clinical practice of blood transfusion. Churchill Livingstone, Edinburgh

37. Blood transfusion in the neonate

E. A. Letsky

All newborn infants, whether term or premature, are more likely to be transfused than any other group of hospitalised individuals. In the majority of instances the need for transfusion in the premature infant arises from the loss of blood withdrawn for laboratory testing. The average daily blood loss per infant in a newborn intensive care unit in the United States has been estimated to be in excess of 3.0 ml/kg. The indications for transfusion and the blood banking procedures to provide for the needs of sick neonates present unique problems for the physicians and blood transfusion serologists providing a service for the nursery. There have been no firm guidelines which have been generally adopted, largely because the regulation of erythropoiesis in the perinatal period is more complex than at any other time in life (see above) and transfusion policy for the anaemia of prematurity depends largely on how the clinician views this condition. Some believe that the fall in haemoglobin is a purely temporary physiological process that should never be interfered with and they emphasise the known hazards of transfusion. In addition, too much oxygen is known to do harm in the neonate and may cause retrolental fibroplasia and bronchopulmonary dysplasia. Raising the haemoglobin may prolong the suppression of marrow erythropoietin activity and delay its reactivation. On the other hand, the anaemia of prematurity has become greatly exaggerated in recent years by improved survival of very small infants and they have been shown to benefit from transfusions in terms of general activity and weight gain.

The following discussion is an attempt to outline the indications for transfusion in the premature infant, to clarify the real risks of transfusion and to suggest the optimal utilisation of blood and blood products which will give maximum efficiency with least risk to the neonate.

Indications

The definition of true anaemia depends on the delivery of oxygen to the tissues, which in turn depends not solely on the level of haemoglobin but on cardiopulmonary function, the oxygen dissociation curve and the ability of the infant to adjust central venous tension in a compensatory fashion. The lack of firm guidelines as to indications for the need for transfusion results largely from the inability to measure all the parameters determining oxygen availability and the need for oxygen in the premature infant.

When considering the need for transfusion it is essential to compare the level of haemoglobin with the expected level in a premature infant of similar birthweight and age.

Haemoglobin levels fall by 1 g/dl per week on average from the second to eighth week of life. A haemoglobin of 8.5 g/dl in an otherwise healthy premature infant at 7 weeks may be within the normal range, but it would obviously be grossly abnormal in an infant of 2–3 weeks of age. Indeed the haemoglobin may fall naturally within the first weeks of life to 7.0 g/dl and in an otherwise healthy premature infant this should cause no concern.

It should be remembered that a blood transfusion given solely on the basis of haemoglobin concentration is likely to be one of a series. The first transfusion will increase the concentration of HbA, shift the oxygen dissociation curve, and lower the oxygen affinity of the circulating haemoglobin. This will then depress red cell production and the haemoglobin will fall to a lower level before erythropoiesis is reactivated.

A very important indication of the need for transfusion is a failure to achieve the expected daily weight gain. This is due to an increase in metabolic needs arising from an increase in oxygen consumption which appears to be an early response to anaemia. It has been shown that regular transfusion in the premature infant will result in improved weight gain in those babes who are lagging behind the expected average.

It has also been shown that clinical anaemia can be associated with haemoglobins as high as 10.5 g/dl, emphasising again that the haemoglobin level taken alone is no indication for giving or withholding transfusion in the premature infant.

Until more precise guidelines are available concerning the expression of true anaemia in the premature infant, the physician caring for infants will have to make decisions based on clinical judgments about the need for blood transfusions. Certain simple measures should be instituted which will avoid unnecessary blood administration and result in essential transfusions only being given. These include the following:

1. All blood taken from the babe should be carefully recorded, and if 5–10% of the babe's blood volume should be removed over a short space of time, it should be replaced with packed red cells.
2. The haemoglobin should be measured on entry to the nursery and at regular, minimum weekly, intervals thereafter; the haemoglobin will drop 1 g/dl (on average) per week. Do not transfuse on level of haemoglobin alone. Although haemoglobin values of 7.0 g/dl or less require explanation, they may not need correction.
3. Evaluate:

   (a) Weight gain
   (b) Fatigue while feeding
   (c) Tachypnoea and tachycardia
   (d) Hypoxia – reflected in elevated levels of lactic and pyruvic acid.

4. Infants with cardiac or pulmonary disease reducing arterial oxygen saturation may need to have the haemoglobin maintained in the range of 16–17 g/dl to ensure sufficient differential between arterial and venous oxygen tension.

COMPLICATIONS OF BLOOD TRANSFUSION IN THE PREMATURE NEONATE

In principle, all of the hazards associated with blood transfusion apply to the newborn but in addition there are special complications and risks which arise from the unique blood-banking needs in the nursery created by the small size of the recipient and the special vulnerability, because of the neonate's immaturity, to transfusion of infections and metabolic disturbances.

Metabolic problems

On storage of blood in the anticoagulant citrate phosphate dextrose (CPD) the pH will fall in the first week from 7.0 to 6.8 and to 6.7 on 3 weeks' storage. The serum potassium level may reach 10 mmol/l by the end of the first week, but the 2,3-DPG levels are maintained

during this time. The adult recipient can quickly adjust these adverse metabolic changes on storage of blood which the immature neonate may find a problem. Massive transfusions, e.g. exchange transfusions, can result in systemic acidosis followed by a rebound alkalosis as excess CO_2 is expired quickly. Occasionally, citrate binding results in symptomatic hypocalcaemia and hypomagnesaemia. Another complication seen after exchange transfusion is hyperglycaemia followed by rebound hypoglycaemia. A further potential source of difficulty is the fact that the serum sodium of CPD stored blood is elevated. Because of these problems with CPD anticoagulation in the newborn, the use of heparin has been advocated, since it does not result in any of these adverse metabolic changes. The major disadvantage is that it has a limited effect as an anticoagulant and in the United Kingdom blood taken into heparin has to be used within 12 hours of donation. This necessitates tests for hepatitis and HIV and for processing the blood being carried out on the donor before the blood is taken. It also results, inevitably, in much wastage of blood. Now that most blood banks make components from a unit of blood, red cells, platelets, fresh frozen plasma, coagulant factor concentrates, etc., they are not enthusiastic about the preparation of heparinised fresh blood which cannot be used for the preparation of component therapy. Therefore, they encourage the use of CPD blood within 24–72 hours of donation when the metabolic changes are at a minimum and the blood has been safely screened for hepatitis B surface antigen, syphylis, CMV, HIV and the group checked before release from the centre.

Necrotising enterocolitis

The exact aetiology of necrotising enterocolitis (NEC) is not defined as yet, but many now believe that the pathogenesis depends on the interaction of three factors:

1. Disturbed intestinal mucosal integrity.

2. Presence of pathogenic bacteria.

3. Availability of substrate to promote growth of bacteria – enteral feeding.

Damage to the intestinal mucosa may be caused by a variety of events and procedures which occur regularly in the intensive care nursery. These include asphyxia, shock, umbilical vessel catheterisation and exchange transfusion. The association of neonatal intestinal perforation and NEC with exchange transfusion was first reported from a number of independent centres in the United Kingdom in the late 1960s. Many argue that this association was a chance one concomitant with more aggressive and successful intensive care in the premature infant, but others have suggested that the explanation may lie in the increased use of plastic perfusion equipment and the widespread adoption at this time of pre-packed gamma-irradiated polyvinyl-chloride (PVC) exchange-transfusion kits in place of the rubber, glass and metal sets.

The plasticisers used in the treatment of PVC bags and catheters can be leached out and do accumulate in the blood during storage. The phthalate ester diethyl-hexyl phthalate (DEHP) may have toxic effects in the neonate. Perfused human umbilical arteries lose physiologic responsiveness after perfusion using PVC apparatus. These responses can be restored after a return to the use of glass and silicon and rubber tubing. DEHP has also been shown to inhibit mitosis and growth of lymphocytes in vitro. There are at least two ways in which the use of PVC catheters during exchange may lead to NEC and intestinal perforations.

1. The leached toxic substances could lead to direct chemical necrosis of the mucosa.
2. The toxic substances may affect the responses of the portal vasculature, exposing it to insults during the exchange.

Attempts to bring these possible potential dangers of the use of PVC catheters in the neonate to the attention of the medical profession at large and the paediatrician in particular have not met with much response.

As nothing seems to have been done in terms of regulation controls of PVC equipment for the neonate, paediatricians should be alert for the possible complications and avoid precipitating factors as far as possible.

Transmission of infection

Post-transfusion hepatitis is probably the most common and serious of all the problems associated with the transfusion of blood and blood products. In the neonate the risk is increased for a chronic carrier state and although blood can be fairly efficiently screened for hepatitis B, the increasing problem of 'non-A non-B' transfusion-transmitted hepatitis remains.

Cytomegalovirus infection

It is known that massive transfusion of blood to an adult immune-suppressed patient may result in infection with a variety of microbiological agents which would normally have little or no effect. Among these is cytomegalovirus, which is widespread in nature. In fact,

approximately 60% of all blood donors are CMV-antibody positive. Unfortunately, this does not necessarily mean that their blood confers passive immunity. Some carry live virus in their white cells which can be reactivated in a suitable milieu. In fact, congenital cytomegalovirus infection has been reported in more than 3% of the offspring of sero-immune women, but it would appear that infants born to CMV-negative mothers are more prone to morbidity induced by neonatal CMV infections. In the healthy immunocompetent child or adult, post-transfusion CMV infection results in sero-conversion with little or no morbidity – and possibly a transient atypical mononuclear cell syndrome.

In contrast, CMV infection in an immuno-incompetent individual, such as patients with malignant disease, transplant patients and premature newborns, may be associated with significant morbidity and even mortality.

Recently there has been an attempt to reduce the potential infectivity of donor blood from some blood banks in special situations, but blood transfusion is only one of many sources of CMV infection in the nursery and other environmental factors must also be taken into consideration.

The ways in which the infectivity of donor blood can be cut down is by selecting CMV-negative donors or by transfusing frozen or leukocyte-depleted red cells. It would appear that it is difficult to identify the potentially dangerous carrier of live virus within the 60% of donors who are antibody-positive; therefore they all have to be rejected if transfusion transmission is to be avoided. However, blood which has been stored at 4°C for 48 hours is much less likely to transmit CMV infection than fresh blood, even if there is live virus in the blood when collected from the donor.

Problems associated with provision of small aliquots of blood

Unique difficulties for the blood transfusion service are created because procedures must be developed to provide unusually small quantities of reasonably fresh blood for transfusion to term and preterm infants, with minimum wastage. Volumes of blood required in the nursery, other than for exchange transfusion, vary between 20 and 100 ml per transfusion. If the usual single unit of 450 ml of freshly donated blood is used for top-up transfusions, then more than three-quarters will be wasted for each transfusion given. In the United Kingdom, many large blood transfusion centres still do not provide smaller sub-units suitable for transfusion to infants.

EXCHANGE TRANSFUSION IN THE NEONATE

In recent years the exchange transfusion rate for hyperbilirubinaemia has fallen dramatically. This depends in part on the following three factors:

1. Although haemolytic disease of the newborn may occur in any situation where a baby carries paternally-derived blood group antigens which the mother lacks, the vast majority of really severe cases were due, in the past, to anti-D antibodies and the number of severely sensitised mothers has fallen dramatically following the introduction of prophylaxis.
2. Successful intra-uterine corrections of anaemia are now carried out prior to delivery in utero with red cells unaffected by the mother's immune antibody.
3. Post-delivery we have learnt to use other optimal methods of preventing kernicterus, such as intensive phototherapy.

In the United States exchange transfusions are carried out frequently in supportive care for babes with the RDS, the principle being that the decreased oxygen affinity of cells containing adult haemoglobin will aid oxygenation of tissues. In the United Kingdom most neonatologists are sceptical about the value of this therapy and conscious of the risks, and they prefer to give small top-up transfusions with adult blood, maintaining a haemoglobin concentration of above 12.5 g/dl at all times.

Complications associated with exchange transfusions

Mortality rate from blood component therapy in the neonate is very low and most transfusion-related deaths are associated with exchange transfusion.

Metabolic

A variety of metabolic complications have been reported to occur during transfusion and in the post-transfusion period.

Hypoglycaemia

This can occur following exchange because the high glucose load in the transfusions stimulates insulin secretion causing rebound hypoglycaemia. This reactive hypoglycaemia is exaggerated in preterm infants who are hypoglycaemic to start with.

Hyperkalaemia

Hyperkalaemia following exchange transfusion has been reported to cause cardiac arrhythmia. However, the contribution of plasma potassium in this situation is probably negligible. The plasma of blood stored for up to 7 days contains less than 3 mg of potassium. Hyperkalaemia may be produced by the infusion of non-viable cells. For this reason, in the United Kingdom, blood stored for less than 5 days is provided for exchange transfusion and usually within 72 hours of donation. Other factors may influence the plasma level of potassium during an exchange transfusion, such as the presence of metabolic alkalosis. It is also possible that stored red cells which are deficient in potassium may absorb potassium from the recipient plasma, thus causing hypokalaemia – a recognised consequence of massive blood transfusion in the adult.

Hypocalcaemia

This may be associated with exchange transfusion but there is good evidence that the neuromuscular effects of citrate are not caused by hypocalcaemia alone. Routine administration of calcium during exchange has led to hypercalcaemia and alkalosis post-transfusion in term infants. On the other hand preterm infants may require calcium administration during the course of an exchange transfusion.

Cardiac and vascular complications

Careful monitoring of input and output during exchange is mandatory to avoid acute hypervolaemia. Small aliquots of 5–10 ml should be used. The haematocrit of the transfused blood should be adjusted to be no greater than 50% to avoid hyperviscosity. Thrombosis of the portal vein may occur as a result of cannulation and can progress to result in portal hypertension and varices appearing within the second year of life.

Air embolism has been reported during the course of exchange transfusion, caused by negative pressure occurring in the umbilical vein, resulting in air entering the exchange transfusion system. Exchange transfusion through the umbilical artery has resulted in spasm of that vessel, causing ischaemia of the lumbar spinal cord, leading to paralysis of the lower extremeties. An alternative to the umbilical vein is the radial artery as outflow and peripheral vein as inflow. The umbilical artery should only be used as a last resort. Hypothermia as a result of not warming the blood properly may result in lethal cardiac arrhythmia.

Haemostatic complications

Thombocytopenia and coagulation factor deficiency may complicate exchange transfusion. Stored blood will lack viable platelets and the labile clotting factors V and VIII. In addition, the newborn has deficiency of the vitamin K-dependent coagulation factors due to immaturity of the liver.

Red cell injury

Non-immunologically-mediated haemolysis is the usual cause of what appears to be a haemolytic transfusion reaction in the neonate. This may be caused by forcing red cells through a fine bore needle or catheter or by excessive heating in a blood warmer. Rarely a true haemolytic transfusion reaction occurs, and when it does it invariably results from a clerical error.

Allo-immunisation to red blood cell and white cell antigens

Recent studies have shown that neonates do not readily form allo-antibodies to either red cell or white cell antigens. It has been suggested that it is probably not necessary to continue red cell cross-matching for neonatal transfusion as this does not result in red cell allo-immunisation. The cross-match is, however, a safeguard in recipient identification as long as rigorous adherence to established procedures is observed.

Graft-versus-host disease (GVHD)

GVHD has been described subsequent to red cell transfusion, plasma exchange and intra-uterine transfusion. In the neonate the clinical picture is one of skin rash, hepatitis and marrow aplasia. GVHD may be an important cause of death following exchange transfusion and can be prevented by irradiation of blood prior to infusion into immunocompromised patients or preterm infants. Although there has been an increased frequency of reports in recent years, GVHD is a rare entity and routine irradiation of blood for simple transfusion to neonates is not indicated, although a case can be made for irradiation of blood products for exchange transfusion.

AIDS AND THE NEONATE

Transmission of HIV

There are only two modes of transmission of HIV infection so far documented in the neonate:

1. Parenteral contact with blood and blood products.

2. Vertical transmission from an infected mother to her infant.

Blood and blood products

The first reported case of neonatally acquired AIDS came from California in 1982. A 20-months-old white boy, born preterm, who had received multiple top-up transfusions in the Special Care Baby Unit developed hepatosplenomegaly, neutropenia, autoimmune haemolytic anaemia, thrombocytopenia, in vitro evidence of T-cell dysfunction and opportunistic infection. One of the donors was a homosexual man who, although symptom-free at the time, subsequently developed AIDS and died.

As outlined below the chance of HIV transmission in blood transfusion is extremely remote.

Vertical transmission

The presence of transplacentally acquired maternal HIV antibody in infants under 15 months of age limits the use of antibody detection tests as evidence of HIV infection in the neonate.

The expense and difficulty of standardising retrovirus cultures make this method impractical for identifying the virus in blood or tissue. Recently developed antigen-detection methods may overcome this difficulty.

Confirmation of HIV infection in the neonate must include clinical signs and symptoms of infection, results of laboratory tests for detection of virus in blood or tissues and any immunological abnormalities. In many cases it is obvious that it may only be possible to identify the newborn infant at risk and positive proof of infection will only be confirmed if the HIV antibody, present at birth, remains positive beyond 15 months of age.

An infant born to a seropositive mother is considered infected if:

1. Virus is detected in blood or tissue – not possible in all centres.
2. There is evidence of reliably diagnosed disease indicative of underlying cellular immunodeficiency, with exclusion of primary immunodeficiency syndromes such as SCID, Wiscott-Aldrich syndrome, ataxia telangiectasia, Di Georgio syndrome, etc.
3. There is persistent reliable HIV antibody detection together with abnormal immune responses.

For practical purposes, in most centres it is not usually possible to be absolutely certain of active infection until some months of life have been negotiated. In the first 4 weeks of life (the defined neonatal period) it is usual only to identify the baby who is potentially at risk by finding a positive HIV antibody test in the baby born to a seropositive mother.

BIBLIOGRAPHY

Alter B P 1979 Perinatal Hematology. Churchill
  Livingstone, Edinburgh
Bove J R 1986 Transfusion transmitted diseases: current
  problems and challenges. Progress in Haematology
  14: 123–147

Isherwood D M, Fletcher K A 1985 Neonatal jaundice:
  investigation and monitoring. Annals of Clinical
  Biochemistry 22: 109–128

38. Adverse effects of transfusion

S. J. Urbaniak

Table 38.1 Adverse effects of transfusion

Symptoms reported			
Chills	– 55%	Nausea and vomiting	– 7%
Fever	– 47%	Lumbar pain	– 5%
Urticaria	– 35%	Red urine	
Tachycardia	– 28%	(haemoglobinuria)	– 5%
Chest tightness	– 7%	Hypotension	– 2%
Breathlessness	– 7%	Jaundice (delayed)	– 1%

NB None of these symptoms alone is pathognomonic of a true haemolytic reaction

Transfusion of blood or blood products is not uncommonly associated with adverse reactions (Table 38.1). As many as 5% of transfusion recipients react in some way to transfusion. Whilst the majority of these reactions are not preventable (in advance), they are mild and not life-threatening.

The difficulty facing the clinician is deciding whether or not the symptoms and signs observed are due to one of the milder types of reaction or the beginning of a severe reaction. Furthermore, most of the symptoms reported are not specific to transfusion per se and may equally be due to the underlying condition of the patient, or other operative procedures.

A further complication is that many transfusions are given peri-operatively when the patient may be anaesthetised, or not able to report symptoms; accurate observation and interpretation of clinical signs become even more important under these circumstances.

The average clinician equates transfusion with the infusion of red blood cells in one form or another, which numerically, form the greatest number of transfusion events. Other blood products or plasma derivatives are not without their own hazards (see Ch. 36), particularly transmission of viral disease and anaphylactic reactions, but the clinical consequences of the acute haemolytic transfusion reaction (HTR) are life-threatening, and constitute an acute medical emergency which must be managed promptly and appropriately. The pre-transfusion testing, administrative check procedures and bedside observations are designed primarily to prevent acute HTR, and to aid rapid diagnosis if it does occur.

It is also not often appreciated by clinicians that there are a number of delayed adverse effects which present some time after the transfusion event, but affect the patient in such a way that the original clinician is not faced with the clinical consequences of the decision to transfuse (e.g. non-A, non-B hepatitis). This apparent dissociation of cause and effect is a factor in the liberal transfusion habits of some clinicians.

Whilst the majority of adverse effects are due to antibodies interacting with blood constituents, a number are due to physical or infectious complications, and it is convenient to classify reactions as immunological or non-immunological, since this also influences management.

Acute reactions may occur within minutes of beginning transfusion or some time during infusion but this is not invariable, even with haemolytic reactions, and delayed haemolysis may begin 3–10 days after infusion. It is customary to define delayed reactions as occurring more than 72 hours after infusion. Acute and delayed transfusion reactions are listed in Table 38.2.

Numerous metabolic, coagulation and respiratory complications can occur as a consequence of rapid transfusion, or massive transfusion (exceeding blood volume in 24 hours) in susceptible individuals, particularly the very young, the very old and very ill individuals whose compensating mechanisms are inadequate. Storage of blood at 4°C in citrate anticoagulant medium results in biochemical changes in the plasma (lowered pH, raised potassium and lactate) which are the consequence of red cell senescence and lysis, and the metabolism of dextrose by RBC to lactic acid. However, even though potassium may be as high as 20 mm/l at the end of the shelf-life of blood, the consequences are minimal, except in renal failure and in exchange transfusions, because the total amount of plasma infused is rather small.

Rapid infusion of cold blood (at 4°C), i.e. faster than

Table 38.2 Classification of transfusion reactions

Acute (during or within 72 hours)

Immunological
Haemolytic:
  – haemolytic transfusion reactions
Non-haemolytic:
  – febrile non-haemolytic reactions
  – allergic reactions – urticarial
                 – anaphylactoid
  – non-cardiac pulmonary oedema

Non-immunological
Circulatory overload
Physical damage:
  – overheating
  – freezing
  – incompatible solutions
Bacteriological contamination
Metabolic effects of stored blood:
  – hypothermia
  – increased O_2 affinity
  – K^+/H^+
  – micro-aggregates
Dilutional coagulation defects

Delayed (after 72 hours)

Immunological
Delayed haemolytic transfusion reaction
Post-transfusion purpura
Graft-versus-host disease
Allo-immunisation (particularly HLA)

Non-immunological
Iron overload
Viral hepatitis (HAV, HBV, NANB)
AIDS
Other transmissible diseases:
  – syphilis
  – malaria
  – CMV, etc.

100 ml/min for 30 mins, can produce cardiac arrhythmias, including arrest, by inducing cardiac hypothermia, and the combined effects of high potassium, low ionised calcium and excess citrate. These complications are minimised by the use of controlled temperature blood warmers. Abnormal bleeding may occur after haemostasis has been achieved, but this is not directly related to the number of units transfused, and abnormal coagulation test results do not correlate with clinical bleeding. Depressed factors V and VIII in stored blood are rarely of consequence unless there is excessive consumption with DIC, or gross liver disease with decreased synthesis. The most common bleeding problem is dilution of platelets which may be below $50 \times 10^9/l$. If there is no bleeding diathesis, abnormal laboratory results are of no significance.

Circulatory overload may also occur if whole blood is given to patients with a normal blood volume (most anaemias), rather than red cell concentrates, and some leukaemia patients (e.g. chronic myeloid leukaemia) with significant leukocytosis are also at risk if blood is not transfused very slowly (over 4 hours). There is also a greater risk in patients who have adapted to a very low haemoglobin level which has developed over a long period of time, particularly megaloblastic anaemias.

The formation of micro-aggregates after 1 week of storage has not been directly related to any pathology except in cardiac bypass where micro-emboli generated during the procedure might adversely affect the brain.

ACUTE EFFECTS OF TRANSFUSIONS

Acute haemolytic reactions

The pathogenesis of these reactions is the consequence of antibody-mediated destruction of incompatible red cells, which involves complement binding, lysis of RBC, and release of anaphylatoxins and thromboplastins which then activate the coagulation system and kinin system. In the case of potent complement-fixing IgM antibodies (e.g. anti-A, anti-B, anti-Lewis), rapid intravascular haemolysis may occur, resulting in the most severe signs and symptoms. Most other red cell antibodies are IgG, and result in less rapid haemolysis, which tends to occur extravascularly in the liver or spleen. Symptoms, whilst they can be severe, tend to be less immediate and dramatic and may result in delayed HTR (see below).

Because of the potency of ABO antibodies and the invariable presence of anti-A and anti-B in the appropriate groups, blood is always ABO-matched. Rh grouping is important due to the immunogenicity of the D antigen, the particular need to avoid immunising females during their reproductive years, and the effectiveness of anti-D in causing haemolysis of Rh(D) positive red cells.

Haemolysis is the most serious *avoidable* acute complication of transfusion, and can result in the death of the patient from acute renal failure (tubular ischaemia) or disseminated intravascular coagulation. In the classical ABO-incompatible transfusion reaction there is a sequence of clinical manifestations which usually begin within minutes of infusion:

– burning sensation at infusion site and along vein
– feeling of discomfort and apprehension with facial flushing, headache
– chill and/or rigor with ensuing fever
– lumbar pain and/or chest tightness
– development of shock and/or diffuse bleeding and/or haemoglobinuria

Under anaesthesia, or when the patient is unable to communicate, the development of hypotension, pyrexia or diffuse microvascular bleeding may be the only warning sign of acute haemolysis.

The symptoms and signs of acute HTR are usually proportional to the volume of blood transfused (and haemolysed) and usually develop within minutes of infusion. There are exceptions, with relatively mild symptoms in some patients developing only after one or more units of incompatible blood have been accidentally transfused.

Management

Although acute HTR's are relatively uncommon (1 per 12 500 units transfused), and the early symptoms may be indistinguishable from milder non-haemolytic reactions, the initial management is designed to identify haemolysis, and to safeguard the patient from its harmful effects (see Appendix I).

The most important decision is whether or not transfusion should continue, and this depends on the initial assessment of the patient's underlying condition. In massive, acute bleeding (e.g. varices) and trauma, the dangers of hypovolaemic shock and undertransfusion are statistically greater than the complication of acute HTR, once more than 40% loss of blood volume has occurred. However, there are few situations where blood volume replacement cannot be maintained by a volume expander until the essential checks have been completed. Since the majority of ABO-incompatible transfusions are due to clerical errors or administrative procedures at the bedside, a rapid check of identity of blood and patient will often reveal the problem.

Rapid confirmation of acute haemolysis can be obtained by simple centrifugation of an anticoagulated blood sample in the ward side-room or laboratory, and examination of the plasma with the naked eye for free haemoglobin (limit of detection 250 mg/l).

Examination of the physical condition of a unit of blood may also indicate if there has been mishandling, such as accidental freezing or overheating leading to haemolysis, the addition of incompatible hypotonic solutions (e.g. dextrose or drugs such as ethacrynic acid), or infection in the blood pack causing haemolysis.

Definitive diagnosis of haemolysis, and whether this is due to physical or imunological causes, requires laboratory investigation of blood samples from the patient, and of all materials used in the transfusion, including the administration set and any unused units.

Whilst investigations are under way, the patient must be observed for symptoms and signs to corroborate the diagnosis and to monitor progress, and emergency treatment must be instituted if required. These measures are primarily to maintain the blood volume, blood pressure and renal blood flow to avoid acute tubular necrosis, to induce diuresis and to monitor coagulation parameters for the development of DIC, which may require treatment with heparin and/or blood components.

The laboratory plan is designed to exclude or establish that a haemolytic reaction has occurred, to exclude bacterial infection of the blood pack, and to identify any physical damage to the blood pack which may cause haemolysis (see Appendix II).

Acute non-haemolytic reactions

The majority of acute reactions are not haemolytic in origin (see Table 38.2), and are generally mild. The definitive diagnosis can only be made by exclusion of haemolysis and laboratory investigation, but the classical clinical presentations of each type of reaction should lead to a presumptive diagnosis in most instances.

The majority of these adverse effects are due to antigen-antibody reactions involving leukocytes or plasma proteins, which are not taken into account in routine compatibility testing, and are also associated with blood components and plasma derivatives which are devoid of RBC. Non-haemolytic reactions of an immunological nature are also seen most frequently in individuals who have been previously transfused and/or are pregnant.

Allergic reactions

Urticarial (Appendix III)

Mild urticarial reactions probably occur much more commonly than realised. Once symptoms have appeared, it is expedient to assess the patient initially as for acute HTR, to rule out any clerical error leading to transfusion of mismatched blood. Experience with plasma exchange and large volume infusion of plasma has shown that slowing the rate of infusion will usually result in abating of symptoms but occasionally antihistamines may be required. The diagnosis can only be made on clinical grounds and by evaluation, as there are no definitive laboratory tests. Absence of pyrexia may be helpful in distinguishing this condition from more severe reactions. A summary of the features of urticarial reactions is given in Appendix III.

Anaphylactic (Appendix IV)

Anaphylactic reactions are acute medical emergencies which must be recognised and managed in the absence of definitive laboratory investigations. These reactions are idiosyncratic and are totally unpredictable in that they are not related to the frequency or the quantity of previous transfusions. In rare instances, potent anti-IgA antibodies appear implicated in IgA-deficient individuals.

Only a small minority of IgA-deficient individuals react in this way, but once they are identified, blood products containing IgA should be avoided if at all possible. Symptoms are dramatic, begin within minutes of infusion, and are related to the massive release of vasoactive amines and their effects on smooth muscle and vascular permeability in the lungs, the gut and the circulation. Although extremely rare, anaphylactic reactions are more commonly associated with rapid infusion of fresh frozen plasma, as seen in plasma exchange, when a large number of individual plasma donations are used, increasing the exposure risk to potential allergenic components.

Febrile reactions (Appendix V)

The development of pyrexia with rigors and chills is associated with several types of transfusion reaction, and may be the first sign of a serious haemolytic reaction or post-transfusion bacterial infection. However, febrile reactions are more commonly associated with immunological reaction to transfused leukocytes or platelets. The initial assessment and management is the same as for a suspected acute HTR, and diagnosis is made by the exclusion of haemolysis and infection, and the presence of lymphocytotoxic (anti-HLA) or leukoagglutinating antibodies in the serum of the recipient.

Typically, the non-haemolytic febrile transfusion reaction (FTR) develops towards the end of the first unit transfused, with development of chills and malaise within 30 minutes to 2 hours post-transfusion. This is followed by tachycardia and abrupt rise in temperature, and in severe cases there may be rigors, hypotension, pulmonary symptoms, myalgia and emesis.

The onset of symptoms is related to the potency of the circulating antibodies, and the number of leukocytes transfused and therefore the rate of infusion; leukocyte-free products do not initiate a classical FTR. In some patients with restricted specificity of HLA antibodies, one or more units of blood may, by chance, be compatible, and symptoms may not develop until the second, or even third unit (containing mismatched leukocytes) is infused.

Classical FTRs occur only in multitransfused or multiparous patients who have been immunised by leukocytes, or in transplant patients who may become immunised by an incompatible graft. Typically, they arise sooner or later in patients with normal immunity

who are sustained by regular transfusions in conditions such as sickle cell disease, thalassaemia and hypoplastic anaemia. Although generally mild, the latter category of patients can develop very severe symptoms, which may progress to non-cardiogenic pulmonary oedema (q.v.), and prophylactic measures are required (see Appendix V).

True febrile reactions occurring during transfusion need to be distinguished from causes of pyrexia due to the patient's underlying condition, such as sepsis. Patients with isolated mild FTRs which occur in the absence of identifiable causes are unlikely to have a repeat reaction on subsequent transfusion (only 1 in 8 do so).

Normally, the development of FTR is a cause for full investigation, as indicated in Appendices I and II. In patients who are on long-term transfusion support, and who have already been investigated for FTR, transfusion may continue provided haemolysis has been ruled out, and the patient is treated symptomatically. Leukocyte-poor transfusions may be indicated for these patients.

It should be noted that infants do not shiver or produce rigors in association with pyrexia as do adults, and other signs such as pallor or restlessness may develop associated with incompatible transfusion.

Non-cardiogenic pulmonary oedema (Appendix VI)

Pulmonary oedema associated with transfusion is most commonly due to circulatory overload or too rapid infusion in patients with cardiac insufficiency. Rarely an acute reaction occurs with the features of pulmonary oedema associated with severe chills, fever, cyanosis and respiratory distress shortly after transfusion, particularly of granulocytes. These reactions can be life-threatening, and patients may require assisted ventilation and other supportive measures. The symptoms resemble a severe form of the classical febrile reaction, with predominantly pulmonary symptoms, and are normally related to the presence of potent anti-leukocyte antibodies, usually passively transferred in the donor plasma.

The reaction is usually self-limiting provided the patient can be supported through the acute phase (see Appendix VI for details).

Initial investigations should exclude acute haemolysis due to mismatched blood, and clinical signs and symptoms should distinguish this condition from the onset of acute anaphylaxis and the development of endotoxaemic shock from infected blood.

Bacterial infection (Appendix VII)

Acute collapse due to infected blood can be distinguished from anaphylactic reactions by the systemic symptoms. Infusion of blood containing endotoxin produced by contaminating gram-negative bacteria produces rapid circulatory collapse with peripheral vasodilation and hypotension, with warm extremities and pyrexia, i.e. the symptoms of endotoxaemic shock. Less immediate, but no less severe, is the development of DIC or septicaemia in the recipient following bacterial growth. The features of bacterial contamination are detailed in Appendix VII. Examination of the container used for transfusion may reveal damage to the exterior (e.g. pinholes) or the closure which have allowed ingress of organisms. The modern pre-sterilised plastic containers used for blood and blood components and disposable glass bottles which are filled under pharmaceutical conditions have reduced bacterial contamination to an extremely rare event. Nevertheless, it does happen (and is usually fatal), and pre-transfusion checks at the bedside must always include visual inspection of blood packs for leaks or evidence of tampering with the seals, and examination of bottles for cracks, etc., as well as inspection of the contents for any abnormalities. Unfortunately, a haemolysed pack of blood is normally indistinguishable from a normal pack of blood until centrifuged.

The development of septicaemia and its complications may occur some time after transfusion has occurred and under these circumstances it is very difficult to prove that the blood is the source of infection, because the original containers are not usually available for inspection, or if they are the packs are already 'open' and contamination/bacterial growth has occurred in residual blood after the completion of transfusion.

DELAYED EFFECTS OF TRANSFUSION

Adverse effects which are made manifest some time after the completion of transfusion are more common than realised, probably because the major complication, transmission of infectious diseases, results in presentation to a different speciality. Haemologists who have long-term responsibility for patients with sickle cell disease, thalassaemia and haemophilia are more aware than most that any transfusion is potentially dangerous, and the problems of allo-immunisation, iron overload and viral transmission are considerable. All blood and its derivatives in the UK are routinely screened for the presence of hepatitis B, anti-HIV and syphilis, and in selected circumstances for CMV. The current AIDS epidemic has been a salutary reminder to those who transfuse without critical thought, and a challenge to the transfusion services to increase standards of screening.

Non-infectious complications

Delayed haemolytic reactions

Haemolytic reactions appearing 72 hours after transfusion occur more frequently than appreciated (1 in 12 000 units transfused) and are underdiagnosed, largely because they present some time after the transfusion event and are not usually associated with symptoms. An unexplained fall in haemoglobin or the appearance of jaundice are the most common findings which lead to the diagnosis. The immunological events are the same as for acute HTR – antibody-mediated destruction of RBC – and the potential consequences are the same, including acute renal failure and DIC. The delay is due to the boosting and emergence of antibodies that were undetectable at the time of transfusion. A rapidly developing antibody is more likely to cause the appearance of symptoms normally associated with acute HTR, such as fever, chills and rigors; a slowly developing antibody is more likely to produce acute anaemia and a raised bilirubin associated with gradual removal of incompatible blood from the circulation.

Delayed HTRs occur only in patients who are already immunised to red cell antigens and therefore occur only in patients who have a history of previous transfusion and/or pregnancy.

The principles, investigation and management of delayed HTRs are the same as for acute HTR, but the situation is usually complicated by the lack of availability of pre-transfusion samples, administration sets and blood pack samples. Clinical acumen and consideration of delayed HTR in the differential diagnosis of unexplained anaemia and jaundice post-transfusion are required to initiate the confirmatory laboratory investigations.

Post-transfusion purpura (Appendix VIII)

This is a rare but serious complication of transfusions which contain platelets. It is characterised by the sudden onset of purpura and thrombocytopenia about a week after transfusion. The pathogenesis is unknown but involves prior immunisation in PL^{A1} negative females, associated with the presence of anti-PL^{A1}. The diagnosis is made largely on circumstantial evidence, substantiated by laboratory findings compatible with the diagnosis. Clinical awareness is required, since thrombocytopenia may be attributed to the patient's underlying pathology, or other complications such as DIC or infection. PTP is a self-limiting disease, and in milder forms no action is required other than observation. In patients with life-threatening thrombocytopenia some form of intervention is required, but there is no clearly established treatment. High dose steroids, removal of antibody by plasma exchange, and high dose intravenous immunoglobulin to block the RE system have all been reported to be effective.

Graft-versus-host-disease (GVHD) (Appendix IX)

GVHD is a rare risk of transfusion to neonates with deficient cell-mediated immunity and to immunocompromised patients; it is also considered in detail in Chapter 21. Outwith the context of BMT, transfusion rarely causes serious GVHD, but it is possibly underdiagnosed in premature low-birth-weight babies who receive intra-uterine or exchange transfusion. Occasionally, adults with leukaemia or lymphomas have sufficiently depressed CMI as to manifest transient GVHD.

Symptoms usually begin 1 2 weeks after transfusion, with the development of fever and an erythematous skin rash which becomes exfoliating in severe cases. In severe cases also, diarrhoea and hepatitis develop 2–4 weeks after transfusion. The diagnosis of severe combined immunodeficiency is not infrequently made following the development of GVHD after transfusion, when it is often fatal. Once GVHD has developed, there is no specific treatment. Prevention, where possible as in bone marrow transplant, is effectively carried out by irradiating the blood components to inactivate the donor lymphocytes.

Iron overload

This is an invariable consequence of long-term transfusion. Each unit of blood contains about 250 mg of iron which is conserved by the body (unless there is blood loss) and causes damage to the myocardium, liver and pancreas, resulting in organ failure in due course. Iron overload can be delayed by the use of iron chelation therapy. Some delay may also be achieved by using relatively fresh red cells so as to minimise premature red cell breakdown, extend the transfusion interval and decrease the frequency of transfusion.

The diagnosis and management of transfusion siderosis is detailed in Chapter 13.

Infectious complications

In theory, any microorganisms present in donor blood could transmit disease to the recipient. However, in practice most candidate diseases cause obvious symptoms so that potential donors are unfit to give blood, or are identified prior to donation by history. In addition, the period of bacteraemia or viraemia is often short-lived in most common infectious diseases. Transmission by blood is favoured by:

1. Long incubation period
2. Prolonged presence in the blood
3. Asymptomatic infection
4. Presence of a 'carrier' state
5. Transmission within cells
6. Stability in stored blood or blood derivatives.

Microorganisms which are recognised as particular hazards of transfusion (even if rarely) are detailed in Table 38.3.

The major risks are presented by transfusion-associated hepatitis, and by transfusion-associated AIDS, and routine screening tests for prevention are mandatory for HBV and HIV-l in the UK. The screening test for syphilis is still mandatory for historical reasons, though its usefulness is dubious.

There is little that can be done at the bedside to avoid infectious complications transmitted in donor blood other than to reduce unnecessary transfusions to a minimum, and to use alternatives which are safe (e.g. volume expanders, haematinics). The onus is on the blood-collecting agencies and plasma-fractionation industry to reduce the risks of disease transmission to an acceptable minimum.

Whilst newer virucidal technologies, such as heat-treatment, are available for plasma fractions, there is as yet no adequate means of sterilising red cell, plasma or platelet products. Safety can only be ensured at present by a combination of donor exclusion on the basis of history and travel to or residence in certain endemic areas of the globe, and screening tests where available. These are summarised in Table 38.3.

The relative importance of types of disease commonly associated with transfusion depends on their prevalence and whether they are endemic to the geographical area, e.g. transfusion-transmitted Chagas' disease is a problem restricted to South America. The prevalence of HBsAg carriage also varies widely between different ethnic groups, and HIV-1 and 2 have a greater prevalence in certain high-risk categories (see Chapter 22).

Non-viral disease does not present a significant problem in the UK, due to the absence, or low prevalence, of the organisms implicated. Exclusion of donors by health questionnaires and the deferral of donors for 1 year after return from tropical areas has reduced transmission to negligible levels.

Viral disease transmission falls into two categories: those associated with a 'carrier' state and persistent antigenaemia (post-transfusion hepatitis and AIDS), and those transmitted by leukocytes (CMV, EBV and HTLV-1).

Table 38.3 Diseases transmissible by transfusion

Agent	Prevention
Bacteria	
Syphilis (*Treponema*)	Screening test used (VDRL/TPHA)
Brucellosis (*Brucella*)	Excluded on donor history
Parasites	
Malaria (*Plasmodium*)	Excluded on donor history Geographical exclusion Serological test available (not routine)
Chagas' disease (*Trypanosoma*)	Excluded on donor history Geographical exclusion Screening test used (endemic areas)
Babesiosis (*Babesia*)	Geographical exclusion (USA)
Toxoplasmosis (*T. gondii*)	
Viruses	
(a) Plasma borne	
Post-transfusion hepatitis	
Hepatitis A (HAV)	Serological test available (not routine)
Hepatitis B (HBV) (and delta agent)	Screening test used (HBsAg)
Non-A non-B hepatitis (NANB)	Risk group exclusion Surrogate tests (ALT; anti-HBc) Specific tests under development (anti-HCV)
AIDS	Risk group exclusion Geographical exclusion
HIV-1	Screening test used (anti-HIV-1)
HIV-2	or under development (anti-HIV-2)
Parvoviruses (type B19)	Serological test available (not routine)
(b) Cell-associated	
Cytomegalovirus (CMV)	Screening test available (anti-CMV)
Epstein-Barr Virus (EBV)	Serological test available (not routine)
Human T-cell leukaemia virus (HTLV-1) or (adult T-cell leukaemia virus (ATLV)	Serological test available (not routine) Screening tests under development (anti-HTLV-1)

Acquired immunodeficiency syndrome (AIDS)

The clinical features and pathogenesis are considered in detail in Chapter 22. Since the adoption of universal screening for anti-HIV-1 in October 1985, the risk of new cases of transfusion-associated AIDS is minimal in the UK. The patient population exposed to the greatest risk are the haemophiliacs, who have received large

amounts of pooled blood products, and a considerable number were infected prior to the introduction of donor screening and heat-treatment for factor VIII. Continued efforts to reduce HIV transmission to a minimum involve:

1. Donor self-exclusion by targeting high risk groups
2. Exclusion at health check
3. Anti-HIV screening
4. Sterilisation of blood products where possible.

Efforts continue to find a sensitive rapid screening test for antigen which will identify those very few individuals who are infectious, but have not yet developed anti-HIV antibodies in the initial stages of infection (1 in 300 000). Screening tests may also require to be introduced for HIV-2 and other strains, should these become prevalent in the UK.

Post-transfusion hepatitis (PTH)

The development of jaundice and liver disease post-transfusion depends on a number of factors:

1. The prevalence of the relevant virus in the donor population
2. The number of donors contributing to the transfusion
3. The donor selection criteria
4. The efficacy of screening tests
5. The efficiency of viral inactivation procedures (if any).

Transmission of hepatitis by blood or plasma derivatives is one of the most serious complications of transfusion, with an appreciable morbidity and mortality worldwide. The clinical expression of PTH ranges from mild, or anicteric disturbance of liver function ('transaminitis') detected only biochemically, to fulminant disease with fatal liver necrosis.

Although HAV, HBV, CMV, EBV and NANB are all associated with hepatitis to some degree, the risks of transmission are dissimilar. HAV is rarely transmitted because the period of viraemia usually coincides with ill health in the donor, and also because of the absence of a carrier state and the high prevalence of naturally immune individuals which rises with age. The highest risk group is the newborn, particularly premature infants requiring regular transfusion support, since they lack natural immunity. The diagnosis should be considered when acute hepatitis develops 2–6 weeks post-transfusion, and may be confirmed by serology tests for IgM anti-HAV; sporadic outbreaks have occurred in intensive care nurseries. CMV and EBV may produce a post-transfusion syndrome with fever, atypical lymphocytosis and splenomegaly, sometimes associated with hepatitis. Individuals with normal immunity are rarely inconvenienced by CMV or EBV transmitted by blood. CMV transmission is the greater problem, with premature neonates and bone marrow transplant patients being particularly susceptible. In susceptible individuals, clinical manifestations usually appear 2–8 weeks following transfusion with a mononucleosis-like illness, representing primary infection; many of these patients succumb to pulmonary complications of CMV. In some cases, the disease may be subclinical, being diagnosed by transaminase elevation, and is distinguished from NANB by serological evidence of CMV or EBV infection. CMV and EBV appear to be transmitted only by blood products containing leukocytes.

A more severe disease is associated with HBV, with an incubation period from 6 weeks to 6 months (more usually 9–10 weeks post-transfusion). The diagnosis is confirmed by serological tests, with the identification of specific markers for HBV antigens and antibodies. All blood is now routinely screened for HBsAg, to detect potentially infectious asymptomatic carriers, and this has reduced HBV transfusion by blood and single donor components to negligible levels. However, there is an enhanced risk with pooled plasma derivatives which are not treated with virucidal methods, particularly coagulation factors, due to limitations in the screening procedures.

PTH due to NANB is diagnosed by exclusion, although a screening test developed by genetic engineering methods is under evaluation (anti-Hepatitis C). It is estimated that some 80–90% of PTH is now associated with NANB, with an overall risk of 1 in 100 units transfused (in contrast to HBV with a risk of 1 in 2–4000 units transfused). Most cases are not clinically apparent but are detected in prospective studies by the elevation of liver transaminases, and in some 40% of cases there is progression to chronic hepatitis, including cirrhosis. Two agents appear to be involved, a short incubation (2–4 weeks) and a long incubation (6–10 weeks) variety. As there is no comprehensive screening test at present, potentially infectious donors are identified by ALT and anti-HBc screening (surrogate screening) in countries where the prevalence is perceived to be high (e.g. USA and W. Germany), and this eliminates some 30% of potentially infectious donors. In the UK, the incidence of donors with persistently raised ALT (0.1–1%) is about one-tenth of that in the USA; 0.5–0.8% of the UK population have antibody to HCV. However, there is no direct correlation between raised ALT or anti-HBc and the new anti-HCV screening test.

APPENDIX I: ACUTE TRANSFUSION REACTIONS

What to do at the bedside:

1. Stop transfusion; maintain i.v. line open; carry out emergency treatment (see below); notify clinician in charge

2. Check for clerical errors, e.g. wrong blood to patient; notify blood bank

3. Check physical condition of unit

4. Take appropriate specimens from patient
   - serology
   - FBC
   - coagulation screen
   - bacterial culture

5. Assess risk of not continuing transfusion immediately

6. Return to the blood bank:
   - unit implicated
   - administration set
   - any untransfused units
   - containers of transfused units
   - post-transfusion samples

7. Get post-transfusion urine sample

8. Blood product support for DIC

Emergency treatment (depends on severity)

1. Record BP, pulse, urine output

2. Catheterise if necessary (to monitor urine output)

3. 200 ml 20% mannitol i.v. (or i.v. frusemide)

4. Saline and/or 5% albumin

5. Insert CVP line if necessary

6. Dopamine

7. ? Heparinise for DIC

8. Blood product support for DIC

APPENDIX II: ACUTE TRANSFUSION REACTIONS – Laboratory Investigation

1. Clerical check of all reports and records

2. Examine post-transfusion sample for haemolysis and notify ward

3. Complete serological evaluation:

Repeat ABO and Rh groups on pre and post
samples and units

Direct antiglobulin test on samples (classically
mixed field – may occasionally be negative)

Repeat crossmatch (NB haemolysis as well as
agglutination)

Antibody screen (including WBC and plasma
protein Abs)

Bacteriology on units

4. Confirmatory investigations – haptoglobin;
bilirubin; plasma Hb etc.

5. Compare pre/post Hb level

6. Examine later samples for antibodies (for delayed
HTR)

APPENDIX III: URTICARIAL REACTIONS

Mild skin reactions associated with plasma-containing
products

Incidence

1–5% of all transfusions

Features

Symptoms start within minutes of transfusion

Rarely serious

Rarely cause pyrexia

Associated with urticaria, erythema, itching

Occur in absence of prior transfusion

Antibodies rarely found

Pathogenesis

Unknown but possibly histamine/serotonin release following (?IgE) antigen-antibody reactions

Management

Slow the transfusion

Assess/administer anti-histamine (piriton)

Continue cautiously if no evidence of haemolysis

APPENDIX IV: ANAPHYLACTIC REACTIONS

Circulatory collapse associated with plasma-containing
products

Incidence

Extremely rare

Features

Usually occur within minutes of transfusion

Occur in the absence of prior sensitisation

Can be life-threatening in severity:
  – flushing
  – wheezing and bronchospasm
  – abdominal cramps and diarrhoea
  – nausea and vomiting
  – hypotension and shock

Pathogenesis

Immediate hypersensitivity reaction (sometimes, but not
always, associated with high titre anti-IgA) with
degranulation of mast cells, massive histamine release,
with vasodilation, increased vascular premeability and
smooth muscle constriction (? leukotriene-mediated)

Management

Emergency resuscitation and supportive measures:
  – oxygen
  – adrenalin
  – antihistamines
  – hydrocortisone

Washed red cells

IgA-deficient products

APPENDIX V: FEBRILE TRANSFUSION REACTIONS

A rapid rise of at least 1°C, associated with
WBC/platelet-containing products

Incidence

Approximately 1% of all transfusions

Features*

Symptoms may begin early, but pyrexia develops
30 min to 2 hours later

Associated with malaise, headache, myalgia, chills

Occasionally result in severe rigors, hypotension

Occur in multitransfused or multiparous patients

(*NB may be early warning of haemolytic reaction)

Pathogenesis

Anti-HLA or leuko-agglutinating antibodies, interacting with leukocytes and resulting in the release of endogenous pyrogen (interleukin 1)

Febrile response depends on:
- strength and breadth of Ab specificity
- number of WBC transfused (threshold 0.5×10^9)
- rate of transfusion

Management

Stop the transfusion; maintain i.v. line

Assess as per haemolytic reaction

Continue if no evidence of haemolysis

Treat pyrexia symptomatically; severe reaction may require steroids

Future transfusions:
- premedicate (anti-pyretics/hydrocortisone)
- leukocyte-poor blood if still symptomatic and evidence of leukocyte antibodies

APPENDIX VI: NON-CARDIOGENIC PULMONARY OEDEMA

Acute onset of respiratory distress in the absence of primary heart failure following whole blood or plasma

Incidence

Extremely rare

Features

Rapid onset

Chills, rigors and fever

Dyspnoea, cyanosis, respiratory distress

Radiological appearances of bilateral pulmonary oedema, with normal-sized heart

No evidence of left heart failure

Can be life-threatening

Symptoms usually subside within 12–24 hours

Pathogenesis

Granulocyte aggregation in pulmonary capillaries secondary to anti-leukocyte antibodies (usually agglutinins) in recipient *or* donor plasma, followed by release of toxic/vaso-active material, resulting in increased capillary permeability and adult respiratory distress syndrome/transfusion-related lung injury (ARDS/TRALI)

Management

Stop transfusion; maintain i.v. line

Exclude acute haemolysis

Supportive measures
- oxygen
- intravenous fluids to maintain cardiac output and BP
- avoidance of diuretics
- high dose steroids

May require assisted ventilation

APPENDIX VII: BACTERIAL CONTAMINATION

Circulatory collapse due to endotoxaemic shock, or septicaemia following infusion of infected blood

Incidence

Extremely rare

Features

Usually within minutes of transfusion

Occur in the absence of prior sensitisation

Can be life-threatening in severity:
- chills, fever
- headache, back pain
- severe gastrointestinal upset
- circulation collapse with peripheral vasodilation
- septicaemia
- DIC

Heavy bacterial contamination of transfusion fluid

Pathogenesis

Acute effects due to endotoxin produced by heavy bacterial growth in the transfusion medium; more delayed effects due to infection of the patient and development of septicaemia. Gram-negative cryophilic bacteria are usually implicated (*Pseudomonads*, *Coliforms*) which enter the bag/bottle through cracks, pinholes, faulty closures due to manufacturing defects, or mishandling of blood.

Management

Stop transfusion; maintain i.v. line

Exclude acute haemolysis

Emergency resuscitation and supportive measures for shock

Appropriate antibiotics for septicaemia

Heparin/blood components for DIC

APPENDIX VIII: POST-TRANSFUSION PURPURA

Incidence

Very rare

Features

Severe thrombocytopaenia 5–10 d post-transfusion with purpura and mucosal bleeding

Associated with blood or platelet concentrates

Almost always females

History of previous transfusion and/or pregnancy

Usually PL^{A1}-negative recipients (less than 2% of population)

Anti-PL^{A1} present, which affects autologous platelets

Spontaneous recovery in 3–5 weeks

Pathogenesis

Unknown but involves immunological mechanisms mediated by antibody

Management

Masterly inactivity

High dose steroids

High dose i.v. immunoglobulin

Plasma exchange

APPENDIX IX: GRAFT-VERSUS-HOST DISEASE

Incidence

Very rare

Features:

Onset 1–4 weeks after transfusion

Associated with lymphocyte-containing products

Occurs in:
- intra-uterine transfusion
- exchange transfusion in premature infants
- primary or secondary immunodeficiency with defective cell-mediated immunity
- allogeneic bone marrow transplants

Clinical features
- fever
- skin rash (erythematous)
- diarrhoea
- hepatitis
- pancytopenia

Often fatal

Pathogenesis

Immunocompetent donor T-lymphocytes which recognise the recipient (host) histocompatibility antigens as being 'foreign' and produce a cell-mediated reaction against sensitive tissues, principally the skin, gastrointestinal tract, liver and bone marrow. Occurs only in recipients who have defective CMI due to primary or secondary causes and cannot eliminate transfused lymphocytes.

Management (see Ch. 21)

Supportive measures in established GVHD

Prevention – irradiation (1500 cGy) of all blood components in bone marrow transplant recipients and congenital immunodeficiencies. (Platelets, WBC, RBC are not affected by this level of irradiation.)

39. Psychological support for the patient

G. G. Lloyd

In clinical haematology, as in any other branch of medicine, management involves providing a considerable amount of psychological support for the patient in dealing with the emotional problems which accompany physical illness. The high prevalence of psychological symptoms among medical patients is well established but it is claimed that they often go unrecognised in clinical practice. Furthermore, there is evidence that failure to deal with the psychological aspects of illness can significantly affect the overall prognosis. Haematologists have only recently assumed full clinical responsibilities but are increasingly aware of the importance of psychological factors in management. In most cases responsibility for dealing with patients' emotional problems rests with the clinician in charge of the case. It is preferable that this continues to be so, because splitting management between different doctors can often cause unnecessary complications. However, for optimum clinical management the haematologist needs to have close links with other professional groups, including nurses, social workers, psychologists and psychiatrists, any of whom can be involved in certain aspects of treatment.

PSYCHOLOGICAL REACTIONS TO MALIGNANT DISEASE

Some of the most difficult problems in clinical haematology concern the management of patients with malignant disease. Recent therapeutic advances have considerably improved the prognosis of patients with lymphomas and leukaemias but, paradoxically, the increased survival period has caused greater psychological problems, not least because of the fear of recurrence, even after several years' remission.

Popular attitudes to malignant disease in general continue to set it apart from other types of illness as an object of fear. It has been claimed that illnesses which may be just as serious and even less amenable to treatment are approached in a much calmer manner, both by the patient and the professional staff concerned.

Psychological assessment of patients with malignant disease poses special problems. Symptoms such as anorexia, weight-loss, fatigue and nausea, which are of diagnostic importance in primary psychiatric disorder, have quite a different significance in the presence of physical illness. It is also important to take into account the effects on mental function of various physical methods of treatment, including cytotoxic drugs and radiotherapy. Furthermore, the intricate association between physical and psychiatric illness means that among any large group of medically ill patients there will be some whose psychiatric illness antedated the onset of their malignancy. It is important that these are distinguished from other patients whose psychological symptoms are a consequence of their malignancy. When it comes to assessing psychological symptoms in the latter group, it should be remembered that there is a continuum of severity. The distinction between a normal and an abnormal response is often arbitrary and difficult to make in clinical practice. The varying rates of psychiatric morbidity reported in cancer patients are influenced by the interviewer's disposition to regard as normal any symptom he considers understandable in the presence of the physical illness. This is a highly subjective phenomenon which varies from one interviewer to another, but it can be overcome if interview methods are derived from those using structured and standardised measures of assessment.

In the light of these comments any classification of psychological reactions to malignant disease must be regarded as speculative, subject to even more controversy than applies to diagnosis in other areas of psychiatry. The following account outlines the patterns observed in physically ill patients in general, with particular emphasis on malignant disease; they can be seen in any type of disease, malignant or benign, serious or trivial.

Factors influencing psychological response

A wide range of factors has to be considered when trying to understand the patient's response to illness. Central to these is the personal meaning which the illness has for the patient. Among the influences on this are:

1. Premorbid personality
2. Social setting at the time of onset
3. Nature of the illness
4. Impact of treatment.

Premorbid personality

Much has been written about the importance of the patient's personality in this context. Clinical observation suggests that people with obsessional traits find illness particularly stressful if there are doubts about the diagnosis, treatment or prognosis; they look for certainty and detailed explanation from their doctor. Dependent personalities, it has been claimed, may partly welcome illness as it permits the gratification of dependency needs. An association has been demonstrated between personality factors and the perception and communication of pain by patients with malignant disease. Patients with neurotic traits have a greater perception of pain, while those of extrovert nature are more likely to complain of it.

Social setting at the time of onset

The role of social factors (including interaction with family and friends) in influencing a patient's emotional response to cancer is not clear-cut. On clinical grounds such factors would be expected to exert an important influence but this expectation is not always borne out by research findings. Perhaps this is because at present we lack sufficiently sensitive methods of measuring the subtleties of interpersonal relationships, job satisfaction and sexual adjustment. Paradoxically, a supportive family circle and network of friends may be sources of distress as well as of comfort. Concern for children or a spouse has often been cited as a cause of mood disturbance in terminally ill patients. It remains to be determined what patterns of family interaction are most supportive and least stressful when one member of the family is suffering from cancer or any other illness with a potentially fatal outcome. One can be more confident when considering other aspects of the social situation. The illness will be more stressful if it involves loss of a job and financial hardship, or if it prevents the achievement of major ambitions. At less crucial times in a person's life the influence of social factors will be correspondingly reduced.

Specific nature of the malignancy

Aspects of the illness which may be responsible for inducing psychological distress have been considered by various authors. Although individual studies have demonstrated an association between severity of the illness in physical terms and ensuing psychological distress, this has not been a consistent finding. Some of the stressful factors which contribute to the need for psychiatric consultation include pain, disfigurement and dependency. These stresses are not, of course, specific to malignant disease but some of them at least may be more frequent in this group of patients, particularly in view of the peculiar attitudes to cancer referred to earlier.

The impact of treatment

It is never possible to separate clearly the emotional response to the disease itself from the response to other associated factors, such as treatment, which in its broadest sense includes the relationship between the patient and those providing the treatment. Nevertheless, there is evidence that both radiotherapy and chemotherapy can have adverse psychological effects, at least temporarily. Steroid medication is well-known for its effect on mood, being capable of inducing manic symptoms as well as severe depression of a psychotic nature. Bone marrow transplantation is especially traumatic. The fear that the graft will be rejected causes considerable anxiety which is obviously much higher when the compatibility between donor and recipient is not close.

The nature of the psychological response.

In spite of the dearth of standardised evaluations, sufficient information has been accumulated to allow certain psychological responses to be identified. Just as the stressful factors associated with the disease are not specific to cancer, so may the various patterns of emotional response be seen in patients with other illnesses. For convenience these patterns are described separately; in practice they overlap considerably with one another in the same patient and frequently change over a period of time. In her well-known account of the terminally ill, Kubler-Ross has suggested that there is a characteristic progression of attitudes from the time of the diagnosis until the time when death is imminent. She has described five stages through which the patient is assumed to pass, beginning with shock and denial, then progressing through anger, bargaining and depression until the final stage of acceptance is reached. It is doubtful, however, that this evolution of attitudes can be applied to all patients with cancer and in the following account no definite psychological sequence is assumed.

Therapeutic adaptation.

This refers to the tendency for patients to appraise their symptoms, seek medical consultation and co-operate with treatment in such a way as to maximise their chances of recovery or their adjustment to the disability caused by the illness. This does not mean that patients who respond in this manner do not perceive their illness as a stress and are emotionally untroubled by the experience, but their affective responses and behavioural changes are not so marked as to be maladaptive. The coping mechanisms are active, appropriate and flexible to the changing course of the illness. Work and leisure activities are modified in accordance with the demands of treatment and the physical limitations imposed by the illness, but are resumed during periods of physical well-being.

Denial

Patients who use this method of coping minimise, ignore or completely reject evidence of disease or its significance. The concept of denial covers a spectrum of attitudes and is not an all-or-none phenomenon. There is evidence that in certain situations denial of illness has a protective function but in the early stages of malignant disease it can be maladaptive by delaying medical consultation and the start of treatment. It may well be that many of those who delay seeking treatment use denial as a habitual method of coping when faced with threatening situations and in this sense the response to the detection of symptoms of disease reflects their previous behaviour. Not all delay can be attributed to denial, however. Ignorance of the significance of the symptoms is another possible cause, as are fears of hospitals and treatment, and concurrent social difficulties.

Even when the diagnosis is confirmed and discussed with the patient, some will still deny that they have been told. This attitude can be maintained during and after treatment but tends to become less common with time.

Anxiety

Anxiety is usually an early response to illness, associated with the perception of unfamiliar symptoms and with the initiation of new treatment. It is prominent when there is uncertainty about the illness, especially before the diagnosis has been clarified. This is one of the reasons why no time should be lost in establishing the diagnosis and explaining it in terms the patient can understand. During the course of treatment somatic symptoms of anxiety can often raise fears of recurrent disease. These symptoms include headaches and other pains, dizziness, nausea and palpitations. Some patients develop anticipatory anxiety on each occasion they attend hospital for treatment. This is almost certainly a conditioned reflex, brought on by the nausea and other unpleasant side effects of chemotherapy. They experience a variety of somatic symptoms, including nausea and vomiting, before treatment is given and in some the anxiety reaches phobic intensity, resulting in a withdrawal from treatment.

Depression

As would be expected, depression and anxiety frequently co-exist in the physically ill. An important aspect of the relationship between depression and cancer is the claim that the affective changes can precede the diagnosis of the malignancy. Several mechanisms could account for this association, the most likely being that depression occurs as a reaction to the weight-loss and general lethargy. Depressive symptoms are common in patients with established malignancy. Guilt and a loss of self-esteem are characteristic features. Some patients tend to blame themselves for having brought on the disease and recall previous habits to which they attribute causal responsibility. It is as if the illness is viewed as a punishment for past sins and indiscretions. Alternatively, guilt may be experienced because malignant disease is considered unclean and spread to relatives and friends is feared. Feelings of anger and irritability towards members of the therapeutic team are another important source of guilt. Even when these feelings are justified, they are usually mixed with a sense of gratitude; the anger is therefore not expressed, and guilt at feeling angry mounts up. Furthermore, the patient may feel guilty at envying healthy relations and friends or because he realises he is becoming increasingly dependent on them.

Anger

This emotional response is seen most strikingly in those who use projection as a defence mechanism. They attribute their illness and its complications to other people, the usual targets for blame being doctors, nurses or relatives. Outbursts of anger accompanied by accusations of neglect or incompetence are directed at those whom the patient holds responsible for his suffering. At its most extreme this response takes the form of a paranoid psychosis with systematised delusions of persecution. Such psychotic reactions, fortunately rare, cause major management problems because the patient may act in accordance with the paranoid beliefs and urgent psychiatric intervention is then required.

Lesser degrees of anger are far more common but they also can create difficulties. The angry patient is regarded as demanding and unco-operative and the doctor-patient relationship deteriorates. Moreover, as mentioned above, feelings of anger towards someone in a therapeutic capacity often elicit guilt and a fear of retaliation. The physician who is able to acknowledge anger in his patient and to allow its expression may alleviate much emotional distress.

Malignant disease in children

The development of malignancy in children poses special problems. While death in old age is accepted as an inevitable and natural process, the prospect of death in childhood arouses quite different sentiments. The child's concept of death also varies at different ages. Children under the age of 6 view death as temporary and reversible; not until 9 or 10 years of age are they aware of the irreversibility of death. In the case of very young children it is the relatives who are most in need of emotional support and reports have shown that many parents become clinically depressed. With increasing age, as more adult attitudes towards death develop, the emotional distress for the patient becomes more marked, being particularly traumatic for the adolescent.

PSYCHOLOGICAL SUPPORT IN MALIGNANCY

The clinician responsible for the patient's management is the crucial figure in co-ordinating emotional support once the diagnosis is made and treatment commenced. The importance of good communication cannot be overemphasised. Much of the anxiety experienced by patients who are told they have a malignancy can be alleviated or contained by a frank discussion of the disease and its treatment. Several studies have shown that the majority of patients wish to know the nature of their disease and it is now the policy in most units to discuss the diagnosis frankly. Exactly how much detail the information should contain will vary from one case to another but the clinician can be guided by the type of questions the patient asks, provided sufficient time is set aside for this purpose. It is important to realise that much of what is said will not be registered at the first interview, particularly if the patient is highly anxious, and the doctor must be prepared to go over the same items of information and be asked the same questions

on several occasions. Information will also have to be given about drugs used in treatment; this should cover their main actions and side effects. Patients are less likely to drop out of treatment if they are warned in advance about the side effects they are likely to experience.

Some centres have established special counselling services for these patients. Counselling is provided by a social worker or nurse who has detailed knowledge of the disease and its psychosocial consequences and who is in regular contact with the clinician responsible for the patient's management. The counsellor can arrange to see the patient regularly or be available as required at times of particular stress. The aims should be to provide an emotionally supportive relationship, to listen to the patient's symptoms and fears and to provide as much information about the illness as the patient wants to know. This can be supplemented by written information. Work of this type is emotionally demanding, particularly when it involves dealing with the terminally ill. Counsellors need to be selected carefully and trained to identify patients who require referral to other specialists. Evidence suggests that those who are likely to function well are flexible and willing to share problems. They should have their own sourcers of emotional support and other interests outside their work, and should be optimistic but realistic about what can be achieved. They should have a regular opportunity to discuss patients who are causing them difficulties.

Anxiolytic drugs, such as diazepam, can be used for brief periods during the course of treatment and are especially helpful for insomnia. Antidepressants have little place at this stage, even though the patient may become significantly depressed as a result of the debilitating effects of chemotherapy or radiotherapy.

The small proportion of patients who develop anticipatory or phobic anxiety before each attendance for treatment can be helped by diazepam given just prior to each treatment or by behaviour therapy, using techniques of desensitisation and muscular relaxation. This should be carried out under the supervision of a clinical psychologist.

In some cases the impact of the illness is so great that the patient remains depressed after treatment has been completed, even when the result appears successful. Antidepressant medication should be considered if the depression persists for several weeks and shows no signs of lifting. The decision should be based on similar criteria to those used in the management of primary depressive illness and in this context it is helpful if the haematologist has the collaboration of a psychiatrist who is familiar with the problems of managing depression in medically ill patients. In addition to a morbidly depressed mood, other symptoms to look for include depressive thoughts, hypochondriasis, anorexia, weight-loss and sleep disturbance. A joint decision will need to be taken that these symptoms can no longer be attributed to the underlying malignancy or any of the treatments used. The somatic symptoms of depression are very similar to those of malignant disease, so it is essential to exclude residual or recurrent disease before a diagnosis of depression is made. Physically ill patients tolerate tricyclic antidepressants poorly and it is therefore preferable to use one of the newer drugs, such as mianserin, which can be given in doses up to 90 mg at night.

Whatever arrangements are made for the psychological support of the patient, it is important that the needs of relatives are not forgotten. This issue is particularly relevant for the parents of young children, who are at considerable risk of developing psychiatric morbidity themselves.

Some centres have established regular group discussions so that relatives can come together to share their experiences and worries. These groups should be held under the supervision of a member of the professional team who has acquired experience in group dynamics. Although evaluation studies have not been carried out systematically, there is no doubt that many relatives derive considerable support from such meetings.

HAEMOPHILIA AND AIDS

The psychological problems of coping with haemophilia are complicated by its genetic transmission (Ch. 31). The responsible gene for either type of haemophilia is sex-linked recessive; consequently in nearly all cases transmission occurs through the mother and only male children are affected clinically. Maternal guilt is common and the mother's ability to cope with this is decisive in influencing her offspring's emotional development. A frequently observed maternal reaction is extreme anxiety and over-protectiveness. The haemophiliac child is then likely to be overdependent, isolated and unable to form healthy relationships in childhood or adult life. He becomes anxious of bleeding episodes and their complications, is unable to express normal aggressive drives and regresses to infantile levels of passivity. Less commonly, parents and child exhibit the defense mechanism of denial which results in inappropriately robust behaviour and excessive risk-taking.

In adult life, depressive episodes are common if joint deformities develop and some clinicians have observed a high prevalence of analgesic dependence and alcohol abuse among their patients.

Counselling about the nature of the condition forms a major part of long-term management. Genetic information also needs to be given carefully so that affected individuals and carriers, together with their partners, can decide whether to try to have children. If they decide to conceive, amniocentesis and fetal blood sampling should be offered; prospective parents may request a termination of the pregnancy if the fetus is shown to have haemophilia or to be a carrier.

The problems of haemophiliacs have been greatly complicated since the recognition of the acquired immune deficiency syndrome (AIDS) in 1981. Haemophiliacs are at risk of contracting the condition through repeated infusions of clotting factor concentrates to control bleeding and those who have been exposed to imported, commercially produced factor VIII are especially at risk.

The majority of haemophiliacs in some centres have been shown to have positive serological tests for the human immunodeficiency virus (HIV) but only a small proportion have developed the clinical syndrome as yet. The fear among high risk groups of developing AIDS has sometimes led to widespread panic with depression, multiple somatic preoccupations and suicidal thoughts. The risk of a suicide attempt and other adverse psychological reactions has prompted the opinion that serological testing should not be carried out unless adequate counselling has been provided beforehand. It is not known what proportion of those who are seropositive will go on to develop the full AIDS syndrome, although the proportion appears to be rising with longer follow-up periods. Anxiety, depression and obsessional thoughts are common. Patients often expect to be rejected by friends and colleagues and may report incidents in which they or their family have been ostracised. Consequently, they can become increasingly isolated and this adds to the existing psychological trauma. Uncertainty about the course of the disease, the prospects of treatment and the possibility of a rapidly fatal outcome all aggravate their distress.

Psychiatric problems also develop as a result of organic brain disease. It is now established that HIV is not only lymphotropic but also neurotropic; thus it can directly infect cells in the central nervous system and it has been suggested that this may occur in the absence of immunosuppression. The commonest type of cerebral pathology is a sub-acute encephalitis which leads to a progressive dementia with cognitive, motor and behavioural dysfunction. In the early stages the complaints of mental slowing, poor concentration and memory impairment may be overlooked or attributed to a depressive disorder. It is thus important to consider cerebral disease in all AIDS patients with psychological symptoms. Psychometric testing, electro-encephalography and computerised tomography can all help elucidate the nature of the symptoms. In some cases organic cerebral involvement can declare itself abruptly as an acute confusional state with impairment of consciousness, disorientation, impaired memory and perceptual disturbances. In addition to encephalitis these symptoms may be due to opportunistic meningeal infection with cryptococcus or herpes virus.

Hospitals which treat many AIDS patients have established special counselling services to provide advice and emotional support. Patients should be helped to understand current information about the disease, particularly its cause, mode of transmission and the treatment available. Specific advice should be given about avoiding transmission to sexual partners, family members and friends and a code of practice for 'safe sex' should be described in detail. Supportive psychotherapy should enable patients to express their anger about the disease and the negative reaction of society and professional staff. This can help them avoid acting out their resentment in a destructive manner.

CONCLUSION

Haematologists now have clinical responsibility for patients with extensive psychological problems resulting from the impact of their illness and its treatment. In most cases these problems manifest as a non-specific neurotic response characterised by anxiety and depression and can be alleviated by good communication between doctor and patient. Continuing emotional support can be provided by specially trained counsellors who work closely with the responsible clinician. Only a minority of patients, perhaps 5–10%, develop specific psychiatric syndromes which require specialist treatment.

BIBLIOGRAPHY

Brewin T B 1977 The cancer patient: communication and morale. British Medical Journal ii: 1623–1627
Fenton T W 1987 AIDS-related psychiatric disorder. British Journal of Psychiatry 151: 579–588
Kubler-Ross E 1970 On death and dying. Tavistock, London.

Lloyd G G 1985 Emotional aspects of physical illness. In: Granville-Grossman (ed) Recent advances in clinical psychiatry – 5. Churchill Livingstone, Edinburgh.
Maguire P 1985 Barriers to psychological care of the dying. British Medical Journal 291: 1711–1713

Index